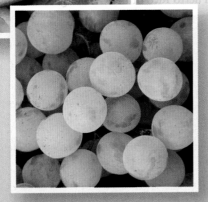

Nutrition Essentials for Nursing Practice

Susan G. Dudek, RD, CDN, BS

Nutrition Instructor, Dietetic Technology Program
Erie Community College
Williamsville, New York

Consultant Dietitian for Employee Assistance
Program of Child and Family Services
Williamsville, New York

SEVENTH EDITION

Wolters Kluwer | Lippincott Williams & Wilkins
Health

Philadelphia · Baltimore · New York · London
Buenos Aires · Hong Kong · Sydney · Tokyo

Acquisitions Editor: David Troy
Product Manager: Maria McAvey
Editorial Assistant: Latisha Ogelsby
Design Coordinator: Holly Reid McLaughlin
Creative Services Director: Doug Smock
Manufacturing Coordinator: Karin Duffield
Prepress Vendor: Absolute Service, Inc.

Seventh Edition

Library of Congress Cataloging-in-Publication Data

Dudek, Susan G.
  Nutrition essentials for nursing practice / Susan G. Dudek. — 7th ed.
    p. ; cm.
  Includes bibliographical references and index.
  ISBN 978-1-4511-8612-3 (alk. paper)
  I. Title.
  [DNLM: 1. Diet Therapy—Handbooks. 2. Diet Therapy—Nurses' Instruction. 3. Nutritional Physiological Phenomena—Handbooks. 4. Nutritional Physiological Phenomena—Nurses' Instruction. WB 39]
  RM216
  615.8'54—dc23
                                                                                      2013007075

In loving memory of my mother, Annie M. Maedl—
everyone should be so lucky to have a mom like her.

Reviewers

Zita Allen, RN, MSN
Professor of Nursing
Alverno College
Milwaukee, Wisconsin

Carmen Bruni, MSN, RN, CAN
Assistant Professor
Texas A&M International University
Laredo, Texas

Ann Cleary, DNS, RN, NP-C
Associate Professor of Nursing
Long Island University, Brooklyn Campus
Brooklyn, New York

Tammie Cohen, RN, BS
Nursing Instructor, Faculty Advisory Committee
    Chairperson
Western Suffolk BOCES
Northport, New York

Janet Goeldner, MSN
Professor
University of Cincinnati—Raymond Walters College
Cincinnati, Ohio

Coleen Kumar, RN, MSN
Associate Professor Nursing
Department Deputy Chairperson
Kingsborough Community College
Brooklyn, New York

Karen Lincoln, RNC, MSN
Nursing Faculty
Montcalm Community College
Sidney, Michigan

Carol Isaac MacKusick, PhDc, MSN, RN, CNN
Adjunct Faculty
Clayton State University
Morrow, Georgia

Marina Martinez-Kratz, RN, BSN, MS
Professor of Nursing
Jackson Community College
Jackson, Michigan

Janet Tompkins McMahon, RN, MSN
Clinical Associate Professor of Nursing
Towson University
Towson, Maryland

Patricia J. Neafsey, RD, PhD
Professor
University of Connecticut School of Nursing
Storrs, Connecticut

Cheryl L. Neudauer, PhD, MEd
Biology Faculty
Center for Teaching and Learning Campus Leader
Minneapolis Community and Technical College
Minneapolis, Minnesota

Christine M. Prince, RN, BSN, CCM
Nursing Faculty
Brown Mackie College Indianapolis
Indianapolis, Indiana

Rhonda Savain, RN, MSN
Nursing Instructor
Ready to Pass Inc.
West Hempstead, New York

Nancy West, RN, MN
Professor of Nursing
Johnson County Community College
Overland Park, Kansas

Preface

Like air and sleep, nutrition is a basic human need essential for survival. Nutrition provides energy and vitality, helps reduce the risk of chronic disease, and can aid in recovery. It is a dynamic blend of science and art, evolving over time and in response to technological advances and cultural shifts. Nutrition at its most basic level is food—for the mind, body, and soul.

Although considered the realm of the dietitian, nutrition is a vital and integral component of nursing care. Today's nurses need to know, understand, apply, analyze, synthesize, and evaluate nutrition throughout the life cycle and along the wellness/illness continuum. They incorporate nutrition into all aspects of nursing care plans, from assessment and nursing diagnoses to implementation and evaluation. By virtue of their close contact with patients and families, nurses are often on the front line in facilitating nutrition. This text seeks to give student nurses a practical and valuable nutrition foundation to better serve themselves and their clients.

NEW TO THIS EDITION

This seventh edition continues the approach of providing the essential information nurses need to know for practice. Building upon this framework, content has been thoroughly updated to reflect the latest evidence-based practice. Examples of content updates that are new to this edition are as follows:

- MyPlate, which replaces MyPyramid as the graphic to illustrate the Dietary Guidelines for Americans
- Recommended Dietary Allowances (RDAs) for calcium and vitamin D
- Inclusion of a validated stand-alone nutrition screening tool for older adults that is appropriate for community settings and in clinical practice
- Expanded coverage of bariatric surgery and obesity in general, particularly with regard to the importance of behavioral strategies for navigating our increasingly obesogenic environment
- The low-FODMAP (fermental oligo-, di-, and monosaccharides and polyols) diet for irritable bowel syndrome and possibly other gastrointestinal disorders
- A shift in focus from single nutrients (e.g., saturated fat) to a food pattern approach (e.g., the DASH diet) for communicating and implementing a heart healthy diet
- Updated 2011 nutrition therapy guidelines for patients with chronic kidney disease who are not on dialysis

ORGANIZATION OF THE TEXT

Unit One is devoted to Principles of Nutrition. It begins with Chapter 1, Nutrition in Nursing, which focuses on why and how nutrition is important to nurses in all settings. Chapters devoted to carbohydrates, protein, lipids, vitamins, water and minerals, and energy balance provide a foundation for wellness. The second part of each chapter highlights health promotion topics and demonstrates practical application of essential information, such as how to increase fiber intake, criteria to consider when buying a vitamin supplement, and the risks and benefits of a vegetarian diet.

Unit Two, Nutrition in Health Promotion, begins with Chapter 8, Guidelines for Healthy Eating. This chapter features the Dietary Reference Intakes, the Dietary Guidelines for Americans, and MyPlate. Other chapters in this unit examine consumer issues and cultural and religious influences on food and nutrition. The nutritional needs associated with the life cycle are presented in chapters devoted to pregnant and lactating women, children and adolescents, and older adults.

Unit Three, Nutrition in Clinical Practice, includes nutrition therapy for obesity and eating disorders, enteral and parenteral nutrition, metabolic and respiratory stress, gastrointestinal disorders, diabetes, cardiovascular disorders, renal disorders, cancer, and HIV/AIDS. Pathophysiology is tightly focused as it pertains to nutrition.

RECURRING FEATURES

This edition retains popular features of the previous edition to facilitate learning and engage students.

- **Check Your Knowledge** presents true/false questions at the beginning of each chapter to assess the students' baseline knowledge. Questions relate to chapter Learning Objectives.
- **Key Terms** are defined in the margin for convenient reference.
- **Quick Bites**—fewer and more condensed to improve layout and readability in the new edition—provide quick nutrition facts, valuable information, and current research.
- **Nursing Process** tables clearly present sample application of nutrition concepts in context of the nursing process.
- **How Do You Respond?** helps students identify potential questions they may encounter in the clinical setting and prepares them to think on their feet.
- A **Case Study** and **Study Questions** at the end of each chapter challenge students to apply what they have learned.
- **Key Concepts** summarize important information from each chapter.

TEACHING AND LEARNING RESOURCES

Instructors and students will find valuable resources to accompany the book on thePoint at **http://thePoint.lww.com/Dudek7e**.

Resources for Instructors

Comprehensive teaching resources are available to instructors upon adoption of this text and include the following materials.

- A free **E-book** on thePoint provides access to the book's full text and images online.
- A **Test Generator** lets instructors put together exclusive new tests from a bank containing NCLEX-style questions.
- **PowerPoint Presentations** provide an easy way to integrate the textbook with the classroom. Multiple-choice and true/false questions are included to promote class participation.
- An **Image Bank** provides the photographs and illustrations from this text for use in course materials.
- Access to all student resources is also provided.

Resources for Students

Students can activate the code in the front of this book at **http://thePoint.lww.com/ activate** to access the following free resources.

- A free **E-book** on thePoint provides access to the book's full text and images online.
- *NEW!* **Practice & Learn Interactive Case Studies** provide realistic case examples and offer students the opportunity to apply nutrition essentials to nursing care.
- **Journal Articles** provided for each chapter offer access to current research available in Lippincott Williams & Wilkins journals.

I hope this text and teaching/learning resource package provide the impetus to embrace nutrition on both a personal and professional level.

Susan G. Dudek, RD, CDN, BS

Acknowledgments

I am humbled and grateful to be still writing this book after six editions. It is a project that has been professionally rewarding, personally challenging, and rich with opportunities to grow. In large part, the success of this book rests with the dedicated and creative professionals at Lippincott Williams & Wilkins. Because of their support and talents, I am able to do what I love—write, create, teach, and learn. I especially thank

- David Troy, Senior Acquisitions Editor, who provided the spark to ignite the project.
- Maria McAvey, Editorial Product Manager, for her meticulous attention to detail and gentle guidance.
- Marian Bellus, Production Project Manager; Holly Reid McLaughlin, Design Coordinator; John Johnson, Education Marketing Manager, Nursing; and Latisha Ogelsby, Editorial Assistant, the behind-the-scene professionals whose efforts help transform an ugly duckling into a beautiful swan.

- The reviewers of the sixth edition, whose insightful comments and suggestions helped shape a new and improved edition.

- My friends and family—my sideline cheerleaders—who so patiently gave me the time and space to work on "my story."

- I am especially thankful to my husband Joe . . . always there through thick and thin.

Contents

Contents

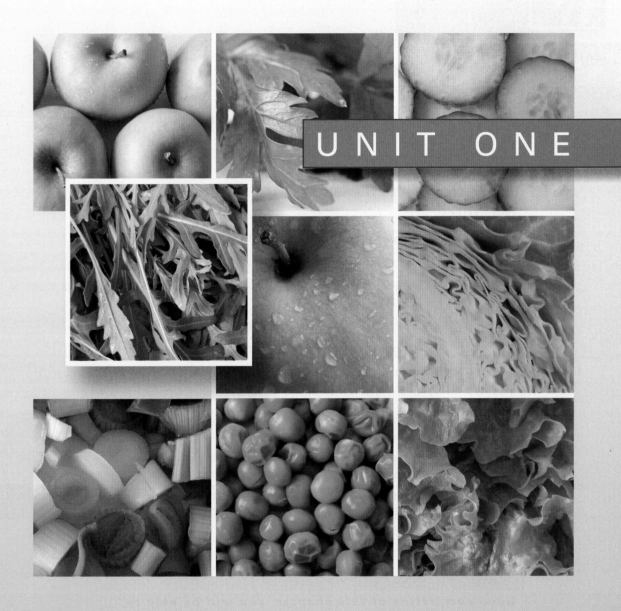

Principles of Nutrition

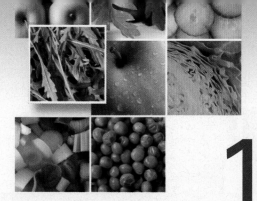

1 Nutrition in Nursing

TRUE	FALSE		
☐	☐	**1**	The nurse's role in nutrition is to call the dietitian.
☐	☐	**2**	Nutrition screening is used to identify clients at risk for malnutrition.
☐	☐	**3**	The Joint Commission stipulates the criteria to be included on a nutritional screen for hospitalized patients.
☐	☐	**4**	Changes in weight reflect acute changes in nutritional status.
☐	☐	**5**	A person can be malnourished without being underweight.
☐	☐	**6**	The only cause of a low serum albumin concentration is protein malnutrition.
☐	☐	**7**	"Significant" weight loss is 5% of body weight in 1 month.
☐	☐	**8**	People who take five or more prescription or over-the-counter medications or dietary supplements are at risk for nutritional problems.
☐	☐	**9**	Obtaining reliable and accurate information on what the client usually eats can help identify intake as a source of nutrition problems.
☐	☐	**10**	Physical signs and symptoms of malnutrition develop only after other signs of malnutrition are apparent (e.g., abnormal lab values, weight change).

LEARNING OBJECTIVES

Upon completion of this chapter, you will be able to

1 Compare nutrition screening to nutrition assessment.
2 Evaluate weight loss for its significance over a 1-month or 6-month interval.
3 Discuss the validity and reliability of using physical signs to support a nutritional diagnosis of malnutrition.
4 Give examples of nursing diagnoses that may use nutrition therapy as an intervention.
5 Demonstrate how nurses can facilitate client and family teaching of nutrition therapy.
6 Explain why an alternative term to "diet" is useful.

Based on Maslow's hierarchy of needs, food and nutrition rank on the same level as air in the basic necessities of life. Obviously, death eventually occurs without food. But unlike air, food does so much more than simply sustain life. Food is loaded with personal, social, and cultural meanings that define our food values, beliefs, and customs. That food nourishes the mind as well as the body broadens nutrition to an art as well as a science. Nutrition is not simply a matter of food or no food but rather a question of what kind, how much, how often, and why. Merging want with need and pleasure with health are keys to feeding the body, mind, and soul.

Although the dietitian is the nutrition and food expert, nurses play a vital role in nutrition care. Nurses may be responsible for screening hospitalized patients to identify patients at nutritional risk. They often serve as the liaison between the dietitian and physician as well as with other members of the health-care team. Nurses have far more contact with the patient and family and are often available as a nutrition resource when dietitians are not, such as during the evening, on weekends, and during discharge instructions. In home care and wellness settings, dietitians may be available only on a consultative basis. Nurses may reinforce nutrition counseling provided by the dietitian and may be responsible for basic nutrition education in hospitalized clients with low to mild nutritional risk. Nurses are intimately involved in all aspects of nutritional care.

This chapter discusses nutrition within the context of nursing, including nutrition screening and how nutrition can be integrated into the nursing care process.

NUTRITION SCREENING

Nutritional Screen: a quick look at a few variables to judge a client's relative risk for nutritional problems. Can be custom designed for a particular population (e.g., pregnant women) or for a specific disorder (e.g., cardiac disease).

Malnutrition: literally "bad nutrition" or any nutritional imbalance including overnutrition. In practice, malnutrition usually means undernutrition or an inadequate intake of protein and/or calories that causes loss of fat stores and/or muscle wasting.

Nutrition screening is a quick look at a few variables to identify individuals who are malnourished or who are at risk for **malnutrition** so that an in-depth nutrition assessment can follow. Screening tools should be simple, reliable, valid, applicable to most patients or clients in the group, and use data that is readily available (Academy of Nutrition and Dietetics, 2012). For instance, a community-based senior center may use a nutrition screen that focuses mostly on intake risks common to that population, such as whether the client eats alone most of the time and/or has physical limitations that impair the ability to buy or cook food (Fig. 1.1). In contrast, common screening parameters in acute care settings include unintentional weight loss, appetite, body mass index (BMI), and disease severity. Advanced age, dementia, and other factors may be considered. There is no universally agreed upon tool that is valid and reliable at identifying risk of malnutrition in all populations at all times.

The Joint Commission, a nonprofit organization that sets health-care standards and accredits health-care facilities that meet those standards, specifies that nutrition screening be conducted within 24 hours after admission to a hospital or other health-care facility—even on weekends and holidays. The Joint Commission allows facilities to determine screening criteria and how risk is defined. For instance, a hospital may use serum creatinine level as a screening criterion, with a level greater than 2.5 mg/dL defined as "high risk" because the majority of their patients are elderly and the prevalence of chronic renal problems is high. The Joint Commission also leaves the decision of who performs the screening up to individual facilities. Because the standard applies 24 hours a day, 7 days a week, staff nurses are often responsible for completing the screen as part of the admission process. Clients who "pass" the initial screen are rescreened after a specified amount of time to determine if their status has changed.

DETERMINE YOUR NUTRITIONAL HEALTH

The warning signs of poor nutritional health are often overlooked. Use this checklist to find out if you or someone you know is at nutritional risk.

Read the statements below. Circle the number in the "yes" column for those that apply to you or someone you know. For each "yes" answer, score the number in the box. Total your nutritional score.

	YES
I have an illness or condition that made me change the kind and/or amount of food I eat.	2
I eat fewer than two meals per day.	3
I eat few fruits or vegetables, or milk products.	2
I have three or more drinks of beer, liquor or wine almost every day.	2
I have tooth or mouth problems that make it hard for me to eat.	2
I don't always have enough money to buy the food I need.	4
I eat alone most of the time.	1
I take three or more different prescribed or over-the-counter drugs a day.	1
Without wanting to, I have lost or gained 10 pounds in the last six months.	2
I am not always physically able to shop, cook and/or feed myself.	2
TOTAL	

Total your nutritional score. If it's –

0-2   Good! Recheck your nutritional score in six months.

3-5   You are at moderate nutritional risk. See what can be done to improve your eating habits and lifestyle. Your office on aging, senior nutrition program, senior citizens center or health department can help. Recheck your nutritional score in three months.

6 or more   You are at high nutritional risk. Bring this checklist the next time you see your doctor, dietitian or other qualified health or social service professional. Talk with them about any problems you may have. Ask for help to improve your nutritional health.

Remember that warning signs suggest risk, but do not represent diagnosis of any condition.

■ **FIGURE 1.1** Determine your nutritional health. American Academy of Family Physicians, the American Dietetic Association, the National Council on the Aging, Inc. The Nutrition Screening Initiative.

Nutritional Assessment: an in-depth analysis of a person's nutritional status. In the clinical setting, nutritional assessments focus on moderate- to high-risk patients with suspected or confirmed protein–energy malnutrition.

NUTRITION CARE PROCESS

Clients considered to be at moderate or high risk for malnutrition through screening are usually referred to a dietitian for a comprehensive **nutritional assessment** to identify specific risks or confirm the existence of malnutrition. Nutritional assessment is more accurately called the nutrition care process, which includes four steps (Fig. 1.2). While nurses use the same problem-solving model to develop nursing or multidisciplinary care plans that

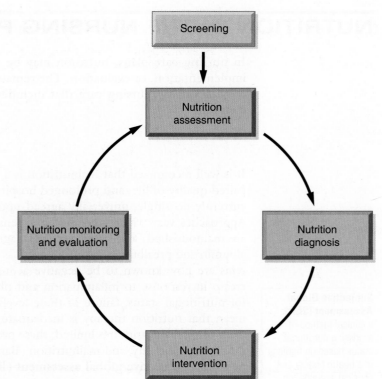

■ FIGURE 1.2   The nutrition care process.
Like the nursing process, the nutrition care
process is a problem-solving method used to
evaluate and treat nutrition-related problems.

may also integrate nutrition, the nutritional plan of care devised by dietitians is specific for nutrition problems. Some obvious differences in focus are described below:

- Dietitians may obtain much of their preliminary information about the patient from the nursing history and physical examination, such as height and weight; skin integrity; usual diet prior to admission; difficulty chewing, swallowing, or self-feeding; chief complaint; medications, supplements, and over-the-counter drugs used prior to admission; and living situation. Dietitians may request laboratory tests to assess vitamin levels when micronutrient deficiencies are suspected.
- Dietitians interview patients and/or families to obtain a nutrition history, which may include information on current dietary habits; recent changes in intake or appetite; intake of snacks; alcohol consumption; food allergies and intolerances; ethnic, cultural, or religious diet influences; nutrition knowledge and beliefs; and use of supplements. A nutrition history can help differentiate nutrition problems caused by inadequate intake from those caused by disease.
- Dietitians usually calculate estimated calorie and protein requirements based on the assessment data and determine whether the diet ordered is adequate and appropriate for the individual.
- Dietitians determine nutrition diagnoses that define the nutritional problem, etiology, and signs and symptoms. While a nursing diagnosis statement may begin with "Altered nutrition: eating less than the body needs," a nutrition diagnosis would be more specific, such as "Inadequate protein–energy intake."
- Dietitians may also determine the appropriate malnutrition diagnosis code for the patient for hospital reimbursement purposes.
- Nutrition interventions may include requesting a diet order change, requesting additional laboratory tests to monitor nutritional repletion, and performing nutrition counseling or education.

NUTRITION IN THE NURSING PROCESS

In nursing care plans, nutrition may be part of the assessment data, diagnosis, plan, implementation, or evaluation. The remainder of this chapter is intended to help nurses provide quality nursing care that includes basic nutrition, not to help nurses become dietitians.

Assessment

It is well recognized that malnutrition is a major contributor to morbidity, mortality, impaired quality of life, and prolonged hospital stays (White et al., 2012). However, there is currently no single, universally agreed upon method to assess or diagnose malnutrition. Approaches vary widely and may lack sensitivity (the ability to diagnose all people who are malnourished) and specificity (misdiagnosing a well-nourished person). For instance, albumin and prealbumin have been used as diagnostic markers of malnutrition. These proteins are now known to be negative acute phase proteins, which means their levels decrease in response to inflammation and physiologic stress. Because they are not specific for nutritional status, failure of these levels to increase with nutrition repletion does not mean that nutrition therapy is inadequate (Fessler, 2008). Although their usefulness in diagnosing malnutrition is limited, these proteins may help identify patients at high risk for morbidity, mortality, and malnutrition (Banh, 2006). BMI and some or all of the components of a **subjective global assessment** (Box 1.1) are commonly used to assess nutrition (Fessler, 2008).

Subjective Global Assessment (SGA): a clinical method of assessing nutritional status based on findings in a health history and physical examination.

Medical History and Diagnosis

The chief complaint and medical history may reveal disease-related risks for malnutrition and whether inflammation is present (Fig. 1.3). Patients with gastrointestinal symptoms or disorders are among those who are most prone to malnutrition, particularly when symptoms such as nausea, vomiting, diarrhea, and anorexia last for more than 2 weeks. Box 1.2 lists psychosocial factors that may impact intake or requirements and help identify nutrition counseling needs.

Box 1.1   CRITERIA INCLUDED IN SUBJECTIVE GLOBAL ASSESSMENT

Weight Change
- Unintentional weight loss and the time period of loss

Dietary Intake
- Change from normal, duration, type of diet consumed

Gastrointestinal Symptoms Lasting Longer than 2 Weeks
- Nausea, vomiting, diarrhea, anorexia

Functional Capacity
- Normal or suboptimal; ambulatory or bedridden

Disease and Its Relation to Nutritional Requirements
- Primary diagnosis; severity of metabolic stress

Physical Signs and Severity of Findings
- Loss of subcutaneous fat (triceps, chest), muscle wasting (quadriceps, deltoids), ankle edema, sacral edema, ascites

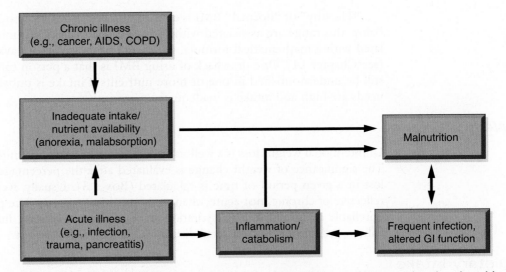

■ **FIGURE 1.3** Factors that may be involved in the etiology of illness-related malnutrition.

Body Mass Index

Body Mass Index:
an index of weight in relation to height that is calculated mathematically by dividing weight in kilograms by the square of height in meters.

Body mass index (BMI) is an index of a person's weight in relation to height used to estimate relative risk of health problems related to weight. Because it is relatively quick and easy to measure height and weight and requires little skill, actual *measures*, not *estimates*, should be used whenever possible to ensure accuracy and reliability. A patient's *stated* height and weight should be used only when there are no other options.

QUICK BITE

Interpreting BMI

<18.5	underweight
18.5–24.9	healthy weight
25–29.9	overweight
30–34.9	obesity class 1
35–39.9	obesity class 2
≥40	obesity class 3

Box 1.2   **PSYCHOSOCIAL FACTORS THAT MAY INFLUENCE INTAKE, NUTRITIONAL REQUIREMENTS, OR NUTRITION COUNSELING**

Psychological Factors
- Depression
- Eating disorders
- Psychosis

Social Factors
- Illiteracy
- Language barriers
- Limited knowledge of nutrition and food safety
- Altered or impaired intake related to culture
- Altered or impaired intake related to religion

- Lack of caregiver or social support system
- Social isolation
- Lack of or inadequate cooking arrangements
- Limited or low income
- Limited access to transportation to obtain food
- Advanced age (older than 80 years)
- Lack of or extreme physical activity
- Use of tobacco or recreational drugs
- Limited use or knowledge of community resources

"Healthy" or "normal" BMI is defined numerically as 18.5 to 24.9. Values above and below this range are associated with increased health risks. Although BMI can be calculated with a mathematical formula, tables and nomograms are available for convenience (see Chapter 14). One drawback of using BMI is that a person can have a high BMI and still be undernourished in one or more nutrients if intake is unbalanced or if nutritional needs are high and intake is inadequate.

Weight Change

Unintentional weight loss is a well-validated indicator of malnutrition (White et al., 2012). The significance of weight change is evaluated after the percentage of usual body weight lost in a given period of time is calculated (Box 1.3). Usually, weight changes are more reflective of chronic, not acute, changes in nutritional status. The patient's weight can be unreliable or invalid due to hydration status. Edema, anasarca, fluid resuscitation, heart failure, and chronic liver or renal disease can falsely inflate weight.

Dietary Intake

A decrease in intake compared to the patient's normal intake may indicate nutritional risk. However, like other data, validity and reliability may be an issue. Although the nurse may only be required to fill in a blank space next to the word "appetite," simply asking the client "How is your appetite?" will probably not provide sufficient information. A better question may be "Has the type or amount of food you eat recently changed? If so, please explain." Consuming only liquids and severely limiting the type or amount of food are risks.

Another question to avoid while obtaining a nursing history is "Are you on a diet?" To many people, diet is synonymous with weight loss diet; they may fail to mention they use nutrition therapy to avoid sodium, modify fat, or count carbohydrates. A better question would be, "Do you avoid any particular foods?" or "Do you watch what you eat in any way?" Even the term "meal" may elicit a stereotypical mental picture. Questions to consider when asking a client about his or her usual intake appear in Box 1.4.

Box 1.3   CALCULATING AND EVALUATING PERCENT WEIGHT CHANGE

Calculating Percent Weight Change

$$\% \text{ weight change} = \frac{(\text{usual body weight} - \text{current body weight})}{\text{usual body weight}} \times 100$$

Significant Unintentional Weight Loss

Time Period	(% of Weight Lost)
1 week	>2
1 month	>5
3 months	>7.5
6 months	>10

Source: Academy of Nutrition and Dietetics. (2012). *Nutrition Care Manual.* Available at http://nutritioncaremanual.org/content.cfm?ncm_content_id=79554. Accessed on 8/16/2012.

Box 1.4   QUESTIONS TO CONSIDER ABOUT INTAKE

How many meals and snacks do you eat in a 24-hour period? This question helps to establish the pattern of eating and identifies unusual food habits such as pica, food faddism, eating disorders, and meal skipping.

Do you have any food allergies or intolerances, and, if so, what are they? The greater the number of foods restricted or eliminated in the diet, the greater the likelihood of nutritional deficiencies. This question may also shed light on the client's need for nutrition counseling. For instance, clients with hiatal hernia who are intolerant of citrus fruits and juices may benefit from counseling on how to ensure an adequate intake of vitamin C.

What types of vitamin, mineral, herbal, or other supplements do you use and why? A multivitamin, multimineral supplement that provides 100% or less of the daily value offers some protection against less than optimal food choices. Folic acid in supplements or fortified food is recommended for women of childbearing age; people older than 50 years are encouraged to obtain vitamin B_{12} from fortified foods or supplements. However, potential problems may arise from other types or amounts of supplements. For instance, large doses of vitamins A, B_6, and D have the potential to cause toxicity symptoms. Iron supplements may decrease zinc absorption and negatively impact zinc status over time.

What concerns do you have about what or how you eat? This question places the responsibility of healthy eating with the client, where it should be. A client who may benefit from nutrition intervention and counseling *in theory* may not be a candidate for such *in practice* depending on his or her level of interest and motivation. This question may also shed light on whether or not the client understands what he or she should be eating and whether the client is willing to make changes in eating habits.

For clients who are acutely ill: How has illness affected your choice or tolerance of food? Sometimes, food aversions or intolerances can shed light on what is going on with the client. For instance, someone who experiences abdominal pain that is relieved by eating may have a duodenal ulcer. Clients with little or no intake of food or liquids are at risk for dehydration and nutrient deficiencies.

Who prepares the meals? This person may need nutritional counseling.

Do you have enough food to eat? Be aware that pride and an unwillingness to admit inability to afford an adequate diet may prevent some clients and families from answering this question. For hospitalized clients, it may be more useful to ask the client to compare the size of the meals they are served in the hospital with the size of meals they normally eat.

How much alcohol do you consume daily? Risk begins at more than one drink daily for women and more than two drinks daily for men.

Physical Findings

Loss of subcutaneous fat, such as in the triceps and chest, muscle wasting in the quadriceps and deltoids, ankle edema, sacral edema, and ascites may be indicative of malnutrition. These abnormal findings are subjectively assessed as mild, moderate, or severe.

Box 1.5 lists other physical findings that may suggest malnutrition. Most physical symptoms cannot be considered diagnostic because evaluation of "normal" versus "abnormal" findings is subjective, and the signs of malnutrition may be nonspecific. For instance, dull, dry hair may be related to severe protein deficiency or to overexposure to the sun or use of hair products such as colorants. In addition, physical signs and symptoms of malnutrition can vary in intensity among population groups because of genetic and environmental differences. Lastly, physical findings occur only with overt malnutrition, not **subclinical** malnutrition.

Subclinical: asymptomatic.

Box 1.5	PHYSICAL SYMPTOMS SUGGESTIVE OF MALNUTRITION

- Hair that is dull, brittle, or dry, or falls out easily
- Swollen glands of the neck and cheeks
- Dry, rough, or spotty skin that may have a sandpaper feel
- Poor or delayed wound healing or sores
- Thin appearance with lack of subcutaneous fat
- Muscle wasting (decreased size and strength)
- Edema of the lower extremities
- Weakened hand grasp
- Depressed mood
- Abnormal heart rate, heart rhythm, or blood pressure
- Enlarged liver or spleen
- Loss of balance and coordination

Nursing Diagnosis

A diagnosis is made after assessment data are interpreted. Nursing diagnoses in hospitals and long-term care facilities provide written documentation of the client's status and serve as a framework for the plan of care that follows. The diagnoses relate directly to nutrition when the pattern of nutrition and metabolism is the problem. Other nursing diagnoses, while not specific for nutrition, may involve nutrition as part of the plan, such as teaching the patient how to increase fiber intake to relieve the nursing diagnosis of constipation. Box 1.6 lists nursing diagnoses with nutritional significance.

Planning: Client Outcomes

Outcomes, or goals, should be measurable, attainable, specific, and client centered. How do you measure success against a vague goal of "gain weight by eating better"? Is "eating better" achieved by adding butter to foods to increase calories or by substituting 1% milk for whole milk because it is heart healthy? Is a 1-pound weight gain in 1 month acceptable or is 1 pound/week preferable? Is 1 pound/week attainable if the client has accelerated metabolism and catabolism caused by third-degree burns?

Client-centered outcomes place the focus on the client, not the health-care provider; they specify where the client is heading. Whenever possible, give the client the opportunity to actively participate in goal setting, even if the client's perception of need differs from yours. In matters that do not involve life or death, it is best to first address the client's concerns. Your primary consideration may be the patient's significant weight loss during the last 6 months of chemotherapy, whereas the patient's major concern may be fatigue. The two issues are undoubtedly related, but your effectiveness as a change agent is greater if you approach the problem from the client's perspective. Commitment to achieving the goal is greatly increased when the client "owns" the goal.

Keep in mind that the goal for all clients is to consume adequate calories, protein, and nutrients using foods they like and tolerate as appropriate. If possible, additional short-term goals may be set to alleviate symptoms or side effects of disease or treatments and to prevent complications or recurrences if appropriate. After short-term goals are met, attention can expand to promoting healthy eating to reduce the risk of chronic diet-related diseases such as obesity, diabetes, hypertension, and atherosclerosis.

Box 1.6	SELECTED NURSING DIAGNOSES WITH NUTRITIONAL SIGNIFICANCE

Pattern Nutrition and Metabolic

High risk for altered nutrition: intake
    exceeds the body's needs
Altered nutrition: intake exceeds the
    body's needs
Altered nutrition: eating less than the
    body needs
Effective breastfeeding
Ineffective breastfeeding
Interrupted breastfeeding
Ineffective infant feeding pattern
High risk of aspiration
Swallowing disorder
Altered oral mucosa
High risk for fluid volume deficits
Fluid volume deficits
Excess fluid volume
High risk for impaired skin integrity
Impaired skin integrity
Impaired tissue integrity
High risk for altered body temperature
Ineffective thermoregulation
Hyperthermia
Hypothermia

**Examples of Other Diagnoses in Which
Nutrition Interventions May Be Part of
the Care Plan**

Altered health maintenance
Ineffective management of therapeutic
    regimen
Infection
Constipation
Diarrhea
Bowel incontinence
Altered urinary excretion
Impaired physical mobility
Fatigue
Self-care deficit: feeding
Household altered
Altered tissue perfusion
Pain
Chronic pain
Alterations sensory/perceptual
Unilateral oblivion
Knowledge deficits
Anxiety
Body image disorder
Social isolation
Ineffective individual coping
Ineffective family coping
Defensive coping

Nursing Interventions

What can you or others do to effectively and efficiently help the client achieve his or her goals? Interventions may include nutrition therapy and client teaching.

Nutrition Therapy

Throughout this book, the heading "Nutrition Therapy" is used in place of "Diet" because, among clients, *diet* is a four-letter word with negative connotations, such as counting calories, deprivation, sacrifice, and misery. A diet is viewed as a short-term punishment to endure until a normal pattern of eating can resume. Clients respond better to terminology that is less emotionally charged. Terms such as *eating pattern*, *food intake*, *eating style*, or *the food you eat* may be used to keep the lines of communication open.

Nutrition therapy recommendations are usually general suggestions to increase/decrease, limit/avoid, reduce/encourage, or modify/maintain aspects of the diet because exact nutrient requirements are determined on an individual basis. Where more precise amounts of nutrients are specified, consider them as a starting point and monitor the client's response. Box 1.7 highlights formulas for calculating calorie and protein requirements.

Nutrition theory does not always apply to practice. Factors such as the client's prognosis, outside support systems, level of intelligence and motivation, willingness to comply, emotional health, financial status, religious or ethnic background, and other medical

Box 1.7 CALCULATING ESTIMATED NEEDS

A "rule-of-thumb" method of estimating calorie requirements:

Multiply weight in kg by

30 cal/kg for most healthy adults
25 cal/kg for elderly adults
20–25 cal/kg for obese adults

Example: For an adult weighing 154 pounds:

$$154 \text{ pounds} \div 2.2 \text{ kg/pound} = 70 \text{ kg}$$

$$70 \text{ kg} \times 30 \text{ cal/kg} = 2100 \text{ cal/day}$$

Estimating protein requirements

$$\text{Healthy adults need } 0.8 \text{ g protein/kg}$$

Example: For an adult weighing 154 pounds:

$$154 \text{ pounds} \div 2.2 \text{ kg/pound} = 70 \text{ kg}$$

$$70 \text{ kg} \times 0.8 \text{ g/kg} = 56 \text{ g protein/day}$$

conditions may cause the optimal diet to be impractical in either the clinical or the home setting. Generalizations do not apply to all individuals at all times. Also, comfort foods (e.g., chicken soup, mashed potatoes, ice cream) are valuable for their emotional benefits if not nutritional ones. Honor clients' requests for individual comfort foods whenever possible. Box 1.8 suggests ways the nurse can promote an adequate intake.

Client Teaching

Compared with "well" clients, patients in a clinical setting may be more receptive to nutritional advice, especially if they feel better by doing so or are fearful of a relapse or complications. But hospitalized patients are also prone to confusion about nutrition messages. The patient's ability to assimilate new information may be compromised by pain, medication, anxiety, or a distracting setting. Time spent with a dietitian or diet technician learning about a "diet" may be

Box 1.8 WAYS TO PROMOTE AN ADEQUATE INTAKE

- Reassure clients who are apprehensive about eating.
- Encourage a big breakfast if appetite deteriorates throughout the day.
- Advocate discontinuation of intravenous therapy as soon as feasible.
- Replace meals withheld for diagnostic tests.
- Promote congregate dining if appropriate.
- Question diet orders that appear inappropriate.
- Display a positive attitude when serving food or discussing nutrition.
- Order snacks and nutritional supplements.
- Request assistance with feeding or meal setup.
- Get the patient out of bed to eat if possible.
- Encourage good oral hygiene.
- Solicit information on food preferences.

Box 1.9   WAYS TO FACILITATE CLIENT AND FAMILY TEACHING

- Listen to the client's concerns and ideas.
- Encourage family involvement if appropriate.
- Reinforce the importance of obtaining adequate nutrition.
- Help the client to select appropriate foods.
- Counsel the client about drug–nutrient interactions.
- Avoid using the term "diet."
- Emphasize things "to do" instead of things "not to do."
- Keep the message simple.
- Review written handouts with the client.
- Advise the client to avoid foods that are not tolerated.

brief or interrupted, and the patient may not even know what questions to ask until long after the dietitian is gone. Box 1.9 suggests ways nurses can facilitate client and family teaching.

Monitoring and Evaluation

In the "Nursing Process" sections of this textbook, monitoring and evaluation are grouped together, even though they are different in practice. In reality, monitoring precedes evaluation as a way to stay on top of progress or difficulties the client is experiencing. Box 1.10 offers general monitoring suggestions. Evaluation assesses whether client outcomes were achieved after the nursing care plan was given time to work. Given the limitations inherent in an abstract nursing care plan, monitoring and evaluation are combined in this textbook.

Ideally, the client's outcomes are achieved on a timely basis, and evaluation statements are client outcomes rewritten from "the client will" to "the client is." In reality, outcomes may be only partially met or not achieved at all; in those instances, it is important to determine why the result was less than ideal. Were the outcomes realistic for this particular client? Were the interventions appropriate and consistently implemented? Evaluation includes deciding whether to continue, change, or abolish the plan.

Consider a male client admitted to the hospital for chronic diarrhea. During the 3 weeks before admission, the client experienced significant weight loss due to malabsorption secondary to diarrhea. Your goal is for the client to maintain his admission weight. Your interventions are to provide small meals of low-residue foods as ordered, to eliminate lactose because of the likelihood of intolerance, to increase protein and calories with appropriate

Box 1.10   MONITORING SUGGESTIONS

- Observe intake whenever possible to judge the adequacy.
- Document appetite and take action when the client does not eat.
- Order supplements if intake is low or needs are high.
- Request a nutritional consult.
- Assess tolerance (i.e., absence of side effects).
- Monitor weight.
- Monitor progression of restrictive diets. Clients who are receiving nothing by mouth (NPO), who are restricted to a clear liquid diet, or who are receiving enteral or parenteral nutrition are at risk for nutritional problems.
- Monitor the client's grasp of the information and motivation to change.

nutrient-dense supplements, and to explain the nutrition therapy recommendations to the client to ease his concerns about eating. You find that the client's intake is poor because of lack of appetite and a fear that eating and drinking will promote diarrhea. You notify the dietitian who counsels the client about low-residue foods, obtains likes and dislikes, and urges the client to think of the supplements as part of the medical treatment, not as a food eaten for taste or pleasure. You document intake and diligently encourage the client to eat and drink everything served. However, the client's weight continues to drop. You attribute this to his reluctance to eat and to the slow resolution of diarrhea related to inflammation. You determine that the goal is still realistic and appropriate but that the client is not willing or able to consume foods orally. You consult with the physician and dietitian about the client's refusal to eat and the plan changes from an oral diet to tube feeding.

HOW DO YOU RESPOND?

Should I save my menus from the hospital to help me plan meals at home? This is not a bad idea if the in-house and discharge food plans are the same, but the menus should serve as a guide, not a gospel. Just because shrimp was never on the menu doesn't mean it is taboo. Likewise, if the client hated the orange juice served every morning, he or she shouldn't feel compelled to continue drinking it. By necessity, hospital menus are more rigid than at-home eating plans.

Can you just tell me what to eat and I'll do it? A black-and-white approach should be used only when absolutely necessary, such as for food allergies or for clients who insist on a rigid plan rather than the freedom to make choices. In most cases, flexible and individualized guidelines and recommendations will promote the greatest chance of compliance. Urge the client not to think of foods as "good" or "bad" but rather "more healthy" and "less healthy," except in situations of food allergy or intolerance. In most other cases, foods are negotiable.

CASE STUDY

Steven is a 44-year-old male who is 5 ft 11 in tall and weighs 182 pounds. Over the last month, he has lost approximately 10 pounds, which he blames on loss of appetite and fatigue. When he went to his family doctor with flu-like symptoms, a blood test revealed a very high white blood cell count, low platelet count, and low hemoglobin. The doctor told him to proceed to the hospital for admission to rule out acute leukemia. Further laboratory tests are pending. Admitting orders include a regular diet. Steven does not have a significant medical history. He is married, has three children, and enjoys a successful career.

Calculate and evaluate Steven's weight according to the following standards:

- BMI
- Percent weight change
- Based on Steven's weight and weight change, is he at nutritional risk?
- Does Steven's possible diagnosis place him at nutritional risk?
- What other criteria would help determine his level of risk?
- Calculate his estimated calorie requirements. Calculate his Recommended Dietary Allowance (RDA) for protein.
- If he is treated for leukemia, his protein need may increase to approximately 1.2 g protein/kg. How much would he then require?
- The hospital's diet manual says that, on average, a regular diet provides 2400 calories and 90 g of protein. Is this diet adequate to meet his needs?

STUDY QUESTIONS

1. Nurses are in an ideal position to
   a. Screen patients for risk of malnutrition
   b. Order therapeutic diets
   c. Conduct comprehensive nutrition assessments
   d. Calculate a patient's calorie and protein needs

2. How much weight would a 200-pound adult need to lose in a month to be considered significant?
   a. It depends on the patient's BMI.
   b. More than 5 pounds
   c. More than 7.5 pounds
   d. More than 10 pounds

3. Which of the following criteria would most likely be on a nutrition screen in the hospital?
   a. Prealbumin value
   b. Weight change
   c. Serum potassium value
   d. Cultural food preferences

4. Which of the following statements is accurate regarding physical signs and symptoms of malnutrition?
   a. "Physical signs of malnutrition appear before changes in weight or laboratory values occur."
   b. "Physical signs of malnutrition are suggestive, not definitive, for malnutrition."
   c. "Physical signs are easily identified as 'abnormal.'"
   d. "All races and genders exhibit the same intensity of physical changes in response to malnutrition."

5. Your patient has a question about the cardiac diet the dietitian reviewed with him yesterday. What is the nurse's best response?
   a. "Ask your doctor when you go for your follow-up appointment."
   b. "What is the question? If I can't answer it, I will get the dietitian to come back to answer it."
   c. "Just do your best. The handout she gave you is simply a list of guidelines, not rigid instructions."
   d. "If I see the dietitian around, I will tell her you need to see her."

6. Which of the following statements is true regarding albumin?
   a. Albumin is a reliable and sensitive indicator of protein status.
   b. An increase in serum albumin accurately reflects the adequacy of nutrition therapy.
   c. An increase in albumin levels means nutrition therapy is adequate.
   d. Low albumin is associated with morbidity, mortality, and risk of malnutrition because it reflects severity of illness.

KEY CONCEPTS

■ Nutrition is an integral part of nursing care. Like air, food is a basic human need.
■ Nutrition screening is used to identify patients or clients who may be at risk for malnutrition. Screening tools are simple, quick, easy to use, and rely on available data.
■ The Joint Commission stipulates that nutrition screens be performed within 24 hours of admission to a health-care facility, but facilities are free to decide what criteria to include on a screen, what findings indicate risk, and who is to conduct the screen.

Screens are often the responsibility of staff nurses because they can be completed during a history and physical examination upon admission.

■ Patients who are identified to be a low or no nutritional risk are rescreened within a specified period of time to determine whether their nutritional risk status has changed.

■ Patients who are found to be a moderate to high nutritional risk at screening receive a comprehensive nutritional assessment by the dietitian that includes the steps of assessment, diagnosis, intervention, and monitoring and evaluation.

■ Dietitians use information from the nursing history and physical examination to begin the assessment process. They may also obtain a nutritional history from the patient, calculate estimated protein and calorie needs, assess the adequacy and appropriateness of the diet order, and identify the patient's diagnostic code for malnutrition, if appropriate.

■ Nurses can integrate nutrition into the nursing care process to develop care plans that address the individual's needs. Nurses are not expected to be dietitians but rather use nutrition to provide quality nursing care.

■ Albumin and prealbumin are not valid criteria for assessing protein status because they become depleted from inflammation and physiologic stress.

■ Accurate height and weight are essential for assessing risk and monitoring progress. They are used to determine BMI and percentage of weight loss. Significant unintentional weight loss is defined according to the length of time over which the loss occurred.

■ Dietary data can help determine whether a nutrition problem is caused by intake or by illness or its treatments. The term *diet* inspires negative feelings in most people. Replace it with *eating pattern, eating style,* or *foods you normally eat* to avoid negative connotations.

■ People with gastrointestinal symptoms, such as nausea, vomiting, diarrhea, and anorexia, that last more than 2 weeks are at risk for malnutrition.

■ Physical signs and symptoms of malnutrition are nonspecific, subjective, and develop slowly and should be considered suggestive, not diagnostic, of malnutrition.

■ Medical–psychosocial history can reveal factors that influence intake, nutritional requirements, or nutrition counseling needs.

■ Medications and nutritional supplements should be evaluated for their potential impact on nutrient intake, absorption, utilization, or excretion.

■ Nursing diagnoses relate directly to nutrition when the pattern of nutrition or metabolism is altered. Many other nursing diagnoses, such as constipation, impaired skin integrity, knowledge deficits, and infection, may include nutrition in some aspect of the plan.

■ A nutrition priority for all clients is to obtain adequate calories and nutrients based on individual needs.

■ Short-term nutrition goals are to attain or maintain adequate weight and nutritional status and (as appropriate) to avoid nutrition-related symptoms and complications of illness. Client-centered outcomes should be measurable, attainable, and specific.

■ Intake recommendations are not always appropriate for all persons; what is recommended in theory may not work for an individual. Clients may revert to comfort foods during periods of illness or stress.

■ Nurses can reinforce nutrition counseling provided by the dietitian and initiate counseling for clients with low or mild risk.

■ Use preprinted lists of "do's" and "don'ts" only if absolutely necessary, such as in the case of food allergies. For most people, actual food choices should be considered in view of how much and how often they are eaten rather than as foods that "must" or "must not" be consumed.

Check Your Knowledge Answer Key

1. **FALSE** The nurse is in an ideal position to provide nutrition information to patients and their families since he or she is the one with the greatest client contact.

2. **TRUE** Nutritional screening uses a small number of factors to identify patients or clients with malnutrition or at risk of malnutrition.

3. **FALSE** Hospitals and health-care facilities are free to decide what criteria they will use to identify risk for malnutrition and what defines risk. For instance, one hospital may use acute pancreatitis as a high-risk diagnosis, whereas another may not.

4. **FALSE** Changes in weight may be slow to occur. Weight changes are more reflective of chronic, not acute, changes in nutritional status.

5. **TRUE** A person can be malnourished without being underweight. Weight does not provide qualitative information about body composition.

6. **FALSE** Low serum albumin levels may be caused by problems other than protein malnutrition, such as injury, infection, overhydration, and liver disease.

7. **TRUE** Weight loss is judged as significant if there is a 5% loss over the course of 1 month.

8. **TRUE** People who take five or more prescription drugs, over-the-counter drugs, or dietary supplements are at increased risk for developing drug-induced nutrient deficiencies.

9. **TRUE** Determining what the patient normally eats can help diagnose the role of intake in the nutritional problem as primary, secondary, or insignificant.

10. **TRUE** Physical signs and symptoms of malnutrition develop only after other signs of malnutrition, such as laboratory values and weight changes, are observed.

Student Resources on thePoint

For additional learning materials, activate the code in the front of this book at
http://thePoint.lww.com/activate

Websites

For more on the nutrition care process used by dietitians, go to **http://www.eatright.org/HealthProfessionals/content.aspx?id=5902**

Find tools to assess dietary intake in well people at **http://fnic.nal.usda.gov/dietary-guidance/dietary-assessment**

References

Academy of Nutrition and Dietetics. (2012). *Nutrition Care Manual.* Available at http://www.nutritioncaremanual.org. Accessed on 8/15/12.

Banh, L. (2006). Serum proteins as markers of nutrition: What are we treating? *Practical Gastroenterology, 30,* 46–64.

Fessler, T. (2008). Malnutrition: A serious concern for hospitalized patients. *Today's Dietitian, 10,* 44–48.

White, J., Guenter, P., Jensen, G., Malone, A., Schofield, M., Academy Malnutrition Work Group, . . . ASPEN Board of Directors. (2012). Consensus statement of the Academy of Nutrition and Dietetics/American Society for Parenteral and Enteral Nutrition: Characteristics recommended for the identification and documentation of adults malnutrition (undernutrition). *Journal of the Academy of Nutrition and Dietetics, 112,* 730–738.

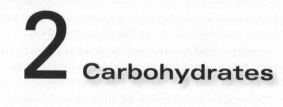

2 Carbohydrates

LEARNING OBJECTIVES

Upon completion of this chapter, you will be able to

1 Classify the type(s) of carbohydrate found in various foods.
2 Describe the functions of carbohydrates.
3 Modify a menu to ensure that the adequate intake for fiber is provided.
4 Calculate the calorie content of a food that contains only carbohydrates.
5 Debate the usefulness of using glycemic load to make food choices.
6 Suggest ways to limit sugar intake.
7 Discuss the benefits and disadvantages of using sugar alternatives.

CARBOHYDRATES

Sugar and starch come to mind when people hear the word "carbs," but carbohydrates are so much more than just table sugar and bread. Foods containing carbohydrates can be empty calories, nutritional powerhouses, or something in between. Globally, carbohydrates provide the majority of calories in almost all human diets.

This chapter describes what carbohydrates are, where they are found in the diet, and how they are handled in the body. Recommendations regarding intake and the role of carbohydrates in health are presented.

Carbohydrate Classifications

Carbohydrates (CHO): a class of energy-yielding nutrients that contain only carbon, hydrogen, and oxygen, hence the common abbreviation of CHO.

Simple Sugars: a classification of carbohydrates that includes monosaccharides and disaccharides; commonly referred to as sugars.

Complex Carbohydrates: a group name for starch, glycogen, and fiber; composed of long chains of glucose molecules.

Monosaccharide: single (mono) molecules of sugar (saccharide); the most common monosaccharides in foods are hexoses that contain six carbon atoms.

Disaccharide: "double sugar" composed of two (di) monosaccharides (e.g., sucrose, maltose, lactose).

Polysaccharides: carbohydrates consisting of many (poly) sugar molecules.

Starch: the storage form of glucose in plants.

Carbohydrates (CHO) are comprised of the elements carbon, hydrogen, and oxygen arranged into basic sugar molecules. They are classified as either **simple sugars** or **complex carbohydrates** (Fig. 2.1).

Simple Sugars

Simple sugars contain only one (mono-) or two (di-) sugar (saccharide) molecules; they vary in sweetness and sources (Table 2.1). **Monosaccharides**, such as glucose, fructose, and galactose, are absorbed "as is" without undergoing digestion; **disaccharides**, such as sucrose (table sugar), maltose, and lactose, must be split into their component monosaccharides before they can be absorbed.

Glucose, also known as dextrose, is the simple sugar of greatest distinction: it circulates through the blood to provide energy for body cells; it is a component of all disaccharides and is virtually the sole constituent of complex carbohydrates; and it is the sugar to which the body converts all other digestible carbohydrates.

Complex Carbohydrates

Complex carbohydrates, also known as **polysaccharides**, are composed of hundreds to thousands of glucose molecules linked together. Despite being made of sugar, polysaccharides do not taste sweet because their molecules are too large to fit on the tongue's taste bud receptors that sense sweetness. Starch, glycogen, and fiber are types of polysaccharides.

Starch. Through the process of photosynthesis, plants synthesize glucose, which they use for energy. Glucose not used by the plant for immediate energy is stored in the form of **starch** in seeds, roots, or stems. Grains, such as wheat, rice, corn, barley, millet, sorghum,

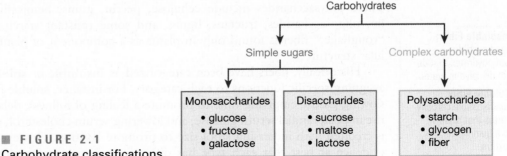

■ **FIGURE 2.1**
Carbohydrate classifications.

Table 2.1 Simple Sugars

	Relative Sweetness	Sources
Monosaccharides		
Glucose (also known as dextrose)	70	Fruit, vegetables, honey, corn syrup, cornstarch
Fructose (also known as fruit sugar)	170	Fruit, honey, some vegetables
Galactose	60	Does not occur in appreciable amounts in foods; significant only as it combines with glucose to form lactose
Disaccharides		
Sucrose (composed of glucose and fructose)	100	Fruit, vegetables Extracted from sugarcane and sugar beets into white, brown, confectioners, and turbinado sugars
Maltose (composed of two glucose molecules)	50	Not found naturally in foods; added to some foods for flavoring (e.g., malted milk shakes) and to beer for coloring Is an intermediate in starch digestion
Lactose (composed of glucose and galactose)	40	"Milk sugar"; used as an additive in many foods and drugs

oats, and rye, are the world's major food crops and the foundation of all diets. Other sources of starch include potatoes, legumes, and other starchy vegetables.

Glycogen: storage form of glucose in animals and humans.

Glycogen. Glycogen is the animal (including human) version of starch; it is stored carbohydrate available for energy as needed. Humans have a limited supply of glycogen stored in the liver and muscles. Liver glycogen breaks down and releases glucose into the bloodstream between meals to maintain normal blood glucose levels and provide fuel for tissues. Muscles do not share their supply of glycogen but use it for their own energy needs. There is virtually no dietary source of glycogen because any glycogen stored in animal tissue is quickly converted to lactic acid at the time of slaughter. Miniscule amounts of glycogen are found in shellfish, such as scallops and oysters, which is why they taste slightly sweet compared to other fish.

Fiber. Although there is no universally accepted definition of fiber, it is generally considered a group name for polysaccharides that cannot be digested by human enzymes. These polysaccharides include cellulose, pectin, gums, hemicellulose, β-glucans, inulin, oligosaccharides, fructans, lignin, and some resistant starch. Often referred to as "roughage," fiber is found only in plants as a component of plant cell walls or intercellular structure.

Insoluble Fiber: nondigestible carbohydrates that do not dissolve in water.

Soluble Fiber: nondigestible carbohydrates that dissolve to a gummy, viscous texture.

Historically, fibers have been categorized as **insoluble** or **soluble** for the purpose of assigning specific functions to each category. For instance, soluble fibers are credited with slowing gastric emptying time to promote a feeling of fullness, delaying and blunting the rise in postprandial serum glucose, and lowering serum cholesterol, whereas insoluble fiber is credited with increasing stool size to promote laxation. However, there is inconsistent evidence at best that each type has different and specific functions (American Dietetic

Association, 2008). In reality, although sources of fiber may be considered either soluble or insoluble, almost all sources of fiber provide a blend of different fibers.

The National Academy of Sciences recommends that the terms insoluble and soluble be phased out in favor of ascribing specific physiologic benefits to a particular fiber. **Dietary fiber** refers to intact and naturally occurring fiber found in plants; **functional fiber** refers to fiber that has been isolated or extracted from plants that has beneficial physiologic effects in the body. The sum of dietary and functional fiber equals **total fiber**. The rationale for discontinuing soluble and insoluble fiber is that the amounts of soluble and insoluble fibers measured in a mixed diet are dependent on methods of analysis that are not able to exactly replicate human digestion.

It is commonly assumed that fiber does not provide any calories because it is not truly digested by human enzymes and may actually trap macronutrients eaten at the same time and prevent them from being absorbed. Yet most fibers, particularly soluble fibers, are fermented by bacteria in the colon to produce carbon dioxide, methane, hydrogen, and short-chain fatty acids, which serve as a source of energy (calories) for the mucosal lining of the colon. Although the exact energy value available to humans from the blend of fibers in food is unknown, current data indicate the value is between 1.5 and 2.5 cal/g (Institute of Medicine, 2005).

Dietary Fiber: carbohydrates and lignin that are natural and intact components of plants that cannot be digested by human enzymes.

Functional Fiber: as proposed by the Food and Nutrition Board, functional fiber consists of extracted or isolated nondigestible carbohydrates that have beneficial physiologic effects in humans.

Total Fiber: total fiber = dietary fiber + functional fiber.

Sources of Carbohydrates

Sources of carbohydrates include natural sugars in fruit and milk; starch in grains, vegetables, legumes, and nuts; and **added sugars** in foods with empty calories. Servings of commonly consumed grains, fruit, and vegetables contain only 1 to 3 g of dietary fiber; legumes are rich in fiber (Table 2.2). Figure 2.2 shows the average carbohydrate and fiber content of each MyPlate food group.

Added Sugars: caloric sugars and syrups added to foods during processing preparation or consumed separately; do not include sugars naturally present in foods, such as fructose in fruit and lactose in milk.

Whole Grains and Whole Grain Flours: contain the entire grain, or seed, which includes the endosperm, bran, and germ.

Phytochemicals: bioactive, nonnutrient plant compounds associated with a reduced risk of chronic diseases.

Refined Grains and Refined Flours: consist of only the endosperm (middle part) of the grain and therefore do not contain the bran and germ portions.

Enrichment: adding back certain nutrients (to specific levels) that were lost during processing.

Grains

This group is synonymous with "carbs" and consists of grains (e.g., wheat, barley, oats, rye, corn, and rice) and products made with flours from grains (e.g., bread, crackers, pasta, and tortillas).

Grains are classified as "whole" or "refined" (Box 2.1). **Whole grains** consist of the entire kernel of a grain (Fig. 2.3). They may be eaten whole as a complete food (e.g., oatmeal, brown rice, or popcorn) or milled into flour to be used as an ingredient in bread, cereal, and baked goods. Even when whole grains are ground, cracked, or flaked, they must have the same proportion of the original three parts:

- The bran, or tough outer coating, which provides antioxidants, iron, zinc, copper, magnesium, B vitamins, fiber, and **phytochemicals**.
- The endosperm, the largest portion of the kernel, which supplies starch, protein, and small amounts of vitamins and minerals.
- The germ (embryo), the smallest portion of the kernel that contains B vitamins, vitamin E, antioxidants, phytochemicals, and unsaturated fat. Its unsaturated fat content makes whole wheat flour more susceptible to rancidity than refined flour.

Bran cereals and wheat germ are not whole grains because they come from only one part of the whole.

"Refined" grains have most of the bran and germ removed. They are rich in starch but lack the fiber, B vitamins, vitamin E, trace minerals, unsaturated fat, and most of the phytochemicals found in whole grains (International Food Information Council, 2009). The process of **enrichment** restores some B vitamins (thiamin, riboflavin, and niacin) and iron to levels

Table 2.2 Fiber Content of Selected Foods

Food	Total Fiber (g)
Breads (1 slice)	
Rye	1.9
White	0.7
Whole wheat	1.9
Cereals (½ cup)	
All-Bran	8.8
Cream of Wheat	0.6
Cornflakes	0.3
Oatmeal	2.0
Puffed rice	0.1
Fruit (1 medium unless otherwise specified)	
Apple with skin	3.3
Banana	3.0
Orange	3.0
Peach	1.5
Strawberries (½ cup)	1.6
Tangerine	1.5
Watermelon (½ cup)	0.3
Legumes (½ cup cooked)	
Baked, vegetarian	5.2
Great northern	6.2
Lentils	7.8
Lima	5.4
Navy	9.5
White	6.3
Nuts (1 oz)	
Almonds (24 nuts)	3.3
Cashews (18 nuts)	0.9
Pistachios (47 nuts)	2.8
Walnuts (14 halves)	1.9
Vegetables (½ cup cooked)	
Asparagus	1.4
Broccoli	2.5
Brussels sprouts	2.0
Cabbage	1.5
Collards	2.4
Mustard greens	1.4
Sweet potato	3.0
Tomatoes	2.4

Source: U.S. Department of Agriculture National Nutrient Database for Standard Reference, Release 24. (n.d.). Available at https://www.ars.usda.gov/SP2UserFiles/Place/12354500/Data/SR24/nutrlist/sr24a291.pdf. Accessed 8/28/2012.

Fortified: adding nutrients that are not naturally present in the food or were present in insignificant amounts.

found prior to processing. Other substances that are lost, such as other vitamins, other minerals, fiber, and phytochemicals, are not replaced by enrichment. Enriched grains are also required to be **fortified** with folic acid, a mandate designed to reduce the risk of neural tube defects. Examples of refined grains include white flour, white bread, white rice, and refined cornmeal.

Whether whole or refined, a serving of grain is estimated to provide 15 g of carbohydrates. Fiber content can range from 0 g in refined grains to 10 g or more per serving

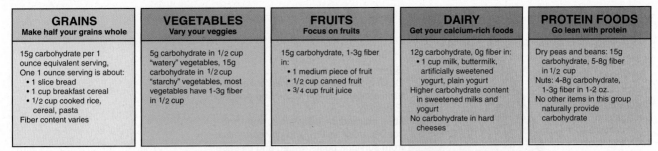

GRAINS Make half your grains whole	VEGETABLES Vary your veggies	FRUITS Focus on fruits	DAIRY Get your calcium-rich foods	PROTEIN FOODS Go lean with protein
15g carbohydrate per 1 ounce equivalent serving, One 1 ounce serving is about: • 1 slice bread • 1 cup breakfast cereal • 1/2 cup cooked rice, cereal, pasta Fiber content varies	5g carbohydrate in 1/2 cup "watery" vegetables, 15g carbohydrate in 1/2 cup "starchy" vegetables, most vegetables have 1-3g fiber in 1/2 cup	15g carbohydrate, 1-3g fiber in: • 1 medium piece of fruit • 1/2 cup canned fruit • 3/4 cup fruit juice	12g carbohydrate, 0g fiber in: • 1 cup milk, buttermilk, artificially sweetened yogurt, plain yogurt Higher carbohydrate content in sweetened milks and yogurt No carbohydrate in hard cheeses	Dry peas and beans: 15g carbohydrate, 5-8g fiber in 1/2 cup Nuts: 4-8g carbohydrate, 1-3g fiber in 1-2 oz. No other items in this group naturally provide carbohydrate

■ **FIGURE 2.2**   Carbohydrate content of MyPlate groups. (**Source:** U.S. Department of Agriculture, Center for Nutrition Policy and Promotion. [2011]. Available at www.choosemyplate.gov)

of high-fiber cereals. Some items in this group, such as sweetened ready-to-eat cereals, muffins, and pancakes, have added sugar.

Vegetables

Starch and some sugars provide the majority of calories in vegetables, but the content varies widely among individual vegetables. A ½ cup serving of the following "starchy" vegetables provides approximately 15 g carbohydrates:

Corn
Legumes (e.g., pinto beans, black beans, garbanzo beans)
Lentils
Peas
Potatoes, sweet potatoes, yams
Winter squash (e.g., acorn, butternut)

Box 2.1   SOURCES OF WHOLE AND REFINED GRAINS

Whole Grains	Refined Grains
Whole wheat grain, including varieties of spelt, emmer, faro, einkorn, bulgur, cracked wheat, and wheat berries	Cream of Wheat, puffed wheat, refined ready-to-eat wheat cereals
Products made with whole wheat flour, such as 100% whole wheat bread, whole wheat pasta, shredded wheat, Wheaties, whole wheat tortillas, whole wheat crackers	Products made with enriched white or wheat flour as found in white or wheat bread, white pasta, flour tortillas, refined crackers
Whole oats, oatmeal, Cheerios	Oat flour
Brown rice	White rice, Rice Krispies, cream of rice, puffed rice
Corn, popcorn	Cornstarch, grits, hominy, cornflakes
Whole-grain barley, whole rye, teff, triticale, millet, amaranth*, buckwheat*, sorghum*, quinoa*, wild rice*	Pearled barley

*Considered whole grains but are technically not cereals but rather pseudocereals.

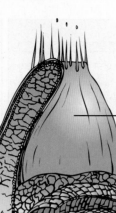

Endosperm
Storage site
for starch; main
source of flour
Provides:
protein, starch,
small amounts
of vitamins,
and trace minerals

Germ
Embryo that
will sprout into
another plant
if fertilized
Provides:
B vitamins,
some protein,
healthy fat, vitamin E,
minerals, antioxidants,
and phytochemicals

Bran
Outer layer that protects rest of kernel
from sunlight, pests, water, and disease
Provides:
fiber, antioxidants, B vitamin, iron, zinc,
copper, magnesium, and phytochemicals
from sunlight, pests, water, and disease

Refined grains:
• made only from endosperm
• are enriched with
  thiamin, riboflavin, niacin,
  and iron lost through processing
• are fortified with folic acid
• are inferior to whole
  grains in vitamin B6, protein,
  pantothenic acid, vitamin E,
  fiber, phytochemicals

■ **FIGURE 2.3** Whole
wheat. The components of the
whole wheat kernel are the
bran, the *germ,* and the
endosperm.

In comparison, "watery" vegetables provide 5 g carbohydrate or less per ½ cup serving:

Asparagus
Bean sprouts
Broccoli
Carrots
Green beans, wax beans
Okra
Tomatoes

The average fiber content of vegetables is 2 to 3 g per serving.

Fruits

Generally, almost all of the calories in fruit come from the natural sugars fructose and glucose. (The exceptions to this are avocado, olives, and coconut, which get the majority of their calories from fat.) A serving of fruit, defined as ¾ cup of juice, 1 piece of fresh fruit, ½ cup of canned fruit, or ¼ cup of dried fruit, provides 15 g carbohydrate and approximately 2 g fiber. Because fiber is located in the skin of fruits, fresh whole fruits provide more fiber than do fresh peeled fruits, canned fruits, or fruit juices. The effect of processing on fiber content is demonstrated in the examples on the left.

	Fiber (g/serving)
Unpeeled fresh apple (1)	3.0
Peeled fresh apple (1)	1.9
Applesauce (½ cup)	1.5
Apple juice (¾ cup)	Negligible

Dairy

Although milk is considered a "protein," more of milk's calories come from carbohydrate than from protein. One cup of milk, regardless of the fat content, provides 12 g of carbohydrate in the form of lactose. Flavored milk and yogurt have added sugars, as do ice cream, ice milk, and frozen yogurt. With the exception of cottage cheese, which has about 6 g of carbohydrate per cup, cheese is virtually lactose free because lactose is converted to lactic acid during production. The carbohydrate content, including both natural and added sugars, of various dairy foods is listed in the box on the left.

	Carbohydrate (g)
Milk, 8 oz	12
Chocolate milk, 8 oz	26
Plain yogurt, 8 oz	15
Strawberry yogurt, 8 oz	48.5
Regular vanilla ice cream, ½ cup	15.6
Swiss cheese, 1 oz	1

Empty Calories

Empty carbohydrate calories are calories that come from added sugars and syrups; these ingredients provide calories with few or no nutrients. Sometimes, 100% of the calories in a food are from added sugar, such as in pancake syrup, sweetened soft drinks, and hard candies. In other products, added sugars account for only some of the calories. For instance, in the chocolate milk listed above, added sugars provide 14 g (56 empty calories) of the 26 g total carbohydrate—the difference between the total carbohydrate in chocolate milk compared to the total carbohydrate (the natural sugar lactose) in plain milk. Only the calories of the added sugar are considered "empty."

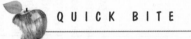

QUICK BITE

Sugar content of selected "extras"

	Sugar (g)
White sugar, 1 tsp	4.0
Brown sugar, 1 tsp	4.5
Jelly, 1 tsp	4.5
Gelatin, ½ cup	19.0
Cola drink, 12 oz	40.0

How the Body Handles Carbohydrates

Digestion

Cooked starch begins to undergo digestion in the mouth by the action of salivary amylase, but the overall effect is small because food is not held in the mouth very long (Fig. 2.4). The stomach churns and mixes its contents, but its acid medium halts any residual effect of the swallowed amylase. Most carbohydrate digestion occurs in the small intestine, where pancreatic amylase reduces complex carbohydrates into shorter chains and disaccharides.

Disaccharidase enzymes (maltase, sucrase, and lactase) on the surface of the cells of the small intestine split maltose, sucrose, and lactose, respectively, into monosaccharides. Monosaccharides are the only form of carbohydrates the body is able to absorb intact and the form all other digestible carbohydrates must be reduced to before they can be absorbed. Normally, 95% of starch is digested usually within 1 to 4 hours after eating.

Absorption

Glucose, fructose, and galactose are absorbed through intestinal mucosa cells and travel to the liver via the portal vein. Small amounts of starch that have not been fully digested pass into the colon with fiber and are excreted in the stools. Fibers may impair the absorption of some minerals—namely, calcium, zinc, and iron—by binding with them in the small intestine.

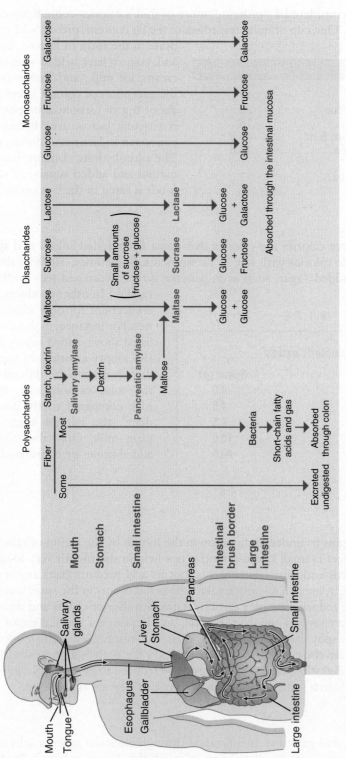

■ **FIGURE 2.4** Carbohydrate digestion. Dietary carbohydrates include the polysaccharides or complex carbohydrates (fiber, starch, and dextrin), the disaccharides (maltose, sucrose, and lactose), and the monosaccharides (glucose, fructose, and galactose). Digestion begins in the *mouth*, where food is chewed into pieces and salivary amylase begins the process of chemical digestion. The *stomach* churns and mixes the carbohydrate, but stomach acids halt residual action of the salivary amylase. The *small intestine* is the site of most carbohydrate digestion, and pancreatic amylase reduces complex carbohydrates into disaccharides. Disaccharide enzymes (maltase, sucrase, and lactase) on the surface of the small intestine cells split maltose, sucrose, and lactose into monosaccharides, thus completing the process of carbohydrate digestion. Fiber is not digested per se, but most is fermented by bacteria in the *large intestine* to yield gas, water, and short-chain fatty acids.

Metabolism

Fructose and galactose are converted to glucose in the liver. The liver releases glucose into the bloodstream, where its level is held fairly constant by the action of hormones. A rise in blood glucose concentration after eating causes the pancreas to secrete insulin, which moves glucose out of the bloodstream and into the cells. Most cells take only as much glucose as they need for immediate energy needs; muscle and liver cells take extra glucose to store as glycogen. The release of insulin lowers blood glucose to normal levels.

In the **postprandial** state, as the body uses the energy from the last meal, the blood glucose concentration begins to drop. Even a slight fall in blood glucose stimulates the pancreas to release glucagon, which causes the liver to release glucose from its supply of glycogen. The result is that blood glucose levels increase to normal.

> **Postprandial:** following a meal.

Glycemic Response

> **Glycemic Response:** the effect a food has on the blood glucose concentration; how quickly the glucose level rises, how high it goes, and how long it takes to return to normal.

It was commonly believed that sugars produce a greater increase in blood glucose levels, or **glycemic response**, than complex carbohydrates because they are rapidly and completely absorbed. This proved to be too simplistic of an assumption, as illustrated by the lower glycemic index of cola (sugar) compared to that of baked potatoes (complex carbohydrate) (Table 2.3). A food's glycemic response is actually influenced by many variables including

Table 2.3 Glycemic Index and Glycemic Load of Selected Foods

Item	Glycemic Index (Glucose = 100)	Glycemic Load/Serving
White spaghetti	58	28
Baked potato	85	26
White bagel	72	25
Cornflakes	92	24
Long-grain white rice	56	24
Snickers Bar	68	23
Jelly beans	78	22
Macaroni	45	22
Sweet corn	60	20
Honey	87	18
Boiled sweet potato	59	18
Shredded wheat	83	17
Coca-Cola	56	16
Steamed brown rice	50	16
Pound cake	54	15
Unsweetened clear apple juice	44	13
Banana	46	12
White bread	70	10
Chickpeas	33	10
All-Bran cereal	38	9
Reduced-fat yogurt	26	8
Watermelon	72	4
Orange	40	4
Premium ice cream	37	4
Low-fat ice cream	50	3
Peanuts	17	1

Source: Foster-Powell, K., Holt, S., & Brand-Miller, J. (2002). International table of glycemic index and glycemic load values: 2002. *The American Journal of Clinical Nutrition, 76,* 50–56.

the amounts of fat, fiber, and acid in the food; the degree of processing; the method of preparation; the amount eaten; the degree of ripeness (for fruits and vegetables); and whether other foods are eaten at the same time.

To assess a food's impact on blood glucose response more accurately, the concept of **glycemic index** was developed. A food's glycemic index is determined by comparing the impact on blood glucose after 50 g of a food sample is eaten to the impact of 50 g of pure glucose or white bread. For instance, a baked potato with a glycemic index of 76 elicits 76% of the blood glucose response as an equivalent amount of pure glucose.

Because the amount of carbohydrate contained in a typical portion of food also influences glycemic response, the concept of **glycemic load** was created to define a food's impact on blood glucose levels more accurately (see Table 2.3). It takes into account both the glycemic index of a food and the amount of carbohydrate in a serving of that food. For example, watermelon has a high glycemic index of 72, but because its carbohydrate content is low (it is mostly water), the glycemic load is only 4.

In a practical sense, glycemic load is not a reliable tool for choosing a healthy diet, and claims that a low glycemic index diet promotes significant weight loss or helps control appetite are unfounded. Soft drinks, candy, sugars, and high-fat foods may have a low to moderate glycemic index, but these foods are not nutritious and eating them does not promote weight loss. In addition, a food's actual impact on glucose levels is difficult to predict because of the many factors influencing glycemic load. However, glycemic index may help people with diabetes fine-tune optimal meal planning (see Chapter 19), and athletes can use the glycemic index to choose optimal fuels for before, during, and after exercise (see Chapter 7).

Glycemic Index: a numeric measure of the glycemic response of 50 g of a food sample; the higher the number, the higher the glycemic response.

Glycemic Load: a food's glycemic index multiplied by the amount of carbohydrate it contains to determine impact on blood glucose levels.

Functions of Carbohydrates

Glucose metabolism is a dynamic state of balance between burning glucose for energy (*catabolism*) and using glucose to build other compounds (*anabolism*). This process is a continuous response to the supply of glucose from food and the demand for glucose for energy needs.

Glucose for Energy

The primary function of carbohydrates is to provide energy for cells. Glucose is burned more efficiently and more completely than either protein or fat, and it does not leave an end product that the body must excrete. Although muscles use a mixture of fat and glucose for energy, the brain is totally dependent on glucose for energy. All digestible carbohydrates—namely, simple sugars and complex carbohydrates—provide 4 cal/g. As a primary source of energy, carbohydrates also spare protein and prevent ketosis.

Protein Sparing

Although protein provides 4 cal/g just like carbohydrates, it has other specialized functions that only protein can perform, such as replenishing enzymes, hormones, antibodies, and blood cells. Consuming adequate carbohydrate to meet energy needs has the effect of "sparing protein" from being used for energy, leaving it available to do its special functions. An adequate carbohydrate intake is especially important whenever protein needs are increased such as for wound healing and during pregnancy and lactation.

Preventing Ketosis

Fat normally supplies about half of the body's energy requirement. Yet glucose fragments are needed to efficiently and completely burn fat for energy. Without adequate glucose, fat

Ketone Bodies: intermediate, acidic compounds formed from the incomplete breakdown of fat when adequate glucose is not available.

oxidation prematurely stops at the intermediate step of **ketone body** formation. Although muscles and other tissues can use ketone bodies for energy, they are normally produced only in small quantities. An increased production of ketone bodies and their accumulation in the bloodstream cause nausea, fatigue, loss of appetite, and ketoacidosis. Dehydration and sodium depletion may follow as the body tries to excrete ketones in the urine.

Using Glucose to Make Other Compounds

After energy needs are met, excess glucose can be converted to glycogen, be used to make nonessential amino acids and specific body compounds, or be converted to fat and stored.

Glycogen. The body's backup supply of glucose is liver glycogen. Liver and muscle cells pick up extra glucose molecules during times of plenty and join them together to form glycogen, which can quickly release glucose in times of need. Typically one-third of the body's glycogen reserve is in the liver and can be released into circulation for all body cells to use, and two-thirds is in muscle, which is available only for use by muscles. Unlike fat, glycogen storage is limited and may provide only enough calories for about a half-day of moderate activity.

Nonessential Amino Acids. If an adequate supply of essential amino acids is available, the body can use them and glucose to make nonessential amino acids.

Carbohydrate-Containing Compounds. The body can convert glucose to other essential carbohydrates such as ribose, a component of ribonucleic acid (RNA) and deoxyribonucleic acid (DNA), keratin sulfate (in fingernails), and hyaluronic acid (found in the fluid that lubricates the joints and vitreous humor of the eyeball).

Fat. Any glucose remaining at this point—after energy needs are met, glycogen stores are saturated, and other specific compounds are made—is converted by liver cells to triglycerides and stored in the body's fat tissue. The body does this by combining acetate molecules to form fatty acids, which then are combined with glycerol to make triglycerides. Although it sounds easy for excess carbohydrates to be converted to fat, it is not a primary pathway; the body prefers to make body fat from dietary fat, not carbohydrates.

Dietary Reference Intakes

Total Carbohydrate

The Recommended Dietary Allowance (RDA) for total carbohydrate (starch, natural sugar, added sugar) is set at 130 g for both adults and children, based on the average *minimum* amount of glucose that is needed to fuel the brain and assuming total calorie intake is adequate (National Research Council, 2005). Yet at this level, total calorie needs are not met unless protein and fat intakes exceed levels considered healthy.

A more useful guideline for determining appropriate carbohydrate intake is the Acceptable Macronutrient Distribution Range (AMDR); it suggests that carbohydrates provide 45% to 65% of total calories consumed (National Research Council, 2005). As illustrated in Figure 2.5, the carbohydrate content using AMDR standards is significantly higher than the minimum of 130 g/day. Table 2.4 estimates the carbohydrate content of a 2000-calorie MyPlate meal pattern. A Tolerable Upper Intake Level (UL) has not been established for total carbohydrates.

According to the National Health and Nutrition Examination Survey (NHANES) 2007–2008 data, the mean carbohydrate intake for men 20 years and older was 296 g or 48% of total calories consumed; for women in the same age category, the mean intake was 256 g or 50% of total calories consumed (U.S. Department of Agriculture, Agricultural Research Service, 2010).

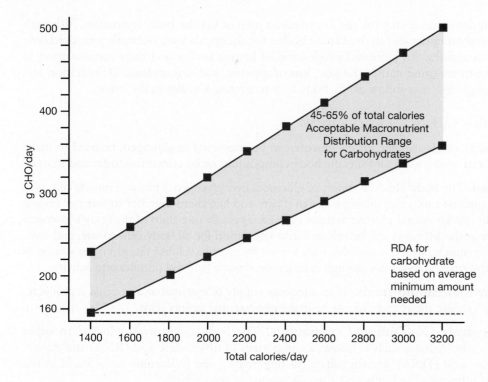

FIGURE 2.5 Amount of total carbohydrates (CHO) appropriate at various caloric levels based on the Acceptable Macronutrient Distribution Range of 45% to 65% of total calories. The dotted line represents the Recommended Dietary Allowance (RDA) for carbohydrate based on average minimum amount needed.

Fiber

An Adequate Intake (AI) for total fiber is set at 14 g/1000 calories or 25 g/day for women and 38 g/day for men (National Research Council, 2005). Fiber is not an essential nutrient that must be consumed through food in order to prevent a deficiency disease; the recommendation is based on intake levels that have been observed to protect against coronary heart disease based on epidemiologic and clinical data. Mean fiber intake among American men and women 20 years and older is 17.7 g and 14.3 g, respectively (U.S. Department

Table 2.4 Carbohydrate Content of the MyPlate 2000-Calorie Food Intake Pattern

Group	Recommended Amount	Average g CHO/Serving[1]	Estimated Total g CHO/Group
Grains[1]	6 ounces	15 g per 1 oz equivalent	90
Vegetables[2]	2.5 cups	5 g per ½ cup	25
Fruits	2 cups	15 g per ½ cup	60
Dairy	3 cups	12 g/cup	36
Protein Foods	5.5 ounces	Only legumes and nuts have CHO; assuming neither were consumed	0
Total estimated grams carbohydrate/day[2]			211 g

[1]Based on the American Diabetes Association, American Dietetic Association Choose Your Foods: Exchange Lists for Diabetes, 2008.

[2]Total carbohydrate does not account for any additional carbohydrate that may come from choosing nuts or legumes from the Protein Foods group or from added sugars in empty calories.

Source: U.S. Department of Agriculture, Center for Nutrition Policy and Promotion. (2011). Available at www.choosemyplate.gov

of Agriculture, Agricultural Research Service, 2010), about half as much fiber as recommended. A UL has not been established for fiber.

CARBOHYDRATES IN HEALTH PROMOTION

Americans, on average, consume an appropriate percentage of their calories from carbohydrate but are urged to choose healthier sources to promote health and reduce the risk of chronic disease (U.S. Department of Agriculture, U.S. Department of Health and Human Services, 2010). The *Dietary Guidelines for Americans, 2010* key recommendations regarding carbohydrate intake appear in Box 2.2. Recommendations regarding whole grains and added sugars are discussed below.

Increase Whole Grains

The *Dietary Guidelines for Americans, 2010* recommend that adults and children consume at least one-half of their grain servings, or a minimum of three servings per day, in the form of whole grains. While whole grains may be best known for their fiber content, the health benefits are likely due to the "whole package" of healthful components, including essential fatty acids, antioxidants, vitamins, minerals, and phytochemicals (International Food Information Council, 2009). Studies show that diets rich in whole grains are associated with a lower risk of cardiovascular disease, certain types of cancer, and type 2 diabetes, and may aid weight management (U.S. Department of Agriculture, U.S. Department of Health and Human Services, 2010; Ye, Chacko, Chou, Kugizaki, and Liu, 2012). Whole grains may be best known for their role in maintaining gastrointestinal function.

Cardiovascular Disease

Epidemiologic studies consistently demonstrate that the intake of whole grains is associated with a reduced risk of cardiovascular disease (Seal and Brownlee, 2010). A meta-analysis of seven prospective cohort studies estimated a 21% lower risk of cardiovascular disease events with a whole-grain intake of 2.5 servings/day versus 0.2 servings/day (Mellen, Walsh, and Herrington, 2008). Although the exact mechanism is unknown, various components of whole grains, including fiber, antioxidants, and phytochemicals, may synergistically work to influence cholesterol levels, blood pressure, blood clotting, and insulin sensitivity.

Cancer

Observational studies in the United States suggest a strong inverse relationship between whole-grain intake and gastrointestinal cancers, certain hormone-related cancers, and pancreatic

Box 2.2	2010 DIETARY GUIDELINES KEY RECOMMENDATIONS REGARDING CARBOHYDRATE INTAKE

- Reduce the intake of calories from solid fats and added sugars.
- Limit the consumption of foods that contain refined grains, especially refined grain foods that contain solid fats, added sugars, and sodium.
- Increase vegetable and fruit intake.
- Consume at least half of all grains as whole grains. Increase whole-grain intake by replacing refined grains with whole grains.

cancer (Jonnalagadda et al., 2011). A prospective study by Schatzkin et al. (2007) showed a 24% lower risk of colorectal cancer in people in the highest quintile of whole-grain intake compared to those in the lowest quintile. The American Cancer Society guidelines on nutrition and physical activity for cancer prevention urge Americans to choose whole grains in preference to refined grain products (Kushi et al., 2012).

Type 2 Diabetes

Epidemiologic studies show an inverse relationship between whole-grain intake and the risk of type 2 diabetes (Jonnalagadda et al., 2011). A prospective cohort study found a significant decrease in type 2 diabetes risk in people in the highest quintile of whole-grain intake compared to those in the lowest, after adjusting for age and calorie intake (Liu, 2002). The American Diabetes Association's nutrition recommendations for the primary prevention of diabetes suggest that half of grain consumption be in the form of whole grains (Bantle et al., 2008).

Weight Management

Cross-sectional and prospective epidemiologic studies show that whole-grain intake is associated with lower risk of obesity and weight gain (Harland and Garton, 2008). Fourteen cross-sectional studies show that a daily intake of approximately three servings of whole grains is associated with lower body mass index in adults (Jonnalagadda et al., 2011). Analyses of both the Physicians' Health Study (Koh-Banerjee et al., 2004) and the Nurses' Health Study (Liu et al., 1999) showed that those who consume more whole grains consistently weigh less than their non–whole grain eating counterparts. Whole grains may help to promote weight management because they are generally less calorically dense than refined foods; are high in bulk, which means they may take longer to consume; and prolong gastric emptying, delaying the return of hunger.

Gastrointestinal Function

The fiber in whole grains is credited with promoting regularity by increasing stool bulk and shortening transit time. Other components of whole grains may lower oxidative stress and inflammation. It is likely that the sum of the parts of whole grains, such as fiber, antioxidant vitamins, phytochemicals, minerals, and prebiotics work synergistically to improve gastrointestinal function and help protect against disease.

Tips for Choosing Whole Grains

The most common whole grains consumed in the United States are wheat, corn, oats, barley, and rice, with wheat as the most prominent grain consumed on a daily basis (Jonnalagadda et al., 2011). However, 95% of Americans do not meet their daily whole-grain intake recommendation; on average, Americans consume only one whole-grain serving per day (Cleveland, Moshfegh, Albertson, and Goldman, 2000; Good, Holschuh, Albertson, and Eldridge, 2008). Factors contributing to the low intake of whole grains include consumers' inability to identify whole grains, a lack of awareness of their health benefits, cost, taste, and unfamiliarity with how to prepare whole grains. Consumers need to understand that the recommendation to eat whole grains is qualified by the advice that whole grains *replace* refined grains, not that they are simply added to usual grain intake. Tips for eating more whole grains appear in Box 2.3.

| Box 2.3 | TIPS FOR INCREASING WHOLE-GRAIN INTAKE |

Substitute
- Whole wheat bread for white bread
- Brown rice for white rice
- Whole wheat pasta or pasta that is part whole wheat, part white flour for white pasta
- Whole wheat pita for white pita
- Whole wheat tortillas for flour tortillas
- Whole grain or bran cereals for refined cereals
- Half of the white flour in pancakes, waffles, muffins, quick breads, and cookies with whole wheat flour or oats
- Whole wheat bread or cracker crumbs for white crumbs as a coating or breading for meat, fish, and poultry
- Whole corn meal for refined corn meal in corn cakes, corn bread, and corn muffins

Add
- Barley, brown rice, or bulgur to soups, stews, bread stuffing, and casseroles
- A handful of oats or whole-grain cereal to yogurt

Snack on
- Ready-to-eat whole-grain cereal, such as shredded wheat or toasted oat cereal
- Whole-grain baked tortilla chips
- Popcorn

Reduce Sugars

Limit All Added Sugars

In foods, sugar adds flavor and interest. Few would question the value brown sugar adds to a bowl of hot oatmeal. Besides its sweet taste, sugar has important functions in baked goods. In yeast breads, sugar promotes fermentation by serving as food for the yeast. Sugar in cakes promotes tenderness and a smooth crumb texture. Cookies owe their crisp texture and light brown color to sugar. In jams and jellies, sugar inhibits the growth of mold; in candy, it influences texture. Sugar has many functional roles in foods including taste, physical properties, antimicrobial purposes, and chemical properties. To some extent, sugar is inaccurately blamed for a variety of health problems. The idea that sugar causes hyperactivity in children has been around for decades, even though there is no supporting evidence, even among children who are reported to be sensitive to sugar. Clinical practice guidelines for the treatment of attention deficit-hyperactivity disorder (ADHD) in children state there is a lack of evidence that removing sugar from the diet of a child with ADHD results in fewer symptoms (Ballard, Hall, and Kaufmann, 2010). Similarly, type 2 diabetes is commonly blamed on a high-sugar diet, even though increasing intakes of sugar are not linked to increasing risk of diabetes. Type 2 diabetes is related to excess body weight, not to eating too much sugar.

High-fructose corn syrup (HFCS) is a commercially made liquid sweetener made from enzymatically treated corn syrup, which is typically 100% glucose. HFCS is composed of glucose and either 42% or 55% fructose, making it similar in composition to sucrose (Fig. 2.6). A review of short-term randomized controlled trials, cross-sectional studies, and review articles consistently found little evidence that HFCS differs uniquely from sucrose and other

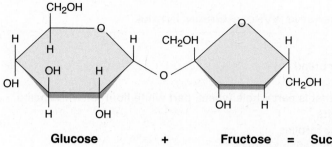

■ **FIGURE 2.6** Sucrose (table sugar) is half glucose and half fructose.

Glucose + Fructose = Sucrose

nutritive sweeteners in metabolic effects (e.g., levels of circulating glucose, insulin, postprandial triglycerides), subjective effects (e.g., hunger, satiety, calorie intake at subsequent meals), and adverse effects such as risk of weight gain (Academy of Nutrition and Dietetics, 2012).

Although sugar may not be the evil it is portrayed to be, limiting the intake of added sugar is a prudent idea. Most health organizations urge Americans to reduce their intake of added sugars because diets high in added sugar are more likely to be inadequate in essential nutrients (if empty calorie foods displace more nutritious ones), excessive in calories (if empty calorie foods are added to the diet), or both. The Dietary Reference Intakes suggestion for added sugar is that it be limited to 25% or less of total calories consumed (National Research Council, 2005). In 2009, the American Heart Association recommended that most American women limit added sugar intake to a maximum of 100 calories per day (25 g or 6 tsp) and that most American men limit their added sugar intake to 150 calories or less per day (38 g or 10 tsp) (Johnson et al., 2009). Ways to limit added sugars appear in Box 2.4.

Using 2007–2008 NHANES data, Welsh, Sharma, Grellinger, and Vos (2011) determined that added sugars account for 14.6% of total calorie intake in a typical American diet. Based on these data, the usual intake of added sugars for Americans aged 19 years and older is 20 tsp/day, with sweetened soft drinks and energy/sports drinks the main contributors to added sugar intake. Figure 2.7 illustrates the sources of added sugar in the typical American diet. Although these recent data show a decrease in added sugar intake from 1999–2000 when sugar provided 18.1% of total calories, added sugar intake is still higher than recommended.

Consider Sugar Alternatives

Polyols: sugar alcohols produced from the fermentation or hydrogenation of monosaccharides or disaccharides; most originate in sucrose or glucose and maltose in starches.

Nonnutritive Sweeteners: synthetically made sweeteners that provide minimal or no carbohydrate and calories; also known as artificial sweeteners.

One way to reduce sugar intake and not forsake sweetened foods is to consume sugar alternatives, such as **polyols** and **nonnutritive sweeteners**, in place of regular sugar.

Polyols. Polyols, or sugar alcohols, are used as sweeteners but are not true sugars; they are derived from hydrogenated sugars and starches (Table 2.5). Although polyols occur naturally in some fruits, vegetables, and fermented foods such as wine and soy sauce, the majority of polyols in the food supply are commercially synthesized. With the exception of xylitol, they are all less sweet than sucrose, so they are often combined with nonnutritive sweeteners in sugarless foods. Sugar alcohols are approved for use in a variety of products, including candies, chewing gum, jams and jellies, baked goods, and frozen confections. Foods containing polyols and no added sugars can be labeled as sugar free (Academy of Nutrition and Dietetics, 2012). Polyols offer some advantages to sugar:

- They are not fermented by mouth bacteria and thus do not cause dental caries. Because they are noncariogenic, they are often used in items held in the mouth, such as chewing gum and breath mints.
- They are considered low-calorie sweeteners because they are incompletely absorbed. Their calorie value ranges from 1.6 to 3.0 cal/g.

Box 2.4   Ways to Limit Added Sugars

Cut Back or Eliminate Sugar-Sweetened Beverages
Because soft drinks are the biggest source of added sugars in many diets, eliminating them can make a big impact on sugar intake. In fact, every 12-oz can of soft drink provides 9 to 10 teaspoons of added sugar. Water, flavored water, and diet sodas are sugar-free alternatives to sweetened soft drinks. Using low-fat milk or 100% fruit juice in place of soft drinks may not impact total calorie intake, but vitamin and mineral intake will increase. Limit fruit juices to no more than 1 serving/day.

Rely on Natural Sugars in Fruit to Satisfy a "Sweet Tooth"
Besides being less concentrated in sugars than candy, cookies, pastries, and cakes, fruits boost nutrient, phytochemical, and fiber intake.

Limit Sweetened Grain-Based and Dairy-Based Desserts and Candy
Pies, cakes, cookies, bars, and chocolate candy provide empty calories from both added sugars and added fats.

Cut Sugar in Home-Baked Products, if Possible
Although reducing the amount of sugar in some foods does not appreciably alter taste or other qualities, in others, it can be disastrous. For instance, because sugar in jams and jellies inhibits the growth of mold, less sugar results in a product that supports mold growth.

Read Labels
"Nutrition Facts" labels (see Chapter 9) list the amount of sugars per serving, but they do not include sugar alcohols and do not distinguish between natural and added sugars.

- In foods that are sources of natural sugars (e.g., milk, plain yogurt, and fruit), the sugars on the label are natural sugars and should not be avoided. They are considered "healthy" sugars.
- For foods that contain little or no milk or fruit, the sugars listed are mostly or all added sugars. Multiplying the grams of sugar per serving yields the number of empty calories from sugar in that food; dividing by 4 reveals the teaspoons of added sugar.
- For foods that contain both natural and added sugars, look at the ingredient list to identify sources of sugar. The more added sugars on the ingredient label and the closer to the beginning of the list they appear, the higher the content of added sugar in that product. Look for these sources of sugar:

Agave syrup	High-fructose corn syrup
Anhydrous dextrose	Honey
Beet juice	Invert sugar
Brown rice syrup	Lactose
Brown sugar	Liquid fructose
Cane juice	Malt syrup
Confectioner's powdered sugar	Maltose
Corn sweetener	Maple syrup
Corn syrup	Molasses
Corn syrup solids	Nectars (e.g., peach nectar, pear nectar)
Crystal dextrose	Pancake syrup
Dextrose	Raw sugar
Evaporated cane juice	Sucrose
Fructose	Sugar cane juice
Fruit juice concentrate	White granulated sugar

(continues on page 36)

Box 2.4   WAYS TO LIMIT ADDED SUGARS (continued)

Consider Using Sugar Alternatives Such as Sugar Alcohols or Nonnutritive Sweeteners
On the plus side, sugar alternatives are low in calories or calorie free; they do not produce a rise in blood glucose levels and do not promote tooth decay because they are not fermented by mouth bacteria. On the downside, the use of sugar alternatives does not guarantee lower calorie intake. Sugar free is not synonymous with calorie free (see section on sugar alternatives).

- Because they are generally slowly and incompletely absorbed and/or metabolized differently than true sugars, they produce a smaller effect on blood glucose levels and insulin response, making them attractive to people with diabetes.
- Polyols that are not fully absorbed in the small intestine enter the large intestine where they function as a prebiotic; they are fermented into short-chain fatty acids, which foster the growth of colonic bacteria.

The disadvantage of polyols is that because they are incompletely absorbed, they can produce a laxative effect (abdominal gas, discomfort, osmotic diarrhea) when they are fermented in the large intestine. Laxation thresholds are included in Table 2.5.

Nonnutritive Sweeteners. Nonnutritive sweeteners are virtually calorie free and are hundreds to thousands of times sweeter than sugar. Sometimes, combinations of nonnutritive sweeteners are used in a food to produce a synergistically sweeter taste, decrease the amount of sweetener needed, and minimize aftertaste. They have different functional properties, which influences how they are used in foods. Because they do not raise blood

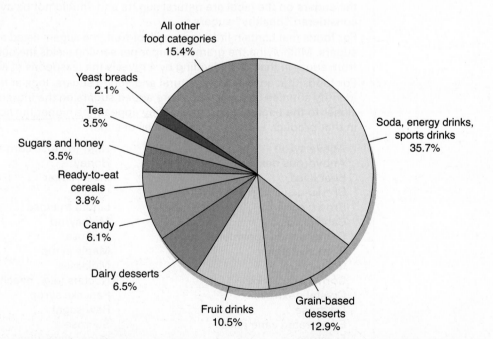

■ FIGURE 2.7 Sources of added sugar in American diets. (**Source:** National Cancer Institute. Sources of added sugars in the diets of the U.S. population ages 2 years and older, NHANES 2005–2006. From U.S. Department of Agriculture, U.S. Department of Health and Human Services. [2010]. *Dietary guidelines for Americans, 2010* [7th ed.]. Washington, DC: U.S. Government Printing Office; p. 29.)

Table 2.5 Polyols

Polyol	Relative Sweetness (Sucrose = 100)	Calories per Gram	Laxation Threshold (per day)	Sources/Uses
Sorbitol	50–70	2.6	50 g	Made from corn syrup or glucose Used in sugar-free candies and chewing gums and sugar-free foods such as frozen desserts and baked goods
Mannitol	50–70	1.6	20 g	Extracted from seaweed or made from mannose Used as dusting powder on chewing gum, in chocolate-flavored coatings for ice cream and candy
Xylitol	100	2.4	50 g	Produced from birch and other hardwood trees Used in chewing gum, hard candies
Maltitol	90	2.1	40–100 g	Made from maltose in corn syrup Used in sugarless hard candies, chewing gum, baked goods, ice cream
Lactitol	30–40	2.0	20–50 g	Derived from lactose Used in low-calorie, low-fat, and/or low-sugar foods such as ice cream, chocolate candy, baked goods, chewing gum
Isomalt	45–65	2.0	40–50 g	Made from sucrose Used in hard candies, toffee, chewing gum, baked goods, nutritional supplements
Hydrogenated starch hydrolysates	25–50	3.0 or less	40–100 g	Produced from partial breakdown of corn, wheat, or potato starch Used in candy, baked goods
Erythritol	60–80	0.2	Because it is rapidly absorbed in the small intestine, it is not likely to produce laxative side effects.	Derived from glucose in corn or wheat starch Used as a bulk sweetener in reduced-calorie foods

Sources: Calorie Control Council. (n.d.). *Polyols information source.* Available at http://www.polyol.org/facts_about_polyols.html. Accessed on 8/24/12; Academy of Nutrition and Dietetics. (2012). Position of the Academy of Nutrition and Dietetics: Use of nutritive and nonnutritive sweeteners. *Journal of the Academy of Nutrition and Dietetics, 112,* 739–758; Canadian Diabetes Association, Nutrition Education Resources Committee. (2009). *Sugar alcohols.* Available at www.diabetes.ca/files/for_professionas/sugar_alcohol.pdf. Accessed on 8/24/12.

glucose levels, nonnutritive sweeteners appeal to people with diabetes. The seven nonnutritive sweeteners approved by the U.S. Food and Drug Administration (FDA) for use in the United States are featured in Table 2.6.

Risks and Benefits of Nonnutritive Sweeteners. At first glance, nonnutritive sweeteners appear to answer Americans' passion for calorie-free sweetness. But are they safe for everyone, including pregnant women and children? Do they help people manage their weight? Are they appropriate for people with diabetes?

Safety. The FDA is responsible for approving the safety of all food additives, including nonnutritive sweeteners. When consumed at levels within the **Acceptable Daily Intake (ADI)**,

Acceptable Daily Intake (ADI): the estimated amount of a food additive that a person can safely consume every day over a lifetime without risk.

Table 2.6 Nonnutritive Sweeteners Approved for Use in the United States

Sweetener	Times Sweeter than Sucrose	Taste Characteristics	Uses	Comments/ADI
Acesulfame K (Sunette, Sweet One)	200	Bitter aftertaste like saccharin	Tabletop sweeteners, dry beverage mixes, and chewing gum	Often mixed with other sweeteners to synergize the sweetness and minimize the aftertaste Not digested; excreted unchanged in the urine ADI: 15 mg/kg BW
Aspartame (NutraSweet, Equal, Spoonful)	160–220	Similar to sucrose; no aftertaste	Tabletop sweeteners, dry beverage mixes, chewing gum, beverages, confections, fruit spreads, toppings, and fillings	Made from the amino acids aspartic acid and phenylalanine; people with PKU must avoid aspartame ADI: 50 mg/kg BW
Luo han guo (Swingle fruit extract)	150–300	Aftertaste at high levels	Intended as tabletop sweetener, a food ingredient, and a component of other sweetener blends	Approved as GRAS (generally recognized as safe), so it is not officially considered a food additive and is exempt from legal requirement to prove safety ADI: not determined
Neotame	7000–13,000	Clean, sugar-like taste; enhances flavors of other ingredients	Rarely used in foods	Made from aspartic acid and phenylalanine but is not metabolized to phenylalanine so a warning label is not required Has the potential to replace both sugar and HFCS ADI: 18 mg/kg BW
Saccharin (Sweet Twin, Sweet'N Low)	300	Persistent aftertaste; bitter at high concentrations	Soft drinks, assorted foods, tabletop sweetener	Potential (weak) carcinogen; the FDA has officially withdrawn its proposed ban so warning labels no longer required ADI: not determined
Stevia (Truvia, Pure Via)	250	Sweet clean taste in usual amounts; may taste bitter in higher amounts	Intended for use in cereal, energy bars, beverages, and as a tabletop sweetener	Refined stevia products are GRAS; whole leaf or crude extracts are not approved because of concerns about health effects. ADI: 4 mg/kg BW
Sucralose (Splenda)	600	Maintain flavor even at high temperatures	Soft drinks, baked goods, chewing gums, and table-top sweeteners	Poorly absorbed; excreted unchanged in the feces ADI: 5 mg/kg BW

ADI, Acceptable Daily Intake; BW, body weight; FDA, U.S. Food and Drug Administration; HFCS, high-fructose corn syrup; PKU, phenylketonuria.

Source: Brown, A. (2008). *Understanding food. Principles and preparation* (3rd ed.). Belmont, CA: Thomson Wadsworth; and Academy of Nutrition and Dietetics. (2012). Position of the Academy of Nutrition and Dietetics: Use of nutritive and non-nutritive sweeteners. *Journal of the Academy of Nutrition and Dietetics, 112,* 739–758.

all FDA-approved nonnutritive sweeteners are safe for use by the general public, including pregnant and lactating women. Although it is difficult to determine the intake of food additives, including nonnutritive sweeteners, data indicate that average intakes by adults are consistently well below their ADIs (Renwick, 2006).

Weight Management. Nonnutritive sweeteners are not a panacea for weight control. In theory, use of nonnutritive sweeteners in place of sugar can save 16 cal/tsp, or 160 calories in a 12-oz can of cola. Eliminating one regularly sweetened soft drink per day for 22 days (160 calories × 22 days = 3520 calories) translates to a 1-pound loss (3500 calories equals 1 pound of body weight) without any other changes in eating or activity. This is because *all* calories in the regular soft drink have been eliminated. But foods whose calories come from a mixture of sugar, starch, protein, and fat still provide calories after sugar calories are reduced or eliminated. For instance, sugar-free cookies can provide as many or more calories than cookies sweetened with sugar. Many people inaccurately believe that low sugar means low calories and will overeat because they overestimate the calories saved by replacing sugar. Evidence that nonnutritive sweeteners are effective in weight management is limited (Academy of Nutrition and Dietetics, 2012).

Appropriateness for Patients with Diabetes Mellitus. Contrary to what was previously believed, regular sugar does not raise blood glucose levels more than complex carbohydrates do; a food's glycemic load is influenced by several factors, not just sugar content. The focus in management of blood glucose levels has shifted from avoiding simple sugars to maintaining a relatively consistent total carbohydrate intake with less emphasis on the source. For that reason, sweets can be included within the context of a nutritious, calorie-appropriate, carbohydrate-controlled diet. However, because most people with type 2 diabetes are overweight, substitution of calorie-free sweets for calorie-containing ones has the potential to improve blood glucose levels by promoting weight management. The full benefit of this is seen when "diet" soft drinks, jellies, syrups, and hard candies replace those containing sugar. The American Diabetes Association 2008 nutrition recommendations state that "Sugar alcohols and nonnutritive sweeteners are safe when consumed within the daily intake levels established by the Food and Drug Administration" (Bantle et al., 2008, p. S64).

Prevent Dental Caries

Feeding on sugars and starches, bacteria residing in the mouth produce an acid that erodes tooth enamel. Although whole-grain crackers and orange juice are more nutritious than caramels and soft drinks, their potential damage to teeth is the same. How often carbohydrates are consumed, what they are eaten with, and how long after eating brushing occurs may be more important than whether or not they are "sticky." Anticavity strategies include the following:

- Choose between-meal snacks that are healthy and teeth friendly, such as fresh vegetables, apples, cheese, and popcorn.
- Limit between-meal carbohydrate snacking including drinking soft drinks.
- Avoid high-sugar items that stay in the mouth for a long time, such as hard candy, suckers, and cough drops.
- Brush promptly after eating.
- Chew gum sweetened with sugar alcohols (e.g., sorbitol, mannitol, and xylitol) or with nonnutritive sweeteners after eating. This may reduce the risk of cavities by stimulating production of saliva, which helps to rinse the teeth and neutralize plaque acids. Unlike sucrose and other nutritive sweeteners, sugar alcohols and nonnutritive sweeteners are not fermented by bacteria in the mouth so they do not promote cavities.
- Use fluoridated toothpaste.

HOW DO YOU RESPOND?

Aren't carbohydrates fattening? At 4 cal/g, carbohydrates are no more fattening than protein and are less than half as fattening as fat at 9 cal/g. Whether or not a food is "fattening" has more to do with frequency and total calories provided than whether the calories are in the form of carbohydrates, protein, or fat.

Is whole "white" wheat bread as nutritious as whole wheat? Whole "white" wheat flour is made from albino wheat that is white in color, not the characteristic bran color of whole wheat. Because it is a whole grain, it is nutritionally comparable to whole wheat. Many people not only prefer its lighter color but also its milder flavor.

"Light" or "diet" breads are high in fiber. Can I use them in place of whole-grain breads? So-called "light breads" usually have processed fiber from peas or other foods substituted for some starch; the result is a lower calorie, higher fiber bread that may help to prevent constipation but lacks the unique "package" of vitamins, minerals, and phytochemicals found in whole grains.

CASE STUDY

Amanda is convinced that white flour and white sugar cause her to overeat, resulting in an extra 30 pounds of weight she is carrying around. To control her impulse to overeat, she has decided to eliminate all foods made with white or whole wheat flour and white sugar from her diet. Her total calorie needs are estimated to be 2000 per day. Yesterday, she ate the following:

Breakfast:	2 scrambled eggs and 2 sausage links 1 cup orange juice lots of black coffee
Snack:	2 ounces of cashews and a diet soft drink
Lunch:	tossed salad with 1 hard cooked egg, 3 ounces of sliced turkey, 2 ounces of sliced cheese, 3 tbsp of Italian dressing 1 can diet soft drink 1 cup of diet gelatin
Snack:	2 ounces of cheese curds and a diet soft drink
Dinner:	6 ounces of fried chicken 1 cup of French fries ½ cup corn ½ cup diet pudding with whipped cream 1 can diet soft drink
Snack:	5 chicken wings with ¼ cup bleu cheese dressing

- What foods did she eat yesterday that contained carbohydrates? Estimate how many grams of carbohydrate she ate. How does her intake compare with the amount of total carbohydrate recommended for someone needing 2000 cal/day? How could she increase her carbohydrate intake within the restrictions she has set for herself?
- What sources of fiber did she consume? Estimate how many grams of fiber she ate. How does her fiber intake compare with the AI amount recommended for women? What would you tell her about her fiber intake?
- What would you tell her about her idea to forsake white and wheat flour and white sugar to manage her weight? What are the benefits and potential problems with her diet? What suggestions would you make about her intake?

STUDY QUESTIONS

1. The nurse knows her explanation of glycemic index was effective when the client says which of the following?
   a. "Choosing foods that have a low glycemic index is an effective way to eat healthier."
   b. "Low glycemic index foods promote weight loss because they do not stimulate the release of insulin."
   c. "Glycemic index may help me choose the best foods to eat before, during, and after training."
   d. "Glycemic index is a term to describe the amount of refined sugar in a food."

2. Which of the following recommendations would be most effective for someone wanting to eat more fiber?
   a. Eat legumes more often.
   b. Eat raw vegetables in place of cooked vegetables.
   c. Use potatoes in place of white rice.
   d. Eat fruit for dessert in place of ice cream.

3. A client asks why sugar should be limited in the diet. Which of the following is the nurse's best response?
   a. "A high sugar intake increases the risk of heart disease and diabetes."
   b. "Foods high in sugar generally provide few nutrients other than calories and may make it hard to consume a diet that has enough of all the essential nutrients."
   c. "There is a direct correlation between sugar intake and the risk of obesity."
   d. "Sugar provides more calories per gram than starch, protein, or fat."

4. Compared to refined grains, whole grains have more
   a. Folic acid
   b. Vitamin A
   c. Vitamin C
   d. Phytochemicals

5. The nurse knows her instructions about choosing dairy products that are lactose free have been effective when the client verbalizes she should consume more
   a. Whole milk
   b. Fat-free milk
   c. Cheddar cheese
   d. Pudding

6. A client who has eaten too many dietetic candies sweetened with sorbitol may experience which of the following?
   a. Diarrhea
   b. Heartburn
   c. Vomiting
   d. Low blood glucose

7. The client wants to eat fewer calories and lose weight by substituting regularly sweetened foods with those that are sweetened with sugar alternatives. Which of the following would be the most effective substitution?
   a. Sugar-free cookies for regular cookies
   b. Sugar-free chocolate candy for regular chocolate candy
   c. Sugar-free soft drinks for regular soft drinks
   d. Sugar-free ice cream for regular ice cream

8. A client is on a low-calorie diet that recommends she test her urine for ketones to tell how well she is adhering to the guidelines of the diet. What does the presence of ketones signify about her intake?
   a. It is too high in protein.
   b. It is too high in fat.
   c. It is too high in carbohydrates.
   d. It is too low in carbohydrates.

KEY CONCEPTS

■ Carbohydrates, which are found almost exclusively in plants, provide the major source of energy in almost all human diets.

■ The two major groups are simple sugars (monosaccharides and disaccharides) and complex carbohydrates (polysaccharides).

■ Monosaccharides and disaccharides are composed of one or two sugar molecules, respectively. They vary in sweetness.

■ Polysaccharides—namely, starch, glycogen, and fiber—are made up of many glucose molecules. They do not taste sweet because their molecules are too large to sit on taste buds in the mouth that perceive sweetness.

■ Fiber, the undigestible part of plant cell walls or intracellular structure, is commonly classified as either water soluble or water insoluble. All foods that contain fiber have a mix of different fibers.

■ The most popular American foods are not rich sources of fiber. Whole grains, bran cereals, legumes, and unpeeled fruits and vegetables are the best sources of fiber.

■ Carbohydrates are found in every MyPlate group except Oils. Starches are most abundant in grains, vegetables, and the plant foods found in the Protein Foods group; natural sugars occur in fruits and in the Dairy group. Added sugars can be found in any food group.

■ The majority of carbohydrate digestion occurs in the small intestine, where disaccharides and starches are digested to monosaccharides. Monosaccharides are absorbed through intestinal mucosal cells and transported to the liver through the portal vein. In the liver, fructose and galactose are converted to glucose. The liver releases glucose into the bloodstream.

■ The glycemic response is based on the glycemic index of a food and the carbohydrate content of that food. Because there are so many variables that influence the rise in blood glucose after eating, glycemic response is hard to predict in practice.

■ The major function of carbohydrates is to provide energy, which includes sparing protein and preventing ketosis. Glucose can be converted to glycogen, used to make nonessential amino acids, used for specific body compounds, or converted to fat and stored in adipose tissue.

■ The RDA for total carbohydrates is set as the minimum amount needed to fuel the brain but not as an amount adequate to satisfy typical energy needs. Most experts recommend that 45% to 65% of total calories come from carbohydrates and that added sugars be limited. Twenty-five and 38 g of fiber is recommended daily for adult women and men, respectively.

■ The *Dietary Guidelines for Americans, 2010* urges Americans to consume at least half of all grains as whole grains, limit refined grains, eat fewer calories from added sugars, and consume more fruits and vegetables.

- Whole grains offer health benefits beyond the benefits of fiber. Whole grains may decrease the risk of heart disease, certain cancers, and type 2 diabetes. Whole grains also promote gastrointestinal health and weight management.
- Added sugar is sugar added to food during processing or preparation. It is considered a source of empty calories. The higher the intake of empty calories, the greater is the risk of an inadequate nutrient intake, an excessive calorie intake, or both.
- Polyols are considered to be low-calorie sweeteners because they are incompletely absorbed and, therefore, provide fewer calories per gram than regular sugar does. Because they do not promote dental decay, they are well suited for use in gum and breath mints that stay in the mouth a long time. Most have a laxation effect depending on the dose consumed.
- Nonnutritive sweeteners provide negligible or no calories. Their use as food additives is regulated by the FDA, which sets safety limits known as ADI. The ADI, a level per kilogram of body weight, reflects an amount 100 times less than the maximum level at which no observed adverse effects have occurred in animal studies. Nonnutritive sweeteners have intense sweetening power, ranging from 180 to 8000 times sweeter than that of sucrose.
- Acids produced from fermentation of sugars and starches in the mouth by bacteria lead to dental decay.

Check Your Knowledge Answer Key

1. **TRUE** Starch, the storage form of carbohydrates in plants, is made from hundreds to thousands of glucose molecules.

2. **FALSE** All digestible carbohydrates—whether sugars or starch—provide 4 cal/g. Insoluble fiber does not provide calories because it is not digested; the mix of fiber in food may provide 1.5 to 2.5 cal/g.

3. **FALSE** The body cannot distinguish between the sugar in fruit and the sugar in candy. However, the *package* of nutrients in fruit (vitamins, minerals, fiber, phytochemicals) is better than the package of nutrients in candy (few to no other nutrients with the possible exception of fat).

4. **FALSE** The most commonly consumed American foods provide 1 to 3 g fiber per serving, which is why most Americans typically eat only about one-half the recommended intake of fiber.

5. **FALSE** Although enrichment returns certain B vitamins and iron lost through processing, other vitamins, minerals, phytochemicals, and fiber are not replaced, so whole wheat bread is nutritionally superior to white or "wheat" bread. Enriched white bread offers the advantage of being fortified with folic acid.

6. **TRUE** Soft drinks contribute more added sugar to the average American diet than any other food or beverage.

7. **TRUE** All fermentable carbohydrates, whether sweet or not, promote dental decay by feeding bacteria in the mouth that damage tooth enamel.

8. **FALSE** Although "Nutrition Facts" labels do not distinguish between natural and added sugars, they do list the total sugar content per serving.

9. **FALSE** Nonnutritive sweeteners approved for use in the United States are safe in amounts within the ADI. The exception is the use of aspartame by people who have phenylketonuria.

10 **FALSE** Sugar has not been proven to cause hyperactivity in children.

Student Resources on thePoint

For additional learning materials, activate the code in the front of this book at
http://thePoint.lww.com/activate

Websites

Learn about grains at **www.wholegrainscouncil.org**

References

Academy of Nutrition and Dietetics. (2012). Position of the Academy of Nutrition and Dietetics: Use of nutritive and non-nutritive sweeteners. *Journal of the Academy of Nutrition and Dietetics, 112*, 739–758.

American Dietetic Association. (2008). Position of the American Dietetic Association: Health implications of dietary fiber. *Journal of the American Dietetic Association, 108*, 1716–1731.

Ballard, W., Hall, M., & Kaufmann, L. (2010). Clinical inquiries. Do dietary interventions improve ADHD symptoms in children? *The Journal of Family Practice, 59*, 234–235.

Bantle, J., Wylie-Rosett, J., Albright, A. L., Apovian, C. M., Clark, N. G., Franz, M. J., . . . Wheeler, M. L. (2008). Nutrition recommendations and interventions for diabetes. A position statement of the American Diabetes Association. *Diabetes Care, 31*(Suppl. 1), S61–S78.

Cleveland, L., Moshfegh, A., Albertson, A., & Goldman, J. (2000). Dietary intake of whole grains. *Journal of the American College of Nutrition, 19*, S331–S338.

Good, C., Holschuh, N., Albertson, A., & Eldridge, A. (2008). Whole grain consumption and body mass index in adult women: An analysis of NHANES 1999–2000 and the USDA Pyramid Serving Database. *Journal of the American College of Nutrition, 27*, 80–87.

Harland, J., & Garton, L. (2008). Whole-grain intake as a marker of healthy body weight and adiposity. *Public Heath Nutrition, 11*, 554–563.

Institute of Medicine. (2005). *Dietary Reference Intakes for energy, carbohydrates, fiber, fat, fatty acids, cholesterol, protein, and amino acids (macronutrients)*. Washington, DC: National Academies Press.

International Food Information Council. (2009). *Whole grains fact sheet*. Available at http://www.foodinsight.org/Resources/Detail.aspx?topic=Whole_Grains_Fact_Sheet. Accessed on 3/12/12.

Johnson, R., Appel, L., Brands, M., Howard, B. V., Lefevre, M., Lustig, R. H., . . . Wylie-Rosett, J. (2009). Dietary sugars intake and cardiovascular health. A scientific statement from the American Heart Association. *Circulation, 120*, 1011–1020.

Jonnalagadda, S., Harnack, L., Lui, R., McKeown, N., Seal, C., Liu, S., & Fahey, G. C. (2011). Putting the whole grain puzzle together: Health benefits associated with whole grains— Summary of American Society for Nutrition 2010 Satellite Symposium. *Journal of Nutrition, 141*, 1011S–1022S.

Koh-Banerjee, P., Franz, M., Sampson, L., Liu, S., Jacobs, D. R., Jr., Spiegelman, D., . . . Rimm, E. (2004). Changes in whole-grain, bran, and cereal fiber consumption in relation to 8-y weight gain among men. *American Journal of Clinical Nutrition, 80*, 1237–1245.

Kushi, L., Doyle, C., McCullough, M., Rock, C. L., Demark-Wahnefried, W., Bandera, E. V., . . . Gansler, T. (2012). American Cancer Society guidelines on nutrition and physical activity for cancer prevention. *CA: A Cancer Journal for Clinicians, 62*, 30–67.

Liu, S. (2002). Intake of refined carbohydrates and whole grain foods in relation to risk of type 2 diabetes mellitus and coronary heart disease. *Journal of the American College of Nutrition, 21*, 298–306.

Liu, S., Stampfer, M., Hu, F., Giovannucci, E., Rimm, E., Manson, J. E., . . . Willett, W. C. (1999). Whole-grain consumption and risk of coronary heart disease: Results from the Nurses' Health Study. *American Journal of Clinical Nutrition, 70*, 412–419.

Mellen, P., Walsh, T., & Herrington, D. (2008). Whole grain intake and cardiovascular disease: A meta-analysis. *Nutrition, Metabolism, and Cardiovascular Diseases, 18*, 283–290.

National Research Council. (2005). *Dietary Reference Intakes for energy, carbohydrate, fiber, fat, fatty acids, cholesterol, protein, and amino acids (macronutrients)*. Washington, DC: The National Academies Press.

Renwick, A. (2006). The intake of intense sweeteners—An updated review. *Food Additives and Contaminants, 23,* 327–338.

Schatzkin, A., Mouw, T., Park, Y., Subar, A. F., Kipnis, V., Hollenbeck, A., . . . Thompson, F. E. (2007). Dietary fiber and whole-grain consumption in relation to colorectal cancer in the NIH-AARP Diet and Health Study. *American Journal of Clinical Nutrition, 85,* 1353–1360.

Seal, C., & Brownlee, I. (2010). Whole grains and health, evidence from observational and intervention studies. *Cereal Chemistry, 87,* 167–174.

U.S. Department of Agriculture, Agricultural Research Service. (2010). *Nutrient intakes from food: Mean amounts consumed per individual, by gender and age. What We Eat in American, NHANES 2007–2008.* Available at www.ars.usda.gov/ba/bhnrc/fsrg. Accessed on 6/9/12.

U.S. Department of Agriculture, U.S. Department of Health and Human Services. (2010). *Dietary guidelines for Americans, 2010* (7th ed.). Available at www.health.gov/dietaryguidelines. Accessed on 2/24/11.

Welsh, J., Sharma, A., Grellinger, L., & Vos, M. (2011). Consumption of added sugars is decreasing in the United States. *American Journal of Clinical Nutrition, 94,* 726–734.

Ye, E., Chacko, S., Chou, E., Kugizaki, M., & Liu, S. (2012). Greater whole-grain intake is associated with lower risk of type 2 diabetes, cardiovascular disease, and weight gain. *Journal of Nutrition, 142,* 1304–1313.

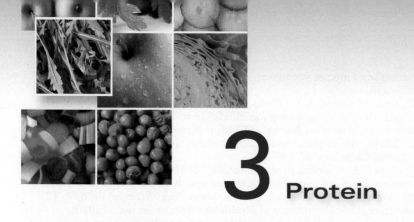

3 Protein

TRUE **FALSE**

☐ ☐ **1** Most Americans eat more protein than they need.

☐ ☐ **2** Protein is the nutrient most likely to be deficient in a purely vegetarian diet.

☐ ☐ **3** The body stores extra amino acids in muscle tissue.

☐ ☐ **4** The quality of soy protein is comparable to or greater than that of animal proteins.

☐ ☐ **5** A high protein intake over time leads to kidney damage.

☐ ☐ **6** A protein classified as "high quality" has the majority of calories provided by protein with few fat or carbohydrate calories.

☐ ☐ **7** Protein is found in all MyPlate groups.

☐ ☐ **8** Healthy adults are in a state of positive nitrogen balance.

☐ ☐ **9** Vegetarian diets are not adequate during pregnancy.

☐ ☐ **10** An Upper Limit (UL) for protein has not been established.

LEARNING OBJECTIVES

Upon completion of this chapter, you will be able to

1 Discuss the functions of protein.
2 Compare complete and incomplete proteins.
3 Explain protein "sparing."
4 Calculate an individual's protein requirement.
5 Estimate the amount of protein in a sample meal plan.
6 Give examples of conditions that increase a person's protein requirement.
7 Select appropriate sources of nutrients that are most likely to be deficient in a vegetarian diet.
8 Describe nitrogen balance and how it is determined.

In Greek, protein means "to take first place," and truly life could not exist without protein. Protein is a component of every living cell: plant, animal, and microorganism. In the adult, protein accounts for 20% of total weight. Dietary protein seems immune to the controversy over optimal intake that surrounds both carbohydrates and fat.

PROTEIN OVERVIEW

This chapter discusses the composition of protein, its functions, and how it is handled in the body. Sources, Dietary Reference Intakes, and the role of protein in health promotion are presented.

Amino Acids

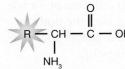

■ **FIGURE 3.1**
Generic amino acid structure.

Amino acids are the basic building blocks of all proteins and the end products of protein digestion. All amino acids have a carbon atom core with four bonding sites: one site holds a hydrogen atom, one an amino group (NH_2), and one an acid group (COOH) (Fig. 3.1). Attached to the fourth bonding site is a side group (R group), which contains the atoms that give each amino acid its own distinct identity. Some side groups contain sulfur, some are acidic, and some are basic. The differences in these side groups account for the differences in size, shape, and electrical charge among amino acids.

There are 20 common amino acids, 9 of which are classified as essential or indispensable because the body cannot make them so they must be supplied through the diet (Box 3.1). The remaining 11 amino acids are classified as nonessential or dispensable because cells can make them as needed through the process of transamination. Some dispensable amino acids may become indispensable when metabolic need is great and endogenous synthesis is not adequate. Note that the terms essential and nonessential refer to whether or not they must be supplied by the diet, not to their relative importance: all 20 amino acids must be available for the body to make proteins.

Box 3.1	AMINO ACIDS		
Essential (Indispensable)	**Nonessential (Dispensable)**	**Conditionally* Essential (Indispensable)**	
Histidine	Alanine	Arginine	
Isoleucine	Asparagine	Cysteine	
Leucine	Aspartic acid	Glutamine	
Lysine	Glutamic acid	Glycine	
Methionine	Serine	Proline	
Phenylalanine		Tyrosine	
Threonine			
Tryptophan			
Valine			

*Under most normal conditions, the body can synthesize adequate amounts of these amino acids. A dietary source is necessary only when metabolic demands exceed endogenous synthesis.

Protein Structure

The types and amounts of amino acids and the unique sequence in which they are joined determine a protein's primary structure. Most proteins contain several dozen to several hundred amino acids: just as the 26 letters of the alphabet can be used to form an infinite number of words, so can amino acids be joined in different amounts, proportions, and sequences to form a great variety of proteins.

Proteins also vary in shape and may be straight, folded, coiled along one dimension, or a three-dimensional shape such as a sphere or globe. Larger proteins are created when two or more three-dimensional polypeptides combine. A protein's shape determines its function.

Functions of Protein

Protein is the major structural and functional component of every living cell. Except for bile and urine, every tissue and fluid in the body contains some protein. In fact, the body may contain as many as 10,000 to 50,000 different proteins that vary in size, shape, and function. Amino acids or proteins are components of or involved in the following:

Body structure and framework. More than 40% of protein in the body is found in skeletal muscle, and approximately 15% is found in each the skin and the blood. Proteins also form tendons, membranes, organs, and bones.

Enzymes. Enzymes are proteins that facilitate specific chemical reactions in the body without undergoing change themselves. Some enzymes (e.g., digestive enzymes) break down larger molecules into smaller ones; others (e.g., enzymes involved in protein synthesis in which amino acids are combined) combine molecules to form larger compounds.

Other body secretions and fluids. Neurotransmitters (e.g., serotonin, acetylcholine), antibodies, and some hormones (e.g., insulin, thyroxine, epinephrine) are made from amino acids, as are breast milk, mucus, sperm, and histamine.

Fluid balance. Proteins help to regulate fluid balance because they attract water, which creates osmotic pressure. Circulating proteins, such as albumin, maintain the proper balance of fluid among the **intravascular**, **intracellular**, and **interstitial** compartments of the body. A symptom of a low albumin level is **edema**.

Acid–base balance. Because amino acids contain both an acid (COOH) and a base (NH_2), they can act as either acids or bases depending on the pH of the surrounding fluid. The ability to buffer or neutralize excess acids and bases enables proteins to maintain normal blood pH, which protects body proteins from being **denatured**.

Transport molecules. **Globular** proteins transport other substances through the blood. For instance, lipoproteins transport fats, cholesterol, and fat-soluble vitamins; hemoglobin transports oxygen; and albumin transports free fatty acids and many drugs.

Other compounds. Amino acids are components of numerous body compounds such as opsin, the light-sensitive visual pigment in the eye, and thrombin, a protein necessary for normal blood clotting.

Some amino acids have specific functions within the body. For instance, tryptophan is a precursor of the vitamin niacin and is also a component of serotonin. Tyrosine is the precursor of melanin, the pigment that colors hair and skin and is incorporated into thyroid hormone.

Fueling the body. Like carbohydrates, protein provides 4 cal/g. Although it is not the body's preferred fuel, protein is a source of energy when it is consumed in excess or when calorie intake from carbohydrates and fat is inadequate.

Intravascular: within blood vessels.

Intracellular: within cells.

Interstitial: between cells.

Edema: the swelling of body tissues secondary to the accumulation of excessive fluid.

Denatured: an irreversible process in which the structure of a protein is disrupted, leading to partial or complete loss of function.

Globular: spherical.

How the Body Handles Protein

Digestion

Chemical digestion of protein begins in the stomach, where hydrochloric acid denatures protein to make the peptide bonds more available to the actions of enzymes (Fig. 3.2). Hydrochloric acid also converts pepsinogen to the active enzyme pepsin, which begins the process of breaking down proteins into smaller polypeptides and some amino acids.

The majority of protein digestion occurs in the small intestine, where pancreatic proteases reduce polypeptides to shorter chains, tripeptides, dipeptides, and amino acids. The enzymes trypsin and chymotrypsin act to break peptide bonds between specific amino acids. Carboxypeptidase breaks off amino acids from the acid (carboxyl) end of polypeptides and dipeptides. Enzymes located on the surface of the cells that line the small intestine complete the digestion: aminopeptidase splits amino acids from the amino ends of short peptides, and dipeptidase reduces dipeptides to amino acids. **Protein digestibility** is 90% to 99% for animal proteins, over 90% for soy and legumes, and 70% to 90% for other plant proteins.

> **Protein Digestibility:** how well a protein is digested to make amino acids available for protein synthesis.

Absorption

Amino acids, and sometimes a few dipeptides or larger peptides, are absorbed through the mucosa of the small intestine by active transport with the aid of vitamin B_6. Intestinal cells release amino acids into the bloodstream for transport to the liver via the portal vein.

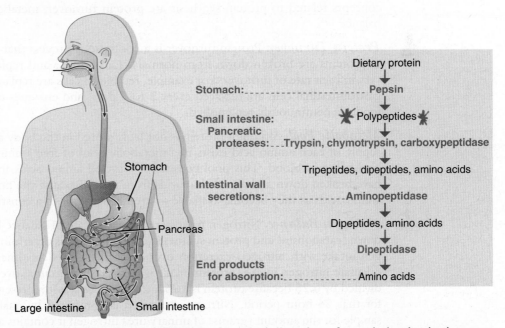

■ **FIGURE 3.2** Protein digestion. Chemical digestion of protein begins in the stomach. Hydrochloric acid converts pepsinogen to the active enzyme pepsin, which begins the process of breaking down proteins into small polypeptides and some amino acids. The majority of protein digestion occurs in the small intestine, where pancreatic proteases reduce polypeptides into shorter chains, tripeptides, dipeptides, and amino acids. Enzymes located on the surface of the cells that line the small intestine complete the digestion: aminopeptidase splits amino acids from the amino ends of short peptides, and dipeptidase reduces dipeptides to amino acids.

Metabolism

The liver acts as a clearinghouse for the amino acids it receives: it uses the amino acids it needs, releases those needed elsewhere, and handles the extra. For instance, the liver

- Retains amino acids to make liver cells, nonessential amino acids, and plasma proteins such as heparin, prothrombin, and albumin
- Regulates the release of amino acids into the bloodstream and removes excess amino acids from the circulation
- Synthesizes specific enzymes to degrade excess amino acids
- Removes the nitrogen from amino acids so that they can be burned for energy
- Converts certain amino acids to glucose, if necessary
- Forms urea from the nitrogenous wastes when protein and calories are consumed in excess of need
- Converts protein to fatty acids that form triglycerides for storage in adipose tissue

Protein Synthesis. Protein synthesis (anabolism) is a complicated but efficient process that quickly assembles amino acids into proteins the body needs, such as proteins lost through normal wear and tear or those needed to support growth and development. Part of what makes every individual unique is the minute differences in body proteins, which are caused by variations in the sequencing of amino acids determined by genetics. Genetic codes created at conception hold the instructions for making all of the body's proteins. Cell function and life itself depend on the precise replication of these codes. Some important concepts related to protein synthesis are protein turnover, metabolic pool, and nitrogen balance.

Protein Turnover. Protein turnover is a continuous process that occurs within each cell as proteins are broken down from normal wear and tear and replenished. Body proteins vary in their rate of turnover. For example, red blood cells are replaced every 60 to 90 days, gastrointestinal cells are replaced every 2 to 3 days, and enzymes used in the digestion of food are continuously replenished.

Metabolic Pool. Although protein is not truly stored in the body as are glucose and fat, a supply of each amino acid exists in a metabolic pool of free amino acids within cells and circulating in blood. This pool consists of recycled amino acids from body proteins that have broken down and also amino acids from food. Because the pool accepts and donates amino acids as they become available or are needed, it is in a constant state of flux.

Nitrogen Balance. Nitrogen balance reflects the state of balance between protein breakdown (catabolism) and protein synthesis (anabolism). It is determined by comparing nitrogen intake with nitrogen excretion over a specific period of time, usually 24 hours. To calculate nitrogen intake, protein intake is measured (in grams) over a 24-hour period and divided by 6.25 because protein is 16% nitrogen. The result represents total nitrogen intake for that 24-hour period. Nitrogen excretion is computed by analyzing a 24-hour urine sample for the amount (grams) of urinary urea nitrogen it contains and adding a coefficient of 4 to this number to account for the estimated daily nitrogen loss in feces, hair, nails, and skin. Comparing grams of nitrogen excretion to grams of nitrogen intake will reveal the state of nitrogen balance, as illustrated in Box 3.2.

A neutral nitrogen balance, or state of equilibrium, exists when nitrogen intake equals nitrogen excretion, indicating protein synthesis is occurring at the same rate as protein breakdown. Healthy adults are in neutral nitrogen balance. When protein synthesis exceeds protein breakdown, as is the case during growth, pregnancy, or recovery from injury, nitrogen balance is positive. A negative nitrogen balance indicates that protein catabolism is

Box 3.2   CALCULATING NITROGEN BALANCE

Mary is a 25-year-old woman who was admitted to the hospital with multiple fractures and traumatic injuries from a car accident. A nutritional intake study indicated a 24-hour protein intake of 64 g. A 24-hour urinary urea nitrogen (UUN) collection result was 19.8 g.

1. Determine nitrogen intake by dividing protein intake by 6.25:

$$64 \text{ g} \div 6.25 = 10.24 \text{ g of nitrogen}$$

2. Determine total nitrogen output by adding a coefficient of 4 to the UUN:

$$19.8 + 4 \text{ g} = 23.8 \text{ g of nitrogen}$$

3. Calculate nitrogen balance by subtracting nitrogen output from nitrogen intake:

$$10.24 \text{ g} - 23.8 \text{ g} = -13.56 \text{ g in 24 hours}$$

4. Interpret the results.

A negative number indicates that protein breakdown is exceeding protein synthesis. Mary is in a catabolic state.

occurring at a faster rate than protein synthesis, which occurs during starvation or the catabolic phase after injury.

Protein Catabolism for Energy. Using protein for energy is a physiologic and economic waste because amino acids used for energy are not available to be used for protein synthesis, a function unique to amino acids. Normally, the body uses very little protein for energy as long as intake and storage of carbohydrate and fat are adequate. If insufficient carbohydrate and fat are available for energy use (e.g., when calorie intake is inadequate), dietary and body proteins are sacrificed to provide amino acids that can be burned for energy. Over time, loss of lean body tissue occurs and, if severe, can lead to decreased muscle strength, altered immune function, altered organ function, and ultimately death. To "spare" protein—both dietary and body—from being burned for calories, an adequate supply of energy from carbohydrate and fat is needed.

Sources of Protein

For most people, protein is synonymous with meat, but protein is also found in dairy, grains, and vegetables (Fig. 3.3). As illustrated in Table 3.1, more than 40% of the protein in a MyPlate 2000-calorie food pattern comes from the Protein Foods group. Although a recommended serving size of meat may be 2½ to 3 oz, restaurant portions may be much larger, such as a 16-oz "king size" steak. Table 3.2 shows the MyPlate recommendations for the Protein Foods group at various calorie levels.

Protein Quality

Dietary proteins differ in quality, based on their content of essential amino acids. For most Americans, protein quality is not important because the amounts of protein and calories consumed are more than adequate. But when protein needs are increased or protein intake is marginal, quality becomes a crucial concern.

Terms that refer to protein quality are complete and incomplete. Complete proteins provide all nine essential amino acids in adequate amounts and proportions needed by the

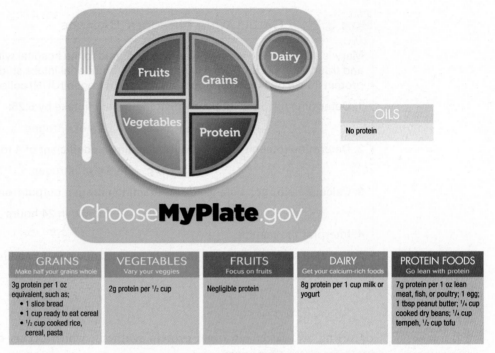

■ FIGURE 3.3   Protein content of MyPlate. (**Source:** U.S. Department of Agriculture, Center for Nutrition Policy and Promotion [2011]. Available at www.choosemyplate.gov)

body for protein synthesis. These high-quality proteins include all animal sources of protein plus soy, the only plant source of complete protein (Box 3.3).

Incomplete proteins also provide all the essential amino acids, but one or more are present in insufficient quantities to support protein synthesis. These amino acids are considered "limiting" in that they limit the process of protein synthesis. All plant proteins, with the exception of soy, are incomplete proteins, as is gelatin.

Different sources of incomplete proteins differ in their limiting amino acids. For instance, grains are typically low in lysine and isoleucine, and legumes are low in methionine and cysteine. Two incomplete proteins that have different limiting amino acids are known as complementary proteins because together they form the equivalent of a

Table 3.1 Protein Content of the MyPlate 2000-Calorie Food Intake Pattern

Group	Amount Recommended in 2000-Calorie Diet	Protein Content per Unit of Measure	Total Protein Content per Group
Grains	6 oz equivalents	3 g/equivalent	18
Vegetables	2½ cups	2 g/½ cup	10
Fruits	2 cups	Negligible	0
Dairy	3 cups	8 g/cup	24
Protein Foods	5.5 oz equivalents	7 g/equivalent	38.5
		Total protein*	90.5

*Total protein does not account for any additional protein in the discretionary calorie category.

Table 3.2 The Amount of Protein Foods Group Equivalents Recommended at Various MyPlate Calorie Levels

Total Daily Calories	Number of oz Equivalents Recommended
1000	2
1200	3
1400	4
1600–1800	5
2000	5.5
2200	6
2400	6.5
2800–3200	7

complete protein. The following are examples of foods that contain complementary proteins:

- Black beans and rice
- Bean tacos
- Pea soup with toast
- Lentils and rice curry
- Falafel sandwich (ground chickpea patties on pita bread)
- Peanut butter sandwich
- Pasta e fagioli (pasta and white bean stew)

Likewise, small amounts of a complete protein combined with any incomplete protein are complementary, such as

- Bread pudding
- Rice pudding
- Corn pudding
- Cereal and milk
- Macaroni and cheese
- French toast
- Cheese sandwich
- Vegetable quiche
- Cheese enchilada

Eating complementary proteins at the same meal is not necessary as long as a variety of incomplete proteins are consumed over the course of a day and calorie intake is adequate.

Box 3.3   SOURCES OF COMPLETE AND INCOMPLETE PROTEINS

Complete/High-Quality Proteins	Incomplete/Lower Quality Proteins
Meat	Grains, items made from grains
Poultry	Vegetables
Seafood	Legumes
Milk, yogurt, cheese	Nuts and seeds
Eggs	Gelatin
Soybeans, soybean products	

Dietary Reference Intakes

The Recommended Dietary Allowance (RDA) for protein for healthy adults is 0.8 g/kg, derived from the absolute minimum requirement needed to maintain nitrogen balance plus an additional factor to account for individual variations and the mixed quality of proteins typically consumed (National Research Council, 2005). This figure also assumes calorie intake is adequate. For the reference adult male who weighs 154 pounds, this translates to 56 g protein/day; the reference female weighing 127 pounds needs 46 g/day. According to the National Health and Nutrition Examination Survey (NHANES) 2007–2008 data, the mean intake for adult men and women aged 20 years and older is 97.7 g/kg and 66.7 g/kg, respectively, an amount well above the RDA (U.S. Department of Agriculture, Agricultural Research Service, 2010).

The Acceptable Macronutrient Distribution Range (AMDR) for protein for adults is 10% to 35% of total calories (National Research Council, 2005). As illustrated in Figure 3.4, the AMDR is a wide range, with the upper end far greater than the both the RDA and median protein intake by American adults cited earlier. From a practical standpoint, grams of protein per day is a more valid standard of adequacy than tracking the percentage of total calories from protein. That is because the RDA for protein is based on enough to fulfill specific protein functions, whereas the AMDR is a range that allows for protein to be used for energy. For both men and women, actual protein intake provides 16% of total calories consumed (U.S. Department of Agriculture, Agricultural Research Service, 2010).

QUICK BITE

To calculate a healthy adult's RDA for protein

1. Divide weight in pounds by 2.2 to determine weight in kilograms.
2. Multiply by 0.8 g/kg.
3. Result is total grams of protein per day.

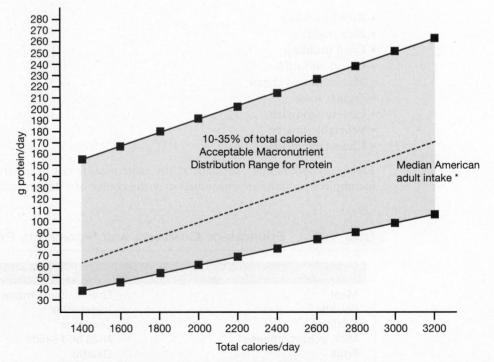

* median American adult intake of 15% of total calories

■ **FIGURE 3.4** Amount of total protein appropriate at various calorie levels based on the Acceptable Macronutrient Distribution Range of 10% to 35% of total calories.

When the RDA Doesn't Apply

The RDA is intended for healthy people only and assumes total calorie intake is adequate. Conditions that require tissue growth or repair increase a person's protein requirement (Box 3.4), as does an inadequate calorie intake. Protein restriction is used for people with severe liver disease (because the liver metabolizes amino acids) and for those who are unable to adequately excrete nitrogenous wastes from protein metabolism due to impaired renal function.

Protein Deficiency

Kwashiorkor: a type of protein–energy malnutrition resulting from a deficiency of protein or infections.

Marasmus: a type of protein–energy malnutrition resulting from severe deficiency or impaired absorption of calories, protein, vitamins, and minerals.

Protein–energy malnutrition (PEM) occurs when protein, calories, or both are deficient in the diet. **Kwashiorkor** and **marasmus** are generally viewed as two distinctly different forms of PEM (Table 3.3), yet there is controversy as to whether kwashiorkor and marasmus simply represent the same disease at different stages. Some studies suggest that marasmus occurs when the body has adapted to starvation and kwashiorkor arises when adaptation to starvation fails due to illness (Shashidhar and Grigsby, 2011).

Although PEM can affect people of any country or age, it is most prevalent in developing countries and in children under the age of 5 years. Approximately 50% of the 10 million annual deaths in developing countries are directly or indirectly blamed on malnutrition in children aged 5 years or younger (Shashidhar and Grigsby, 2011). In the United States, PEM occurs secondary to chronic diseases, such as cancer, AIDS, and chronic pulmonary disease. It may also be seen among homeless people, fad dieters, adults who are addicted to drugs or alcohol, and people with eating disorders. Some studies show that PEM affects 30% to 40% of elderly in long-term care and 50% of hospitalized elderly people (Scheinfeld, Mokashi, and Lin, 2012).

In both children and adults, nutrition therapy begins with correcting fluid and electrolyte imbalances and treating infection (Scheinfeld et al., 2012). Within 48 hours, macronutrients are provided at a level the patient tolerates; the diet is gradually advanced as tolerated. Actual protein and calorie needs may be double that of normal.

Box 3.4   CONDITIONS THAT INCREASE THE NEED FOR PROTEIN

When calorie intake is inadequate so that protein is being used for energy

- Very-low-calorie weight loss diets
- Starvation
- Protein–energy malnutrition

When the body needs to heal itself

- Hypermetabolic conditions such as burns, sepsis, major infection, and major trauma
- Postsurgically
- Acute inflammation such as inflammatory bowel disease
- Skin breakdown
- Multiple fractures
- Hepatitis

When excessive protein losses need replacement

- Peritoneal dialysis
- Protein-losing renal diseases
- Malabsorption syndromes such as protein-losing enteropathy and short bowel syndrome

When periods of normal tissue growth occur

- Pregnancy
- Lactation
- Infancy through adolescence

Table 3.3 Comparison Between Kwashiorkor and Marasmus

	Kwashiorkor	Marasmus
Intake	Fair to normal calorie intake; inadequate protein intake	Inadequate calorie and protein intake
Cause	Acute critical illness or infections that cause loss of appetite while increasing nutrient requirements and losses. Stressors in children in developing countries may be measles or gastroenteritis; in American adults, trauma or sepsis	Severe prolonged starvation may occur in children from chronic or recurring infections with marginal food intake; in adults from developed countries, may occur secondary to chronic illness
Onset	Rapid, acute; may develop in a matter of weeks	Slow, chronic; may take months or years to develop
Edema	Present	Absent
Appearance	Some muscle wasting, retention of some body fat	"Skin and bones" due to severe muscle loss with virtually no body fat
Weight loss	Some	Severe
Other clinical symptoms that may be present	Skin lesions Hair loss, loss of hair color, easy pluckability Enlarged fatty liver	Dry, thin skin that easily wrinkles Hair is sparse; easy pluckability No fatty liver

Protein Excess

There are no proven risks from eating an excess of protein. Data are conflicting as to whether high-protein diets increase the risk of osteoporosis or renal stones. Although a UL has not been established, this does not mean there is no potential for adverse effects from a high protein intake from food or supplements (National Research Council, 2005).

PROTEIN IN HEALTH PROMOTION

The three key recommendations regarding protein in the *2010 Dietary Guidelines for Americans* (see Chapter 8) are more about helping Americans modify their *fat* intake than about consuming the correct amount or type of *protein* (Box 3.5). Eating a variety of

---

Box 3.5   **2010 DIETARY GUIDELINES KEY RECOMMENDATIONS REGARDING PROTEIN INTAKE**

- Choose a variety of protein foods, which include seafood, lean meat and poultry, eggs, beans and peas, soy products, and unsalted nuts and seeds.
- Increase the amount and variety of seafood consumed by choosing seafood in place of some meat and poultry.
- Replace protein foods that are higher in solid fats with choices that are lower in solid fats and calories and/or are sources of oils.

protein sources (including plant proteins), eating more seafood, and choosing sources of protein that are lower in solid fats and calories help to lower fat and saturated fat intake and to increase unsaturated fat intake (U.S. Department of Agriculture, U.S. Department of Health and Human Services, 2010). Very lean and lean options from the Protein Foods group are featured in Table 3.4.

Many leading health organizations, including the American Institute for Cancer Research (World Cancer Research Fund, American Institute for Cancer Research, 2007) and the American Cancer Society (Kushi et al., 2012), recommend a plant-based diet, which means replacing some or most animal sources of protein with vegetable sources, such as soy, legumes, nuts, and seeds. The American Institute for Cancer Research also advises consumers to eat no more than 18 oz (cooked weight) per week of red meats, such as beef,

Table 3.4 Very Lean and Lean Choices from the Protein Foods Group

Item	Very Lean Choices (0–1 g fat/oz)	Lean Choices (3 g fat/oz)
Beef		Select or choice grades of trimmed round, sirloin, and flank steak; tenderloin; rib, chuck, and rump roast; T-bone, porterhouse, and cubed steak; ground round
Pork		Fresh ham; canned, cured, or boiled ham; Canadian bacon; tenderloin, center loin chop
Lamb		Roast, chop, or leg
Veal		Lean chop, roast
Poultry	Skinless white meat chicken or turkey Skinless Cornish hen	Skinless dark meat chicken or turkey White meat with skin Skinless domestic duck or goose
Fish	Cod, flounder, haddock, halibut, trout, smoked salmon, fresh or canned-in-water tuna	Smoked herring, oysters, fresh or canned salmon, catfish, sardines, tuna canned in oil
Shellfish	Clams, crab, lobster, scallops, shrimp, imitation shellfish	
Game	Skinless duck or pheasant, venison, buffalo, ostrich	Skinless goose, rabbit
Cheese	Fat-free or low-fat cottage cheese Fat-free cheese	4.5% cottage cheese Grated parmesan Cheese with 3 g of fat or less per ounce
Processed meats	Those with 1 g of fat or less per ounce, such as turkey ham	Those with 3 g of fat or less per ounce, such as turkey pastrami
Other	Egg whites, egg substitutes Kidney Sausage with 1 g of fat or less per ounce Legumes, lentils (cooked)	Hot dogs with 3 g of fat or less per ounce Liver, heart

pork, and lamb, and to avoid processed meat, such as ham, bacon, salami, hot dogs, and sausages, based on evidence that red meat increases the risk of colorectal cancer (World Cancer Research Fund, American Institute for Cancer Research, 2007). The health benefits of a plant-based diet may come from eating less of certain substances (such as saturated fat and cholesterol), eating more of others (such as fiber, antioxidants, and phytochemicals), or a combination of the two.

Vegetarian Diets

Vegetarian eating patterns range from complete elimination of all animal products to simply avoiding red meat. With a foundation of grains, vegetables, fruit, legumes, seeds, and nuts, categories of vegetarian restrictions are

- Vegan, or total vegetarian, which excludes all animal products
- Lacto-ovo vegetarian, which includes milk and eggs
- Lacto-vegetarian, which includes milk
- Ovo-vegetarian, which includes eggs

Within each defined category of vegetarianism, individuals differ as to how strictly they adhere to their eating style. For instance, some vegans do not eat refried beans that contain lard because lard is an animal product, but other vegans do not avoid animal products so conscientiously. Flexitarians primarily follow a plant-based diet but occasionally allow themselves meat, fish, poultry, or dairy foods. Whatever the level of restriction, properly planned vegetarian and vegan diets are nutritionally adequate during all phases of the life cycle, including pregnancy, lactation, infancy, childhood, and adolescence, and for athletes (American Dietetic Association [ADA], 2009b).

Results of an evidence-based review show that a vegetarian diet is associated with a lower risk of death from ischemic heart disease (ADA, 2009b). Other advantages include lower blood cholesterol levels, lower blood pressure, and lower risk of hypertension and type 2 diabetes (ADA, 2009b). People who consume a vegetarian diet tend to have a lower body mass index and lower overall cancer rate. These health advantages may be attributed to the nutrient content of a vegetarian diet: lower in saturated fat and cholesterol and higher in fiber, magnesium, potassium, vitamin C, vitamin E, folate, and phytochemicals. Vegetarian diets are not automatically healthier than nonvegetarian diets. Poorly planned vegetarian diets may lack certain essential nutrients, which endangers health. Also, vegetarian diets can be excessive in fat and cholesterol if whole milk, whole-milk cheeses, eggs, and high-fat desserts are used extensively. Whether a vegetarian diet is healthy or detrimental to health depends on the actual food choices made over time. Tips for vegetarians appear in Box 3.6.

Nutrients of Concern

Most vegetarian diets, even vegan ones, meet or exceed the RDA for protein despite containing less total protein and more lower quality protein than nonvegetarian diets. Vegetarian sources of protein include legumes, nuts, nut butters, and soy products such as soy milk, tofu, tempeh, and veggie burgers. A glossary of soy products is listed in Box 3.7.

Iron, zinc, calcium, vitamin D, omega-3 fatty acids, and iodine are nutrients of concern not because they cannot be obtained in sufficient quantities from plants but because they may not be adequately consumed, depending on an individual's food choices. Vitamin B_{12} is of concern because it does not occur naturally in plants. Table 3.5 lists vegetarian sources of these nutrients of concern.

Box 3.6   TIPS FOR FOLLOWING A VEGETARIAN DIET

Eat a variety of foods including whole grains, vegetables, fruits, legumes, nuts, seeds, and if desired, dairy products and eggs. Consider meatless versions of familiar favorites, such as vegetable pizza, vegetable lasagna, vegetable stir-fry, vegetable lo mein, and vegetable kabobs.

Experiment with meat substitutes made from vegetables. For variety, try soy sausage patties or links, veggie burgers, or soy hot dogs.

Eat enough calories. Adequate calories are necessary to avoid using amino acids for energy, which could lead to a shortage of amino acids for protein synthesis.

Consume a rich source of vitamin C at every meal. Eating a good source of vitamin C at every meal helps to maximize iron absorption from plants. Try orange and citrus fruits, tomatoes, kiwi, red and green peppers, broccoli, Brussels sprouts, cantaloupe, and strawberries.

Include two servings daily of fats that supply omega-3 fats. A serving is 1 tsp flaxseed oil, 1 tbsp canola or soybean oil, 1 tbsp ground flaxseed, or ¼ cup walnuts. Nuts and seeds may be used as substitutes from the Fat group.

Don't go overboard on high-fat cheese as a meat substitute. Full-fat cheese has more saturated fat and calories than many meats.

Experiment with ethnic cuisines. Many Asian, Middle Eastern, and Indian restaurants offer a variety of meatless dishes.

Supplement nutrients that are lacking from food. For vegans, this means vitamin B_{12} (unless reliable fortified foods are consumed) and perhaps vitamin D. The adequacy of calcium, iron, and zinc intake is evaluated on an individual basis.

Protein for Muscle Building: Not the Limiting Factor

As previously stated, in healthy adults with a stable muscle mass, protein synthesis occurs at the same rate as protein breakdown; the net balance between the two opposing processes is neutral. Muscle mass increases when protein anabolism is greater than protein catabolism, resulting in a net positive balance. Both exercise and nutrition impact net balance.

Box 3.7   GLOSSARY OF SOY PRODUCTS

Edamame: parboiled fresh soybeans, usually in the pod, sold refrigerated or frozen

Meat analogs: imitation burgers, hot dogs, bacon, chicken fingers, etc., made from soy, not meat

Miso: fermented soybean paste

Soy cheese: cheese made from soy milk; can substitute for sour cream, cream cheese, or other cheese

Soy milk: the liquid from soaked, ground, strained soybeans; available in plain and in chocolate and vanilla flavors.

Soy nuts: whole soybeans that have been soaked in water and then baked

Soy nut butter: crushed soy nuts blended with soy oil to resemble peanut butter

Soy sprouts: sprouted soybeans

Tofu: soybean curd

Tempeh: caked fermented soybeans

Textured vegetable protein (TVP): soy flour modified to resemble ground beef when rehydrated

Table 3.5 Sources of Nutrients of Concern in Vegan Diets

Nutrient	Vegetarian Sources	Comments
Iron	Iron-fortified bread and cereals Baked potato with skin Kidney beans, black-eyed peas, and lentils Cooked soybeans Tofu Veggie "meats" Dried apricots, prunes, and raisins Cooking in a cast iron pan, especially with acidic foods such as tomatoes	Because of the lower bioavailability of iron from plants, it is recommended that vegetarians consume 1.8 times the normal iron intake.
Zinc	Whole grains Legumes Zinc-fortified cereals Soybean products Pumpkin seeds Nuts	Zinc from plants is not absorbed as well as zinc from meats. Vegetarians are urged to meet or exceed the RDA for zinc.
Calcium	Bok choy Broccoli Chinese/Napa cabbage Collard greens Kale Calcium-fortified fruit juice Calcium-set tofu Calcium-fortified soy milk, breakfast cereals	Spinach, beet greens, and Swiss chard are also high in calcium, but their oxalate content interferes with calcium absorption. Calcium supplements are recommended for people who do not meet their calcium requirement through food.
Vitamin D	Sunlight Fortified milk Fortified ready-to-eat cereals Fortified soy milk Fortified nondairy milk products	Supplements may be necessary depending on the quality of sunlight exposure and adequacy of food choices.

Omega-3 fatty acids	Fortified foods, such as breakfast cereals, soy milk, and yogurt
	Sources of alpha-linolenic acid are
	  Ground flaxseed and flaxseed oil
	  Walnuts and walnut oil
	  Canola oil
	  Soy
		Diets that exclude fish, eggs, and sea vegetables do not contain a direct source of omega-3 fatty acids.
		The body can convert small amounts of alpha-linolenic acid into one of the omega-3 fatty acids (docosahexaenoic acid [DHA]).

Iodine	Iodized salt; sea vegetables	Sea salt and kosher salt are generally not iodized; iodine content of sea vegetables varies greatly
Vitamin B_{12}	Fortified soy milk, breakfast cereals, and veggie burgers	Seaweed, algae, spirulina, tempeh, miso, beer, and other fermented foods contain a form of vitamin B_{12} that the body cannot use. Supplemental vitamin B_{12} through food or pills is recommended for all people over the age of 50 years regardless of the type of diet they consume because absorption decreases with age.

Exercise in the form of resistance training, also called weight or strength training, is necessary to increase muscle mass. To improve muscle strength and power in most healthy adults, the American College of Sports Medicine recommends two to four sets of 8 to 10 repetitions each of strength-training exercises of all major muscle groups at least twice a week (Garber et al., 2011). When an increase in muscular endurance is the goal, 15 to 20 repetitions are recommended. Athletes and body builders do more.

Protein and amino acids are commonly believed to be the most important factor in building muscle mass because muscle is composed of protein. While protein is vital to the process, the amount needed to stimulate exercise-related muscle anabolism is relatively small: as little as 6 g of essential amino acids consumed before or after exercise results in a positive net balance (Hartman, Moore, and Phillips, 2006). Although a little is good, more is not necessarily better. Data show that an intake greater than 10 g of protein is associated with diminishing increases in muscle anabolism. Protein eaten in excess of need does not build muscles quicker; excess protein is catabolized for energy.

Protein recommendations for athletes are controversial. The American College of Sports Medicine and ADA recommend that endurance and strength-training athletes consume 1.2 to 1.7 g protein/kg/day (ADA, 2009a). This amount of protein can generally be met through diet alone, without the need for protein or amino acid supplements. Lay publications and physical trainers often recommend higher intakes, such as 2.0 g/kg/day, even though supporting evidence is lacking.

The type of protein consumed may impact muscle anabolism. Only essential amino acids in food stimulate protein synthesis, and leucine in particular may be the essential amino acid that has the most impact on muscle protein synthesis (Pasiakos et al., 2011). Animal proteins—namely, eggs, dairy, lean meats, and seafood—provide all essential amino acids in balanced proportions; whey protein, which makes up 20% of the protein in milk, has the highest concentration of leucine. However, current evidence shows that when calorie intake is adequate, protein and amino acid supplements are no more or no less effective than food for increasing muscle mass (Tipton and Witard, 2007).

Nutritionally, the most important factor for increasing muscle mass is calories. If calorie intake meets or exceeds need, muscle growth can occur over a range or protein intakes (Tipton and Witard, 2007). When calorie intake is inadequate, an increase in muscle mass is not likely (ADA, 2009a). A high calorie intake needed to support intense training generally provides adequate protein for muscle anabolism.

How Do You Respond?

Is ground turkey a low-fat alternative to ground beef? Not necessarily. Ground turkey most likely contains skin, dark meat, and fat along with the breast, making it a higher fat product than 95% lean ground beef. Ground turkey breast and ground chicken breast are made only from white meat and are much lower in fat (0.5 g/3 oz cooked) than all varieties of ground beef (5.5–17 g fat/3 oz cooked).

Isn't a high-protein diet better than a high-carbohydrate diet in promoting weight loss? This may be true. A study by Krieger, Sitren, Daniels, and Langkamp-Henken (2006) showed that protein intake is a significant predictor of lean mass retention during calorie-restricted diets. In fact, a daily protein intake of more than 1.05 g/kg was associated with greater muscle retention than was a protein intake closer to the RDA. In other words, protein eaters lost significantly more fat-to-muscle tissue than the carbohydrate eaters; obviously, the loss of fat tissue is more desirable than the loss of muscle. A study

(continues on page 62)

HOW DO YOU RESPOND? (continued)

in postmenopausal women had similar results (Bopp et al., 2008). Clients who choose a high-protein, low-calorie diet should be reminded to choose low-fat sources of protein to keep calories under control.

Does "vegetarian" on the label mean the product is also low fat? No, vegetarian is not synonymous with low fat, particularly for items like vegetarian hot dogs, soy cheese, soy yogurt, and refried beans. Advise clients to read the "Nutrition Facts" label to determine if a vegetarian item is a good nutritional buy.

CASE STUDY

For ethical reasons, Emily does not eat meat, eggs, or milk, although she is not so strict as to avoid baked goods that may contain milk or eggs. Over the last 6 months, she has gained 15 pounds, although she actually expected to lose weight. She needs 2000 cal/day according to MyPlate. A typical daily intake for her is as follows:

Breakfast:	A smoothie made with soy milk, tofu, and fresh fruit A glazed doughnut
Snack:	Potato chips and soda
Lunch:	A peanut butter sandwich Soy yogurt Oatmeal cookies Soda
Snack:	A candy bar
Dinner:	Stir-fried vegetables over rice Bread with margarine A glass of soy milk Apple pie
Snack:	Buttered popcorn

- What kind of vegetarian is Emily? What sources of protein is she consuming? Is she consuming enough protein? How does her daily intake compare to MyPlate recommendations for a 2000-calorie diet? What suggestions would you make to her to improve the quality of her diet?
- Is Emily at risk of any nutrient deficiencies? If so, what would you recommend she do to ensure nutritional adequacy?
- What would you tell Emily about her weight gain? What foods would you recommend she eat less of if she wants to lose weight? What could she substitute for those foods?

STUDY QUESTIONS

1. What is the RDA for protein for a healthy adult who weighs 165 pounds?
   a. 60 g
   b. 75 g
   c. 100 g
   d. 165 g

2. The client asks what foods are rich in protein and are less expensive than meat. Which of the following foods would the nurse recommend she eat more of?
   a. Breads and cereals
   b. Legumes
   c. Fruit and vegetables
   d. Fish and shellfish

3. Which of the following sources of protein would be most appropriate on a low-fat diet?
   a. Eggs
   b. Ground chicken
   c. Boiled ham
   d. Turkey breast without skin

4. Which statement indicates the client understands vegetarian diets?
   a. "Vegetarians need to eat more calories than nonvegetarians in order to spare protein."
   b. "Vegetarian diets are always healthier than nonvegetarian diets."
   c. "Vegetarians usually do not consume enough protein."
   d. "Vegetarians may need to take supplements of iron, vitamin B_{12}, and calcium."

5. A client who is in a positive nitrogen balance is most likely to be
   a. A healthy adult
   b. Starving
   c. Pregnant
   d. Losing weight

6. An adult in the hospital has been diagnosed with marasmus. Which of the following would you expect?
   a. The client has experienced severe weight loss.
   b. The client denies hunger.
   c. The client has edema and a swollen abdomen.
   d. The onset of the deficiency was rapid.

7. The nurse knows that instructions have been effective when the client verbalizes that a source of complete, high-quality protein is found in
   a. Peanut butter
   b. Black-eyed peas
   c. Soy burgers
   d. Corn

8. A client says that she doesn't eat much meat. After teaching the client about serving sizes, the nurse determines that the teaching has been effective when the client states that an ounce of meat provides approximately the same amount of protein as which of the following?
   a. 8 oz of milk
   b. 8 oz of nuts
   c. 2 oz of cheese
   d. 2 eggs

KEY CONCEPTS

■ Protein is a component of every living cell. Protein in the body provides structure and framework. Amino acids are also components of enzymes, hormones, neurotransmitters, and antibodies. Proteins play a role in fluid balance and acid–base balance and are used to transport substances through the blood. Protein provides 4 cal/g of energy.

■ Amino acids, which are composed of carbon, hydrogen, oxygen, and nitrogen atoms, are the building blocks of protein. Of the 20 common amino acids, 9 are considered essential because the body cannot make them. The remaining 11 amino acids are no less important but are considered nonessential because they can be made by the body if nitrogen is available. Some of these are considered conditionally essential under certain circumstances.

■ Amino acids are joined in different amounts, proportions, and sequences to form the thousands of different proteins in the body.

■ The small intestine is the principal site of protein digestion; amino acids and some di-peptides are absorbed through the portal bloodstream.

■ In the body, amino acids are used to make proteins, nonessential amino acids, and other nitrogen-containing compounds. Some amino acids can be converted to glucose. Amino acids consumed in excess of need are burned for energy or converted to fat and stored.

■ Healthy adults are in nitrogen balance, which means that protein synthesis is occurring at the same rate as protein breakdown. Nitrogen balance is determined by compar-ing the amount of nitrogen consumed with the amount of nitrogen excreted in urine, feces, hair, nails, and skin.

■ Except for the Fruits and Oils, all MyPlate groups provide protein in varying amounts.

■ The quality of proteins varies. Complete proteins provide adequate amounts and pro-portions of all essential amino acids needed for protein synthesis. Animal proteins and soy protein are complete proteins. Incomplete proteins lack adequate amounts of one or more essential amino acids. Except for soy protein, all plants are sources of incom-plete proteins. Gelatin is also an incomplete protein.

■ The RDA for protein for adults is 0.8 g/kg of body weight. The AMDR for protein among adults is 10% to 35% of total calories. Most Americans consume more protein than they need.

■ Pure vegans eat no animal products. Most American vegetarians are lacto-vegetarians or lacto-ovo vegetarians, whose diets include milk products or milk products and eggs, respectively.

■ Most vegetarian diets meet or exceed the RDA for protein and are nutritionally ade-quate across the life cycle. Pure vegans who do not have reliable sources of vitamin B_{12} and vitamin D need supplements.

■ To gain muscle mass, resistance exercise is necessary. The small increase in protein that is needed can be easily met by an increase in calorie intake. Nutritionally, adequate calories are the most important factor for increasing muscle mass.

Check Your Knowledge Answer Key

1. **TRUE** Most Americans consume more protein than they need.

2. **FALSE** Over the course of a day, if the food consumed is varied and contains sufficient calories, most vegetarian diets meet or exceed the RDA for protein.

3. **FALSE** Unlike glucose and fat, the body is not able to store excess amino acids for later use.

4. **TRUE** Soy protein is complete. It is a high biologic value protein and is comparable in quality to animal protein.

5. **FALSE** There are no proven risks to having a high protein intake.

6. **FALSE** The quality of a protein is determined by the balance of essential amino acids provided.

7. **FALSE** Fruits generally provide negligible protein, and oils are protein free.

8. **FALSE** Healthy adults are in neutral nitrogen balance: protein synthesis is occurring at the same rate as protein breakdown.

9. **FALSE** Properly planned vegetarian diets are nutritionally adequate during all phases of pregnancy and lactation.

10. **TRUE** Due to lack of sufficient data, a UL has not been established for protein or any of the amino acids. However, the Institute of Medicine warns against using any single amino acid in amounts significantly higher than those found in food.

Student Resources on thePoint

For additional learning materials, activate the code in the front of this book at
http://thePoint.lww.com/activate

Websites

Food and Nutrition Information Center, U.S. Department of Agriculture at **http://fnic.nal.usda.gov/**
Vegan Health at **www.veganhealth.org**
The Vegan Society at **www.vegansociety.com**
Vegetarian Nutrition Dietetic Practice Group at **www.vegetariannutrition.net**
Vegetarian Resource Group at **www.vrg.org**
The Vegetarian Society of the United Kingdom at **www.vegsoc.org/health/**
Seventh-Day Adventist Dietetic Association at **www.sdada.org/health_tips.htm**
Soyfoods Association of North America at **www.soyfoods.org**
United Soybean Board at **www.soyconnection.com**

References

American Dietetic Association. (2009a). Position of the American Dietetic Association, Dietitians of Canada, and the American College of Sports Medicine: Nutrition and athletic performance. *Journal of the American Dietetic Association, 109,* 509–529.

American Dietetic Association. (2009b). Position of the American Dietetic Association: Vegetarian diets. *Journal of the American Dietetic Association, 109,* 1266–1282.

Bopp, M., Houston, D., Lenchik, L., Easter, L., Kritchevsky, S. B., & Nicklas, B. J. (2008). Lean mass loss is associated with low-protein intake during dietary-induced weight loss in postmenopausal women. *Journal of the American Dietetic Association, 108,* 1216–1220.

Garber, C., Blissmer, B., Deschenes, M., Franklin, B. A., Lamonte, M. J., Lee, I. M., . . . Swain, D. P. (2011). Quantity and quality of exercise for developing and maintaining cardiorespiratory, musculoskeletal, and neuromotor fitness in apparently healthy adults: Guidance for prescribing exercise. *Medicine and Science in Sports and Exercise, 43,* 1334–1359.

Hartman, J., Moore, D., & Phillips, S. (2006). Resistance training reduces whole-body protein turnover and improves net protein retention in untrained young males. *Applied Physiology, Nutrition, and Metabolism, 31,* 557–564.

Krieger, J., Sitren, H., Daniels, M., & Langkamp-Henken, B. (2006). Effects of variation in protein and carbohydrate intake on body mass and composition during energy restriction: A meta-regression. *American Journal of Clinical Nutrition, 83,* 260–274.

Kushi, L., Doyle, C., McCullough, M., Rock, C. L., Demark-Wahnefried, W., Bandera, E. V., . . . Gansler, T. (2012). American Cancer Society guidelines on nutrition and physical activity for cancer prevention. *CA: A Cancer Journal For Clinicians, 62,* 30–67.

National Research Council. (2005). *Dietary Reference Intakes for energy, carbohydrate, fiber, fat, fatty acids, cholesterol, protein, and amino acids (macronutrients).* Washington, DC: The National Academies Press.

Pasiakos, S., McClung, H., McClung, J., Margolis, L. M., Andersen, N. E., Cloutier, G. J., . . . Young, A. J. (2011). Leucine-enriched essential amino acid supplementation during moderate steady state exercise enhances postexercise muscle protein synthesis. *The American Journal of Clinical Nutrition, 94,* 809–818.

Scheinfeld, N., Mokashi, A., & Lin, A. (2012). *Protein-energy malnutrition.* Available at http://emedicine.medscape.com/article/1104623-overview. Accessed on 8/30/12.

Shashidhar, H., & Grigsby, D. (2011). *Malnutrition.* Available at http://emedicine.medscape.com/article/985140-overview. Accessed on 8/30/2012.

Tipton, K., & Witard, O. (2007). Protein requirements and recommendations for athletes: Relevance of ivory tower arguments for practical recommendations. *Clinics in Sports Medicine, 26,* 17–36.

U.S. Department of Agriculture, Agricultural Research Service. (2010). *Nutrient intakes from food: Mean amounts consumed per individual, by gender and age. What We Eat in American, NHANES 2007–2008.* Available at www.ars.usda.gov/ba/bhnrc/fsrg. Accessed on 6/9/12.

U.S. Department of Agriculture, U.S. Department of Health and Human Services. (2010). *Dietary guidelines for Americans* (7th ed.). Available at www.health.gov/dietaryguidelines. Accessed on 2/24/11.

World Cancer Research Fund, American Institute for Cancer Research. (2007). *Food, nutrition, physical activity, and the prevention of cancer: A global perspective.* Washington, DC: American Institute for Cancer Research.

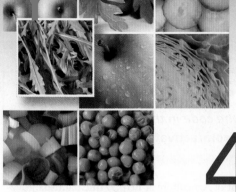

4 Lipids

CHECK YOUR KNOWLEDGE

TRUE   FALSE

☐   ☐   **1** Fat provides more than double the amount of calories as an equivalent amount of carbohydrate or protein.

☐   ☐   **2** All fats are bad fats.

☐   ☐   **3** The body makes two to three times more cholesterol than the typical American consumes.

☐   ☐   **4** In a "healthy" diet, no foods derive more than 30% of their calories from fat.

☐   ☐   **5** Butter is healthier than margarine.

☐   ☐   **6** All sources of fat are a blend of saturated and unsaturated fatty acids.

☐   ☐   **7** Saturated fatty acids are found only in animal products.

☐   ☐   **8** Menu items described as being "cooked in vegetable oil" are trans fat free.

☐   ☐   **9** "Fish oils" are essential in the diet.

☐   ☐   **10** The most effective dietary strategy for lowering serum cholesterol is to limit cholesterol intake.

LEARNING OBJECTIVES

Upon completion of this chapter, you will be able to

1 Compare saturated, monounsaturated, and polyunsaturated fatty acids.
2 Propose ways to improve the type of fat present in a sample meal plan.
3 Explain the functions of fat in the body.
4 Discuss the digestion and absorption of fat.
5 Give examples of foods that provide omega-3 fatty acids.
6 Calculate the amount of calories from fat in various foods.
7 Explain why there is no Recommended Dietary Allowance for total fat, trans fat, and saturated fat.

"Eat less fat" has long been a nutritional mantra. But decades of study have shown that the relationship between fat and chronic disease is far more complex than that simple advice implies. Eating less fat without regard to total calorie intake does not guarantee weight loss. And although obesity increases the risk of certain cancers, the risk may come from an excess of calories, not specifically dietary fat. With heart disease and stroke, the type of fat may be more important than the amount of fat. The bottom line is that while all fats are calorically dense, some fats are "good" (unsaturated) and should be eaten in moderation, and other fats are "bad" (saturated fat and trans fats) and should be limited.

There are three classes of **lipids**, which are referred to as fat throughout the rest of this chapter and book: triglycerides (fats and oils), which account for 98% of the fat in food; phospholipids (e.g., lecithin); and sterols (e.g., cholesterol). This chapter describes fats, their dietary sources, and how they are handled in the body. The functions of fat are presented, as are recommendations regarding intake.

> **Lipids:** a group of water-insoluble, energy-yielding organic compounds composed of carbon, hydrogen, and oxygen atoms.

TRIGLYCERIDES

> **Triglycerides:** a class of lipids composed of a glycerol molecule as its backbone with three fatty acids attached.

Chemically, **triglycerides** are made of the same elements as carbohydrates, namely, carbon, hydrogen, and oxygen; but because there are proportionately more carbon and hydrogen atoms to oxygen atoms, they yield more calories per gram than carbohydrates. Structurally, triglycerides are composed of a three-carbon atom glycerol backbone with three fatty acids attached (Fig. 4.1). An individual triglyceride molecule may contain one, two, or three different types of fatty acids.

Fatty Acids

Fatty acids are basically chains of carbon atoms with hydrogen atoms attached (Fig. 4.2). At one end of the chain is a methyl group (CH_3), and at the other end is an acid group (COOH). Fatty acids are commonly abbreviated by a C followed by the number of carbon atoms, a colon, and the number of double bonds. For example, stearic acid, an 18-carbon length fatty acid with no double bonds, is abbreviated as C18:0. The most common fatty acids and their sources are listed in Box 4.1.

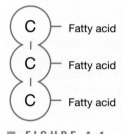

■ **FIGURE 4.1** Generic triglyceride molecule.

> **Fatty Acids:** organic compounds composed of a chain of carbon atoms to which hydrogen atoms are attached. An acid group (COOH) is attached at one end and a methyl group (CH_3) at the other end.

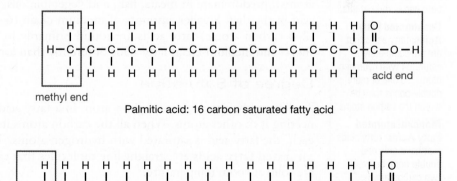

Palmitic acid: 16 carbon saturated fatty acid

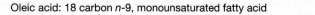

■ **FIGURE 4.2**   Fatty acid configurations.

Oleic acid: 18 carbon *n*-9, monounsaturated fatty acid

Box 4.1   The Most Common Fatty Acids in Food

	Chemical Abbreviation	Common Food Sources
Saturated fatty acids		
Palmitic acid	C16:0	Meat, poultry, eggs, dairy, butter
Stearic acid	C18:0	Animal fats, cocoa butter
Monounsaturated fatty acid		
Oleic acid	C18:1	Meats; canola, peanut, and olive oil; most nuts
n-3 Polyunsaturated fatty acids		
Alpha-linolenic acid	C18:3	Walnuts; flaxseed oil, soybean oil, canola oil
Eicosapentaenoic acid (EPA)	C20:5	Fatty fish, such as salmon, herring, mackerel, tuna
Docosahexaenoic acid (DHA)	C22:6	Fatty fish; marine algae–fortified foods, such as juice
n-6 Polyunsaturated fatty acids		
Linoleic acid	C18:2	Corn, safflower, soybean, cottonseed, and sunflower oils
Arachidonic acid	C20:4	Meat, poultry, eggs

Glycerol: a three-carbon atom chain that serves as the backbone of triglycerides.

Saturated Fatty Acids: fatty acids in which all the carbon atoms are bonded to as many hydrogen atoms as they can hold, so no double bonds exist between carbon atoms.

Unsaturated Fatty Acids: fatty acids that are not completely saturated with hydrogen atoms, so one or more double bonds form between the carbon atoms.

Monounsaturated Fatty Acids: fatty acids that have only one double bond between two carbon atoms.

Polyunsaturated Fatty Acids: fatty acids that have two or more double bonds between carbon atoms.

Fatty acids attach to **glycerol** molecules in various ratios and combinations to form a variety of triglycerides within a single food fat. The types and proportions of fatty acids present influence the sensory and functional properties of the food fat. For instance, butter tastes and acts differently from corn oil, which tastes and acts differently from lard. Fatty acids vary in the length of their carbon chain and in the degree of unsaturation.

Carbon Chain Length

Almost all naturally occurring fatty acids have an even number of carbon atoms in their chain, generally between 4 and 24. Long-chain fatty acids (containing 12 or more carbon atoms), predominate in meats, fish, and vegetable oils, are the most common length fatty acid in the diet. Smaller amounts of medium-chain (6–10 carbon atoms) and short-chain (2–4 carbon atoms) fatty acids are found primarily in dairy products. The body absorbs short- and medium-chain fatty acids differently than long-chain fatty acids.

Degree of Saturation

As dictated by nature, each carbon atom in a fatty acid chain must have four bonds connecting it to other atoms. When all the carbon atoms in a fatty acid have four single bonds each, the fatty acid is saturated with hydrogen atoms. The majority of naturally occurring **saturated fatty acids** are straight-line molecules that can pack tightly together; thus, they are solid at room temperature.

An **"unsaturated" fatty acid** does not have all the hydrogen atoms it can potentially hold; therefore, one (**monounsaturated**) or more (**polyunsaturated**) double bonds form between carbon atoms in the chain. Because of the double bond, unsaturated fatty acids are physically kinked and unable to pack together tightly; they are liquid at room temperature and are referred to as "oils."

All food fats contain a mixture of saturated, monounsaturated, and polyunsaturated fatty acids. When applied to sources of fat in the diet, "unsaturated" and "saturated" are not absolute terms used to describe the only types of fatty acids present; rather, they are relative descriptions that indicate which kinds of fatty acids are present in the largest proportion (Fig. 4.3).

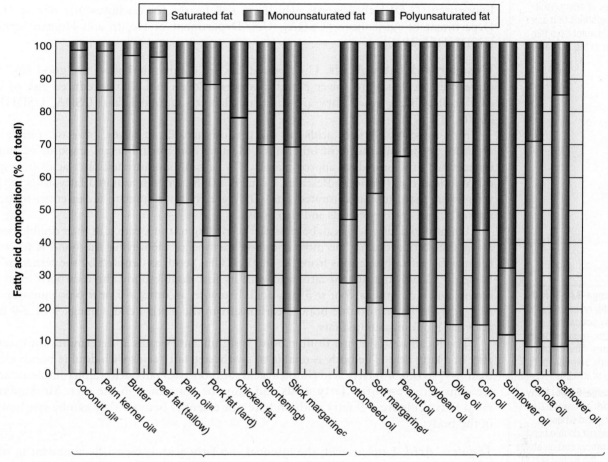

a. Coconut oil, palm kernel oil, and palm oil are called oils because they come from plants. However, they are semi-solid at room temperature due to their high content of short-chain saturated fatty acids. They are considered solid fats for nutritional purposes.
b. Partially hydrogenated vegetable oil shortening, which contains *trans* fats.
c. Most stick margarines contain partially hydrogenated vegetable oil, a source of *trans* fats.
d. The primary ingredient in soft margarine with no *trans* fats is liquid vegetable oil.

■ FIGURE 4.3   Fatty acid profiles of common fats and oils. (**Source:** *Dietary Guidelines for Americans, 2010.* U.S. Department of Agriculture, Agricultural Research Service, Nutrient Data Laboratory. *USDA National Nutrient Database for Standard Reference, Release 22, 2009.* [2009]. Available at http://www.ars.usda.gov/ba/bhnrc/ndl. Accessed 7/19/10.)

Saturated Fats. Fats with a high percentage of saturated fatty acids are referred to as solid fats because they are solid at room temperature. Saturated fatty acids occur to the greatest extent in animal fats—the fat in meats, whole-milk dairy products, and egg yolks. The only vegetable fats that are saturated are palm oil, palm kernel oil, and coconut oil.

Saturated fat is commonly known as a "bad" fat. A strong body of evidence shows that a high intake of most saturated fatty acids is linked with high total and **low-density lipoprotein (LDL) cholesterol**, which are risk factors for cardiovascular disease (U.S. Department of Agriculture [USDA], U.S. Department of Health and Human Services [USDHHS], 2010).

Unsaturated Fatty Acids. Unsaturated fats are commonly known as "good fats" because they are linked to lower blood cholesterol levels and thus a reduced risk of cardiovascular disease when they are eaten in place of saturated fats (USDA, USDHHS, 2010).

Monounsaturated fatty acids are the predominate fat in olives, olive oil, canola oil, avocado, peanut oil, and most other nuts. Meat fat contains moderate amounts of monounsaturated fats, providing approximately 50% of monounsaturated fatty acids in a typical American diet (National Research Council, 2005). Polyunsaturated fatty acids are less ubiquitous than monounsaturated fats. They are the predominate fat in corn, soybean, safflower, and cottonseed oils and also in fish.

Unsaturated fatty acids can be classified according to the location of their double bonds along the carbon chain. The most common method of identifying the bond is to count the number of carbon atoms from the methyl (CH_3) end, as denoted by the terms "*n*" or "omega." A polyunsaturated fatty acid with its first double-bond three carbons from the methyl end is an **omega-3** or *n-3* fatty acid. Likewise, an **omega-6** or *n-6* polyunsaturated fatty acid has its first double-bond 6 carbons from the methyl end. Omega-9 or *n-9* fatty acids are monounsaturated fats.

The location of the first double bond is significant because it determines the essentiality of a fatty acid. The body is unable to synthesize fatty acids with double bonds closer than *n-9*, so one *n-6* fatty acid (linoleic acid) and one *n-3* fatty acid (alpha-linolenic acid) are considered **essential fatty acids** and must be consumed in the diet. Monounsaturated fatty acids are *n-9* fatty acids and are not essential because they can be synthesized in the body.

Linoleic Acid. Linoleic acid, the essential *n-6* fatty acid, is especially abundant in plant oils, such as safflower, sunflower, corn, and soybean oils; poultry fat, nuts, and seeds are also sources. The body can make other *n-6* fatty acids from linoleic acid, such as arachidonic acid. However, if a deficiency of linoleic acid develops, arachidonic acid becomes "conditionally essential" because the body is unable to synthesize it without a supply of linoleic acid.

Alpha-Linolenic Acid. Alpha-linolenic acid, the essential *n-3* fatty acid, is the most prominent *n-3* fatty acid in most Western diets. It is found in flaxseed, canola, soybean, and walnut oils and in nuts, especially walnuts. To a very limited extent, humans can convert alpha-linolenic acid to the *n-3* fatty acids eicosapentaenoic acid (EPA) and docosahexaenoic acid (DHA). These two *n-3* fatty acids are commonly referred to as **"fish oils"** because they are primarily found in fatty fish, especially salmon, anchovy, sardines, herring, lake trout, and mackerel. Cardioprotective benefits of *n-3* fatty acids are attributed to EPA and DHA (International Food Information Council Foundation [IFICF], 2011).

Low-Density Lipoprotein (LDL) Cholesterol: the major class of atherogenic lipoproteins that carry cholesterol from the liver to the tissues.

Omega-3 (*n-3*) Fatty Acid: an unsaturated fatty acid whose endmost double bond occurs three carbon atoms from the methyl end of its carbon chain.

Omega-6 (*n-6*) Fatty Acid: an unsaturated fatty acid whose endmost double bond occurs six carbon atoms from the methyl end of its carbon chain.

Essential Fatty Acids: fatty acids that cannot be synthesized in the body and thus must be consumed through food.

Fish Oils: a common term for the long-chain, polyunsaturated omega-3 fatty acids eicosapentaenoic acid (EPA) and docosahexaenoic acid (DHA) found in the fat of fish, primarily in cold-water fish.

Stability of Fats. Although all fats can become oxidized when exposed to light and oxygen over time, the greater the number of double bonds, the greater is the susceptibility to **rancidity**. Therefore, polyunsaturated fats are most susceptible to rancidity, saturated fats are least susceptible, and monounsaturated fats are somewhere in between.

To help extend the shelf life of foods, manufacturers may add antioxidants, such as butylated hydroxyanisole (BHA) and butylated hydroxytoluene (BHT), to polyunsaturated fat–rich foods and oils. Another commercial method to make oils more stable is hydrogenation.

Hydrogenation. **Hydrogenation** is a process that adds hydrogen atoms to polyunsaturated oils to saturate some of the double bonds so that the resulting product is less susceptible to rancidity and has improved function. Hydrogenation varies in degrees from "light" to "partial" according to the desired outcome. Lightly hydrogenated oils are more stable than polyunsaturated oils because they have fewer double bonds but are still in liquid form. Partial hydrogenation results in a more solid (more saturated) product, such as stick margarine and shortening, yet still maintains some unsaturated (double) bonds. Fully hydrogenated products are virtually completely saturated and do not contain trans fats.

Initially, hydrogenated fats appeared to be superior to both saturated and unsaturated fats, albeit for different reasons. Compared to the saturated fats in butter and lard, hydrogenated fats seemed more heart healthy because they still provide some unsaturated fatty acids. And compared to liquid oils, products made with partially hydrogenated fats have a longer shelf life and better overall quality. Hydrogenated fats make pie crusts flakier, French fries crispier, and frosting creamier. Seemingly a have-your-cake-and-eat-it-too type of product, partially hydrogenated fats permeated the food supply and quickly became a dietary staple in the 1970s.

However, the process of hydrogenation changes the placement of the hydrogen atoms around the remaining double bonds from the natural **cis** position to the rare trans position (Fig. 4.4). Only small amounts of **trans fats** occur naturally in some animal foods, such as beef, lamb, and dairy products.

Partially hydrogenated oils and foods made with partially hydrogenated oils, such as stick margarine, shortening, French fries, potato chips, baked goods, and crackers, provide significant amounts of synthetic trans fat. In fact, most of these products contain more trans fat than saturated fat.

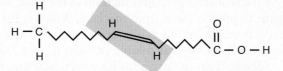

Trans-position: H on opposite sides of double bond

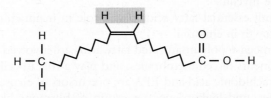

Cis-position: H on same side of double bond

■ FIGURE 4.4   Cis and trans fatty acid configuration.

Trans Fats. Over the last two decades, mounting evidence revealed that trans fats, like saturated fat, raise LDL cholesterol. It is now known that ounce for ounce, trans fats are more unhealthy than saturated fats. However, because we consume so much less trans fat (an average of 2.6% of total calories among American adults) than saturated fat (an average of 11% of total calories), it is inaccurate to assume that cutting trans fat is a higher priority than reducing saturated fat intake.

Since January 1, 2006, trans fatty acid content must be listed on the "Nutrition Facts" label. However, because amounts less than 0.5 g/serving can be rounded down to zero, the label can claim to have "zero trans fats" even if partially hydrogenated oils or shortenings appear on the ingredient list. And while 0.5 g trans fat per serving may sound insignificant, it can add up. For instance, most people will eat 3 cups of microwave popcorn at a time, which is actually three servings according to the label. At 0.5 g trans fat per serving, the total trans fat intake comes to 1.5 g. Only when the label says "no trans fats" is it actually free of trans fat.

Numerous cities around the United States, beginning with New York City, have banned the use of trans fats in restaurants and other food service establishments. The unhealthy image of trans fats has prompted food manufacturers to seek healthier alternatives, and as a result, trans fat–free products are more commonplace on grocery store shelves. Likewise, many fast-food restaurants, hotel chains, cruise ship lines, and even the Disney theme parks have reformulated their recipes to virtually eliminate trans fats. In some items, such as French fries, partially hydrogenated fats (shortening) have been replaced with trans fat–free soybean oil. Ironically, in other products, the choice of fat has come full circle, and saturated fats are being used in place of partially hydrogenated fats.

FUNCTIONS OF FAT IN THE BODY

The primary function of fat is to fuel the body. At rest, fat provides about 60% of the body's calorie needs. All fat, whether saturated or unsaturated, cis or trans, provides 9 cal/g, more than double the amount of calories as an equivalent amount of either carbohydrate or protein. Although fat is an important energy source, it cannot meet all of the body's energy needs because certain cells, such as brain cells and cells of the central nervous system, normally rely solely on glucose for energy.

Fat has other important functions in the body. Fat deposits insulate and cushion internal organs to protect them from mechanical injury. Fat under the skin helps to regulate body temperature by serving as a layer of insulation against the cold. And dietary fat facilitates the absorption of the fat-soluble vitamins A, D, E, and K when consumed at the same meal.

Specific types of fatty acids have particular functions in the body. For instance,

- Saturated fatty acids provide structure to cell membranes and facilitate normal function of proteins.
- Monounsaturated fatty acids are components of lipid membranes, especially nervous tissue myelin.
- Both essential fatty acids play a role in maintaining healthy skin and promoting normal growth in children.
- Omega-6 polyunsaturated fatty acids are involved in the synthesis of fatty acids, are components of cell membranes, and play a role in cell signaling pathways.
- Arachidonic acid and EPA are precursors of eicosanoids (e.g., prostaglandins, thromboxanes, and leukotrienes), a group of hormone-like substances that help regulate blood pressure, blood clotting, and other body functions. Eicosanoids derived from EPA have

more health benefits than those from arachidonic acid; EPA eicosanoids help lower blood pressure, prevent blood clot formation, protect against arrhythmia, and reduce inflammation (Rolfes, Pinna, and Whitney, 2009). Prostaglandins made from arachidonic acid are responsible for the inflammatory response (IFICF, 2011).

- EPA and DHA may play a role in preventing and treating heart disease through their anti-inflammatory, antiarrhythmic, and anticlotting effects (IFICF, 2009). They are essential for normal growth and development. DHA, in particular, is abundant in the structural lipids in the brain and in retinal membranes.

Phospholipids

Phospholipids: a group of compound lipids that is similar to triglycerides in that they contain a glycerol molecule and two fatty acids. In place of the third fatty acid, phospholipids have a phosphate group and a molecule of choline or another nitrogen-containing compound.

Emulsifier: a stabilizing compound that helps to keep both parts of an emulsion (oil and water mixture) from separating.

Like triglycerides, **phospholipids** have a glycerol backbone with fatty acids attached. What makes them different from triglycerides is that a phosphate group replaces one of the fatty acids. Although phospholipids occur naturally in almost all foods, they make up a very small percentage of total fat intake.

Phospholipids are both fat soluble (because of the fatty acids) and water soluble (because of the phosphate group), a unique feature that enables them to act as **emulsifiers**. This role is played out in the body as they emulsify fats to keep them suspended in blood and other body fluids. As a component of all cell membranes, phospholipids not only provide structure but also help to transport fat-soluble substances across cell membranes. Phospholipids are also precursors of prostaglandins.

Lecithin is the best-known phospholipid. Claims that it lowers blood cholesterol; improves memory; controls weight; and cures arthritis, hypertension, and gallbladder problems are unfounded. Studies show no benefit from taking supplements because lecithin is digested in the gastrointestinal tract into its component parts and is not absorbed intact to perform super functions. Lecithin is not even an essential nutrient because it is synthesized in the body. Many people who take lecithin supplements do not realize that they provide 9 cal/g, just like all other fats.

Cholesterol

Sterols: one of three main classes of lipids that include cholesterol, bile acids, sex hormones, the adrenocortical hormones, and vitamin D.

Cholesterol is a **sterol**, a waxy substance whose carbon, hydrogen, and oxygen molecules are arranged in a ring. Cholesterol occurs in the tissues of all animals. It is found in all cell membranes and in myelin. Brain and nerve cells are especially rich in cholesterol. The body synthesizes bile acids, steroid hormones, and vitamin D from cholesterol. Although cholesterol is made from acetyl-coenzyme A (acetyl-CoA), the body cannot break down cholesterol into CoA molecules to yield energy, so cholesterol does not provide calories.

 QUICK BITE

Cholesterol content of selected foods

	Cholesterol (mg)		Cholesterol (mg)
Beef brains, 3 oz	1746	Shrimp, 4	37
Beef liver, 3 oz	375	Whole milk, 1 cup	30
Beef kidney, 3 oz	329	2% milk, 1 cup	15
Egg yolk, 1	213	Butter, 1 tbsp	12
Broiled lobster, 1 cup	110	Nonfat milk, 1 cup	7
Broiled steak, 4 oz	71	Egg whites	0

Cholesterol is found exclusively in animals, with organ meats and egg yolks the richest sources. The cholesterol in food is just cholesterol; descriptions of "good" and "bad" cholesterol refer to the lipoprotein packages that move cholesterol through the blood (see Chapter 20). You cannot eat more "good" cholesterol, but you can make lifestyle changes, such as quitting smoking, exercising, and losing weight if overweight, that increase the amount of "good" cholesterol in the blood.

Because all body cells are capable of making enough cholesterol to meet their needs, cholesterol is not an essential nutrient. In fact, daily endogenous cholesterol synthesis is approximately two to three times more than average cholesterol intake. When dietary cholesterol decreases, endogenous cholesterol production increases to maintain an adequate supply. The body makes cholesterol from acetyl-CoA, which can originate from carbohydrates, protein, fat, or alcohol. Thus, eating an excess of calories, regardless of the source, can increase cholesterol synthesis.

Dietary cholesterol increases total and LDL cholesterol, but the effect is reduced when saturated fat intake is low. Dietary cholesterol may have an independent effect on heart disease risk beyond its effect on serum cholesterol.

HOW THE BODY HANDLES FAT

Digestion

A minimal amount of chemical digestion of fat occurs in the mouth and stomach through the action of lingual lipase and gastric lipases, respectively (Fig. 4.5).

Fat entering the duodenum stimulates the release of the hormone cholecystokinin, which in turn stimulates the gallbladder to release bile. Bile, an emulsifier produced in the liver from bile salts, cholesterol, phospholipids, bilirubin, and electrolytes, prepares fat for digestion by suspending the hydrophobic molecules in the watery intestinal fluid. Emulsified fat particles have enlarged surface areas on which digestive enzymes can work.

Monoglyceride: a glyceride molecule with only one fatty acid attached.

Most fat digestion occurs in the small intestine. Pancreatic lipase, the most important and powerful lipase, splits off one fatty acid at a time from the triglyceride molecule, working from the outside in until two free fatty acids and a **monoglyceride** remain. Usually, the process stops at this point, but sometimes digestion continues and the monoglyceride splits into a free fatty acid and a glyceride molecule. The end products of digestion—mostly monoglycerides with free fatty acids and little glycerol—are absorbed into intestinal cells. It is normal for a small amount of fat (4–5 g) to escape digestion and be excreted in the feces.

The digestion of phospholipids is similar, with the end products being two free fatty acids and a phospholipid fragment. Cholesterol does not undergo digestion; it is absorbed as is.

Absorption

Micelles: fat particles encircled by bile salts to facilitate their diffusion into intestinal cells.

Chylomicrons: lipoproteins that transport absorbed lipids from intestinal cells through the lymph and eventually into the bloodstream.

About 95% of consumed fat is absorbed, mostly in the duodenum and jejunum. Small fat particles, such as short- and medium-chain fatty acids and glycerol, are absorbed directly through the mucosal cells into capillaries. They bind with albumin and are transported to the liver via the portal vein.

The absorption of larger fat particles—namely, monoglycerides and long-chain fatty acids—is more complex. Although they are insoluble in water, monoglycerides and long-chain fatty acids dissolve into **micelles**, which deliver fat to the intestinal cells. Once inside the intestinal cells, the monoglycerides and long-chain fatty acids combine to form triglycerides. The reformed triglycerides, along with phospholipids and cholesterol, become encased in protein to form **chylomicrons**. Chylomicrons distribute dietary lipids throughout the body.

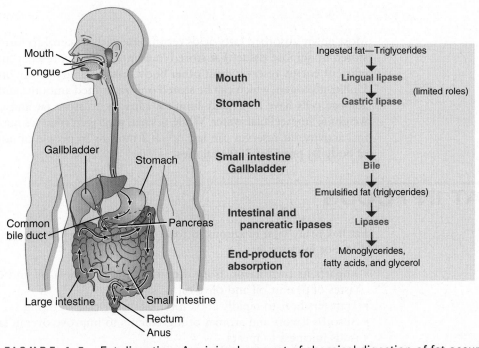

■ FIGURE 4.5 Fat digestion. A minimal amount of chemical digestion of fat occurs in the mouth and stomach through the action of lingual lipase and gastric lipases, respectively. As fat enters the duodenum, it stimulates the release of the hormone cholecystokinin, which in turn stimulates the gallbladder to release bile. Bile prepares fat for digestion by suspending the hydrophobic molecules in the watery intestinal fluid. Most fat digestion occurs in the small intestine. Pancreatic lipase splits off one fatty acid at a time from the triglyceride molecule, working from the outside in until two free fatty acids and a monoglyceride remain. Usually, the process stops at this point, but sometimes digestion continues and the monoglyceride splits into a free fatty acid and glyceride molecule. The end products of digestion—mostly monoglycerides with free fatty acids and little glycerol—are absorbed into intestinal cells. It is normal for a small amount of fat (4–5 g) to escape digestion and be excreted in the feces.

Their job done, most of the released bile salts are reabsorbed in the terminal ileum, transported back to the liver, and recycled (enterohepatic circulation). Some bile salts become bound to fiber in the intestine and are excreted in the feces.

Fat Catabolism

Whether from the most recent meal or from storage, triglycerides that are needed for energy are split into glycerol and fatty acids by lipoprotein lipase and are released into the bloodstream to be picked up by cells.

The catabolism of fatty acids increases when carbohydrate intake is inadequate (e.g., while on a very-low-calorie diet) or unavailable (e.g., in the case of uncontrolled diabetes). Without adequate glucose, the breakdown of fatty acids is incomplete, and ketones are formed. Eventually ketosis and acidosis may result.

Because fatty acids break down into two-carbon molecules, not three-carbon molecules, they cannot be reassembled to make glucose. Only the glycerol component of triglycerides can be used to make glucose, making fat an inefficient choice of fuel for glucose-dependent brain cells, nerve cells, and red blood cells. Fortunately, most body cells can use fatty acids for energy.

Fat Anabolism

Most newly absorbed fatty acids recombine with glycerol to form triglycerides that end up stored in adipose tissue. Fat stored in adipose cells represents the body's largest and most efficient energy reserve; most other body cells are able to store only minute amounts of fat. Unlike glycogen, which can be stored only in limited amounts and is accompanied by water, adipose cells have a virtually limitless capacity to store fat and carry very little additional weight as intracellular water. While normal glycogen reserves may last for half a day of normal activity, fat reserves can last up to 2 months in people of normal weight. Each pound of body fat provides 3500 calories.

FAT IN FOODS

Fat has many vital functions in food and serves to improve the overall palatability of the diet. For instance, it

- Imparts its own flavor, from the mild taste of canola oil and corn oil to the distinctive tastes of peanut oil and olive oil
- Transfers heat to rapidly cook food, as in the case of frying
- Absorbs flavors and aromas of ingredients to improve overall taste
- Adds juiciness to meats
- Creates a creamy and smooth "mouth feel" in items such as ice cream, desserts, and cream soups
- Adds texture or body to many foods, such as flakiness, tenderness, elasticity, and viscosity (e.g., milk is watery and cheese is rubbery when fat is removed)
- Imparts tenderness and moisture in baked goods, such as cookies, pies, and cakes, and delays staling
- Is insoluble in water and thus provides a unique flavor and texture to foods such as salad dressings

The fat content in MyPlate varies greatly among groups and between selections within each group (Fig. 4.6). It is recommended that people choose the lowest fat selections from each group. When higher fat choices are made, the extra calories from the fat are considered "empty calories." For instance, if a person chooses a Belgian waffle (made with added eggs and butter, providing 368 calories per waffle) instead of toast (considered fat free and about 80 calories per slice), the extra 288 calories in the waffle theoretically are empty calories.

Generally, three MyPlate food groups provide little or no fat. Grains naturally contain very little fat, although some items within this group provide significant fat, such as granola cereals, crackers, biscuits, and waffles. Unadulterated vegetables contain little or no fat; vegetables that are fried, creamed, served with cheese, or mixed with mayonnaise provide significant fat. With the exception of avocado, coconut, and olives, fruits are naturally fat free. It is the other three groups—Dairy, Protein Foods, and Oils—that may provide significant fat.

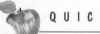 QUICK BITE

Added fats add up

	Fat (g)		Fat (g)
Boiled potato, ½ cup	trace	French fries, 10	8
Mashed potatoes, ½ cup	4.4	Potato salad, ½ cup	10.3
Scalloped potatoes, ½ cup	4.5	Homemade hash browns, ½ cup	10.8

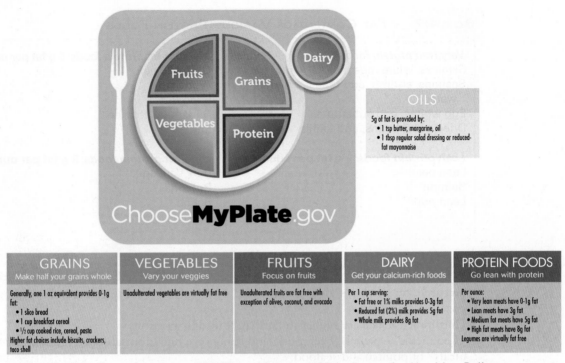

GRAINS Make half your grains whole	VEGETABLES Vary your veggies	FRUITS Focus on fruits	DAIRY Get your calcium-rich foods	PROTEIN FOODS Go lean with protein
Generally, one 1 oz equivalent provides 0-1g fat: • 1 slice bread • 1 cup breakfast cereal • ½ cup cooked rice, cereal, pasta Higher fat choices include biscuits, crackers, taco shell	Unadulterated vegetables are virtually fat free	Unadulterated fruits are fat free with exception of olives, coconut, and avocado	Per 1 cup serving: • Fat free or 1% milks provides 0-3g fat • Reduced fat (2%) milk provides 5g fat • Whole milk provides 8g fat	Per ounce: • Very lean meats have 0-1g fat • Lean meats have 3g fat • Medium fat meats have 5g fat • High fat meats have 8g fat Legumes are virtually fat free

■ **FIGURE 4.6**   Fat content of MyPlate. (**Source:** USDA, Center for Nutrition Policy and Promotion. [2011]. Available at www.choosemyplate.gov)

Dairy

The fat content of milk and yogurt ranges from 0 to 8 g per serving:

- Whole milk provides 8 g fat/cup.
- Reduced-fat milk (2% milk) provides 5 g fat/cup.
- Low-fat milk (1% milk) provides 3 g fat/cup.
- Fat-free milk (nonfat, skim milk) is virtually fat free.

Because the fat in dairy products is predominately saturated and full-fat products have more cholesterol than lower fat options, low-fat and fat-free items are recommended. Reduced- and low-fat milks have some of the fat and cholesterol removed yet retain some of the "mouth feel" characteristic of whole milk. For this reason, reduced-fat milk is suggested as a transition when switching from whole milk to fat-free milk.

Protein Foods

Like the dairy group, the amount of fat in items from the protein foods group varies from virtually fat free to more than 8 g/oz (Box 4.2). Details worth noting are as follows:

- The 1-oz size cited in MyPlate is simply a reference, not a serving size or a portion size. Typically, a *serving size* (the amount recommended for a meal) is 3 or 4 oz, and a *portion size* (the amount actually eaten at one time) may be much larger. For instance, the portion size of meat in a fast-food triple cheeseburger is approximately 9 oz.
- Fat added during cooking, such as frying or basting with fat, increases the overall fat content and counts as choices from the Oils group. It is recommended that meats be

Box 4.2   FAT CONTENT OF VARIOUS PROTEIN FOODS

Very lean protein foods: 0–1 g fat per ounce
Skinless, white meat chicken and turkey
Scallops, shrimp, and tuna canned in
  water
Egg whites, egg substitutes
Dried peas, beans, and lentils

Lean protein foods: 3 g fat per ounce
Lean beef
Salmon
Lean pork

Medium-fat protein foods: 5 g fat per ounce
Ground beef
Prime rib
Fried fish
Dark meat chicken
Egg yolk

High-fat protein foods: 8 g fat per ounce
Pork sausage
Bologna
Bacon
Peanut butter

prepared by methods that do not add fat, such as baked, roasted, broiled, grilled, poached, or boiled.
- Untrimmed meats are higher in fat than lean-only portions.
- "Red meats"—namely, beef, pork, and lamb—are higher in saturated fat than the "white meats" of poultry and seafood.
- White poultry meat is lower in fat than dark meat; removing poultry skin removes significant fat.
- Fat content varies among different cuts of meat. The leanest cuts are beef loin and round, veal and lamb from the loin or leg, and pork tenderloin or center loin chop.
- Beef grades can be used as a guide to fat content because grades are based largely on the amount of **marbling**. Beef graded "prime," sold mostly to restaurants, is the most heavily marbled grade and thus the fattiest. In retail stores, within any cut, "choice" has more marbling and higher fat content than "select."
- Shellfish are very low in fat but have cholesterol.
- Most wild game is very lean. The fat content in bison, venison, elk, ostrich, pheasant (without skin), rabbit, and squirrel ranges from 2 to 5 g per 3-oz serving.
- Processed meats, such as sausage and hot dogs, may provide more fat calories than protein calories.
- Nuts have many healthy attributes; they contain plant protein, fiber, vitamin E, selenium, magnesium, zinc, phosphorus, and potassium in a low–saturated fat, cholesterol-free package. Their high fat content of 13 to 20 g/oz comes mostly from monounsaturated fats and polyunsaturated fats. Walnuts are a rich source of alpha-linolenic acid.
- Egg yolks have approximately 186 mg of cholesterol. The cholesterol content of typical cuts of beef, pork, lamb, and poultry is generally around 70 mg/3 oz. Veal averages slightly more at about 90 mg/3 oz. The exceptions are organ meats, which are very high in cholesterol. Egg whites, legumes, and nuts are cholesterol free.

Marbling: fat deposited in the muscle of meat.

Oils

Oil allowances are small, usually 5 to 7 tsp/day for adults, depending on their total calorie needs. This group includes not only vegetable oils like canola, corn, and olive but also oil-rich foods such as margarine and mayonnaise. Some other items on the oil list, such as avocado and nuts, are also listed in other groups (fruit and protein foods, respectively), but because the overwhelming majority of their calories comes from fat, their fat content is supposed to be counted as part of the oil allowance. For instance, avocado is a fruit, yet 80% of its calories come from fat. Eating half of a medium avocado counts as a serving of fruit *and* as three teaspoons of oil, which is about half of a typical adult's daily oil allowance. Other examples of oil equivalents are as follows:

	Equivalent to this amount of oil
1 tbsp vegetable oil	3 tsp
1 tbsp soft margarine	2½ tsp
2 tbsp Italian dressing	2 tsp
2 tbsp peanut butter	4 tsp
1 oz nuts	3–4 tsp
½ oz sunflower seeds	3 tsp

DIETARY REFERENCE INTAKES

The issue of how much of each particular type of fat is needed, how much is optimal, and how much is too much is complex and in some cases controversial. Fats that the body can synthesize—namely, saturated fatty acids, monounsaturated fatty acids, and cholesterol—do not need to be consumed through food. Trans fats provide no known health benefits, and so they are not essential. As such, neither an Adequate Intake (AI) nor Recommended Dietary Allowance (RDA) exists for any of these fats. The reference values that have been set are discussed later in the text.

Total Fat

Neither an AI nor RDA is set for total fat due to insufficient data to define a level of total fat intake at which risk of deficiency or prevention of chronic disease occurs (National Research Council, 2005). An Acceptable Macronutrient Distribution Range (AMDR) is estimated to be 20% to 35% of total calories for adults (Fig. 4.7). Generally as total fat intake increases, the amount of saturated fat increases; therefore, limiting total fat intake to 35% of total calories or less is prudent in order to limit saturated fat intake.

According to National Health and Nutrition Examination Survey (NHANES) 2007–2008 data, the average intake of total fat for both men and women aged 20 years and older is 34% of total calories (USDA, Agricultural Research Service [ARS], 2010). This translates to a mean intake of 95.3 g/day for men and 67.3 g/day for women.

Saturated and Trans Fat

The National Research Council, Institute of Medicine recommends that the intake of both saturated fat and trans fat be as low as possible within the context of a nutritionally adequate diet (National Research Council, 2005). Because the risk of heart disease increases incrementally as saturated fat and trans fat intake increase, a Tolerable Upper Intake Level (UL) could not be defined.

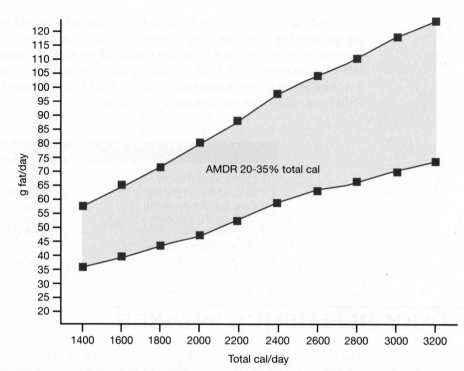

FIGURE 4.7 Amount of total fat appropriate at various calorie levels based on Acceptable Macronutrient Distribution Range of 20% to 35% of total calories.

Essential Fatty Acids

Both an AMDR and AI have been set for the essential fatty acids linoleic acid and alpha-linolenic acid (Table 4.1). The AI values are based on the observed median intake in the United States, where fatty acid deficiencies do not exist in healthy people. AI should not be confused with RDA nor should it be assumed to be an optimal level of intake that confers the lowest risk of disease. Insufficient data exist to set a UL for either of the essential fatty acids.

Cholesterol

Cholesterol intake, like saturated fat and trans fat, is recommended to be as low as possible while consuming a nutritionally adequate diet.

Table 4.1 Dietary Reference Intakes for Essential Fatty Acids

	Acceptable Macronutrient Distribution Range		Adequate Intake	
	Percent of Total Calories from Linoleic Acid (%)	Percent of Total Calories from Alpha-Linolenic Acid (%)	Linolenic Acid (g/day)	Alpha-Linolenic Acid (g/day)
Adult men	5–10	0.6–1.2	17	1.6
Adult women	5–10	0.6–1.2	12	1.1

Fat Deficiency

Although the body cannot make essential fatty acids, it does store them, making deficiencies extremely rare in people eating a mixed diet. Those at risk for deficiency include infants and children consuming low-fat diets (their need for essential fatty acids is proportionately higher than that of adults), clients with anorexia nervosa, and people receiving lipid-free parenteral nutrition for long periods. People with fat malabsorption syndromes are also at risk. Symptoms of essential fatty acid deficiency include growth failure, reproductive failure, scaly dermatitis, and kidney and liver disorders.

FAT IN HEALTH PROMOTION

For decades, fat has virtually been public health enemy number 1, blamed for causing heart disease, cancer, and obesity. For years, eating no more than 30% of total calories from fat was touted by various governmental and health agencies as the way to improve Americans' health. It now appears that the message to eat less fat was too simplistic because it ignored the different health effects produced by different types of fat. Multiple studies have shown that the type of fat in the diet can affect serum lipids more than the total amount of fat (Zarraga and Schwarz, 2006). Other study results about the role of fat in disease are summarized in Box 4.3.

Box 4.3   FAT AND DISEASE: WHAT'S THE CONNECTION?

Total Fat and Heart Disease
Results from the large and long Women's Health Initiative Dietary Modification Trial (WHI DMT) showed that eating a low-fat diet for 8 years did not reduce the risk of coronary heart disease events or stroke (Howard et al., 2006b), but critics argue that it is very difficult to actually achieve a low-fat intake and that study participants may not reduce fat intake enough to see positive results. Also, it may be that risk reduction takes longer to observe than the 8-year-long WHI DMT.

Type of Fat and Heart Disease
Results from the Nurses' Health Study show that replacing only 30 calories (7 g) of carbohydrates every day with 30 calories (4 g) of trans fats nearly doubled the risk for heart disease (Willett et al., 1993). Saturated fat also increased the risk but not as much.

Fat and Cancer
The role of total fat in promoting cancer is controversial. Results from the WHI DMT showed that although a low–total fat diet did not prevent cancer, it did not rule out a potential modest benefit against breast cancer (Prentice et al., 2006). Evidence that certain types of fat promote cancer is suggestive, not conclusive, and the impact of total fat is questionable.

Fat and Weight
Additional results from the WHI DMT show that women assigned to a low-fat diet did not lose, or gain, any more weight than women eating a "usual" diet (Howard et al., 2006a). In theory, cutting fat can cut calories and therefore promote weight loss; in practice, low-fat diets are no more effective in promoting weight loss than are high-fat, low-carbohydrate diets. The key to managing weight is total calories, not the proportion of calories from carbohydrates, protein, or fat.

Box 4.4   DIETARY GUIDELINES FOR AMERICANS, 2010: KEY RECOMMENDATIONS REGARDING FAT INTAKE

- Consume less than 10% of calories from saturated fatty acids by replacing them with monounsaturated and polyunsaturated fatty acids.
- Consume less than 300 mg/day of dietary cholesterol.
- Keep trans fatty acid consumption as low as possible by limiting foods that contain synthetic sources of trans fats, such as partially hydrogenated oils, and by limiting other solid fats.
- Reduce the intake of calories from solid fats.

Although the optimal amount of total fat is controversial, most leading health authorities recommend that Americans limit saturated fat to less than 10% of total calories, cholesterol intake to 200 to 300 mg/day, and trans fat intake to be as low as possible. According to data from NHANES 2007–2008, saturated fat represents 11% of total calories in an average American adult's diet. Among adults 20 years and older, mean intake of cholesterol is 362 mg/day for men and 230 mg/day for women (USDA, ARS, 2010).

The *Dietary Guidelines for Americans, 2010* (USDA, USDHHS, 2010) key recommendations regarding fat intake appear in Box 4.4. Highlights are discussed in the following sections.

What to Limit: Saturated Fat, Trans Fat, Cholesterol, and Solid Fats

The most effective way to limit saturated fat, trans fats, cholesterol, and solids fats is to eat less animal (solid) fats and processed foods containing hydrogenated and partially hydrogenated oils. A healthy fat profile is achieved with a diet rich in a wide variety of fruits and vegetables, whole grains, fat-free and low-fat dairy products, legumes, nuts, poultry, lean meats, and fish (at least twice a week). In place of solid fats, such as butter and margarine, vegetable oils such as canola, olive, soybean, and corn are recommended. Strategies for lowering solid fat and increasing oils appear in Box 4.5.

Increase the Amount and Variety of Seafood

According to the *Dietary Guidelines for Americans, 2010*, mean seafood intake in the United States is approximately 3.5 oz/week, slightly less than half the amount recommended (USDA, USDHHS, 2010). Moderate evidence shows that 8 oz of seafood per week (less for young children) from a variety of seafood sources, which provides an average daily intake of 250 mg/day of EPA and DHA, is associated with reduced cardiac deaths in people with or without cardiovascular disease (USDA, USDHHS, 2010). Current American intake of EPA and DHA is approximately 150 mg/day (IFICF, 2011). Many experts think the daily intake should be approximately 500 mg/day.

Consistent with the *Dietary Guidelines for Americans, 2010*, the American Heart Association recommends that people without coronary heart disease eat a variety of fish, preferably oily fish such as salmon, tuna, mackerel, herring, and trout, at least twice a week (Gidding et al., 2009). For people with documented heart disease, the recommendation is to consume about 1 g/day of fish oils, preferably from oily fish, although

Box 4.5   STRATEGIES FOR REDUCING SOLID FATS AND INCREASING OILS

Reduce Solid Fats

Eat Less Meat

- Eat occasional meatless meals such as bean burritos, meatless chili, vegetable soup with salad, and spaghetti with plain sauce.
- Limit meat to 5 oz/day; a recommended portion is the size of a deck of cards or smaller.

Eat Lean Meats

- Eat meat, fish, and poultry that is baked, broiled, grilled, or roasted instead or fried. Drain fat.
- Remove the skin from chicken before eating.
- Choose "select" grades of beef, which have less marbling than "choice" grades.
- Trim all visible fat from meat.
- Choose ground beef that is at least 90% lean as indicated on the label.
- Choose beef cuts labeled "loin" or "round."
- Limit egg yolks to two to three per week.
- Limit processed meats.

Choose Foods Prepared with Little or No Solid Fats

- Use 1% or nonfat milk.
- Use low-fat or nonfat yogurt.
- Choose cheese with 3 g or less per serving.
- Try sherbet, reduced-fat ice cream, nonfat ice cream, and yogurt.
- Use nonstick spray in place of oil, margarine, or butter to sauté foods and "butter" pans.
- Use imitation butter spray to season vegetables and hot air popcorn.
- When you eat foods with solid fats, limit portion sizes. Foods high in solid fat include cakes, cookies, desserts, pizza, cheese, fatty meats, and ice cream.

Reduce Hydrogenated Fat Intake

- Use soft margarine (liquid or tub) in place of butter or stick margarine. Look for margarine that is "trans fat free," contains no more than 2 g saturated fat per table-spoon, and has liquid vegetable oil as the first ingredient.
- Look for processed foods made with unhydrogenated oil rather than partially hydrogenated or saturated fat.
- Avoid French fries, doughnuts, cookies, and crackers unless they are labeled fat free.
- Avoid fried fast foods that are made with hydrogenated shortenings and oils.

Replace Fatty Foods with Fruit and Vegetables

- Eat fruit for dessert.
- Snack on raw vegetables or fresh fruit instead of snack chips.
- Double up on your usual portion of vegetables.

(continues on page 84)

Box 4.5	STRATEGIES FOR REDUCING SOLID FATS AND INCREASING OILS (continued)

Increase Oils

- Use oils instead of butter or shortening for cooking and baking.
- Eat fatty fish twice a week.
- Eat nuts and nut butters that are rich in monounsaturated fats: walnuts, almonds, hazelnuts, pecans, pistachios, and pine nuts. Walnuts also contain alpha-linolenic acid. Cashews and macadamia nuts are higher in saturated fats.
- Sprinkle flaxseed (1–2 tbsp/day) over cereal or yogurt or use as a fat substitute in many recipes: 3 tbsp of ground flaxseed can replace 1 tbsp of fat or oil.
- Read the Nutrition Facts label to identify oils with the highest unsaturated fat content.

Methyl Mercury: mercury is a heavy metal that occurs naturally in the environment and is released into the air through industrial pollution. It changes to methyl mercury when it falls from the air into the water. Almost all fish contain minute amounts of methyl mercury that are not harmful to humans. Pregnant and lactating women and children younger than age 8 years are vulnerable to the toxic effects of mercury because it can damage the developing brain and spinal cord.

supplements may be considered in consult with a physician. Likewise, the American Diabetes Association recommends two or more servings of fish per week, with the exception of commercially fried fish filets (Bantle et al., 2008). The health risks associated with eating fish contaminated with **methyl mercury** are outweighed by the benefits of consuming 8 oz of fish per week, even for women who are or may become pregnant, lactating women, and young children (USDA, USDHHS, 2010). However, these groups are advised to avoid shark, swordfish, king mackerel, and tilefish to minimize exposure to methyl mercury. Likewise, state and local advisories should be adhered to for locally caught fish. Table 4.2 lists the amount of *n*-3 fatty acids and mercury in various types of seafood.

Despite widespread recommendations to eat more fatty fish, the role of *n*-3 in preventing chronic disease is far from certain. Interest in *n*-3 fatty acids began back in the early 1970s when researchers observed that populations with a high intake of fish, such as Eskimos and Japanese, have lower rates of cardiovascular disease than populations who eat less. Omega-3 fatty acids, in particular EPA and DHA, were credited with protecting against cardiovascular disease, fatal heart attacks, and arrhythmia through their anti-inflammatory and anticoagulant effects (IFICF, 2011). However, promising observations are not the same as clinical trials. A recent meta-analysis of 20 randomized clinical trials found that *n*-3 supplementation was not associated with a lower risk of all-cause mortality, cardiac death, sudden death, myocardial infarction, or stroke (Rizos, Ntzani, Bika, Kostapanos, and Elisaf, 2012). A study by Quinn et al. (2010) found that compared with a placebo, supplementation with DHA did not slow the rate of cognitive and functional decline in patients with mild to moderate Alzheimer disease.

A large randomized clinical trial, the VITAL (*VIT*amin D and Omeg*A*-3 Tria*L*) Study, is currently under way to determine whether taking daily dietary supplements of vitamin D or *n*-3 fatty acids reduces the risk for developing cancer, heart disease, and stroke in people who do not have a prior history of these illnesses (Liebman, 2009). Ancillary studies will also be conducted to determine whether either of these supplements provides other benefits, such as lowering the risk for diabetes, hypertension, memory loss or cognitive decline, autoimmune diseases, infections, asthma, depression, macular degeneration, and others. The controversy over the role of *n*-3 fatty acids in maintaining health is likely to continue.

Table 4.2 Estimated EPA and DHA and Mercury Content in 4 oz of Selected Seafood Varieties

Common Seafood Varieties	EPA+DHA[a] (mg/4 oz)[b]	Mercury[c] (μg/4 oz)[d]
Salmon[e]: Atlantic[f], Chinook[f], Coho[f]	1200–2400	2
Anchovies[e,f], Herring[e,f], and Shad[e]	2300–2400	5–10
Mackerel: Atlantic and Pacific (not King)	1350–2100	8–13
Tuna: Bluefin[e,f] and Albacore[e]	1700	54–58
Sardines[e]: Atlantic[f] and Pacific[f]	1100–1600	2
Trout: Freshwater	1000–1100	11
Tuna: White (Albacore) canned	1000	40
Salmon[e]: Pink[f] and Sockeye[f]	700–900	2
Pollock[e]: Atlantic[f] and Walleye[f]	600	6
Crab[g]: Blue[e], King[e,f], Snow[e], Queen[f], and Dungeness[f]	200–550	9
Tuna: Skipjack and Yellowfin	150–350	31–49
Flounder[e,f], Plaice[e], and Sole[e,f] (Flatfish)	350	7
Tuna: Light canned	150–300	13
Catfish	100–250	7
Cod[e]: Atlantic[f] and Pacific[f]	200	14
Scallops[e,g]: Bay[f] and Sea[f]	200	8
Lobster[g,h]: Northern[e,f] American[e]	200	47
Tilapia	150	2
Shrimp[g]	100	0
Seafood varieties that should not be consumed by women who are pregnant or breastfeeding[i]		
Shark	1250	151
Tilefish[f]: Gulf of Mexico[e,j]	1000	219
Swordfish	1000	147
Mackerel: King	450	110

[a]A total of 1750 mg of eicosapentaenoic acid (EPA) and docosahexaenoic acid (DHA) per week represents an average of 250 mg/day, which is the goal amount to achieve at the recommended 8 oz of seafood per week for the general public.

[b]EPA and DHA values are for the cooked, edible portion rounded to the nearest 50 mg. Ranges are provided when values are comparable. Values are estimates.

[c]A total of 39 μg of mercury per week would reach the EPA reference dose limit (0.1 μg/kg/day) for a woman who is pregnant or breastfeeding and who weighs 124 pounds (56 kg).

[d]Mercury was measured as total mercury and/or methyl mercury. Mercury values of zero were below the level of detection. Values for mercury adjusted to reflect 4-oz weight after cooking, assuming 25% moisture loss. Canned varieties not adjusted; mercury values gathered from cooked forms. Values are rounded to the nearest whole number. Ranges are provided when values are comparable. Values are estimates.

[e]Seafood variety is included in mercury value(s) reported.

[f]Seafood variety is included in EPA+DHA value(s) reported.

[g]Cooked by moist heat.

[h]Spiny lobster has approximately 550 mg of EPA+DHA and 14 μg mercury per 4 oz.

[i]Women who are pregnant or breastfeeding should also limit white (albacore) tuna to 6 oz/week.

[j]Values are for tilefish from the Gulf of Mexico; does not include Atlantic tilefish, which have approximately 22 μg of mercury per 4 oz.

Sources: U.S. Department of Agriculture, U.S. Department of Health and Human Services. (2010). *Dietary guidelines for Americans, 2010* (7th ed.). Available at www.health.gov/dietaryguidelines. Accessed on 2/24/11; U.S. Department of Agriculture, Agricultural Research Service, Nutrient Data Laboratory. (2010). *USDA National Nutrient Database for Standard Reference, Release 23.* Available at http://www.ars.usda.gov/ba/bhnrc/ndl; U.S. Food and Drug Administration. (2011). *Mercury levels in commercial fish and shellfish.* Available at http://www.fda.gov/Food/FoodSafety/Product-SpecificInformation/Seafood/FoodbornePathogensContaminants/Methylmercury/ucm115644.htm; National Marine Fisheries Service. (1978). *National Marine Fisheries Service survey of trace elements in the fishery resource.* Silver Spring, MD: National Marine Fisheries Service; and Environmental Protection Agency. (2000). *The Occurrence of mercury in the fishery resources of the Gulf of Mexico.* Washington, DC: Environmental Protection Agency.

HOW DO YOU RESPOND?

Is coconut oil healthier than butter? Emerging research shows that not all saturated fatty acids have the same impact on cholesterol levels in the blood. Palmitic acid, the main fatty acid in butter, appears more atherogenic than other fatty acids. Lauric acid, the main fatty acid in coconut oil, has the negative effect of raising LDL cholesterol, but it also raises high-density lipoprotein levels, the "good" cholesterol. Until research proves otherwise, canola oil and olive oil, which provide 1 and 2 g saturated fat per tablespoon, respectively, are better choices than either butter (7 g saturated fat per tablespoon) or coconut oil (12 g saturated fat per tablespoon).

What is flaxseed? Flaxseed is derived from the flax plant, the same plant used to make linen. It is a nutritional powerhouse, providing essential fatty acids, fiber, and lignans. Specifically, 57% of its fat is from alpha-linolenic acid, the essential *n*-3 fatty acid. The fiber in flaxseed is predominately soluble, which helps to lower cholesterol levels and improves glucose levels in people with diabetes. Flaxseed contains 100 to 800 times more lignans than other grains; lignans, a group of plant estrogens, may help to reduce the risk of breast and prostate cancers. While flaxseed oil and flaxseed oil pills provide the benefits of alpha-linolenic acid, they lack the fiber found in the whole grain, and the lignan content is variable. However, humans are unable to digest the tough outer coating, so flaxseeds must be eaten ground, not whole. Because they are high in polyunsaturated fat, they are prone to rancidity. Ground flaxseed should be refrigerated and used within a few weeks.

Is it a good idea to substitute foods made with fat replacers for full-fat foods? Although some foods can be made low fat by simply reducing the fat content (e.g., milk), others use fat replacers to simulate the functional properties of fat while reducing total fat, saturated fat, and calories. They are derived from carbohydrates, protein, or fat, and thus their calorie content varies. Considering all the functional properties of fat in food, it is easy to understand that not all fat replacers are appropriate for all types of food. For instance, prune puree can substitute as fat in brownies by imparting moistness and some tenderness, but it cannot be used as a substitute for oil in frying French fries.

Whether fat replacers actually help Americans to eat less fat and fewer calories depends on whether they are used in addition to foods normally eaten or take the place of regular fat foods that would otherwise be eaten. Furthermore, diets low in fat are not guaranteed to be low in calories. For instance, even if the fat content of coffee cake is reduced, there are still considerable calories provided by starch and sugar. People who choose to use fat replacers should do so with the understanding that they are only one component of a total diet and as such, they alone cannot transform an "unhealthy" diet into a healthy one.

CASE STUDY

Michael is a 40-year-old man who lost about 25 pounds 10 years ago by reducing his fat intake. He has slowly regained the weight and now wants to go back to a low-fat diet to manage his weight. He gives you a sample of his usual intake:

Breakfast:	3 cups of coffee with sugar and nondairy creamer
On the way to work:	A bagel with low-fat cream cheese and jelly
Snack before lunch:	Low-fat coffee cake; more coffee with sugar and nondairy creamer
Lunch:	Usually a burger, large order of French fries, and a diet soda from the fast-food restaurant near his office
Snack before dinner:	A glass of wine with cheese and crackers
Dinner:	Meat, potato, and vegetable; often double portions of meat A salad with Italian dressing Bread and butter Sherbet for dessert
Snack:	A bowl of cornflakes with 2% milk and sugar

- What foods and beverages did Michael eat that contain fat? What sources of saturated fat did he eat? What sources of unsaturated fat? What sources of *n*-3 fats? What sources of cholesterol? What specific suggestions would you make for him to eat less fat and/or improve the type of fat he eats?
- What would you tell Michael about cutting fat intake to lose weight? What would you suggest he do to "eat healthier"?

STUDY QUESTIONS

1. The client asks if the cholesterol in shrimp is the "good" or "bad" type. Which of the following would be the nurse's best response?
   a. "All cholesterol is bad cholesterol."
   b. "Bad and good refer to how cholesterol is packaged for transport through the blood. The cholesterol in food is unpackaged and neither bad nor good."
   c. "Good cholesterol is found in plants; bad cholesterol is found in animal sources."
   d. "Shrimp has good cholesterol because it is low in saturated fat; foods high in cholesterol and saturated fat are a bad source of cholesterol."

2. When developing a teaching plan for a client who needs to limit saturated fat, which of the following foods would the nurse suggest the client limit?
   a. Seafood and poultry
   b. Nuts and seeds
   c. Olive oil and canola oil
   d. Red meat and full-fat dairy products

3. What is the primary function of fat?
   a. To facilitate protein metabolism
   b. To provide energy
   c. To promote the absorption of fat-soluble vitamins
   d. To facilitate carbohydrate metabolism

4. The nurse knows that instructions have been effective when the client verbalizes that the sources of synthetic trans fats are
   a. Red meat and full-fat dairy products
   b. Commercial baked goods and stick margarine
   c. Pretzels and nuts
   d. Butter and lard

5. A client asks why lowering saturated fat intake is necessary for lowering serum cholesterol levels. Which of the following is the nurse's best response?
   a. "Saturated fats raise the 'bad' cholesterol levels more than any other fat in the diet."
   b. "Sources of saturated fat also provide monounsaturated fat, and both should be limited to control blood cholesterol levels."
   c. "Saturated fat is high in calories, and excess calories from any source increase the risk of high blood cholesterol levels."
   d. "Saturated fats make blood more likely to clot, increasing the risk of heart attack."

6. What should the nurse tell a client who likes fish but refuses to eat it because of fear of mercury poisoning?
   a. "You are justified to be concerned. To be safe, use fish oil supplements instead."
   b. "You can eat as much fish as you want because most fish are not contaminated with even small amounts of mercury."
   c. "The benefits of eating 8 oz/week of a variety of fish outweigh any potential risks from mercury."
   d. "As a compromise, eat 4 oz of fish per week instead of 8 oz."

7. Which statement indicates the client understands about choosing low-fat foods from MyPlate?
   a. "All items within a food group have approximately the same amount of fat."
   b. "You don't have to consciously select low-fat items because the empty calorie allowance will account for higher fat choices."
   c. "It is best to eliminate as much fat from the diet as possible."
   d. "Within each food group, the foods lowest in fat should be chosen most often."

8. Which of the following are the best sources of omega-3 fatty acids?
   a. Salmon and trout
   b. Flaxseed and walnuts
   c. Olive and canola oils
   d. Cod fish and haddock

KEY CONCEPTS

- Ninety-eight percent of lipids consumed in the diet are triglycerides, which are composed of one glyceride molecule and three fatty acids. Phospholipids and sterols are the other two types of dietary lipids.
- Saturation refers to each carbon atom in the fatty acid chain having four single bonds with hydrogen atoms. In saturated fats, each carbon is "saturated" with as much hydrogen as it can hold. Unsaturated fats have one (monounsaturated) or more than one (polyunsaturated) double bond between carbon atoms.

- All fats in foods contain a mixture of saturated, monounsaturated, and polyunsaturated fats. When used to describe food fats, these terms are relative descriptions of the type of fatty acid present in the largest amount.
- Generally, saturated fats are "bad" because they raise total and LDL cholesterol. Unsaturated fats are "good" because they lower total and LDL cholesterol when consumed in place of saturated fats.
- Trans fatty acids are produced through the process of hydrogenation. They are chemically unsaturated fats; however, like saturated fat, they raise total and LDL cholesterol.
- Linoleic acid (*n*-6) and alpha-linolenic acid (*n*-3) are essential fatty acids because they cannot be made by the body. They are important constituents of cell membranes, are involved in eicosanoid synthesis, and function to maintain healthy skin and promote normal growth.
- The major function of fat is to provide energy; 1 g of fat supplies 9 calories of energy. Fat also provides insulation, protects internal organs from mechanical damage, and promotes absorption of the fat-soluble vitamins.
- Fish oils lower the risk of heart disease by lowering serum lipids and triglycerides and by helping to regulate blood pressure. Although they may also be beneficial in preventing other health problems, the evidence is currently inconclusive or lacking.
- The best sources of *n*-3 fatty acids are fatty cold-water fish such as salmon, trout, herring, swordfish, sardines, and mackerel. Walnuts, soybeans, flaxseed, and canola oil are plant sources of the *n*-3 fatty acid alpha-linolenic acid, but alpha-linolenic acid may not have the same cardioprotective benefits as fish oils.
- Phospholipids are structural components of cell membranes that facilitate the transport of fat-soluble substances across cell membranes. They are widespread but appear in small amounts in the diet.
- Cholesterol, a sterol, is a constituent of all cell membranes and is used to make bile acids, steroid hormones, and vitamin D. Cholesterol is found in all foods of animal origin except egg whites. Most Americans eat about half as much cholesterol as the body makes each day.
- Fat digestion occurs mostly in the small intestine. Short- and medium-chain fatty acids and glycerol are absorbed through mucosal cells into capillaries leading to the portal vein. Larger fat molecules—namely, cholesterol, phospholipids, and reformed triglycerides made from monoglycerides and long-chain fatty acids—are absorbed in chylomicrons and transported through the lymph system.
- Grains, fruits, and vegetables are generally fat free or low in fat, although certain preparation methods can add fat. Dairy, protein foods, and the oil food groups provide fat, with the type and quantity of fat varying considerably among items within each group.
- The AMDR for total fat is set at 20% to 35% of total calories. The intake of saturated fat, trans fat, and cholesterol should be as low as possible within the context of a nutritionally adequate diet. Most leading health authorities recommend that Americans limit trans fat intake as much as possible, saturated fat to less than 10% of total calories, and cholesterol intake to 200 to 300 mg/day.
- Deficiencies of essential fatty acids are nonexistent in healthy people.
- To achieve a more optimal fat intake, a plant-based diet rich in fruit, vegetables, whole grains, legumes, and nuts is recommended with adequate amounts of fat-free dairy products and lean meats. Fats, such as in margarine and salad dressings, should be trans fat free, and these products should preferably be made with canola or olive oil. A total of 8 oz or more of seafood per week is suggested.

Check Your Knowledge Answer Key

1. **TRUE** All fats, whether saturated or unsaturated, provide 9 cal/g compared to 4 cal/g from carbohydrates and protein.

2. **FALSE** "Good" fats—namely, polyunsaturated and monounsaturated fats—may help to lower LDL cholesterol when used in place of saturated fat. Omega-3 fish oils are also "good": they lower triglyceride levels; decrease platelet aggregation; and may decrease inflammation in rheumatoid arthritis, Crohn disease, and ulcerative colitis.

3. **TRUE** Endogenous cholesterol synthesis is generally two to three times higher than the average cholesterol intake in the United States.

4. **FALSE** The 30% guideline refers to the total diet, not individual foods. Over the course of the day, high-fat items (e.g., canola oil, peanut butter) are balanced by low-fat and fat-free items (nonfat milk, grains, vegetables, and fruit).

5. **FALSE** Even though some margarines contain more trans fats than butter, the combined amount of "bad" fat (saturated fat plus trans fat) is higher in butter than in margarine, even stick margarine. In addition, butter contains cholesterol; margarine generally does not.

6. **TRUE** All food fats are a blend of saturated, polyunsaturated, and monounsaturated fatty acids. The description of a fat as "saturated" means that there are more saturated fatty acids than polyunsaturated or monounsaturated fatty acids in that source, not that saturated fatty acids are the only fatty acids present.

7. **FALSE** Saturated fatty acids are found in varying proportions in all sources of fat. A fat labeled as "saturated" has saturated fatty acids providing the biggest percentage of fat in that item. Animal products (meat and full-fat dairy items) and coconut, palm kernel, and palm oils are considered saturated fats.

8. **FALSE** Vegetable oils are still vegetable oils, even when they are lightly or partially hydrogenated; therefore, the term "vegetable oil" is not synonymous with trans fat free.

9. **FALSE** Fish oils are not essential in the diet because the body can convert alpha-linolenic acid to EPA and DHA, although only in limited quantities. Vegetarians do not appear to suffer adverse effects from eliminating fish from their diets.

10. **FALSE** Eating less saturated fat has a greater impact on lowering serum cholesterol than does simply limiting cholesterol intake.

***Student Resources on* the**Point**

For additional learning materials, activate the code in the front of this book at
http://thePoint.lww.com/activate

Websites

American Heart Association at **www.heart.org**
American Oil Chemist's Society at **www.aocs.org**
Calorie Control Council's glossary of fat replacers at **www.caloriecontrol.org/articles-and-**
   video/feature-articles/glossary-of-fat-replacers
Institute of Shortening and Edible Oils at **www.iseo.org**
International Food Information Council at **www.foodinsight.org/**
National Heart, Lung, and Blood Institute at **www.nhlbi.nih.gov**

References   Bantle, J., Wylie-Rosett, J., Albright, A. L., Apovian, C. M., Clark, N. G., Franz, M. J., . . .
Wheeler, M. L. (2008). Nutrition recommendations and the interventions for diabetes: A position statement of the American Diabetes Association. *Diabetes Care, 1*(Suppl. 1), S61–S78.

Gidding, S., Lichtenstein, A., Faith, M., Karpyn, A., Mennella, J. A., Popkin, B., . . . Whitsel, L.
(2009). Implementing American Heart Association pediatric and adult nutrition guidelines.
Circulation, 119, 1161–1175.

Howard, B. V., Manson, J. E., Stefanick, M. L., Beresford, S. A., Frank, G., Jones. B., . . .
Prentice, R. (2006a). Low-fat dietary pattern and weight change over 7 years: The Women's
Health Initiative Dietary Modification Trial. *Journal of the American Medical Association, 295,*
39–49.

Howard, B. V., Van Horn, L., Hsia, J., Manson, J. E., Stefanick, M. L., Wassertheil-Smoller,
S., . . . Kotchen, J. M. (2006b). Low-fat dietary pattern and risk of cardiovascular disease: The
Women's Health Initiative Randomized Controlled Dietary Modification Trial. *Journal of the
American Medical Association, 295,* 655–666.

International Food Information Council Foundation. (2009). *Functional foods fact sheet: Omega-3
fatty acids.* Available at www.foodinsight.org/Resources/Detail.aspx?topic+Functional_Foods_
Fact_Sheet_Omega_3_Fatty_Acid. Accessed on 9/6/12.

International Food Information Council Foundation. (2011). *Food insight interviews: Dr. Bill
Harris on omega-3 and omega-6 fatty acids.* Available at http://www.foodinsight.org/
Newsletter/Detail.aspx?topic=Food_Insight_Interviews_Dr_Bill_Harris. Accessed on 9/11/12.

Liebman, B. (2009). From sun and sea. New study puts vitamin D and omega-3s to the test.
Nutrition Action Health Letter, 1, 3–7.

National Research Council. (2005). *Dietary reference intakes for energy, carbohydrate, fiber, fat,
fatty acids, cholesterol, protein, and amino acids (macronutrients).* Washington, DC: The
National Academies Press.

Prentice, R. L., Caan, B., Chlebowski, R. T., Patterson, R., Kuller, L. H., Ockene, J. K., . . .
Henderson, M. M. (2006). Low-fat dietary pattern and risk of invasive breast cancer: The
Women's Health Initiative Randomized Controlled Dietary Modification Trial. *Journal of the
American Medical Association, 295,* 629–642.

Quinn, J., Raman, R., Thomas, R., Yurko-Mauro, K., Nelson, E. B., Van Dyck, C., . . . Aisen, P. S.
(2010). Cognitive decline in Alzheimer disease: A randomized trial. *Journal of the American
Medical Association, 304,* 1903–1911.

Rizos, E., Ntzani, E., Bika, E., Kostapanos, M. S., & Elisaf, M. S. (2012). Association between
omega-3 fatty acid supplementation and risk of major cardiovascular disease events. A systematic
review and meta-analysis. *Journal of the American Medical Association, 308,* 1024–1033.

Rolfes, S., Pinna, K., & Whitney, E. (2009). *Understanding normal and clinical nutrition*
(8th ed.). Belmont, CA: Wadsworth.

U.S. Department of Agriculture, Agricultural Research Service. (2010). *Nutrient intakes from food:
Mean amounts consumed per individual, by gender and age. What We Eat in American,
NHANES 2007–2008.* Available at www.ars.usda.gov/ba/bhnrc/fsrg. Accessed on 6/9/12.

U.S. Department of Agriculture, U.S. Department of Health and Human Services. (2010). *Dietary
guidelines for Americans, 2010* (7th ed.). Available at www.health.gov/dietaryguidelines.
Accessed on 2/24/11.

Willett, W. C., Stampfer, M. J., Manson, J. E., Colditz, G. A., Speizer, F. E., Rosner, B. A., . . .
Hennekens, C. H. (1993). Intake of trans fatty acids and risk of coronary heart disease among
women. *Lancet, 341,* 581–585.

Zarraga, I., & Schwarz, E. (2006). Impact of dietary patterns and interventions on cardiovascular
health. *Circulation, 114,* 961–973.

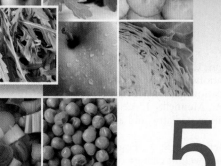

5 Vitamins

LEARNING OBJECTIVES

Upon completion of this chapter, you will be able to

1 Compare and contrast fat- and water-soluble vitamins.
2 Describe general functions and uses of vitamins.
3 Judge when vitamin supplements may be necessary.
4 Evaluate a vitamin supplement label.
5 Give examples of food sources for individual vitamins.
6 Identify characteristics to look for when choosing a vitamin supplement.

In 1913, thiamin was discovered as the first vitamin, the "vital amine" necessary to prevent the deficiency disease beriberi. Today, 13 vitamins have been identified as important for human nutrition; vitamin deficiency diseases are rare in the United States, and vitamin research focuses on whether consuming various vitamins above the minimum basic requirement can reduce the risk of heart disease, cancer, cataracts, cognitive decline in the elderly, and other chronic diseases.

This chapter describes vitamins and their uses. Generalizations about fat- and water-soluble vitamins are presented. Unique features of each vitamin are covered individually, and criteria for selecting a vitamin supplement are discussed.

UNDERSTANDING VITAMINS

Vitamins are organic compounds made of carbon, hydrogen, oxygen, and sometimes, nitrogen or other elements. They differ in their chemistry, biochemistry, function, and availability in foods. Vitamins facilitate biochemical reactions within cells to help regulate body processes such as growth and metabolism. They are essential to life. Unlike the organic compounds covered previously in this unit (carbohydrates, protein, and fat), vitamins

Micronutrients: nutrients that are needed in very small amounts.

- Are individual molecules, not long chains of molecules linked together
- Do not provide energy but are needed for the metabolism of energy
- Are needed in microgram or milligram quantities, not gram quantities, and so are called **micronutrients** (Fig. 5.1)

Vitamins Are Chemically Defined

Vitamins are extremely complex chemical substances that differ widely in their structures. Because vitamins are defined chemically, the body cannot distinguish between natural vitamins extracted from food and synthetic vitamins produced in a laboratory. However, the absorption rates of natural and synthetic vitamins sometimes differ because of different chemical forms of the same vitamin (e.g., synthetic folic acid is better absorbed than natural folate in foods) or because the synthetic vitamins are "free," not "bound" to other components in food (e.g., synthetic vitamin B_{12} is not bound to small peptides as natural vitamin B_{12} is).

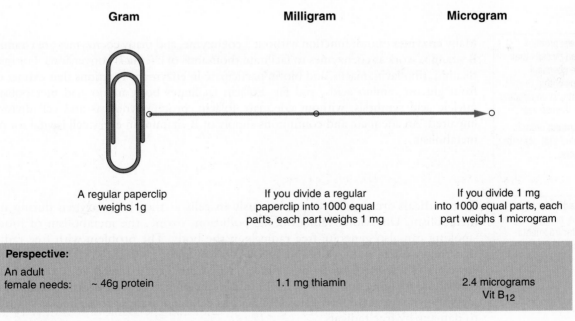

Gram	Milligram	Microgram
A regular paperclip weighs 1g	If you divide a regular paperclip into 1000 equal parts, each part weighs 1 mg	If you divide 1 mg into 1000 equal parts, each part weighs 1 microgram

Perspective: An adult female needs:	~ 46g protein	1.1 mg thiamin	2.4 micrograms Vit B_{12}

■ **FIGURE 5.1**   Representative sizes of 1 g, 1 mg, and 1 μg.

Vitamins Are Susceptible to Destruction

Oxidation: a chemical reaction in which a substance combines with oxygen; the loss of electrons in an atom.

As organic substances, vitamins in food are susceptible to destruction and subsequent loss of function. Individual vitamins differ in their vulnerability to heat, light, **oxidation**, acid, and alkalis. For instance,

- Thiamin is heat sensitive and is easily destroyed by high temperatures and long cooking times.
- Riboflavin is resistant to heat, acid, and oxidation but is quickly destroyed by light. That is why riboflavin-rich milk is sold in opaque, not transparent, containers.
- From 50% to 90% of folate in foods may be lost during preparation, processing, and storage.
- Vitamin C is destroyed by heat, air, and alkalis.

Thiamin = θ heat
Riboflavin = θ light
Vit. C = θ heat, θ air, θ alkalis

Vitamins May Exist in More than One Form

Provitamins: precursors of vitamins.

Many vitamins exist in more than one active form. Different forms perform different functions in the body. For instance, vitamin A exists as retinol (important for reproduction), retinal (needed for vision), and retinoic acid (acts as a hormone to regulate growth). Some vitamins have **provitamins**, an inactive form found in food that the body converts to the active form. Beta-carotene is a provitamin of vitamin A. Dietary Reference Intakes take into account the biologic activity of vitamins as they exist in different forms.

Vitamins Are Essential

Vitamins are essential in the diet because, with a few exceptions, the body cannot make them. The body can make vitamin A, vitamin D, and niacin if the appropriate precursors are available. Microorganisms in the gastrointestinal (GI) tract synthesize vitamin K and vitamin B_{12} but not in amounts sufficient to meet the body's needs.

Some Vitamins Are Coenzymes

Enzymes: proteins produced by cells that catalyze chemical reactions within the body without undergoing change themselves.

Coenzymes: organic molecules that activate an enzyme.

Many **enzymes** cannot function without a **coenzyme**, and many coenzymes are vitamins. All B vitamins work as coenzymes to facilitate thousands of chemical conversions. For instance, thiamin, riboflavin, niacin, and biotin participate in enzymatic reactions that extract energy from glucose, amino acids, and fat. Folacin facilitates both amino acid metabolism and nucleic acid synthesis; without adequate folacin, protein synthesis and cell division are impaired. An adequate and continuous supply of B vitamins in every cell is vital for normal metabolism.

Some Vitamins Are Antioxidants

Free Radicals: highly unstable, highly reactive molecular fragments with one or more unpaired electrons.

Free radicals are produced continuously in cells as they burn oxygen during normal metabolism. Ultraviolet radiation, air pollution, ozone, the metabolism of food, and smoking can also generate free radicals in the body. The problem with free radicals is that they oxidize body cells and DNA in their quest to become stable by gaining an electron. These structurally and functionally damaged oxidized cells are believed to contribute to aging and various health problems such as cancer, heart disease, and cataracts. Polyunsaturated fatty acids (PUFAs) in cell membranes are particularly vulnerable to damage by free radicals.

(handwritten left margin)
Antioxidant Vitamins:
1. Vit C
2. Vit E
3. Beta-carotene

Box 5.1   RICH SOURCES OF ANTIOXIDANTS

Beverages: coffee, green and black tea, red wine
Fruits: bilberries, black currants, wild strawberries, blackberries, goji berries, cranberries, dried apples, dried plums, dried apricots, prunes
Vegetables: kale, red and green chili
Spices and herbs: cloves, peppermint, allspice, cinnamon, oregano, thyme, sage, rosemary
Other: dark chocolate, walnuts and pecans with pellicle

Source: Carlsen, M., Halvorsen, B., Holte, K, Bøhn, S. K., Dragland, S., Sampson, L., . . . Blomhoff, R. (2010). The total antioxidant content of more than 3100 foods, beverages, spices, herbs and supplements used worldwide. *Nutrition Journal.* Available at http://www.biomedcentral.com/content/pdf/1475-2891-9-3.pdf. Accessed on 9/18/12.

Antioxidants: substances that donate electrons to free radicals to prevent oxidation.

Food Additives: substances added intentionally or unintentionally to food that affect its character.

Enrich: to add nutrients back that were lost during processing; for example, white flour is enriched with B vitamins lost when the bran and germ layers are removed.

Fortified: to fortify is to add nutrients to a food that were either not originally present or were present in insignificant amounts.

Megadoses: amounts at least 10 times greater than the Recommended Dietary Allowance (RDA).

Antioxidants protect body cells from being oxidized (destroyed) by free radicals by undergoing oxidation themselves, which renders free radicals harmless. Vitamins and other substances in fruits, vegetables, and other plant-based food provide dozens, if not hundreds, of antioxidants (Box 5.1). Vitamins that function as major antioxidants are vitamin C, vitamin E, and beta-carotene. Each has a slightly different role, so one cannot completely substitute for another. For instance, water-soluble vitamin C works within cells to disable free radicals, and fat-soluble vitamin E functions within fat tissue. Whether high doses of individual antioxidants offer the same health benefits as the package of substances found in food sources is an area of ongoing research.

Some Vitamins Are Used as Food Additives

Some vitamins are used as **food additives** in certain foods to boost their nutritional content; examples include vitamin C–**enriched** fruit drinks, vitamin D–**fortified** milk, and enriched flour and breads. Other foods have certain vitamins added to them to help preserve quality. For instance, vitamin C is added to frozen fish to help prevent rancidity and to luncheon meats to stabilize the red color. Vitamin E helps retard rancidity in vegetable oils, and beta-carotene adds color to margarine.

Vitamins as Drugs
(handwritten) → at least 10× more than RDA

In **megadoses**, vitamins function like drugs, not nutrients. Large doses of niacin are used to lower cholesterol, low-density lipoprotein (LDL) cholesterol, and triglycerides in people with hyperlipidemia who do not respond to diet and exercise. Tretinoin (retinoic acid, a form of vitamin A) is used as a topical treatment for acne vulgaris and orally for acute promyelocytic leukemia. Gram quantities of vitamin C promote healing in patients with impaired bone and wound healing.

VITAMIN CLASSIFICATIONS BASED ON SOLUBILITY

(handwritten left margin)
Fat-soluble Vit
1. Vit A
2. Vit D
3. Vit E
4. Vit K

Vitamins are classified according to their solubility. Vitamins A, D, E, and K are fat soluble. Vitamin C and the B vitamins (thiamin, riboflavin, niacin, folate, B_6, B_{12}, biotin, and pantothenic acid) are water soluble. Solubility determines vitamin absorption, transportation, storage, and excretion.

(handwritten)
Water-soluble Vit:
1. Vit C
2. Vit B →   1. Thiamine 2. Ribof. 3. Niacin 4. B6 5. B12 6. Pantothenic acid

Fat-Soluble Vitamins

Group characteristics of fat-soluble vitamins are summarized in Table 5.1. Table 5.2 highlights recommended intakes, sources, functions, deficiency symptoms, and toxicity symptoms of each fat-soluble vitamin. The complete table of Dietary Reference Intakes for vitamins appears in Appendix 2. Additional features of individual fat-soluble vitamins follow.

Vitamin A

Preformed Vitamin A: the active form of vitamin A.

Carotenoids: a group name of retinol precursors found in plants.

In its preformed state, vitamin A exists as an alcohol (retinol), aldehyde (retinaldehyde), or acid (retinoic acid). **Preformed vitamin A** is found only in animal sources such as liver, whole milk, and fish. Low-fat milk, skim milk, margarine, and ready-to-eat cereals are fortified with vitamin A.

The term vitamin A also includes provitamin A **carotenoids**, natural plant pigments found in deep yellow and orange fruits and vegetables and most dark green leafy vegetables. Although there are over 600 different carotenoids, only a few are considered precursors of retinol. Beta-carotene, lutein, and lycopene are among the most commonly known carotenoids. Carotenoids account for about one-quarter to one-third of the usual intake of vitamin A.

Vitamin A is best known for its roles in normal vision, reproduction, growth, and immune system functioning. It is a relatively poor antioxidant. In contrast, beta-carotene is a major antioxidant in the body, prompting researchers to study whether it can prevent heart disease and cancer. Results of trials with beta-carotene supplements have varied from showing no effect on cancer incidence (Green et al., 1999; Lee, Cook, Manson, Buring, and Hennekens, 1999) to a surprising increase in lung cancer incidence and deaths in smokers and male asbestos workers (The Alpha-Tocopherol, Beta-Carotene Cancer Prevention Study Group, 1994; Omenn et al., 1996).

Table 5.1 Group Characteristics of Fat-Soluble and Water-Soluble Vitamins

Characteristic	Fat-Soluble Vitamins	Water-Soluble Vitamins
Sources	The fat and oil portion of foods	The watery portion of foods
Absorption	With fat encased in chylomicrons that enter the lymphatic system before circulating in the bloodstream	Directly into the bloodstream
Transportation through the blood	Attach to protein carriers because fat is not soluble in watery blood	Move freely through the watery environment of blood and within cells
When consumed in excess of need	Are stored—primarily in the liver and adipose tissue	Are excreted in the urine, although some tissues may hold limited amounts of certain vitamins
Safety of consuming high intakes through supplements	Can be toxic; this applies primarily to vitamins A and D; large doses of vitamins E and K are considered relatively nontoxic	Are generally considered non-toxic, although side effects can occur from consuming very large doses of vitamin B_6 over a prolonged period
Frequency of intake	Generally do not have to be consumed daily because the body can retrieve them from storage as needed	Must be consumed daily because there is no reserve in storage

Table 5.2 Summary of Fat-Soluble Vitamins

Vitamin and Sources	Functions	Deficiency/Toxicity Signs and Symptoms
Vitamin A **Adult RDA:** **Men: 900 μg** **Women: 700 μg** ■ Retinol: beef, liver, milk, butter, cheese, cream, egg yolk, fortified milk, margarine, and ready-to-eat cereals ■ Beta-carotene: "greens" (turnip, dandelion, beet, collard, mustard), spinach, kale, broccoli, carrots, peaches, pumpkin, red peppers, sweet potatoes, winter squash, mango, apricots, cantaloupe	The formation of visual purple, which enables the eye to adapt to dim light Normal growth and development of bones and teeth The formation and maintenance of mucosal epithelium to maintain healthy functioning of skin and membranes, hair, gums, and various glands Important role in immune function	**Deficiency** Slow recovery of vision after flashes of bright light at night is the first ocular symptom; can progress to xerophthalmia and blindness Bone growth ceases; bone shape changes; enamel-forming cells in the teeth malfunction; teeth crack and tend to decay Skin becomes dry, scaly, rough, and cracked; keratinization or hyperkeratosis develops; mucous membrane cells flatten and harden: eyes become dry (xerosis); irreversible drying and hardening of the cornea can result in blindness Decreased saliva secretion → difficulty chewing, swallowing → anorexia Decreased mucous secretion of the stomach and intestines → impaired digestion and absorption → diarrhea, increased excretion of nutrients Impaired immune system functioning → increased susceptibility to respiratory, urinary tract, and vaginal infections increases **Toxicity** Headaches, vomiting, double vision, hair loss, bone abnormalities, liver damage, which may be reversible or fatal Can cause birth defects during pregnancy

Vitamin D
Adult RDA:
Up to age 70 years:
  15 μg/day
≥71 years: 20 μg/day
■ Sunlight on the skin
■ Cod liver oil, oysters, mackerel, most fish, egg yolks, fortified milk, some ready-to-eat cereals, and margarine
	Maintains serum calcium concentrations by
	Stimulating GI absorption
	Stimulating the release of calcium from the bones
	Stimulating calcium absorption from the kidneys
		Deficiency
		① Rickets (in infants and children)
		  Retarded bone growth
		  Bone malformations (bowed legs)
		  Enlargement of ends of long bones (knock-knees)
		  Deformities of the ribs (bowed, with beads or knobs)
		  Delayed closing of the fontanel → rapid enlargement of the head
		  Decreased serum calcium and/or phosphorus
		  Malformed teeth; decayed teeth
		  Protrusion of the abdomen related to relaxation of the abdominal muscles
		  Increased secretion of parathyroid hormone
		② Osteomalacia (in adults)
		  Softening of the bones → deformities, pain, and easy fracture
		  Decreased serum calcium and/or phosphorus, increased alkaline phosphatase
		  Involuntary muscle twitching and spasms
		
		Toxicity
		① Kidney stones, irreversible kidney damage, muscle and bone weakness, excessive bleeding, loss of appetite, headache, excessive thirst, calcification of soft tissues (blood vessels, kidneys, heart, lungs), death

(continues on page 98)

Table 5.2 Summary of Fat-Soluble Vitamins (continued)

Vitamin and Sources	Functions	Deficiency/Toxicity Signs and Symptoms
Vitamin E **Adult RDA: 15 mg** ■ Vegetable oils, margarine, salad dressing, other foods made with vegetable oil, nuts, seeds, wheat germ, dark green vegetables, whole grains, fortified cereals	Acts as an antioxidant to protect vitamin A and polyunsaturated fatty acids from being destroyed Protects cell membranes	**Deficiency** Increased red blood cell hemolysis In infants, anemia, edema, and skin lesions **Toxicity** Relatively nontoxic High doses enhance action of anticoagulant medications
Vitamin K **Adult AI:** **Men: 120 μg** **Women: 90 μg** ■ Bacterial synthesis ■ Brussels sprouts, broccoli, cauliflower, Swiss chard, spinach, loose leaf lettuce, carrots, green beans, asparagus, eggs	Synthesis of blood clotting proteins and a bone protein that regulates blood calcium	**Deficiency** Hemorrhaging **Toxicity** No symptoms have been observed from excessive intake of vitamin K

The body can store up to a year supply of vitamin A, 90% of which is in the liver. Because deficiency symptoms do not develop until body stores are exhausted, it may take 1 to 2 years for them to appear. Although severe vitamin A deficiency is rare in the United States, a large percentage of adults may have suboptimal liver stores of vitamin A even though they are not clinically deficient. Worldwide, vitamin A deficiency is a major health problem; an estimated 250,000 to 500,000 vitamin A–deficient children become blind every year. Half of them die within a year of losing their sight from common infections such as diarrheal disease and measles (World Health Organization, 2012).

Only preformed vitamin A, the form found in animal foods, fortified foods, and supplements, is toxic in high doses. The risk of toxicity is much greater when supplements of vitamin A are consumed. Extremely high doses (at least 30,000 μg/day) consumed over months or years may cause central nervous system (CNS) changes, bone and skin changes, and liver abnormalities that range from reversible to fatal. At high doses during pregnancy, such as three to four times the recommended intake, vitamin A is teratogenic. Supplementation is not recommended during the first trimester of pregnancy unless there is specific evidence of vitamin A deficiency.

Beta-carotene is nontoxic because the body makes vitamin A from it only as needed and the conversion is not rapid enough to cause hypervitaminosis A. Instead, carotene is stored primarily in adipose tissue and may accumulate under the skin to the extent that it causes the skin color to turn yellowish orange, a harmless condition known as hypercarotenemia. The Tolerable Upper Intake Level (UL) for vitamin A does not apply to vitamin A derived from carotenoids.

Vitamin D

Vitamin D is unique in that the body has the potential to make all the vitamin D it needs if exposure to sunlight is optimal and liver and kidney functions are normal. The process starts in the liver, which converts cholesterol into 7-dehydrocholesterol, a precursor of vitamin D. Sunlight on the skin converts 7-dehydrocholesterol to cholecalciferol also known as vitamin D_3, a prohormone. Whether synthesized in the skin or originating from food, cholecalciferol is converted to the active form of vitamin D (1,25-dihydroxyvitamin D_3) through a series of reactions involving the liver and kidneys. Because it can be endogenously synthesized, vitamin D is not an **essential nutrient**.

Another distinctive feature of vitamin D is that it acts like a hormone because it is synthesized in one part of the body (skin) and stimulates functional activity elsewhere (e.g., GI tract, bones, kidneys) through vitamin D receptors. The primary function of vitamin D is to maintain normal blood concentrations of calcium and phosphorus by

- Stimulating calcium and phosphorus absorption from the GI tract
- Mobilizing calcium and phosphorus from the bone as needed to maintain normal serum levels
- Stimulating the kidneys to retain calcium and phosphorus

> **Essential Nutrient:**
> a nutrient that must be supplied by the diet because it is not synthesized in the body. Essentiality does not refer to importance, merely to the need for a dietary source.

In addition to its role in bone health, emerging evidence suggests vitamin D may have the potential to protect against cancer (Davis, 2008; Garland et al., 2006; Gorham et al., 2007), metabolic syndrome (Fung et al., 2012; Hypponen, Boucher, Berry, and Power, 2008), diabetes (Palomer, Gonzalex-Clemente, Blanco-Vaca, and Mauricio, 2008; Tai, Need, Horowitz, and Chapman, 2008), hypertension (Pilz, Tomaschitz, Ritz, and Pieber, 2009), multiple sclerosis (Ascherio, Munger, and Simon, 2010; Munger, Levin, Hollis, Howard, and Ascherio, 2006), and depression (Bertone-Johnson et al., 2011). However, the 2011 Institute of Medicine report on dietary requirements for calcium and vitamin D concluded that evidence linking vitamin D with extraskeletal outcomes, including cancer, cardiovascular disease, diabetes, and autoimmune disorders, is inconsistent, inconclusive, and insufficient to use in determining nutrient requirements (Institute of Medicine, 2011). Additional research, including large-scale, randomized clinical trials, is needed (Ross et al., 2011). The basis for determining vitamin D requirement continues to be its cause-and-effect relationship with bone health.

It is possible to fulfill the vitamin D requirement by taking a daily 15-minute walk in the sun under optimal conditions. However, significant rates of low vitamin D status are documented in studies of healthy adults and children in the United States and other countries. A study by Bailey, Fulgoni, Keast, and Dwyer (2012) revealed that 90% of adults who did not use vitamin supplements failed to meet the recommended intake levels for vitamin D; even with supplement use, vitamin D intakes were still low. Winter, living in northern latitudes, dark skin pigmentation, air pollution, clothing, and older age are associated with low vitamin D synthesis (Toner, Davis, and Milner, 2010). During the winter months in northern latitudes, the angle of the sun is such that most ultraviolet B rays are absorbed by the earth's ozone layer, preventing most or all endogenous vitamin D synthesis. People living north of the line connecting San Francisco to Philadelphia are not likely to make adequate vitamin D. Elderly persons are particularly at risk for vitamin D deficiency because of various risk factors, including inadequate intake, limited sun exposure, reduced skin thickness, impaired GI absorption, and impaired activation by the liver and kidneys. A dietary source is considered necessary because few people meet optimal conditions.

Vitamin D_2 (ergocalciferol) is a plant version of vitamin D; vitamin D_3 (cholecalciferol) is an animal version. Vitamin D occurs naturally in only a few foods: liver, fatty fish, and egg yolks. Fortified foods are important sources: all milks, most ready-to-eat cereals, and a few brands of orange juice, yogurt, margarine, and hot cereals.

Previously, there was insufficient evidence to establish a Recommended Dietary Allowance (RDA) for vitamin D, so the recommendations were an estimate of Adequate Intake (AI). With more high-quality studies now available, the Institute of Medicine was able to set RDAs for vitamin D in 2011, which are higher than the previous recommendation

IU: International Units, the former unit of measure of vitamin D that has been replaced by micrograms of cholecalciferol, the active form of vitamin D. To convert micrograms of vitamin D to IU, multiply micrograms by 40.

QUICK BITE

Vitamin D content of selected items

	Micrograms of Vitamin D
3 oz sockeye salmon	11.2
2 oz canned tuna in oil	5.8
1 cup milk	3.1
1 oz pasteurized, processed cheese fortified with vitamin D	2.1
1 hard cooked egg	1.1
1 beef frankfurter	0.4
1 tbsp butter	0.2
1 oz Swiss cheese	0.15

but lower than those proposed by some researchers (Ross et al., 2011). The current RDA is 15 μg/day (600 IU/day) for children and adults through age 70 years and 20 μg/day (800 IU/day) for adults age 71 years and older. These levels are based on the assumption of minimal or no sun exposure.

According to National Health and Nutrition Examination Survey (NHANES) 2007–2008 data, mean intake of vitamin D in Americans 20 years and older is 5 μg/day (200 IU) for men and 3.8 μg/day (152 IU) for women. A meta-analysis indicates that supplements of vitamin D_3 are more efficacious at increasing serum 25-hydroxyvitamin D concentrations than is vitamin D_2 (Tripkovic et al., 2012).

Overt deficiency of vitamin D causes poor calcium absorption, leading to a calcium deficit in the blood that the body corrects by releasing calcium from bone. In children, the result is **rickets**, a condition characterized by abnormal bone shape and structure. Children at risk include breastfed infants who do not receive vitamin D supplements, toddlers given unfortified soy and rice beverages in place of milk, and children who replace milk with soft drinks. In adults, vitamin D deficiency can result in **osteomalacia**, a softening of the bones.

Rickets: vitamin D deficiency disease in children, most prominently characterized by bowed legs.

Osteomalacia: adult rickets characterized by inadequate bone mineralization due to the lack of vitamin D.

The current UL for vitamin D is set at 100 μg/day (4000 IU/day) for ages 9 years and older. Factors considered in determining the UL included hypercalcemia, hypercalciuria, vascular and soft tissue calcification, and emerging evidence of a U-shaped relationship for all-cause mortality, cardiovascular disease, certain cancers, falls, and fractures (Ross et al., 2011). Because the body destroys excess vitamin D produced from overexposure to the sun, there has never been a reported case of vitamin D toxicity from too much sun (Food and Nutrition Board, Institute of Medicine, 1997).

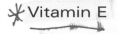

Vitamin E

QUICK BITE

Oils containing active form of vitamin E (in descending order)
Wheat germ oil
Walnut oil
Sunflower oil
Cottonseed oil
Safflower oil
Palm oil
Canola oil
Sesame oil
Peanut oil
Olive oil
Corn oil
Soybean oil

Vitamin E is a generic term that describes a group of at least eight structurally related, naturally occurring compounds. Alpha-tocopherol is considered the most biologically active form of vitamin E, although other forms also have important roles in maintaining health. As a group, vitamin E functions as the primary fat-soluble antioxidant in the body, protecting PUFAs and other lipid molecules, such as LDL cholesterol, from oxidative damage. By doing so, it helps to maintain the integrity of PUFA-rich cell membranes, protects red blood cells against hemolysis, and protects vitamin A from oxidation. Vitamin E also has several important functions independent of its antioxidant activity, such as inhibiting cell division, enhancing immune system functioning, regulating gene expression, inhibiting platelet aggregation, and suppressing tumor angiogenesis (Traber and Atkinson, 2007).

The need for vitamin E increases as the intake of PUFA increases. Fortunately, vitamin E and PUFA share many of the same food sources, particularly vegetable oils and products made from oil such as margarine, salad dressings, and other prepared foods. However, not all oils are rich in alpha-tocopherol, the active form of vitamin E. Soybean oil, the most commonly used oil in food processing, ranks low in alpha-tocopherol content.

Observational studies suggest an inverse relationship between dietary and supplemental vitamin E intakes and the incidence of several chronic diseases, including cardiovascular disease and cancer (Gaziano, 2004; Sung et al., 2003). A prospective cohort study of the Finnish male smokers who participated in the Alpha-Tocopherol, Beta-Carotene Cancer Prevention (ATBC) study revealed a significantly lower total and cause-specific mortality in older male smokers who had circulating concentrations of alpha-tocopherol at the high end of normal, whether from dietary intake, low-dose vitamin E supplements, or both (Wright et al., 2006). However, the relationship between vitamin E status and overall mortality remains controversial: a meta-analysis of randomized trials suggested a small increase in the risk of all-cause mortality with high-dose supplements of vitamin E (Miller et al., 2005). Similarly, the Selenium and Vitamin E Cancer Prevention Trial (SELECT) showed that vitamin E supplementation significantly increased the risk of prostate cancer in healthy men (Klein et al., 2011). Clearly, more randomized clinical trials are needed to determine the safety and efficacy of using vitamin E supplements.

Vitamin E deficiency is rare and more likely to occur secondary to fat malabsorption syndromes, such as cystic fibrosis and short bowel syndrome, than from an inadequate intake. Premature infants who have not benefited from the transfer of vitamin E from mother to fetus in the last weeks of pregnancy are at risk for red blood cell hemolysis. The breaking of their red blood cell membranes is caused by oxidation; vitamin E corrects red blood cell hemolysis by preventing oxidation. Prolonged vitamin E deficiency symptoms include peripheral neuropathy, ataxia, and impaired vision and speech.

Vitamin E has been used for fibrocystic breast disease and intermittent claudication with inconsistent results. Large amounts of vitamin E are relatively nontoxic but can interfere with vitamin K action (blood clotting) by decreasing platelet aggregation. Large doses may also potentiate the effects of blood-thinning drugs, increasing the risk of hemorrhage. The UL is 66 times higher than the RDA.

Vitamin K

Vitamin K occurs naturally in two forms: phylloquinone, found in plants, and menaquinones, which are synthesized in the intestinal tract by bacteria. Relatively few foods contribute to the dietary phylloquinone intake of most people: collards, spinach, salad greens, broccoli, Brussels sprouts, and cabbage.

Vitamin K is a coenzyme essential for the synthesis of prothrombin and at least 6 of the other 13 proteins needed for normal blood clotting. Without adequate vitamin K, life is threatened: even a small wound can cause someone deficient in vitamin K to bleed to death. Vitamin K also activates at least three proteins involved in building and maintaining bone.

Newborns are prone to vitamin K deficiency because their sterile GI tracts cannot synthesize vitamin K, and it may take weeks for bacteria to establish themselves in the newborn's intestines. To prevent hemorrhagic disease, a single intramuscular dose of vitamin K is given prophylactically at birth.

Clinically significant vitamin K deficiency is defined as vitamin K–responsive hypoprothrombinemia and is characterized by an increase in prothrombin time. Vitamin K deficiency does not occur from inadequate intake but may occur secondary to malabsorption syndromes or to the use of certain medications that interfere with vitamin K metabolism or synthesis, such as anticoagulants and antibiotics. Anticoagulants, such as warfarin (Coumadin), interfere with hepatic synthesis of vitamin K–dependent clotting factors. People who take anticoagulants do not need to avoid vitamin K, but they should try to maintain a consistent intake so that the effect on coagulation time is as constant and as predictable as possible. Antibiotics kill the intestinal bacteria that synthesize vitamin K.

Due to the lack of data to estimate an average requirement, an AI, not an RDA, has been set. A UL has not been set because no adverse effects are associated with vitamin K intake from food or supplements.

Water-Soluble Vitamins

Group characteristics of water-soluble vitamins are summarized in Table 5.1. Table 5.3 highlights sources, functions, deficiency symptoms, and toxicity symptoms of each water-soluble vitamin. The complete table of Dietary Reference Intakes for vitamins appears in Appendix 2. Additional features of individual water-soluble vitamins are summarized in the following sections.

Thiamin

Thiamin (vitamin B_1) is a coenzyme in the metabolism of carbohydrates and branched-chain amino acids. In addition to its role in energy metabolism, thiamin is important in nervous system functioning.

In the United States and other developed countries, the use of enriched breads and cereals has virtually eliminated the thiamin deficiency disease known as beriberi. Today, thiamin deficiency is usually seen only in alcoholics with limited food consumption because chronic alcohol abuse impairs thiamin intake, absorption, and metabolism. Edema occurs in wet beriberi; muscle wasting is prominent in dry beriberi. Cardiac and renal complications can be fatal.

No adverse effects have been noted from high intakes of thiamin from food or supplements, so a UL has not been set.

Riboflavin

Riboflavin (vitamin B_2) is an integral component of the coenzymes flavin adenine dinucleotide (FAD) and flavin mononucleotide (FMN) that function to release energy from nutrients in all body cells. Flavin coenzymes are also involved in the formation of some vitamins and their coenzymes and in the conversion of **homocysteine** to **methionine**. Riboflavin is unique among water-soluble vitamins in that milk and dairy products contribute the most riboflavin to the diet.

Homocysteine: an amino acid correlated with increased risk of heart disease.

Methionine: an essential amino acid.

Biochemical signs of an inadequate riboflavin status can appear after only a few days of a poor intake. The elderly and adolescents are at greatest risk for riboflavin deficiency. Riboflavin deficiency interferes with iron handling and contributes to anemia when iron intake is low. Other deficiency symptoms include sore throat, cheilosis, stomatitis, glossitis, and dermatitis, many of which may be related to the effect riboflavin deficiency has on the metabolism of folate and vitamin B_6. Certain diseases, such as cancer, heart disease, and diabetes, precipitate or exacerbate riboflavin deficiency.

Niacin

Niacin (vitamin B_3) exists as nicotinic acid and nicotinamide. The body converts nicotinic acid to nicotinamide, which is the major form of niacin in the blood. All protein foods provide niacin, as do whole-grain and enriched breads and fortified ready-to-eat cereals.

Table 5.3 Summary of Water-Soluble Vitamins

Vitamin and Sources	Functions	Deficiency/Toxicity Signs and Symptoms

Thiamin (vitamin B$_1$)
Adult RDA
Men: 1.2 mg
Women: 1.1 mg
▪ Whole-grain and enriched breads and cereals, liver, nuts, wheat germ, pork, dried peas and beans
	Coenzyme in energy metabolism
	Promotes normal appetite and nervous system functioning
		Deficiency
		Beriberi
		   Mental confusion, decrease in short-term memory
		   Fatigue, apathy
		   Peripheral paralysis
		   Muscle weakness and wasting
		   Painful calf muscles
		   Anorexia, weight loss
		   Edema
		   Enlarged heart
		   Sudden death from heart failure
		
		Toxicity
		No toxicity symptoms reported

Riboflavin (vitamin B$_2$) **Adult RDA** **Men: 1.3 mg** **Women: 1.1 mg** ▪ Milk and other dairy products; whole-grain and enriched breads and cereals; liver, eggs, meat, spinach	Coenzyme in energy metabolism Aids in the conversion of tryptophan into niacin	**Deficiency** Dermatitis Cheilosis Glossitis Photophobia Reddening of the cornea **Toxicity** No toxicity symptoms reported

Niacin (vitamin B$_3$)
Adult RDA
Men: 16 mg
Women: 14 mg
▪ All protein foods, whole-grain and enriched breads and cereals
	Coenzyme in energy metabolism
	Promotes normal nervous system functioning
		Deficiency
		Pellagra: 4 Ds
		   Dermatitis (bilateral and symmetrical) and glossitis
		   Diarrhea
		   Dementia, irritability, mental confusion → psychosis
		   Death, if untreated
		
		Toxicity (from supplements/drugs)
		Flushing, liver damage, gastric ulcers, low blood pressure, diarrhea, nausea, vomiting

Vitamin B$_6$ **Adult RDA** **Men: 1.3–1.7 mg** **Women: 1.3–1.5 mg** ▪ Meats, fish, poultry, fruits, green leafy vegetables, whole grains, nuts, dried peas and beans	Coenzyme in amino acid and fatty acid metabolism Helps convert tryptophan to niacin Helps produce insulin, hemoglobin, myelin sheaths, and antibodies	**Deficiency** Dermatitis, cheilosis, glossitis, abnormal brain wave pattern, convulsions, and anemia **Toxicity** Depression, fatigue, irritability, headaches; sensory neuropathy characteristic
Folate **Adult RDA: 400 μg** ▪ Liver, okra, spinach, asparagus, dried peas and beans, seeds, orange juice; breads, cereals, and other grains are fortified with folic acid	Coenzyme in DNA synthesis; therefore vital for new cell synthesis and the transmission of inherited characteristics	**Deficiency** Glossitis, diarrhea, macrocytic anemia, depression, mental confusion, fainting, fatigue **Toxicity** Too much can mask B$_{12}$ deficiency

(continues on page 104)

Table 5.3 Summary of Water-Soluble Vitamins (continued)

Vitamin and Sources	Functions	Deficiency/Toxicity Signs and Symptoms
Vitamin B$_{12}$ **Adult RDA: 2.4 μg** ■ Animal products: meat, fish, poultry, shellfish, milk, dairy products, eggs ■ Some fortified foods	Coenzyme in the synthesis of new cells Activates folate Maintains nerve cells Helps metabolize some fatty acids and amino acids	**Deficiency** GI changes: glossitis, anorexia, indigestion, recurring diarrhea or constipation, and weight loss Macrocytic anemia: pallor, dyspnea, weakness, fatigue, and palpitations Neurologic changes: paresthesia of the hands and feet, decreased sense of position, poor muscle coordination, poor memory, irritability, depression, paranoia, delirium, and hallucinations **Toxicity** No toxicity symptoms reported
Pantothenic Acid **Adult AI: 5 mg** ■ Widespread in foods ■ Meat, poultry, fish, whole-grain cereals, and dried peas and beans are among best sources	Part of coenzyme A used in energy metabolism	**Deficiency** Rare; general failure of all body systems **Toxicity** No toxicity symptoms reported, although large doses may cause diarrhea
Biotin **Adult AI: 30 μg** ■ Widespread in foods ■ Eggs, liver, milk, and dark green vegetables are among best choices ■ Synthesized by GI flora	Coenzyme in energy metabolism, fatty acid synthesis, amino acid metabolism, and glycogen formation	**Deficiency** Rare; anorexia, fatigue, depression, dry skin, heart abnormalities **Toxicity** No toxicity symptoms reported

Vitamin C
Adult RDA
Men: 90 mg
Women: 75 mg
■ Citrus fruits and juices, red and green peppers, broccoli, cauliflower, Brussels sprouts, cantaloupe, kiwifruit, mustard greens, strawberries, tomatoes
	Collagen synthesis
	Antioxidant
	Promotes iron absorption
	Involved in the metabolism of certain amino acids
	Thyroxin synthesis
	Immune system functioning
		Deficiency
		Bleeding gums, pinpoint hemorrhages under the skin
		Scurvy, characterized by
		  Hemorrhaging
		  Muscle degeneration
		  Skin changes
		  Delayed wound healing: reopening of old wounds
		  Softening of the bones →
		    malformations, pain, easy fractures
		  Soft, loose teeth
		  Anemia
		  Increased susceptibility to infection
		  Hysteria and depression
		
		Toxicity
		Diarrhea, mild GI upset

Niacin Equivalents (NEs): the amount of niacin available to the body including that made from tryptophan.

A unique feature of niacin is that the body can make it from the amino acid tryptophan: approximately 60 mg of tryptophan is used to synthesize 1 mg of niacin. Because of this additional source of niacin, niacin requirements are stated in **niacin equivalents (NEs)**. Median intake in the United States generously exceeds the RDA.

Niacin is part of the coenzymes nicotinamide adenine dinucleotide (NAD) and nicotinamide adenine dinucleotide phosphate (NADP), which are involved in energy transfer reactions in the metabolism of glucose, fat, and alcohol in all body cells. Reduced NADP is used in the synthesis of fatty acids, cholesterol, and steroid hormones.

Pellagra, the disorder caused by severe niacin deficiency, is rare in the United States and usually is seen only in alcoholics. However, pellagra is widespread in areas that rely on corn as a staple, such as parts of Africa and Asia, because corn is low in niacin and tryptophan. Before grain products were enriched with niacin in the early 20th century, pellagra was also common in the southern United States.

Niacin deficiency may be treated with niacin, tryptophan, or both. Because a deficiency of niacin rarely occurs alone, treatment is most effective when other B-complex vitamins are also given, especially thiamin and riboflavin.

Large doses of niacin in the form of nicotinic acid (1–6 g/day) are used therapeutically to lower total cholesterol and LDL cholesterol and raise high-density lipoprotein (HDL) cholesterol. Flushing is a common side effect caused by vasodilation. Large doses, which may cause liver damage and gout, should be used only with a doctor's supervision. The UL of 35 mg of NE does not apply for clinical applications using niacin as a drug.

Vitamin B$_6$

Vitamin B$_6$ and pyridoxine are group names for six related compounds that include pyridoxine, pyridoxal, and pyridoxamine. All forms can be converted to the active form, pyridoxal phosphate, which is involved in nearly 100 enzymatic reactions.

Vitamin B$_6$ plays a role in the synthesis, catabolism, and transport of amino acids and in the conversion of tryptophan to niacin. It is involved in the formation of heme for hemoglobin and in the synthesis of myelin sheaths and neurotransmitters. It facilitates the transfer of carbon groups for DNA synthesis. Vitamin B$_6$ helps to regulate blood glucose levels by assisting in the release of stored glucose from glycogen and is important in the maintenance of cellular immunity. Unlike other B vitamins, vitamin B$_6$ is stored extensively in muscle tissue.

Low concentrations of vitamin B$_6$, folic acid, and vitamin B$_{12}$ are associated with an increase in blood homocysteine levels, a nonessential amino acid linked to an increased risk of stroke (Lonn et al., 2006), coronary heart disease (Humphrey, Fu, Rogers, Freeman, and Helfand, 2008), cognitive decline (Elias et al., 2005), and vascular disease (McCully, 2007). Findings from three major studies, the HOPE2 trial (Lonn et al., 2006), NORVIT trial (Bønaa et al., 2006), and VISP trial (Toole et al., 2004), showed that the combination of vitamin B$_6$, vitamin B$_{12}$, and folic acid lowers homocysteine levels in people with advanced vascular disease but has little effect on recurrent heart attack or stroke. Independently, vitamin B$_6$ had no effect on lowering plasma homocysteine in a meta-analysis of intervention trials (Clarke and Armitage, 2000). The American Heart Association (AHA) has not defined hyperhomocysteinemia a major risk factor for cardiovascular disease nor does it recommend widespread use of folic acid and B vitamin supplements to reduce the risk of heart disease and stroke (AHA, 2012).

The role of vitamin B$_6$ in disease prevention and control is actively studied (Mooney, Leuendorf, Hendrickson, and Hellmann, 2009). A meta-analysis of prospective studies showed an inverse relationship between vitamin B$_6$ intake and blood levels and the risk of colorectal cancer (Larsson, Orsini, and Wolk, 2010). Doses of 50 to 200 mg/day of vitamin B$_6$ have been shown to have an antiemetic effect, and there is some evidence that it helps treat morning sickness in pregnancy (Jewell and Young, 2003). Several studies have shown that supplements of 50 to 100 mg/day of vitamin B$_6$ normalize glucose tolerance in gestational diabetes but that they have no effect on glucose tolerance in nonpregnant women (Bennink and Schreurs, 1975; Spellacy, Buhi, and Birk, 1977).

Supplements of vitamin B$_6$ in amounts ranging from 25 to 500 mg/day have been advocated for treating a variety of other conditions in which it seems reasonable that vitamin B$_6$ may play a protective role based on its known functions, such as in steroid hormone–dependent cancers, depression, and hypertension (Bender, 2011). However, large-scale, controlled trials are lacking. Evidence from randomized controlled trials shows no benefit to using vitamin B_6 for cognitive function, dementia, autism, or carpal tunnel syndrome.

High intakes of vitamin B_6 from food do not pose any danger. Long-term use of high-dose supplements (1000–4000 mg/day) is associated with neuropathy that is reversible with discontinuation (Institute of Medicine, 1998).

Deficiencies of vitamin B_6 are uncommon but are usually accompanied by deficiencies of other B vitamins. Secondary deficiencies are related to alcohol abuse (the metabolism of alcohol promotes the destruction and excretion of vitamin B_6) and to other drug therapies such as isoniazid, the antituberculosis drug that acts as a vitamin B_6 antagonist.

Folate

Dietary Folate Equivalents (DFEs):
DFE = microgram of food folate + (1.7 × micrograms synthetic folic acid).

Folate is the generic term for this B vitamin that includes both synthetic folic acid found in vitamin supplements and fortified foods and naturally occurring folate in foods such as green leafy vegetables, legumes, seeds, liver, and orange juice. **Dietary folate equivalents (DFEs)**, used in establishing folate requirement, are based on the assumption that natural food folate is approximately only half as available to the body as synthetic folic acid. A more recent study showed that bioavailability of food folate may be as high as 80% of synthetic folic acid (Winkels, Brouwer, Siebelink, Katan, and Verhoef, 2007).

As part of the coenzymes tetrahydrofolate (THF) and dihydrofolate (DHF), folate's major function is in the synthesis of DNA. With the aid of vitamin B_{12}, folate is vital for synthesis of new cells and transmission of inherited characteristics. Folate is also involved in homocysteine metabolism.

Because folate is recycled through the intestinal tract (much like the enterohepatic circulation of bile), a healthy GI tract is essential to maintain folate balance. When GI integrity is impaired, as in malabsorption syndromes, failure to reabsorb folate quickly leads to folate deficiency. GI cells are particularly susceptible to folate deficiency because they are rapidly dividing cells that depend on folate for new cell synthesis. Without the formation of new cells, GI function declines and widespread malabsorption of nutrients occurs.

Folate deficiency impairs DNA synthesis and cell division and results in macrocytic anemia and other clinical symptoms. It is prevalent in all parts of the world. In developing countries, folate deficiency commonly is caused by parasitic infections that alter GI integrity. In the United States, alcoholics are at highest risk of folate deficiency because of alcohol's toxic effect on the GI tract. Groups at risk because of poor intake include the elderly, fad dieters, and people of low socioeconomic status. Because new tissue growth increases folate requirements, infants, adolescents, and pregnant women may have difficulty consuming adequate amounts.

Studies show that an adequate intake of folate before conception and during the first trimester of pregnancy reduces the risk of neural tube defects (e.g., spina bifida) in infants (Medical Research Council Vitamin Study Research Group, 1991). This discovery prompted the U.S. Public Health Service to recommend that all women of childbearing age who are capable of becoming pregnant consume 400 µg of synthetic folic acid from fortified food and/or supplements in addition to folate from a varied diet. Mandatory folic acid fortification of enriched bread and grain products began on January 1, 1998.

As mentioned in the section on vitamin B_6, studies using supplements of folic acid to lower homocysteine levels and the risk of cardiovascular disease have failed to show a benefit. However, a meta-analysis of randomized trials showed that folic acid significantly reduced the risk of stroke overall by 18% and up to 25% in people with no history of stroke or when homocysteine-lowering effect was great (Wang et al., 2007). Tighe et al. (2011) found that as little as 200 µg/day taken for 6 months effectively lowers homocysteine concentration and that higher doses may not be necessary or appropriate due to potential adverse effects of long-term high folic acid intakes. However, more studies are needed to determine whether folic acid alone is optimal or whether additional benefits are possible when folic acid is combined with vitamin B_{12}.

The UL for folic acid is 1000 µg/day from fortified food or supplements, exclusive of food folate. Long-term exposure to synthetic folic acid may mask vitamin B_{12} deficiency, which can cause permanent neurologic damage if left untreated (Reynolds, 2006). Other potential risks of high folic acid intakes may include an increased risk of cognitive decline in older people with a low vitamin B_{12} status (Morris, Jacques, Rosenberg, and Selhub, 2007), increased tumorigenesis in patients with pre-existing lesions (Cole et al., 2007), and increased risk of cancer in general (Ebbing et al., 2009).

Vitamin B_{12}

Vitamin B_{12} (cobalamin) has several interesting features. First, vitamin B_{12} has an interdependent relationship with folate: each vitamin must have the other to be activated. Because it activates folate, vitamin B_{12} is involved in DNA synthesis and maturation of red blood cells. Like folate, vitamin B_{12} functions as a coenzyme in homocysteine metabolism. Unlike folate, vitamin B_{12} has important roles in maintaining the myelin sheath around nerves. For this reason, large doses of folic acid can alleviate the anemia caused by vitamin B_{12} deficiency (a function of both vitamins), but folic acid cannot halt the progressive neurologic impairments that only vitamin B_{12} can treat. Nervous system damage may be irreversible without early treatment with vitamin B_{12}.

Vitamin B_{12} also holds the distinction of being the only water-soluble vitamin that does not occur naturally in plants. Fermented soy products and algae may be enriched with vitamin B_{12}, but it is in an inactive, unavailable form. Some ready-to-eat cereals are fortified with vitamin B_{12}. All animal foods contain vitamin B_{12}.

Another unique feature of vitamin B_{12} is that it requires an intrinsic factor, a glycoprotein secreted in the stomach, to be absorbed from the terminal ileum. But before it can bind to the intrinsic factor, vitamin B_{12} must first be separated from the small peptides to which it is bound in food sources. Separation is accomplished by pepsin and gastric acid.

Vitamin B_{12} deficiency symptoms may take 5 to 10 years or longer to develop because the liver can store relatively large amounts of B_{12} and the body recycles B_{12} by reabsorbing it.

Dietary deficiencies of vitamin B_{12} are rare and are likely to occur only in strict vegans who consume no animal products and do not adequately supplement their diet. A more frequent cause of deficiency is the lack of intrinsic factor, which prevents absorption of vitamin B_{12} regardless of intake; this condition is known as pernicious anemia. People with pernicious anemia, which can occur secondary to gastric surgery or gastric cancer, require parenteral injections of vitamin B_{12}. Most commonly, B_{12} deficiency arises from inadequate gastric acid secretion, which prevents protein-bound vitamin B_{12} in foods from being freed. An estimated 6% to 15% of older adults have vitamin B_{12} deficiency, and another 20% are estimated to have marginal status due to pernicious anemia, atrophic gastritis, or inadequate intake (Allen, 2009). Other factors that increase the risk of B_{12} deficiency include gastric resection, use of medications that suppress gastric acid secretion, and gastric infection with *Helicobacter pylori* (McCully, 2007). Because people with protein-bound vitamin B_{12} deficiency are able to absorb synthetic (free) vitamin B_{12}, the National Academy of Sciences Institute of Medicine recommends that people older than age 50 years obtain most of their requirement from fortified foods or supplements (Food and Nutrition Board, Institute of Medicine, 1998).

Other B Vitamins

Pantothenic acid is part of coenzyme A (CoA), the coenzyme involved in the formation of acetyl-CoA and in the TCA (tricarboxylic acid) cycle. Pantothenic acid participates in more than 100 different metabolic reactions. It is widespread in the diet. The best sources of pantothenic acid are meat, fish, poultry, whole-grain cereals, and dried peas and beans.

As a coenzyme, biotin is involved in the TCA cycle, gluconeogenesis, fatty acid synthesis, and chemical reactions that add or remove carbon dioxide from other compounds. Biotin is widely distributed in nature, and significant amounts are synthesized by GI flora, but it is not known how much is available for absorption. It is assumed that the average American diet provides adequate amounts of both pantothenic acid and biotin.

Non–B Vitamins

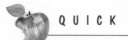

QUICK BITE

Substances often falsely promoted as B vitamins
Para-aminobenzoic acid (PABA)
Bioflavonoids
Vitamin P
Hesperidin
Ubiquinone
Vitamin B_{15}
Vitamin B_{17}

Other substances, such as inositol and carnitine, are sometimes inaccurately referred to as B vitamins because they are coenzymes. Research is needed to determine whether these substances are essential in the diet.

Choline plays important roles in the metabolism and functioning of cells and was assigned an AI value in 1998. Since then, studies have shown potential deleterious effects of choline deficiencies (Hollenbeck, 2010). Although its essentiality is currently uncertain, it may eventually be classified as a B vitamin.

Vitamin C

Vitamin C (ascorbic acid), most notably found in citrus fruits and juices, may be the most famous vitamin. Its long history dates back more than 250 years when it was determined that something in citrus fruits prevents scurvy, a disease that killed as many as two-thirds of sailors on long journeys. Years later, British sailors acquired the nickname "Limeys" because of Great Britain's policy to prevent scurvy by providing limes to all navy men. It wasn't until 1932 that the antiscurvy agent was identified as vitamin C. Since then, vitamin C has been touted as a cure for a variety of ills, including cancer, colds, and infertility.

Vitamin C prevents scurvy by promoting the formation of collagen, the most abundant protein in fibrous tissues, such as connective tissue, cartilage, bone matrix, tooth dentin, skin, and tendon. Without adequate vitamin C, the integrity of collagen is compromised; muscles degenerate, weakened bones break, wounds fail to heal, teeth are lost, and infection occurs. Hemorrhaging begins as pinpoints under the skin and progresses to massive internal bleeding and death. Even though scurvy is deadly, it can be cured within a matter of days with moderate doses of vitamin C.

Vitamin C is a water-soluble antioxidant that protects vitamin A, vitamin E, PUFA, and iron from destruction. As an antioxidant, vitamin C is being studied for its ability to prevent heart disease, certain cancers, cataracts, and asthma. It is involved in many metabolic reactions including the promotion of iron absorption, the formation of some neurotransmitters, the synthesis of thyroxine, the metabolism of some amino acids, and normal immune system functioning.

The newest RDA for vitamin C represents an increase from the previous recommendation. Cigarette smokers are advised to increase their intake by 35 mg/day because smoking increases oxidative stress and metabolic turnover of vitamin C (Food and Nutrition Board, Institute of Medicine, 2000). The need for vitamin C also increases in response to other stresses such as fever, chronic illness, infection, and wound healing as well as from chronic use of certain medications such as aspirin, barbiturates, and oral contraceptives. There is no evidence that mental stress increases the need for vitamin C.

There is no clear and convincing evidence that large doses of vitamin C prevent colds, although it is possible that supplements may benefit those with low plasma vitamin C stores or those experiencing oxidative stress from intense physical exercise, such as ultramarathon runners (Peters, Goetzsche, Grobbelaar, and Noakes, 1993). Efficacy is difficult to measure because it may be influenced by how much, how often, and how long supplements are used and by which outcome it is measured, such as frequency of colds, length of cold, and severity of symptoms (Fragakis and Thomson, 2007).

Phytochemicals

Phytochemicals: bioactive, nonnutrient plant compounds associated with a reduced risk of chronic diseases.

Phytochemicals are literally plant ("phyto" in Greek) chemicals, a broad class of non-nutritive compounds that plants produce to protect themselves against viruses, bacteria, and fungi. In foods, phytochemicals impart color, taste, aroma, and other characteristics. When eaten in the "package" of fruit, vegetables, whole grains, or nuts, these chemicals work together with nutrients and fiber to promote health, for example, by acting as antioxidants, detoxifying enzymes, stimulating the immune system, and regulating hormones or by inactivating bacteria and viruses. Often their actions in the body are complementary and overlapping. Table 5.4 lists possible effects and sources of selected phytochemicals.

Table 5.4 Possible Effects and Sources of Selected Phytochemicals

Phytochemical (Name or Class)	Possible Effects	Sources
Lycopene	Potent antioxidant that may reduce the risk of prostate cancer and heart disease	Red fruits and vegetables, such as tomatoes, tomato products, red grapefruit, red peppers, watermelon
Allyl sulfides	Boost levels of naturally occurring enzymes that may help to maintain healthy immune system	Garlic, onions, leeks, chives
Isoflavones (genistein and daidzein)	Antiestrogen activity, which may decrease the risk of estrogen-dependent cancers; may inhibit the formation of blood vessels that enable tumors to grow	Soybeans, soy flour, soy milk, tofu, other legumes
Ellagic acid	May reduce the risk of certain cancers and decrease cholesterol levels	Red grapes, strawberries, raspberries, blueberries, kiwifruit, currants
Limonene	Boosts levels of body enzymes that may destroy carcinogens	Oranges, grapefruit, tangerines, lemons, and limes
Polyphenols (catechins)	May help to prevent DNA damage by neutralizing free radicals	Onions, apples, tea, red wine, grapes, grape juice, strawberries, green tea
Lignans	Act as a phytoestrogen; may reduce the risk of certain kinds of cancer	Flaxseed, whole grains
Phytic acid	May inhibit oxidative reactions in the colon that produce harmful free radicals	Whole wheat
Lutein	Acts as an antioxidant; may reduce the risk of heart disease, age-related eye diseases, and cancer	Kale, spinach, collard greens, kiwifruit, broccoli, Brussels sprouts, Swiss chard, romaine
Zeaxanthin	May help prevent macular degeneration and certain types of cancer	Corn, spinach, winter squash
Resveratrol	May reduce the risk of heart disease, cancer, and stroke by improving blood flow to the heart and brain and preventing blood clots	Red grapes, red grape juice, red wine

Phytochemicals are an emerging area of nutrition research. At this time, researchers simply do not know all the components in plants, how they function, which ones are beneficial, which ones are potentially harmful, and the ideal combination and concentration of these chemicals to be able to create a pill to substitute for a varied diet rich in plants. More than likely, it is the total package and balance of nutrients and nonnutritive substances that make fruits and vegetables so healthy. Until science catches up to nature, the best advice is to eat a diet rich in plants. Variety is important because different plants supply different types and amounts of the hundreds of phytochemicals that have already been identified.

VITAMINS IN HEALTH PROMOTION

A premise of the *Dietary Guidelines for Americans, 2010* is that nutrients should come primarily from food, not supplements (Fig. 5.2). MyPlate (Chapter 8) and the DASH Eating Plan (Chapter 20) translate the Dietary Guidelines into food plans aimed at ensuring nutrient adequacy. Generally, a food group approach, rather than actual intake calculations, is "good enough" to assess vitamin adequacy because

- Food composition data may be inaccurate (as in the case of vitamin E, which includes all types of E, not just the active form) or limited (e.g., biotin and pantothenic acid content of food is scarce).
- An individual's intake varies from day to day, so "usual" intake is hard to define.
- People tend to underreport their actual food intake.
- An individual's actual nutrient requirements are unknown; the RDAs are intended to meet the needs of 97% to 98% of all healthy people but not necessarily individuals.

The only population-wide recommendation in the *Dietary Guidelines for Americans, 2010* that concerns vitamins is that Americans choose foods that provide more vitamin D. Additional population-specific recommendations regarding the use of vitamin supplements

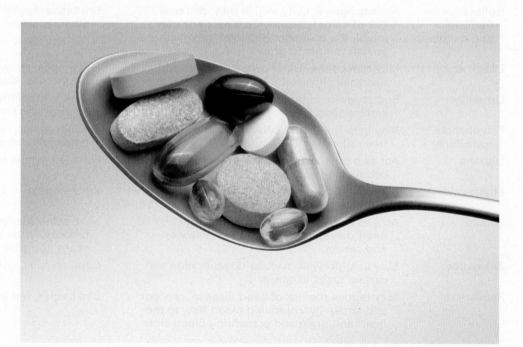

■ FIGURE 5.2   Nutrients are best obtained from food, not pills.

Box 5.2   2010 DIETARY GUIDELINES KEY RECOMMENDATIONS FOR SPECIFIC POPULATION GROUPS REGARDING VITAMINS

Individuals Age 50 Years and Older

Consume foods fortified with vitamin B_{12}, such as fortified cereals, or dietary supplements. Men and women older than age 50 years are urged to consume most of their RDA for vitamin B_{12} via fortified cereals or supplements because they may not adequately absorb adequate B_{12} from protein-bound food sources.

Women Capable of Becoming Pregnant

Consume 400 μg daily of synthetic folic acid (from fortified foods and/or supplements) in addition to food forms of folate from a varied diet. Women who consume folic acid–fortified cereal do not need a supplement; in fact, they may be at risk for an excessive folic acid intake if they consume both. Although fortified cereals only provide 400 μg of folic acid per serving, actual portion sizes eaten are usually much bigger.

Women Who Are Pregnant (Including Adolescents)

Consume 600 μg/day of dietary folate equivalents from all sources (natural and synthetic).

Source: U.S. Department of Agriculture, U.S. Department of Health and Human Services. (2010). *Dietary guidelines for Americans, 2010* (7th ed.). Available at www.health.gov/dietaryguidelines. Accessed on 2/24/11.

and/or fortified foods are made for women who are capable of becoming pregnant (folic acid) and adults age 50 years and older (vitamin B_{12}) (Box 5.2). However, the Dietary Guidelines identify vitamins E, A, and C as vitamins of concern in adults (U.S. Department of Agriculture, U.S. Department of Health and Human Services, 2010). The newest NHANES data show that adult mean intakes of vitamin A (which includes beta-carotene) and vitamin E fall below the Dietary Reference Intakes (Table 5.5). Although all MyPlate

Table 5.5 Comparison Between Mean Nutrient Intakes Among Adults and Dietary Reference Intakes*

Vitamin	Men Age 20 Years and Older Mean Intake	Recommended Adult Intake	Women Age 20 Years and Older Mean Intake	Recommended Adult Intake
Vitamin A (μg RAE)	**649**	900	**580**	700
Vitamin E (mg alpha-tocopherol)	**8.3**	15	**6.9**	15
Vitamin K (μg)	**103.7**	120	95.7	90
Thiamin (mg)	1.9	1.2	1.37	1.1
Riboflavin (mg)	2.54	1.3	1.86	1.1
Niacin (mg)	29.9	16	20.4	14
Vitamin B_6 (mg)	2.32	1.3–1.7	1.66	1.3–1.5
Folate (μg, dietary folate equivalents)	613	400	463	400
Vitamin B_{12} (μg)	6.32	2.4	4.32	2.4
Vitamin C (mg)	91.3	90	77.9	75

Numbers in bold represent nutrients whose mean intake falls below the recommended intake.

RAE, retinol activity equivalents.

*Dietary Reference Intakes are Recommended Dietary Allowances for vitamins A, E, thiamin, riboflavin, niacin, vitamin B_6, folate, vitamin B_{12}, and vitamin C. Recommended intake is an Adequate Intake for vitamin K.

Source: U.S. Department of Agriculture, Agricultural Research Service. (2010). *Nutrient intakes from food: Mean amounts consumed per individual, by gender and age. What We Eat in American, NHANES 2007–2008.* Available at www.ars.usda.gov/ba/bhnrc/fsrg. Accessed on 6/9/12.

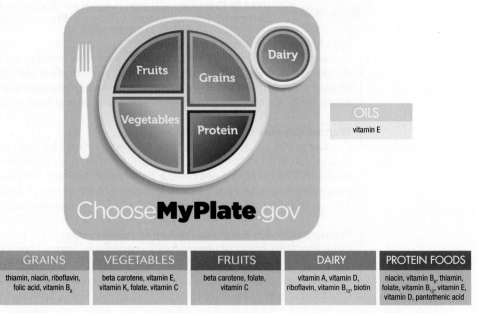

GRAINS	VEGETABLES	FRUITS	DAIRY	PROTEIN FOODS
thiamin, niacin, riboflavin, folic acid, vitamin B_6	beta carotene, vitamin E, vitamin K, folate, vitamin C	beta carotene, folate, vitamin C	vitamin A, vitamin D, riboflavin, vitamin B_{12}, biotin	niacin, vitamin B_6, thiamin, folate, vitamin B_{12}, vitamin E, vitamin D, pantothenic acid

■ FIGURE 5.3   Vitamins in MyPlate food groups. (*Source:* U.S. Department of Agriculture, Center for Nutrition Policy and Promotion. [2011]. Available at www .choosemyplate.gov)

groups provide a mixture of vitamins in varying amounts (Fig. 5.3), the vitamins of concern are found almost exclusively in plants.

- Beta-carotene (and vitamin C) are found exclusively in fruits and vegetables. The amounts of fruits and vegetables recommended at various MyPlate calorie levels appear in Table 5.6. According to food consumption data, an estimated 32.5% of adults consume fruits two or more times daily, and approximately 27% eat vegetables three or more times daily (Grimm, Blanck, Scanlon, Moore, and Grummer-Strawn, 2010). The variety of fruits and vegetables eaten is also limited, with apples, oranges, and bananas accounting for almost 50% of the fruit consumed in the United States. The most commonly eaten vegetables are potatoes and iceberg lettuce. Tips for boosting fruit and vegetable intake appear in Box 5.3.

Table 5.6 Amounts of Fruits and Vegetables Recommended at Various MyPlate Calorie Levels

Total Calorie Intake	Amount of Fruit Recommended/Day (in cups)	Amount of Vegetables Recommended/Day (in cups)
1600	1.5	2
1800	1.5	2.5
2000	2	2.5
2200–2400	2	3
2600	2	3.5
2800	2.5	3.5
3000–3200	2.5	4

| Box 5.3 | TIPS FOR BOOSTING FRUIT AND VEGETABLE INTAKE |

- Eat at least five servings of fruits and vegetables every day. More is even better. Five servings of fruits and vegetables per day may provide more than 200 mg of vitamin C, far more than the RDA of 75 mg for adult women and 90 mg for adult men.
- Concentrate on variety and color. Aim for at least one green, one orange, one red, one citrus, and one legume serving every day.
- Make an effort to preserve the vitamin content of vegetables: store them in the refrigerator (except for onions, tomatoes, winter squash, and potatoes), prepare them with minimal peeling, and cook for as short a time as possible in as little water as necessary. Microwaving is a better option than boiling.
- Start at least one meal each day with a fresh salad.
- Eat raw vegetables or fresh fruits for snacks.
- Add vegetables to other foods, such as zucchini to spaghetti sauce, grated carrots to meat loaf, and spinach to lasagna.
- Double the normal portion size of vegetables.
- Buy a new fruit or vegetable when you go grocery shopping.
- Eat occasional meatless entrees such as pasta primavera, vegetable stir fry, or black beans and rice.
- Order a vegetable when you eat out.
- Choose 100% fruit juice at breakfast and during the day instead of drinks, cocktails, "-ades" (e.g., lemonade), and/or carbonated beverages.
- Eat fruit for dessert.
- Make fruits and vegetables more visible. Leave a bowl of fruit on the center of your table. Keep fresh vegetables on the top shelf of the refrigerator in plain view.

- Vitamin E is found mostly in vegetable oils, nuts, seeds, wheat germ, and green leafy vegetables. Some seafood, such as sardines, blue crab, and herring, also provide vitamin E. Although vitamin E is mentioned as a vitamin of concern, average intake among Americans may be underestimated because of (1) underreporting of total fat intake, (2) difficulty in estimating the amount of fat used in the food preparation (e.g., frying), and (3) vague ingredient lists that state "may contain one or more of the following oils" because vegetable oils differ in their vitamin E content. It is noteworthy that deficiency symptoms have never been reported in healthy people eating a low–vitamin E diet.

What About Supplements?

An estimated 54% of American adults use dietary supplements, primarily in the form of multivitamins with or without minerals (Bailey et al., 2012). This represents a slight increase in use since 1999–2000. Ironically, supplement users tend to have higher intakes of some vitamins from food than people who do not use supplements (Sebastian, Cleveland, Goldman, and Moshfegh, 2007). Data from NHANES 2003–2006 (Bailey et al., 2012) reveal that

- Supplement use is lowest among obese and overweight individuals.
- Supplement use is highest among non-Hispanic whites, older adults, and those with more than a high-school education.
- Most people who take supplements use only one; however, approximately 10% of Americans take more than five dietary supplements.
- The most commonly taken vitamins are B_6, B_{12}, C, A, and E.

Except for the population groups cited earlier, healthy people who eat a variety of nutritious foods are able to obtain an adequate and balanced intake of vitamins, other essential nutrients, and healthy food components for which no recommendations have been made. Population groups that many benefit from a multivitamin supplement include the following:

- Dieters who consume fewer than 1200 calories. Even with optimal food choices, it may not be possible to consume adequate amounts of all nutrients on a low-calorie diet.
- Vegans, who eat no animal products, need supplemental B_{12} because it is found naturally only in animal products. They may also need vitamin D if sunlight exposure is inadequate because the only plant sources of vitamin D are some fortified margarines and some fortified cereals.
- Finicky eaters and people who eliminate one or more food groups from their typical diet. For instance, someone who cannot tolerate citrus juices because of gastric reflux may not consistently obtain adequate vitamin C without the use of a vitamin supplement.
- A large proportion of adults age 51 years and older do not consume adequate amounts of many nutrients from food alone (Sebastian et al., 2007). Risk factors in this population include limited food budget, impaired chewing and swallowing, social isolation, physical limitations that make shopping or cooking difficult, or a decreased sense of taste leading to poor appetite. In addition, their vitamin requirements may be elevated as a result of chronic disease or as a side effect of certain medications. Low-dose multivitamin and mineral supplements can help meet recommended intake levels in the elderly when dietary selection is limited (Academy of Nutrition and Dietetics, 2012).
- Alcoholics, because alcohol alters vitamin intake, absorption, metabolism, and excretion; the nutrients most profoundly affected are thiamin, riboflavin, niacin, folic acid, and pantothenic acid.
- People who are food insecure, meaning they may not always have sufficient money or other resources for food for all household members.
- People with chronic illness or chronic use of a medication that impairs nutrient absorption or increases metabolism or excretion (American Dietetic Association, 2009).

Are Supplements a Good Idea?

While there is little scientific evidence to suggest that vitamin supplements can benefit the average person, there is also little evidence of harm from low-dose multivitamin or multivitamin and mineral supplements. Because vitamins work best together and in balanced proportions, a multivitamin that provides no more than 100% of the daily value (DV) is usually better than single-vitamin supplements that tend to provide doses much greater than the RDA. Remember that pills are not a substitute for healthy food: "supplement" means "add to," not "replace."

The U.S. Food and Drug Administration (FDA) requires a standardized "Supplement Facts" label on all supplements (Fig. 5.4). Like the "Nutrition Facts" label, the supplement label is intended to provide consumers with better information. However, beware of label claims: because the FDA does not closely regulate the supplement industry, manufacturers' claims may be less than reliable and not defined (Box 5.4). In fact, the term "multivitamin" does not have a standard regulatory definition (Yetley, 2007).

Although multivitamins are generally safe, excessive intakes of certain vitamins can be potentially harmful. According to NHANES 2003–2006 data, supplement users had

Cost is not an indication of quality. Large retail chains are high volume customers and can demand their own top-quality, private label supplements that are comparable to brand name varieties in quality and content.

For most people, choose a multivitamin that provides no more than 100% Daily Value for the 13 vitamins (and 8 minerals) for which there are established Daily Values. Note: Daily Values are the same as the 1968 USRDA and may not accurately reflect current DRI's.

USP on the label means the product passes tests for disintegration, dissolution, strength and purity. Does not ensure that the supplement is safe or beneficial to health.

Complete ingredient list must be stated.

Made to U.S. Pharmacopia (USP) quality, purity, and potency standards. Laboratory tested to dissolve within 60 minutes.

Serving size (and calories per serving, if any) must be stated.

Ingredients: Cellulose, Ascorbic acid, cornstarch, dl-Alpha Tocophenyl acetate, Niacinamide, Stearic acid, Maltodextrin, Gelatin, d-Calcium Panthothenate, Pyridoxine hydrochloride, Sucrose, Riboflavin, Vitamin A acetate, Thiamine mononitrate, Lycopene, Folic Acid, Beta Carotene, dl-Alpha Tocopherol, Biotin, Cyanocobalamin, Ergocalciferol.

Supplement Facts
Serving Size 1 Tablet

Each Tablet Contains		% DV
Vitamin A	3500 iu	70%
14% as beta carotene		
Vitamin C	90 mg	150%
Vitamin D	400 iu	100%
Vitamin E	45 iu	150%
Vitamin K	20 mcg	25%
Thiamin (B_1)	1.2 mg	80%
Riboflavin (B_2)	1.7 mg	100%
Niacin (B_3)	16 mg	80%
Vitamin B_6	3 mg	150%
Folic Acid	400 mcg	100%
Vitamin B_{12}	18 mcg	300%
Biotin	30 mcg	10%
Pantothenic Acid	5 mg	50%
Lycopene	0.6 mg	*

* Daily Value not established

Median US intake of these B vitamins meets or exceeds recommendations; they aren't dangerous but probably aren't necessary.

Deficiencies of these vitamins almost never occur. They are not necessary.

Ingredients not proven to be important to health must appear at the bottom and be separated from established nutrients by a solid line.

dl-Alpha Tocopherol is the synthetic form of Vitamin E and is less well absorbed than natural Vitamin E labeled d-Alpha Tocopherol.

The amount of nutrient present and the % Daily Value must be listed.

FRESHNESS AND POTENCY GUARANTEED THROUGH JUN 2017

Beyond this date the ingredients may no longer meet standards of purity, strength, and/or quality.

Manufacturers are free to put in or leave out whatever nutrients they choose

For ingredients that do not have a Daily Value, an asterisk must be used to indicate there is no official recommendation for that substance.

■ FIGURE 5.4   Sample supplement label.

Box 5.4   SUPPLEMENT LABELING LINGO

"High potency," at least to the FDA, means that at least two-thirds of the product's nutrients are provided at 100% of the DV. To most people, high potency means more than the DV.

"Advanced," "Complete," or "Maximum" formulas are not defined; manufacturers can use those terms as desired.

"Clinically proven" is also not defined.

"Mature" or "50+" formulas usually have less iron and vitamin K. While seniors do need less iron, the need for vitamin K does not decrease with aging. In fact, vitamin K may help prevent hip fractures. However, people using anticoagulants should strive for a consistent vitamin K intake.

"Women's" formulas have 18 mg of iron, which is appropriate for premenopausal women. Postmenopausal women need around 8 mg, which is the same amount of iron as men need.

"Energy" multivitamins may contain caffeine for "energy" or simply B vitamins based on the industry-promoted myth that B vitamins provide extra energy.

a higher prevalence of excessive intakes for vitamin A and folic acid (Bailey et al., 2012). Excess vitamin A is associated with headaches, liver damage, and reduced bone strength; excess folic acid can mask the hematologic signs of a vitamin B_{12} deficiency, perhaps delaying the diagnosis of B_{12} deficiency until neurologic impairments are irreversible. With vitamins, more is not necessarily better.

HOW DO YOU RESPOND?

Is it better to take vitamin supplements with meals or between meals? In general, it is better to take supplements with meals because food enhances the absorption of some vitamins.

Should I choose vitamin-fortified foods over those that are not fortified? For the most part, fortified foods are a good bet. Fortified milk and fortified cereals provide nutrients (vitamin D and iron, respectively) that otherwise may not be consumed in adequate amounts by some people. On the other hand, a vitamin-fortified candy bar is still a candy bar. Be aware of slick marketing techniques that might lead you to believe that junk food with vitamins is healthy.

I am under a lot of emotional stress. Should I take stress vitamins? Although significant physical stress (e.g., thermal injury, trauma) increases the requirements for certain vitamins, mental stress does not. Misleading advertising is to blame for this widespread misconception.

▣ CASE STUDY

Michael is a 22-year-old college student who lives off campus. Although he has a kitchen in his apartment, he has neither the time nor the interest in making his own food or stocking his own kitchen. All three of his daily meals come from fast-food restaurants. A typical day's intake is as follows:

Breakfast:	Two egg and bacon sandwiches on English muffins Large coffee with creamer and sugar
Lunch:	Two cheeseburgers with catsup Large French fries Soft drink Cookies
Dinner:	A foot-long submarine with cold cuts, cheese, mayonnaise, lettuce, tomato, onion, and pickles Bag of potato chips Soft drink
Snacks:	Chocolate bar Chips and salsa Popcorn

- What vitamins is Michael probably lacking in his diet? What vitamins is he probably getting enough of?
- Are there better choices he could make at fast-food restaurants that would improve his vitamin intake?
- What suggestions would you make for keeping "quick" and "easy" food in his apartment that would improve his vitamin intake without being too much "bother"?
- How would you respond to this question from Michael: "Can I just take a multivitamin so I don't have to make changes in my eating habits?"

STUDY QUESTIONS

1. When developing a teaching plan for a client who is on warfarin (Coumadin), which of the following foods would the nurse suggest the client consume a consistent intake of because of their vitamin K content?
   a. Liver, milk, and eggs
   b. Brussels sprouts, cauliflower, and spinach
   c. Fortified cereals, whole grains, and nuts
   d. Dried peas and beans, wheat germ, and seeds

2. A client asks if it is better to consume folic acid from fortified foods or from a vitamin pill. Which of the following is the nurse's best response?
   a. "It is better to consume folic acid through fortified foods because it will be better absorbed than through pill form."
   b. "It is better to consume folic acid through vitamin pills because it will be better absorbed than through fortified foods."
   c. "Fortified foods and vitamin pills have the same form of folic acid, so it does not matter which source you use because they are both well absorbed."
   d. "It is best to consume naturally rich sources of folate because that form is better absorbed than the folic acid in either fortified foods or vitamin pills."

3. Which population is at risk for combined deficiencies of thiamin, riboflavin, and niacin?
   a. Pregnant women
   b. Vegetarians
   c. Alcoholics
   d. Athletes

4. Which vitamin is given in large doses to facilitate wound and bone healing?
   a. Vitamin A
   b. Vitamin D
   c. Vitamin C
   d. Niacin

5. Which statement indicates that the client understands the instruction about using a vitamin supplement?
   a. "USP on the label guarantees safety and effectiveness."
   b. "Natural vitamins are always better for you than synthetic vitamins."
   c. "Vitamins are best absorbed on an empty stomach."
   d. "Taking a multivitamin cannot make up for poor food choices."

6. The client asks if taking supplements of beta-carotene will help reduce the risk of cancer. Which of the following would be the nurse's best response?
   a. "Supplements of beta-carotene may help reduce the risk of heart disease but not of cancer."
   b. "Supplements of beta-carotene have not been shown to lower the risk of cancer and may even promote cancer in certain people."
   c. "Although evidence is preliminary, taking beta-carotene supplements is safe and may prove to be effective against cancer in the future."
   d. "Natural supplements of beta-carotene are generally harmless; synthetic supplements of beta-carotene may increase cancer risk and should be avoided."

7. A client is diagnosed with pernicious anemia. What vitamin is he not absorbing?
   a. Folic acid
   b. Vitamin B_6
   c. Vitamin B_{12}
   d. Niacin

8. A client with hyperlipidemia is prescribed niacin. The client asks if he can just include more niacin-rich foods in his diet and forgo the need for niacin in pill form. Which of the following would be the nurse's best response?
   a. "The dose of niacin needed to treat hyperlipidemia is far more than can be consumed through eating a niacin-rich diet."
   b. "You can't get the therapeutic form of niacin through food."
   c. "Niacin from food is not as well absorbed as niacin from pills."
   d. "If you are able to consistently choose niacin-fortified foods in your diet, your doctor may allow you to forgo the pills and rely on dietary sources of niacin."

KEY CONCEPTS

■ Vitamins do not provide energy (calories), but they are needed for metabolism of energy. Most vitamins function as coenzymes to activate enzymes.

■ The body needs vitamins in small amounts (microgram or milligram quantities). Vitamins are essential in the diet because they cannot be made by the body or they are synthesized in inadequate amounts.

■ Fortification and enrichment have virtually eliminated vitamin deficiencies in healthy Americans.

■ It is assumed that if a variety of nutritious foods are consumed, the diet's vitamin content will generally be adequate for most people.

■ Vitamins are organic compounds that are soluble in either water or fat; their solubility determines how they are absorbed, transported through the blood, stored, and excreted.

■ Vitamins A, D, E, and K are the fat-soluble vitamins. Because they are stored in liver and adipose tissue, they do not need to be consumed daily. Vitamins A and D are toxic when consumed in large quantities over a long period.

■ The B-complex vitamins and vitamin C are water-soluble vitamins. Although some tissues are able to hold limited amounts of certain water-soluble vitamins, they are not generally stored in the body, so a daily intake is necessary. Because they are not stored, they are considered nontoxic; however, adverse side effects can occur from taking megadoses of certain water-soluble vitamins over a prolonged period.

■ Phytochemicals are substances produced by plants to protect them from bacteria, viruses, and fungi. They add color, flavor, and aroma to foods. In the body, they impart important physiologic effects that may reduce the risk of chronic diseases.

■ Not enough is known about phytochemicals to elevate them to the status of essential nutrients. Research is needed to determine which phytochemicals are protective, what quantity is optimal for health, and how they interact with other substances. Until then, the best advice is to eat a varied diet rich in fruits and vegetables.

■ Antioxidant vitamins in foods are suspected of being beneficial, but high-dose supplements have not been proven to prevent disease and may disrupt nutrient balances. Long-term safety has not been established; some reports indicate that single-nutrient supplements may actually increase, not decrease, health risks.

■ It is recommended that women who are capable of becoming pregnant consume 400 μg of folic acid through supplements or fortified food daily. People older than the age of 50 years are urged to consume most of their B_{12} requirement from supplements or fortified food. Vegans need supplemental vitamin D, if exposure to sunshine is inadequate, and also supplemental vitamin B_{12}.

■ Multivitamin supplements provide a limited safeguard when food choices are less than optimal. Other groups who may benefit from taking a daily multivitamin are the elderly, dieters, finicky eaters, and alcoholics.

■ People who choose to take an all-purpose multivitamin should select one that provides 100% of the DV for vitamins with an established DV. The USP stamp ensures the quality but not safety or benefits. High-cost supplements are not necessarily superior to lower cost ones.

Check Your Knowledge Answer Key

1. **FALSE** In theory, most healthy adults should be able to obtain all the nutrients they need by choosing a varied diet of nutrient-dense foods. Exceptions include the following: (1) people older than 50 years should consume synthetic vitamin B_{12} from fortified food or supplements, (2) women who are capable of becoming pregnant need synthetic folic acid, and (3) anyone who obtains insufficient sunlight exposure needs supplemental vitamin D.

2. **FALSE** Vitamins are needed to release energy from carbohydrates, protein, and fat but are not a source of energy (calories).

3. **FALSE** Adverse side effects can occur from taking large doses of certain water-soluble vitamins over a long period of time. For instance, adverse effects can be seen from large doses of B_6 (neuropathy) and niacin (flushing).

4. **TRUE** Vitamins differ in their vulnerability to air, heat, light, acids, and alkalis. Proper food handling and storage, especially of fruits and vegetables, are needed to preserve vitamin content.

5. **FALSE** Cost and quality are not necessarily related.

6. **FALSE** "Natural" vitamins are not naturally better.

7. **TRUE** Under optimal conditions, such as exposing unprotected skin to the sun for several minutes, the body can make all the vitamin D it needs provided that kidney and liver functions are normal. However, sunscreen, smog, dark skin, clothing, and dense cloud cover hinder vitamin D synthesis.

8. **FALSE** Natural folate in foods is only half as available to the body as synthetic folic acid.

9. **FALSE** USP on a vitamin label means that the product passes tests that evaluate disintegration, dissolution, strength, and purity. It does not mean the product is safe. For instance, large doses of vitamin A are not safe, but they may have USP on the label.

10. **FALSE** Because fat-soluble vitamins are stored, a daily intake is not considered essential. It is recommended that water-soluble vitamins be consumed daily because they are not stored in the body.

Student Resources on thePoint

For additional learning materials, activate the code in the front of this book at
http://thePoint.lww.com/activate

Websites

Dietary Reference Intakes from the Institute of Medicine at **www.nap.edu**
Produce for Better Health Foundation at **www.fruitsandveggiesmorematters.org**
U.S. Department of Agriculture National Nutrient Database for Standard Reference Nutrient Lists at **http://www.nal.usda.gov/fnic/foodcomp/Data/SR15/wtrank/wt_rank.html**

References

Academy of Nutrition and Dietetics. (2012). Position of the Academy of Nutrition and Dietetics: Food and nutrition for older adults: Promoting health and wellness. *Journal of the Academy of Nutrition and Dietetics, 112*, 1255–1277.

Allen, L. (2009). How common is B12 deficiency? *American Journal of Clinical Nutrition, 89*, 712S–716S.

The Alpha-Tocopherol, Beta-Carotene Cancer Prevention Study Group. (1994). The effect of vitamin D and beta carotene on the incidence of lung cancer and other cancers in small smokers. *The New England Journal of Medicine, 330*, 1029–1035.

American Dietetic Association. (2009). Position of the American Dietetic Association: Nutrient supplementation. *Journal of the American Dietetic Association, 109*, 2073–2085.

American Heart Association. (2012). *Homocysteine, folic acid and cardiovascular disease.* Available at www.heart.org/HEARTORG/GettingHealthy/NutritionCenter/Homocysteine-Folic-Acid-and-Cardiovascular-Disease_UCM_305997_Article.jsp. Accessed on 9/14/12.

Ascherio, A., Munger, K., & Simon, K. (2010). Vitamin D and multiple sclerosis. *Lancet Neurology, 6*, 599–612.

Bailey, R., Fulgoni, V., Keast, D., & Dwyer, J. (2012). Examination of vitamin intakes among US adults by dietary supplement use. *Journal of the Academy of Nutrition and Dietetics, 112*, 657–663.

Bender, D. (2011). Vitamin B6: Beyond adequacy. *Journal of Evidence-Based Complementary and Alternative Medicine, 16*, 29–39.

Bennink, H., & Schreurs, W. (1975). Improvement of oral glycose tolerance in gestational diabetes by pyridoxine. *British Medical Journal, 3*, 13–15.

Bertone-Johnson, E., Powers, S., Spangler, L., Brunner, R. L., Michael, Y. L., Larson, J. C., . . . Manson, J. E. (2011). Vitamin D intake from foods and supplements and depressive symptomsin a diverse population of older women. *American Journal of Clinical Nutrition, 94*, 1104–1112.

Bønaa, K., Njølstad, I., Ueland, P., Schirmer, H., Tverdal, A., Steigen, T., . . . Rasmussen, K. (2006). Homocysteine lowering and cardiovascular events after acute myocardial infarction. *The New England Journal of Medicine, 354*, 1578–1588.

Clarke, R., & Armitage, J. (2000). Vitamin supplements and cardiovascular risk: Review of the randomized trials of homocysteine-lowering vitamin supplements. *Seminars in Thrombosis Hemostasis, 26*, 341–348.

Cole, B., Baron, J., Sandler, R., Haile, R. W., Ahnen, D. J., Bresalier, R. S., . . . Greenberg, E. R. (2007). Folic acid for the prevention of colorectal adenomas: A randomized clinical trial. *Journal of the American Medical Association, 297*, 2351–2359.

Davis, C. (2008). Vitamin D and cancer: Current dilemmas and future research needs. *American Journal of Clinical Nutrition, 88*, 565S–569S.

Ebbing, M., Bonaa, K., Nygard, O., Arnesen, E., Ueland, P. M., Nordrehaug, J. E., . . . Vollset, S. E. (2009). Cancer incidence and mortality after treatment with folic acid and vitamin B12. *Journal of the American Medical Association, 302*, 2119–2126.

Elias, M., Sullivan, L., D'Agostino, R., Elias, P. K., Jacques, P. F., Selhub, J., . . . Wolf, P. A. (2005). Homocysteine and cognitive performance in the Framingham offspring study: Age is important. *American Journal of Epidemiology, 162*, 644–653.

Food and Nutrition Board, Institute of Medicine. (1997). *Dietary Reference Intakes for calcium, phosphorus, magnesium, vitamin D, and fluoride.* Washington, DC: National Academies Press.

Food and Nutrition Board, Institute of Medicine. (1998). *Dietary Reference Intakes for thiamin, riboflavin, niacin, vitamin B$_6$, folate, vitamin B$_{12}$, pantothenic acid, biotin, and choline.* Washington, DC: National Academies Press.

Food and Nutrition Board, Institute of Medicine. (2000). *Dietary Reference Intakes for vitamin C, vitamin E, selenium, and carotenoids.* Washington, DC: National Academies Press.

Fragakis, A., & Thomson, C. (2007). *The health professional's guide to popular dietary supplements* (3rd ed.). Chicago, IL: American Dietetic Association.

Fung, G., Steffan, L., Zhou, X., Harnack, L., Tang, W., Lutsey, P. L., . . . Van Horn, L. V. (2012). Vitamin D intake is inversely related to risk of developing metabolic syndrome in African American and white men and women over 20 y: The Coronary Artery Risk Development in Young Adults study. *American Journal of Clinical Nutrition, 96*, 24–29.

Garland, C., Garland, F., Gorham, E., Lipkin, M., Newmark, H., Mohr, S. B., & Holick, M. F. (2006). The role of vitamin D in cancer prevention. *American Journal of Public Health, 96*, 252–261.

Gaziano, J. (2004). Vitamin E and cardiovascular disease: Observational studies. *Annals of the New York Academy of Science, 1031*, 280–291.

Gorham, E., Garland, C., Garland, F., Grant, W. B., Mohr, S. B., Lipkin, M., . . . Holick, M. F. (2007). Optimal vitamin D status for colorectal cancer prevention: A quantitative meta-analysis. *American Journal of Preventive Medicine, 32*, 210–216.

Green, A., Williams, G., Neale, R., Hart, V., Leslie, D., Parsons, P., . . . Russell, A. (1999). Daily sunscreen application and beta-carotene supplementation in prevention of basal-cell and squamous-cell carcinomas of the skin: A randomized controlled trial. *The Lancet, 354*, 723–729.

Grimm, K., Blanck, H., Scanlon, K., Moore, L., & Grummer-Strawn, L. (2010). State-specific trends in fruit and vegetable consumption among adults—United States, 2000–2009. *Morbidity and Mortality Weekly Report, 59*, 1125–1130.

Hollenbeck, C. (2010). The importance of being choline. *Journal of the American Dietetic Association, 110*, 1162–1165.

Humphrey, L., Fu, R., Rogers, K., Freeman, M., & Helfand, M. (2008). Homocysteine level and coronary heart disease incidence: A systematic review and meta-analysis. *Mayo Clinic Proceedings, 83*, 1203–1212.

Hypponen, E., Boucher, B., Berry, D., & Power, C. (2008). 25-Hydroxyvitamin D, IGF-1, and metabolic syndrome at 45 years of age: A cross-sectional study in the 1958 British Birth Cohort. *Diabetes, 57*, 298–305.

Institute of Medicine. (1998). *Dietary Reference Intakes for thiamin, riboflavin, niacin, vitamin B$_6$, pantothenic acid, biotin, and choline.* Washington, DC: National Academies Press.

Institute of Medicine. (2011). *Dietary reference intakes for calcium and vitamin D.* Washington, DC: National Academies Press.

Jewell, D., & Young, G. (2003). Interventions for nausea and vomiting in early pregnancy. *Cochrane Database of Systematic Reviews, 4*, CD000145.

Klein, E., Thompson, I., Tangen, C., Crowley, J. J., Lucia, M. S., Goodman, P. J., . . . Baker, L. H. (2011). Vitamin E and the risk of prostate cancer: The Selenium and Vitamin E Cancer Prevention Trial (SELECT). *Journal of the American Medical Association, 306*, 1549–1556.

Larsson, S., Orsini, N., & Wolk, A. (2010). Vitamin B6 and risk of colorectal cancer: A meta-analysis of prospective studies. *Journal of the American Medical Association, 303*, 1077–1083.

Lee, I., Cook, N., Manson, J., Buring, J. E., & Hennekens, C. H. (1999). Beta-carotene supplementation and incidence of cancer and cardiovascular disease: The Women's Health Study. *Journal of the National Cancer Institute, 91*, 2101–2106.

Lonn, E., Yusuf, S., Arnold, M. J., Sheridan, P., Pogue, J., Micks, M., . . . Genest, J., Jr. (2006). Homocysteine lowering with folic acid and B vitamins in vascular disease. *The New England Journal of Medicine, 354*, 1567–1577.

McCully, L. (2007). Homocysteine, vitamins, and vascular disease prevention. *American Journal of Clinical Nutrition, 86*, 1563S–1568S.

Medical Research Council Vitamin Study Research Group. (1991). Prevention of neural tube defects: Results of the Medical Research Council Vitamin Study. *The Lancet, 338*, 131–137.

Miller, E. R., III, Pastor-Barriuso, R., Dalal, D., Riemersma, R. A., Appel, L. J., & Guallar, E. (2005). Meta-analysis: High-dosage vitamin E supplementation may increase all-cause mortality. *Annals of Internal Medicine, 142*, 37–46.

Mooney, S., Leuendorf, J., Hendrickson, C., & Hellmann, H. (2009). Vitamin B6: A long known compound of surprising complexity. *Molecules, 14*, 329–351.

Morris, M., Jacques, P., Rosenberg, I., and Selhub, J. (2007). Folate and vitamin B12 status in relation to anemia, macrocytosis, and cognitive impairment in older Americans in the age of folic acid fortification. *American Journal of Clinical Nutrition, 85*, 193–200.

Munger, K., Levin, L., Hollis, B., Howard, N. S., & Ascherio, A. (2006). Serum 25-hydroxyvitamin D levels and risk of multiple sclerosis. *Journal of the American Medical Association, 296*, 2832–2838.

Omenn, G. S., Goodman, G. E., Thornquist, M. D., Balmes, J., Cullen, M. R., Glass, A., . . . Hammar, S. (1996). Effects of a combination of beta carotene and vitamin A on lung cancer and cardiovascular disease. *The New England Journal of Medicine, 334*, 1150–1155.

Palomer, X., Gonzalex-Clemente, J., Blanco-Vaca, F., & Mauricio, D. (2008). Role of vitamin D in the pathogenesis of type 2 diabetes mellitus. *Diabetes, Obesity, and Metabolism, 10*, 185–197.

Peters, E. M., Goetzsche, J. M., Grobbelaar, B., & Noakes, T. D. (1993). Vitamin C supplementation reduces the incidence of postrace symptoms of upper-respiratory-tract infection in ultramarathon runners. *American Journal of Clinical Nutrition, 57*, 170–174.

Pilz, S., Tomaschitz, A., Ritz, E., & Pieber, T. (2009). Vitamin D status and arterial hypertension: A systematic review. *Nature Reviews Cardiology, 6*, 621–630.

Reynolds, E. (2006). Vitamin B12, folic acid, and the nervous system. *Lancet Neurology, 5*, 949–960.

Ross, A., Manson, J., Abrams, S., Aloia, J. F., Brannon, P. M., Clinton, S. K., . . . Shapses, S. A. (2011). The 2011 report on Dietary Reference Intakes for calcium and vitamin D from the Institute of Medicine: What clinicians need to know. *Journal of Clinical Endocrinology and Metabolism, 96*, 53–58.

Sebastian, R., Cleveland, L., Goldman, J., & Moshfegh, A. (2007). Older adults who use vitamin/mineral supplements differ from nonusers in nutrient intake adequacy and dietary attitudes. *Journal of the American Dietetic Association, 107*, 1322–1332.

Spellacy, W., Buhi, W., & Birk, S. (1977). Vitamin B6 treatment of gestational diabetes mellitus: Studies of blood glucose and plasma inulin. *American Journal of Obstetrics and Gynecology, 127*, 599–602.

Sung, L., Greenberg, M., Koren, G., Tomlinson, G. A., Tong, A., Malkin, D., & Feldman, B. M. (2003). Vitamin E: The evidence for multiple roles in cancer. *Nutrition and Cancer, 46*, 1–14.

Tai, K., Need, A., Horowitz, M., & Chapman, I. (2008). Vitamin D, glucose, insulin, and insulin sensitivity. *Nutrition, 24*, 279–285.

Tighe, P., Ward, M., McNulty, H., Finnegan, O., Dunne, A., Strain, J., . . . Scott, J. M. (2011). A dose-finding trial of the effect of long-term folic acid intervention: Implications for food fortification policy. *American Journal of Clinical Nutrition, 93*, 11–18.

Toner, C., Davis, C., & Milner, J. (2010). The vitamin D and cancer conundrum: Aiming at a moving target. *Journal of the American Dietetic Association, 110*, 1492–1500.

Toole, J., Malinow, M., Chambless, L., Spence, J. D., Pettigrew, L. C., Howard, V. J., . . . Stampfer, M. (2004). Lowering homocysteine in patients with ischemic stroke to prevent recurrent stroke, myocardial infarction, and death. The Vitamin Intervention for Stroke Prevention (VISP) randomized controlled trial. *Journal of the American Medical Association, 291*, 565–575.

Traber, M., & Atkinson, J. (2007). Vitamin E, antioxidant and nothing more. *Free Radical Biology and Medicine, 43*, 4–15.

Tripkovic, L., Lambert, H., Hart, K., Smith, C. P., Bucca, G., Penson, S., . . . Lanham-New, S. (2012). Comparison of vitamin D2 and vitamin D3 supplementation in raising serum 25-hydroxyvitamin D status: A systematic review and meta-analysis. *American Journal of Clinical Nutrition, 95*, 1357–1364.

U.S. Department of Agriculture, U.S. Department of Health and Human Services. (2010). *Dietary guidelines for Americans, 2010* (7th ed.). Available at www.health.gov/dietaryguidelines. Accessed on 2/24/11.

Wang, X., Zin, S., Demirtas, J., Li, J., Mao, G., Huo, Y., . . . Xu, X. (2007). Efficacy of folic acid supplementation in stroke prevention: A meta-analysis. *The Lancet, 369*, 1876–1882.

Winkels, R. M., Brouwer, I. A., Siebelink, E., Katan, M. B., & Verhoef, P. (2007). Bioavailability of food folates is 80% of that of folic acid. *American Journal of Clinical Nutrition, 85*, 465–473.

World Health Organization. (2012). *Micronutrient deficiencies. Vitamin A deficiency.* Available at www.who.int/nutrition/topics/vad/en/#. Accessed on 9/13/12.

Wright, M., Lawson, K., Weinstein, S., Pietinen, P., Taylor, P. R., Virtamo, J., & Albanes, D. (2006). Higher baseline serum concentrations of vitamin D are associated with lower total and cause-specific mortality in the Alpha-Tocopherol, Beta-Carotene Cancer Prevention Study. *American Journal of Clinical Nutrition, 84*, 1200–1207.

Yetley, E. (2007). Multivitamin and multimineral dietary supplements: Definitions, characterization, bioavailability, and drug interactions. *American Journal of Clinical Nutrition, 85*, 269S–276S.

6 Water and Minerals

CHECK YOUR KNOWLEDGE

TRUE FALSE

☐ ☐ **1** Most people have an inadequate intake of fluid.

☐ ☐ **2** All minerals consumed in excess of need are excreted in the urine.

☐ ☐ **3** Sodium is the most plentiful mineral in the body.

☐ ☐ **4** An increase in sodium intake is associated with an increase in blood pressure.

☐ ☐ **5** Calcium supplements are a safe and effective way to ensure an adequate calcium intake.

☐ ☐ **6** Foods high in sodium tend to be low in potassium, and foods high in potassium tend to be low in sodium.

☐ ☐ **7** Major minerals are more important for health than trace minerals.

☐ ☐ **8** For most people, thirst is a reliable indicator of fluid needs.

☐ ☐ **9** Trace mineral balance is strongly influenced by interactions with other minerals and dietary factors.

☐ ☐ **10** A chronically low intake of calcium leads to hypocalcemia.

LEARNING OBJECTIVES

Upon completion of this chapter, you will be able to

1 Calculate a person's fluid requirement.
2 Evaluate the adequacy of fluid intake in a healthy adult.
3 Give examples of mechanisms by which the body maintains mineral homeostasis.
4 Identify sources of minerals.
5 Predict potential consequences of mineral deficiencies or toxicities.
6 Compare characteristics of minerals to those of vitamins.

W ater is fundamental to life. It is the single largest constituent of the human body, averaging approximately 60% of the total body weight. It is the medium in which all biochemical reactions take place. Although most people can survive 6 weeks or longer without food, death occurs in a matter of days without water.

OVERVIEW OF WATER

Water occupies essentially every space within and between body cells and is involved in virtually every body function. Water

- *Provides shape and structure to cells.* Approximately two-thirds of the body's water is located within cells (intracellular fluid). Muscle cells have a higher concentration of water (70%–75%) than fat, which is only about 25% water. Men generally have more muscle mass than women and, therefore, have a higher percentage of body water.
- *Regulates body temperature.* Because water absorbs heat slowly, the large amount of water contained in the body helps to maintain body temperature homeostasis despite fluctuations in environmental temperatures. Evaporation of water (sweat) from the skin cools the body.
- *Aids in the digestion and absorption of nutrients.* Approximately 7 to 9 L of water is secreted in the gastrointestinal tract daily to aid in digestion and absorption. Except for the approximately 100 mL of water excreted through the feces, all of the water contained in the gastrointestinal secretions (saliva, gastric secretions, bile, pancreatic secretions, and intestinal mucosal secretions) is reabsorbed in the ileum and colon.
- *Transports nutrients and oxygen to cells.* By moistening the air sacs in the lungs, water allows oxygen to dissolve and move into blood for distribution throughout the body. Approximately 92% of blood plasma is water.
- *Serves as a solvent for vitamins, minerals, glucose, and amino acids.* The solvating property of water is vital for health and survival.
- *Participates in metabolic reactions.* For instance, water is used in the synthesis of hormones and enzymes.
- *Eliminates waste products.* Water helps to excrete body wastes through urine, feces, and expirations.
- *Is a major component of mucus and other lubricating fluids.* Water reduces friction in joints where bones, ligaments, and tendons come in contact with each other, and it cushions contacts between internal organs that slide over one another.

Water Balance

Water balance is the dynamic state between water output and water intake. Under normal conditions, output and intake are approximately equal (Fig. 6.1).

Water Output

Insensible Water Loss: immeasurable losses.

Sensible Water Loss: measurable losses.

On average, adults lose approximately 1750 to 3000 mL of water daily. Extreme environmental temperatures (very hot or very cold), high altitude, low humidity, and strenuous exercise increase **insensible water losses** from respirations and the skin. Water evaporation from the skin is also increased by prolonged exposure to heated or recirculated air, for example, during long airplane flights. **Sensible water losses** from urine and feces make up the remaining water loss. Because the body needs to excrete a minimum of 500 mL of urine daily to rid itself of metabolic wastes, the minimum daily total fluid output is approximately 1500 mL. To maintain water balance, intake should approximate output.

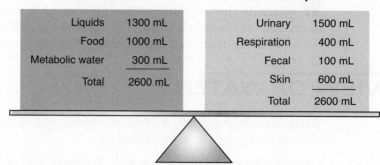

FIGURE 6.1 Water balance approximations.

Water Intake

Metabolic Water: water produced as a by-product from the breakdown of carbohydrates, protein, and fat for energy.

Total water intake averages about 2½ liters per day, of which approximately 80% is from fluids and 20% from solid food (Institute of Medicine [IOM], 2005). Box 6.1 describes various types of bottled water. Except for oils, almost all foods contain water, with fruits and vegetables providing the most (Fig. 6.2). The body also produces a small amount of water from normal metabolism: the catabolism of carbohydrates, protein, and fat for energy yields carbon and hydrogen atoms that combine with oxygen to form water and carbon dioxide. On average, 250 to 350 mL of **metabolic water** is produced daily, depending on total calorie intake.

Box 6.1	STANDARDS OF IDENTITY FOR COMMON TYPES OF BOTTLED WATER

- *Artesian water* originates from a well and is collected without mechanical pumping. The well must tap a confined aquifer, and the water level must stand at some height above the top of the aquifer. An aquifer is an underground layer of rock or sand with water.
- *Fluoridated water* has fluoride added within the limits established by the U.S. Food and Drug Administration.
- *Ground water* is from an underground source that is under pressure greater than or equal to atmospheric pressure.
- *Mineral water* contains at least 250 ppm total dissolved solids (minerals) that are naturally present, not added.
- *Purified water* is produced by distillation, deionization, reverse osmosis, or other suitable processes to remove minerals and other solids. It may also be referred to as "demineralized" water. Purified is not synonymous with "sterile."
- *Sparkling water* contains a "fizz" from carbon dioxide that was either present in the water when it emerged from its source or was present, removed in processing, and then replaced. Carbon dioxide levels cannot exceed the amount present in the original water. Seltzer, tonic water, and club soda are carbonated soft drinks that contain sugar and calories; they are not types of sparkling water.
- *Spring water* comes from an underground source that flows naturally to the surface. It must be collected at the spring or through a bored hole that taps the spring underground.
- *Sterile water* meets U.S. Pharmacopoeia (USP) requirements under "sterility tests."
- *Well water* is collected with a mechanical pump from an underground aquifer.

Source: National Science Foundation Consumer Information. (n.d.). *Types and treatment of bottled water.* Available at www.nsf.org/consumer/bottled_water/bw_types.asp?program+Bottledwat. Accessed on 9/28/12.

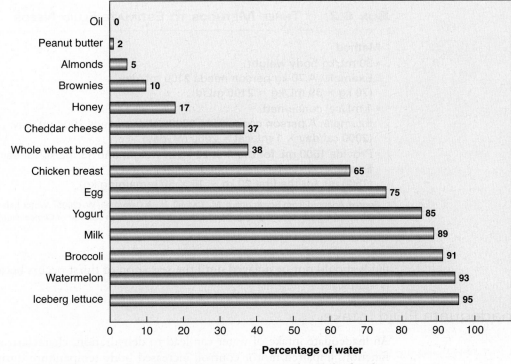

■ **FIGURE 6.2**   Percentage of water content of various foods.

Water Recommendations

Water is an essential nutrient because the body cannot produce as much water as it needs. The Dietary Reference Intake (DRI) committee on fluid and electrolytes did not establish a Recommended Dietary Allowance (RDA) for water because of insufficient evidence linking a specific amount of water intake to health; actual requirements vary depending on diet, physical activity, environmental temperatures, and humidity.

The Adequate Intake (AI) for total water, which includes water from liquids and solids, is based on the median total water intake from U.S. food consumption survey data (IOM, 2005). For men age 19 to older than 70 years, the AI is 3.7 L/day, which includes 3 L as fluids. For women of the same age, the AI is 2.7 L, which includes approximately 2.2 L from fluids. Similar to AIs set for other nutrients, daily intakes below the AI may not be harmful to healthy people because normal hydration is maintained over a wide range of intakes. Amounts higher than the AI are recommended for rigorous activity in hot climates. Because the body cannot store water, it should be consumed throughout the day.

The IOM did not specify how much of total fluid intake should come specifically from water. For healthy people, the universal, age-old advice has been to drink at least eight 8-oz glasses of water daily. Although that may be excellent advice, there is little scientific evidence to support this recommendation (Valtin, 2002). For healthy people, hydration is unconsciously maintained with ad lib access to water. In healthy adults, thirst is usually a reliable indicator of water need, and fluid intake is assumed to be adequate when the color of urine produced is pale yellow. In some conditions and for some segments of the population, the sensation of thirst is blunted and may not be a reliable indicator of need. For the elderly and children, and during hot weather or strenuous exercise, drinking

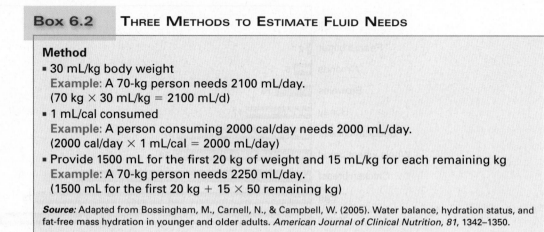

fluids should not be delayed until the sensation of thirst occurs because by then fluid loss is significant.

Inadequate Fluid Intake

An inadequate intake of water can lead to dehydration, characterized by impaired mental function, impaired motor control, increased body temperature during exercise, increased resting heart rate when standing or lying down, and an increased risk of life-threatening heat stroke. A net water loss of 1% to 2% of body weight causes thirst, fatigue, weakness, vague discomfort, and loss of appetite. A loss of 7% to 10% leads to dizziness, muscle spasticity, loss of balance, delirium, exhaustion, and collapse. Left untreated, dehydration ends in death.

Clinical situations in which water losses are increased—and thus water needs are elevated—include vomiting, diarrhea, fever, thermal injuries, uncontrolled diabetes, hemorrhage, certain renal disorders, and the use of drainage tubes. Fluid needs can be estimated by several methods (Box 6.2). Intake and output records are used to assess adequacy of intake.

Excessive Fluid Intake

A chronic high intake of water has not been shown to cause adverse effects in healthy people who consume a varied diet as long as intake approximates output (IOM, 2005). An excessive water intake may cause hyponatremia, but it is rare in healthy people who consume a typical diet. People most at risk include infants; psychiatric patients with excessive thirst; women who have undergone surgery using a uterine distention medium; and athletes in endurance events who drink too much water, fail to replace lost sodium, or both. Symptoms of hyponatremia include lung congestion, muscle weakness, lethargy, and confusion. Hyponatremia can progress to convulsions and prolonged coma. Death can result.

KEYS TO UNDERSTANDING MINERALS

Although minerals account for only about 4% of the body's total weight, they are found in all body fluids and tissues. Calcium, phosphorus, magnesium, sulfur, sodium, potassium, and chloride are considered major minerals because they are present in the body in amounts greater than 5 g (the equivalent of 1 tsp). Iron, iodine, zinc, selenium, copper, manganese, fluoride, chromium, and molybdenum are classified as trace minerals, or trace elements, because they are present in the body in amounts less than 5 g, not because they are less important than major minerals. Both groups are essential for life. As many as 30 other potentially harmful minerals are present in the body, including lead, gold, and mercury. Their presence appears to be related to environmental contamination.

General Chemistry

Inorganic: not containing carbon or concerning living things.

Unlike the energy nutrients and vitamins, minerals are **inorganic** elements that originate from the earth's crust, not from plants or animals. Minerals do not undergo digestion nor are they broken down or rearranged during metabolism. Although they combine with other elements to form salts (e.g., sodium chloride) or with organic compounds (e.g., iron in hemoglobin), they always retain their chemical identities.

Unlike vitamins, minerals are not destroyed by light, air, heat, or acids during food preparation. In fact, when food is completely burned, minerals are the ash that remains. Minerals are lost only when foods are soaked in water.

General Functions

Minerals function to provide structure to body tissues and to regulate body processes such as fluid balance, acid–base balance, nerve cell transmission, muscle contraction, and vitamin, enzyme, and hormonal activities (Table 6.1).

Table 6.1 General Functions of Minerals

Functions	Examples
Provide structure	Calcium, phosphorus, and magnesium provide structure to bones and teeth. Phosphorus, potassium, iron, and sulfur provide structure to soft tissues. Sulfur is a constituent of skin, hair, and nails.
Fluid balance	Sodium, potassium, and chloride maintain fluid balance.
Acid–base balance	Sodium hydroxide and sodium bicarbonate are part of the carbonic acid–bicarbonate system that regulates blood pH. Phosphorus is involved in buffer systems that regulate kidney tubular fluids.
Nerve cell transmission and muscle contraction	Sodium and potassium are involved in transmission of nerve impulses. Calcium stimulates muscle contractions. Sodium, potassium, and magnesium stimulate muscle relaxation.
Vitamin, enzyme, and hormone activity	Cobalt is a component of vitamin B_{12}. Magnesium is a cofactor for hundreds of enzymes. Iodine is essential for the production of thyroxine. Chromium enhances the action of insulin.

Mineral Balance

The body has several mechanisms by which it maintains mineral balance, depending on the mineral involved, such as

- *Releasing minerals from storage for redistribution*. Some minerals can be released from storage and redistributed as needed, which is what happens when calcium is released from bones to restore normal serum calcium levels.
- *Altering rate of absorption*. For example, normally only about 10% of the iron consumed is absorbed, but the rate increases to 50% when the body is deficient in iron.
- *Altering rate of excretion*. Virtually all of the sodium consumed in the diet is absorbed. The only way the body can rid itself of excess sodium is to increase urinary sodium excretion. For most people, the higher the intake of sodium, the greater is the amount of sodium excreted in the urine. Excess potassium is also excreted in the urine.

Mineral Toxicities

Minerals that are easily excreted, such as sodium and potassium, do not accumulate to toxic levels in the body under normal circumstances. Stored minerals can produce toxicity symptoms when intake is excessive, but excessive intake is not likely to occur from eating a balanced diet. Instead, mineral toxicity is related to excessive use of mineral supplements, environmental or industrial exposure, human errors in commercial food processing, or alterations in metabolism. For instance, in 2008, 200 Americans met the definition of selenium poisoning after taking an improperly manufactured dietary supplement that contained 200 times the labeled concentration of selenium (MacFarquhar et al., 2010).

Mineral Interactions

Mineral balance is influenced by hundreds of interactions that occur among minerals and between minerals and other dietary components. For instance, caffeine promotes calcium excretion, whereas vitamin D and lactose promote its absorption. Mineral status must be viewed as a function of the total diet, not just from the standpoint of the quantity consumed.

Sources of Minerals

Generally, unrefined or unprocessed foods have more minerals than refined foods. Trace mineral content varies with the content of soil from which the food originates. Within most food groups, processed foods are high in sodium and chloride. Drinking water contains varying amounts of calcium, magnesium, and other minerals; sodium is added to soften water. Fluoride may be a natural or added component of drinking water.

Mineral supplements, alone or combined with vitamins, contribute to mineral intake. As with vitamins, people who take mineral supplements have higher intakes of minerals from food than do people who do not take supplements (Baily, Fulgoni, Keast, and Dwyer, 2011). With some minerals—namely, calcium, iron, zinc, and magnesium—supplements may contribute to potentially excessive intakes (Baily et al., 2011).

MAJOR ELECTROLYTES

Sodium, chloride, and potassium are major minerals that are also major electrolytes in the body. Salient features for each electrolyte are presented in the following paragraphs.

Table 6.2 details their recommended intakes, sources, functions, and signs and symptoms of deficiency and toxicity.

Sodium

By weight, salt (sodium chloride) is approximately 40% sodium; 1 tsp of salt (5 g) provides approximately 2300 mg of sodium. It is estimated that approximately 75% of the sodium consumed in the typical American diet comes from salt or sodium preservatives added to foods by food manufacturers. Only 12% of total sodium intake is from sodium that occurs naturally in foods such as milk, meat, poultry, vegetables, tap water, and bottled water (IOM, 2005). Salt added during cooking or at the table accounts for the remaining sodium intake. Box 6.3 defines various types of salt. Wide variations in sodium intake exist between cultures and between individuals within a culture. Variations are related to the amount of processed foods consumed.

Table 6.2 Summary of Major Electrolytes

Electrolyte and Sources	Functions	Deficiency/Toxicity Signs and Symptoms
Sodium (Na) Adult AI: 19–50 yr: 1.5 g 50–70 yr: 1.3 g 71+ yr: 1.2 g Adult UL: 2.3 g ▪ Processed foods; canned meat, vegetables, soups; convenience foods; restaurant and fast foods	Fluid and electrolyte balance, acid–base balance, maintains muscle irritability, regulates cell membrane permeability and nerve impulse transmission	*Deficiency* Rare, except with chronic diarrhea or vomiting and certain renal disorders; nausea, dizziness, muscle cramps, apathy *Toxicity* Hypertension, edema
Potassium (K) Adult AI: 4.7 g No UL ▪ Canned tomato products, sweet potatoes, soy nuts, pistachios, prunes, clams, molasses, yogurt, tomato juice, prune juice, baked potatoes, cantaloupe, legumes, orange juice, bananas, peanuts, artichokes, fish, beef, lamb, avocados, apple juice, raisins, plantains, spinach, asparagus, kiwifruit, apricots	Fluid and electrolyte balance, acid–base balance, nerve impulse transmission, catalyst for many metabolic reactions, involved in skeletal and cardiac muscle activity	*Deficiency* Muscular weakness, paralysis, anorexia, confusion (occurs with dehydration) *Toxicity (from supplements/drugs)* Muscular weakness, vomiting
Chloride (Cl) Adult AI: 19–50 yr: 2.3 g 50–70 yr: 2.0 g 71+ yr: 1.8 g Adult UL: 3.6 g ▪ 1 tsp salt = 3600 mg Cl ▪ Same sources as sodium	Fluid and electrolyte balance, acid–base balance, component of hydrochloric acid in stomach	*Deficiency* Rare, may occur secondary to chronic diarrhea or vomiting and certain renal disorders: muscle cramps, anorexia, apathy *Toxicity* Normally harmless; can cause vomiting

Box 6.3   TYPES OF SALT

Table salt is a fine-grained salt from salt mines that is refined until it is pure sodium chloride. It is mainly used in cooking and at the table and may or may not contain iodine. It often contains calcium silicate to keep it free flowing.

Kosher salt is a coarse-grain salt that does not contain any additives. It is used in the preparation of kosher meat according to Jewish dietary laws. Although the terms "kosher salt" and "sea salt" are often used interchangeably, kosher salt does not necessarily originate from the sea.

Sea salt may be fine or coarse grained. It has a slightly different flavor than table salt due to its mineral content. Although it is often promoted as a healthier alternative to table salt, the sodium content is essentially the same. The advantage is that people may use less sea salt than table salt because of its more pronounced flavor. Examples include Mediterranean sea salt, Alaea (Hawaiian) sea salt, and Black salt—salts named after the originating sea.

Pickling salt is a fine-grained salt used for making pickles and sauerkraut. It does not contain additives or anticlumping agents.

Specialty salts, such as popcorn salt, come in various grains and textures and are intended for specific purposes. Generally, table salt can be substituted for these salts.

Seasoned salt is a blend of salt, herbs, and other seasoning ingredients. Examples include celery salt, onion salt, and garlic salt. The actual sodium content is lower than table salt because other ingredients dilute the concentration of sodium.

Salt substitutes have some or all of the sodium replaced with another mineral, such as potassium or magnesium. They are also referred to as lite salt. They may have a bitter or metallic aftertaste.

Rock salt is a nonedible salt of large crystals used to deice driveways and walkways. When combined with regular ice in home ice cream makers, it helps freeze homemade ice cream more quickly by absorbing heat.

Source: International Food Information Council. (2010). *IFIC review: Sodium in food and health.* Available at http://www.foodinsight.org/Resources/Detail.aspx?topic=IFIC_Review_Sodium_in_Food_and_Health. Accessed on 9/28/12.

 QUICK BITE

Examples of sodium additives
To enhance flavor
  Sodium chloride
  Monosodium glutamate (MSG)
  Soy sauce
  Teriyaki sauce
To preserve freshness
  Brine
  Sodium sulfite (for dried fruits)
To prevent the growth of yeast and/or bacteria
  Sodium benzoate
  Sodium nitrate or sodium nitrite
  Sodium lactate
  Sodium diacetate

To prevent the growth of mold
  Sodium propionate
As an antioxidant
  Sodium erythorbate
As a sweetener
  Sodium saccharin
As a binder/thickener
  Sodium caprate
  Sodium caseinate
As a leavening agent
  Sodium bicarbonate (baking soda)
  Baking powder
As a stabilizer
  Sodium citrate
  Disodium phosphate

As the major extracellular cation, sodium is largely responsible for regulating fluid balance. It also regulates cell permeability and the movement of fluid, electrolytes, glucose, insulin, and amino acids. Sodium is pivotal in acid–base balance, nerve transmission, and muscular irritability. Although sodium plays vital roles, under normal conditions, the amount actually needed is very small, maybe even less than 200 mg/day.

Almost 98% of all sodium consumed is absorbed, yet humans are able to maintain homeostasis over a wide range of intakes, largely through urinary excretion. A salty meal causes a transitory increase in serum sodium, which triggers thirst. Drinking fluids dilutes the sodium in the blood to normal concentration, even though the volume of both sodium and fluid are increased. The increased volume stimulates the kidneys to excrete more sodium and fluid together to restore normal blood volume. Conversely, low blood volume or low extracellular sodium stimulates the hormone aldosterone to increase sodium reabsorption by the kidneys. In people who have minimal sweat losses, sodium intake and sodium excretion are approximately equal.

An AI for sodium is set at 1500 mg/day for young adults to ensure that the total diet provides adequate amounts of other essential nutrients and to compensate for sodium lost in sweat in unacclimatized people who are exposed to high temperatures or who become physically active. For men and women aged 50 to 70 years, the AI is 1300 mg, and after age 70 years, AI decreases to 1200 mg. An Upper Limit (UL) for adults is set at 2300 mg/day.

Regardless of age or gender, Americans consume more sodium than recommended (U.S. Department of Agriculture [USDA], U.S. Department of Health and Human Services [USDHHS], 2010). According to National Health and Nutrition Examination Survey (NHANES) 2007–2008 data, mean intake of sodium among adult men and women age 20 years and older is 4043 and 2884 mg/day, respectively. Figure 6.3 shows the relationship between the AI and UL for sodium and the sodium content of selected foods.

Potassium

Most of the body's potassium is located in the cells as the major cation of the intracellular fluid. The remainder is in the extracellular fluid, where it works to maintain fluid balance, maintain acid–base balance, transmit nerve impulses, catalyze metabolic reactions, aid in carbohydrate metabolism and protein synthesis, and control skeletal muscle contractility.

Potassium is naturally present in most foods, such as fruits, vegetables, whole grains, meats, milk, and yogurt. Processed foods, such as cheeses, processed meats, breads, soups, fast foods, pastries, and sugary items, have a higher sodium-to-potassium ratio (Bussemaker, Hillebrand, Hausberg, Pavenstädt, and Oberleithner, 2010). Unlike sodium, potassium content is not required on the Nutrition Facts label, eliminating the option of comparison shopping.

The AI for potassium is set at 4.7 g/day for all adults, a level believed necessary to maintain lower blood pressure levels, lessen the adverse effects of high sodium intake on blood pressure, reduce the risk of kidney stones, and possibly reduce bone loss. Indeed, moderate potassium deficiency, which typically occurs without hypokalemia, is characterized by increased blood pressure, increased salt sensitivity, increased risk of kidney stones, and increased bone turnover (IOM, 2005). An inadequate potassium intake may also increase the risk of cardiovascular disease, particularly stroke. Most American adults consume only half to two-thirds of the recommended potassium intake: mean intake is 3026 mg for men and 2290 mg for women (USDA, Agricultural Research Service [ARS], 2010). In healthy people with normal kidney function, a high intake of potassium does not lead to

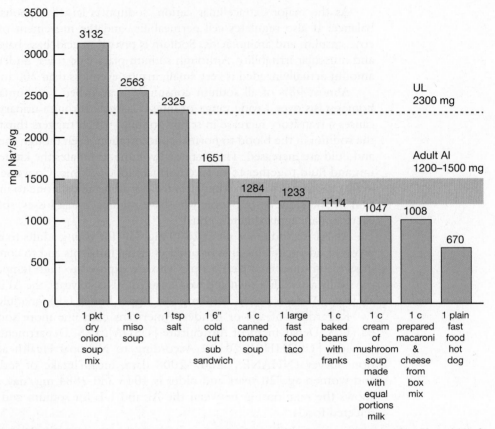

FIGURE 6.3 The sodium content of selected foods compared to the AI and UL for sodium.

an elevated serum potassium concentration because the hormone aldosterone promotes urinary potassium excretion to keep serum levels within normal range. Therefore, a UL has not been set. However, when potassium excretion is impaired (e.g., secondary to diabetes, chronic kidney insufficiency, end-stage kidney disease, severe heart failure, or adrenal insufficiency), high potassium intakes can lead to hyperkalemia and life-threatening cardiac arrhythmias.

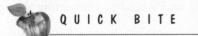

QUICK BITE

Average potassium content by food group

	mg K/serving
Grains (except bran or whole wheat)	35 mg/1 slice bread or ¾ cup most ready-to-eat cereals
Vegetables	0–350 mg/½ cup of most
Fruit	0–350 mg/½ cup or 1 small to medium piece fresh fruit
Milk	370 mg/cup
Meat (not including dried peas and beans)	100 mg/oz
Butter, margarine, oil	10 mg/tsp

Chloride

Chloride is the major anion in the extracellular fluid, where it helps to maintain fluid and electrolyte balance in conjunction with sodium. Chloride is an essential component of hydrochloric acid in the stomach and, therefore, plays a role in digestion and acid–base balance. Its concentration in most cells is low.

Because almost all the chloride in the diet comes from salt (sodium chloride), the AI for chloride is set at a level equivalent (on a molar basis) to that of sodium. The AI for younger adults is 2.3 g/day, the equivalent to 3.8 g/day of salt or 1500 mg sodium. Sodium and chloride share dietary sources, conditions that cause them to become depleted in the body, and signs and symptoms of deficiency.

MAJOR MINERALS

The remaining major minerals are calcium, phosphorus, magnesium, and sulfur. They are summarized in Table 6.3; additional salient information appears in the following section.

Calcium

Calcium is the most plentiful mineral in the body, making up about half of the body's total mineral content. Almost all of the body's calcium (99%) is found in bones and teeth, where it combines with phosphorus, magnesium, and other minerals to provide rigidity and structure. Bones serve as a large, dynamic reservoir of calcium that readily releases calcium when serum levels drop; this helps to maintain blood calcium levels within normal limits when calcium intake is inadequate. The remaining 1% of calcium in the body is found in plasma and other body fluids, where it has important roles in blood clotting, nerve transmission, muscle contraction and relaxation, cell membrane permeability, and the activation of certain enzymes. Calcium balance—or, more accurately, calcium balance in the blood—is achieved through the action of vitamin D and hormones. When blood calcium levels fall, the parathyroid gland secretes parathormone (PTH), which promotes calcium reabsorption in the kidneys and stimulates the release of calcium from bones. Vitamin D has the same effects on the kidneys and bones and additionally increases the absorption of calcium from the gastrointestinal tract. Together, the actions of PTH and vitamin D restore low blood calcium levels to normal, even though bone calcium content may fall. A chronically low calcium intake compromises bone integrity without affecting blood calcium levels. When blood calcium levels are too high, the thyroid gland secretes calcitonin, which promotes the formation of new bone by taking excess calcium from the blood. A high calcium intake does not lead to hypercalcemia but rather maximizes bone density. Abnormal blood concentrations of calcium occur from alterations in the secretion of PTH.

An adequate calcium intake throughout the first three decades of life is needed to attain peak bone mass as determined by genetics. A dense bone mass offers protection against the inevitable net bone loss that occurs in all people after the age of about 35 years. In the United States, an estimated 72% of calcium intake comes from milk, cheese, yogurt, and foods containing dairy products, such as pizza (IOM, 2011). People who avoid dairy products are challenged to consume adequate calcium because although calcium is well absorbed from some plants, the total amount of calcium provided is much lower than in dairy foods. Fortified ready-to-eat breakfast cereals and calcium-fortified orange juice are excellent sources of calcium.

Table 6.3 Summary of Major Minerals

Mineral and Sources	Functions	Deficiency/Toxicity Signs and Symptoms
Calcium (Ca) *Adult RDA* 19–50 yr: 1000 mg 51–70 yr (men): 1000 mg 51–70 yr (women): 1200 mg 71+ yr: 1200 mg Adult UL: 19–50 yr: 2500 mg 51+ yr: 2000 mg ▪ Milk, yogurt, hard natural cheese, bok choy, broccoli, Chinese/Napa cabbage, collards, kale, okra, turnip greens, fortified breakfast cereal, fortified orange juice, legumes, fortified soy milk, almonds Less well-absorbed sources: spinach, beet greens, Swiss chard	Bone and teeth formation and maintenance, blood clotting, nerve transmission, muscle contraction and relaxation, cell membrane permeability, blood pressure	*Deficiency* Children: impaired growth Adults: osteoporosis *Toxicity* Constipation, increased risk of renal stone formation, impaired absorption of iron and other minerals
Phosphorus (P) *Adult RDA* Men and women: 700 mg Adult UL: To age 70: 4 g/day 70+ yr: 3 g/day ▪ All animal products (meat, poultry, eggs, milk), ready-to-eat cereal, dried peas and beans; bran and whole grains; raisins, prunes, dates	Bone and teeth formation and maintenance, acid–base balance, energy metabolism, cell membrane structure, regulation of hormone and coenzyme activity	*Deficiency* Unknown *Toxicity* Low blood calcium

Magnesium (Mg)
Adult RDA
Men:
  19–30 yr: 400 mg
  31+ yr: 420 mg
Women:
  19–30 yr: 310 mg
  31+ yr: 320 mg
Adult UL: 350 mg/day from supplements only (does not include intake from food and water)
▪ Spinach, beet greens, okra, Brazil nuts, almonds, cashews, bran cereal, dried peas and beans, halibut, tuna, chocolate, cocoa
	Bone formation, nerve transmission, smooth muscle relaxation, protein synthesis, carbohydrate metabolism, enzyme activity	*Deficiency*
		Weakness, confusion; growth failure in children
		Severe deficiency: convulsions, hallucinations, tetany
		Toxicity
		No toxicity demonstrated from food
		Supplemental Mg can cause diarrhea, nausea, and cramping.
		Excessive Mg from magnesium in Epsom salts causes diarrhea.

Sulfur (S) No recommended intake or UL ▪ All protein foods (meat, poultry, fish, eggs, milk, dried peas and beans, nuts)	Component of disulfide bridges in proteins; component of biotin, thiamin, and insulin	*Deficiency* Unknown *Toxicity* In animals, excessive intake of sulfur-containing amino acids impairs growth.

The RDA for calcium is 1300 mg for adolescents up to 18 years of age, 1000 mg for women between the ages of 19 and 50 years, and 1200 mg thereafter (IOM, 2011). The RDA for men is 1000 mg between the ages of 19 and 70 years and 1200 mg after age 70 years. Mean intake among Americans age 20 years and older is 1038 mg for men and 833 mg for women (USDA, ARS, 2010).

Phosphorus

After calcium, the most abundant mineral in the body is phosphorus. Approximately 85% of the body's phosphorus is combined with calcium in bones and teeth. The rest is distributed in every body cell, where it performs various functions, such as regulating acid–base balance (phosphoric acid and its salts), metabolizing energy (adenosine triphosphate), and providing structure to cell membranes (phospholipids). Phosphorus is an important component of RNA and DNA and is responsible for activating many enzymes and the B vitamins.

Normally about 60% of natural phosphorus from food sources is absorbed, but absorption of phosphorus from food preservatives (e.g., phosphoric acid) is almost 100% (Bell, Draper, Tzeng, Shin, and Schmidt, 1977). As with calcium, phosphorus absorption is enhanced by vitamin D and regulated by PTH. The major route of phosphorus excretion is in the urine.

Because phosphorus is pervasive in the food supply, dietary deficiencies of phosphorus do not occur. Animal proteins, dairy products, and legumes are rich natural sources of phosphorus; soft drinks contain phosphoric acid. Phosphate additives—which are often added to commercially prepared foods to extend shelf life, improve taste, improve texture, or retain moisture—can be significant sources of phosphorus. Mean intake in Americans age 20 years and older is 1550 mg/day among men and 1123 mg in women, which are amounts significantly higher than the RDA of 700 mg (USDA, ARS, 2010). Because most food databases do not count phosphorus derived from food additives, the total amount of phosphorus consumed by the average person in the United States is unknown.

Magnesium

Magnesium is the fourth most abundant mineral in the body; approximately 50% of the body's magnesium content is deposited in bone with calcium and phosphorus. The remaining magnesium is distributed in various soft tissues, muscles, and body fluids. Magnesium is a cofactor for more than 300 enzymes in the body, including those involved in energy metabolism, protein synthesis, and cell membrane transport. There is increasing interest in the role magnesium may play in preventing hypertension and managing cardiovascular disease and diabetes (Office of Dietary Supplements, National Institutes of Health, 2009).

Mean magnesium intake among American adults is approximately 80% of the RDA. A low magnesium intake is related to the intake of refined grains over whole-grain breads and cereals because magnesium that is lost in the refining process is not added back through routine enrichment. However, food consumption data do not include the magnesium content of water, which is significant in water classified as "hard." Despite chronically low intakes, deficiency symptoms are rare and appear only in conjunction with certain disorders, such as alcohol abuse, protein malnutrition, renal impairments, endocrine disorders, and prolonged vomiting or diarrhea.

Sulfur

Sulfur does not function independently as a nutrient, but it is a component of biotin, thiamin, and the amino acids methionine and cysteine. The proteins in skin, hair, and nails are made more rigid by the presence of sulfur.

There is neither an RDA nor an AI for sulfur, and no deficiency symptoms are known. Although food and various sources of drinking water provide significant amounts of sulfur, the major source of inorganic sulfate for humans is body protein turnover of methionine and cysteine. The need for sulfur is met when the intake of sulfur amino acids is adequate. A sulfur deficiency is likely only when protein deficiency is severe.

TRACE MINERALS

Although the presence of minerals in the body is small, their impact on health is significant. Each trace mineral has its own range over which the body can maintain homeostasis (Fig. 6.4). People who consume an adequate diet derive no further benefit from supplementing their intake with minerals and may induce a deficiency by upsetting the delicate balance that exists between minerals. Even though too little of a trace mineral can be just as deadly as too much, routine supplementation is not recommended. Factors that complicate the study of trace minerals are as follows:

- The high variability of trace mineral content of foods. The mineral content of the soil from which a food originates largely influences trace mineral content. For instance, grains, vegetables, and meat raised in South Dakota, Wyoming, New Mexico, and Utah are high in selenium, whereas foods grown in the southern states and from both coasts of the United States have much less selenium. Other factors that influence a food's trace mineral content are the quality of the water supply and food processing. Because of these factors, the trace mineral content listed in food composition tables may not represent the actual amount in a given sample.
- Food composition data are not available for all trace minerals. Food composition tables generally include data on the content of iron, zinc, manganese, selenium, and copper, but data on other trace minerals, such as iodine, chromium, and molybdenum, are not readily available.
- Bioavailability varies within the context of the total diet. Even when trace element intake can be estimated, the amount available to the body may be significantly less because the

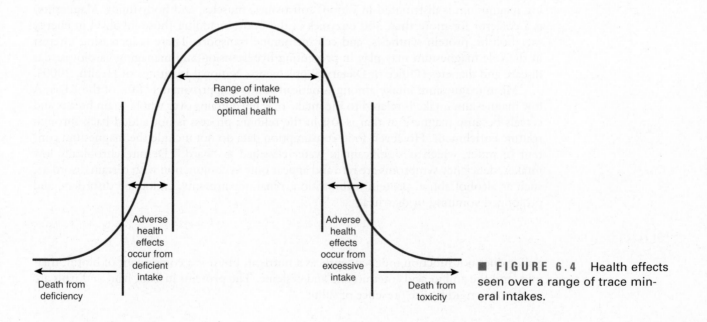

■ **FIGURE 6.4** Health effects seen over a range of trace mineral intakes.

absorption and metabolism of individual trace elements is strongly influenced by mineral interactions and other dietary factors. An excess of one trace mineral may induce a deficiency of another. For instance, a high intake of zinc impairs copper absorption. Conversely, a deficiency of one trace mineral may potentiate toxic effects of another, as when iron deficiency increases vulnerability to lead poisoning.

- Reliable and valid indicators of trace element status (e.g., measured serum levels, results of balance studies, enzyme activity determinations) are not available for all trace minerals, so assessment of trace element status is not always possible.

Table 6.4 summarizes the sources, functions, recommended intakes, and signs and symptoms of deficiency and toxicity of trace minerals that have either an RDA or AI. Additional salient features are presented in the following sections.

Iron

Approximately two-thirds of the body's 3 to 5 g of iron is contained in the heme portion of hemoglobin. Iron is also found in transferrin, the transport carrier of iron, and in enzyme systems that are active in energy metabolism. Ferritin, the storage form of iron, is located in the liver, bone marrow, and spleen.

Iron in foods exists in two forms: heme iron, found in meat, fish, and poultry, and nonheme iron, found in plants such as grains, vegetables, legumes, and nuts. The majority of iron in the diet is nonheme iron.

Normally the overall rate of iron absorption, which includes both heme and nonheme iron, is only 10% to 15% of total intake. In times of need, such as during growth, pregnancy, or iron deficiency, iron is absorbed more efficiently to boost the overall absorption rate to as high as 50%.

QUICK BITE

Nonheme iron absorption
Nonheme iron absorption is *enhanced* when consumed at the same time as
Vitamin C–rich foods, such as orange juice or tomato products
Heme iron found in meat, fish, and poultry
Nonheme iron absorption is *impaired* when consumed at the same time as
Coffee
Tea
Calcium
Phytates found in dried peas and beans, rice, and grains
Oxalates found in spinach, chard, berries, and chocolate

The bioavailability of heme and nonheme iron differs greatly. The rate of heme iron absorption is normally about 15% and is influenced only by need, not by dietary factors. In contrast, nonheme iron absorption is enhanced or inhibited by numerous dietary factors. Nonheme iron absorption is enhanced when it is consumed with heme iron or vitamin C-rich foods, such as orange juice or tomatoes. For instance, consuming 50 mg of vitamin C with a meal, which is the amount of vitamin C found in one small orange, can increase nonheme iron absorption three to six times above normal. Nonheme iron absorption is impaired when it is consumed at the same time as coffee, calcium, phytates (found in legumes and grains), or oxalates (found in spinach, chard). Tea is a potent inhibitor that can reduce nonheme iron absorption in a meal by 60%. When plant foods are consumed as a single food, only 1% to 7% of nonheme iron is absorbed.

Based on average absorption rates and to compensate for daily (and monthly) iron losses, the RDA for iron is set at 8 mg for men and postmenopausal women and 18 mg for

Table 6.4 Summary of Trace Minerals

Mineral and Sources	Functions	Deficiency/Toxicity Signs and Symptoms

Iron (Fe)
Adult RDA
Men: 8 mg
Women:
   19–50 yr: 18 mg
   51+ yr: 8 mg
Adult UL: 45 mg
■ Beef liver, red meats, fish, poultry, clams, tofu, oysters, lentils, dried peas and beans, fortified cereals, bread, dried fruit
	Oxygen transport via hemoglobin and myoglobin; constituent of enzyme systems	***Deficiency***
		Impaired immune function, decreased work capacity, apathy, lethargy, fatigue, itchy skin, pale nail beds and eye membranes, impaired wound healing, intolerance to cold temperatures
		Toxicity
		Increased risk of infections, apathy, fatigue, lethargy, joint disease, hair loss, organ damage, enlarged liver, amenorrhea, impotence
		Accidental poisoning in children causes death.

Zinc (Zn) *Adult RDA* Men: 11 mg Women: 8 mg Adult UL: 40 mg ■ Oysters, red meat, poultry, dried peas and beans, fortified breakfast cereals, yogurt, cashews, pecans, milk	Tissue growth and wound healing, sexual maturation and reproduction; constituent of many enzymes in energy and nucleic acid metabolism; immune function; vitamin A transport, taste perception	***Deficiency*** Growth retardation, hair loss, diarrhea, delayed sexual maturation and impotence, eye and skin lesions, anorexia, delayed wound healing, taste abnormality, mental lethargy ***Toxicity*** Anemia, elevated low-density lipoprotein, lowered high-density lipoprotein, diarrhea, vomiting, impaired calcium absorption, fever, renal failure, muscle pain, dizziness, reproductive failure
Iodine *Adult RDA* 150 µg Adult UL: 1100 µg ■ Iodized salt, seafood, bread, dairy products	Component of thyroid hormones that regulate growth, development, and metabolic rate	***Deficiency*** Goiter, weight gain, lethargy During pregnancy may cause severe and irreversible mental and physical retardation (cretinism) ***Toxicity*** Enlarged thyroid gland, decreased thyroid activity
Selenium (Se) *Adult RDA* Men and women: 55 µg Adult UL: 400 µg/day ■ Brazil nuts, tuna, beef, cod, turkey, egg, cottage cheese, rice, enriched and whole wheat bread	Component of antioxidant enzymes, immune system functioning, thyroid gland activity	***Deficiency*** Enlarged heart, poor heart function, impaired thyroid activity ***Toxicity*** Rare; nausea, vomiting, abdominal pain, diarrhea, hair and nail changes, nerve damage, fatigue
Copper (Cu) *Adult RDA* 900 µg Adult UL: 10,000 µg ■ Organ meats, seafood, nuts, seeds, whole grains, cocoa products, drinking water	Used in the production of hemoglobin; component of several enzymes; used in energy metabolism	***Deficiency*** Rare; anemia, bone abnormalities ***Toxicity*** Vomiting, diarrhea, liver damage

Table 6.4 Summary of Trace Minerals (continued)

Mineral and Sources	Functions	Deficiency/Toxicity Signs and Symptoms
Manganese (Mn) *Adult AI* Men: 2.3 mg Women: 1.8 mg Adult UL: 11 mg • Widely distributed in foods; best sources are whole grains, oat bran, tea, pineapple, spinach, dried peas and beans	Component of enzymes involved in the metabolism of carbohydrates, protein, and fat, and in bone formation	***Deficiency*** Rare ***Toxicity*** Rare; nervous system disorders
Fluoride (Fl) *Adult AI* Men: 4 mg Women: 3 mg Adult UL: 10 mg • Fluoridated water, water that naturally contains fluoride, tea, seafood	Formation and maintenance of tooth enamel, promotes resistance to dental decay, role in bone formation and integrity	***Deficiency*** Susceptibility to dental decay; may increase risk of osteoporosis ***Toxicity*** Fluorosis (mottling of teeth), nausea, vomiting, diarrhea, chest pain, itching

Chromium (Cr)
Adult AI
Men:
  19–50 yr: 35 µg
  51+ yr: 30 µg
Women:
  51+ yr: 30 µg
  19–50 yr: 25 µg
Adult UL:
Undetermined
• Broccoli, grape juice, whole grains, red wine
	Cofactor for insulin	***Deficiency***
		Insulin resistance, impaired glucose tolerance
		
		Toxicity
		Dietary toxicity unknown
		Occupational exposure to chromium dust damages skin and kidneys.

Molybdenum (Mo) *Adult RDA* 45 µg Adult UL: 2000 µg • Milk, legumes, bread, grains	Component of many enzymes; works with riboflavin to incorporate iron into hemoglobin	***Deficiency*** Unknown ***Toxicity*** Occupational exposure to molybdenum dust causes gout-like symptoms.

premenopausal women. Iron requirements increase during growth and in response to heavy or chronic blood loss related to menstruation, surgery, injury, gastrointestinal bleeding, or aspirin abuse. Iron recommendations for vegetarians are 1.8 times higher than those for nonvegetarians because of the lower bioavailability of iron from a vegetarian diet (IOM, 2001). Most adult men and postmenopausal women consume adequate amounts of iron. Women of childbearing age, pregnant women, and breastfeeding women generally do not consume the recommended amounts of iron.

Iron deficiency anemia, a **microcytic**, **hypochromic** anemia, occurs when total iron stores become depleted, leading to a decrease in hemoglobin. Clinical manifestations include fatigue, decreased work capacity, impaired cognitive function, and poor pregnancy outcome, such as premature delivery, low birth weight, and increased perinatal infant mortality, and maternal death. According to the World Health Organization (WHO), iron

Microcytic: small blood cells.

Hypochromic: pale red blood cells related to the decrease in hemoglobin pigment.

deficiency is the most common and widespread nutritional disorder in the world, affecting more than 30% of the world's population (WHO, 2012). In developing countries, iron deficiency is exacerbated by worm infections, malaria, and other infectious diseases such as HIV and tuberculosis (WHO, 2012).

In the United States, about 10% of the population is iron deficient. Because the typical American diet provides only 6 to 7 mg of iron per 1000 calories, many menstruating women simply do not consume enough calories to satisfy their iron requirement. In fact, NHANES data show mean iron intake among women 20 years and older is 13.0 mg, well below the RDA of 18 mg (USDA, ARS, 2010). Other groups most likely to have iron deficiency from an inadequate intake are older infants and toddlers, adolescent girls, and pregnant women. Some people with iron deficiency anemia practice **pica**, which impairs iron absorption. Nonnutritional risk factors for iron deficiency, particularly among older populations, include blood loss, medication use, and renal insufficiency (Tussing-Humphreys and Braunschweig, 2011). Obesity is also linked to iron deficiency anemia, although the exact mechanism is unclear. Because symptoms of iron deficiency are similar to iron overload—namely, apathy, lethargy, and fatigue—iron supplements should not be taken on the basis of symptoms alone.

Because very little iron is excreted from the body, the potential for toxicity is moderate to high. Although repeated blood transfusions, rare metabolic disorders, and megadoses of supplemental iron can cause iron overload, the most frequent cause is hemochromatosis, one of the most common genetic disorders in the United States. The absorption of excessive amounts of iron leads to iron accumulation in body tissues, especially the liver, heart, brain, joints, and pancreas. Left untreated, excess iron can cause heart disease, cancer, cirrhosis, diabetes, and arthritis. Phlebotomies are used to reduce body iron. Given the prevalence of iron enrichment and iron fortification in the U.S. food supply, a low-iron diet is not recommended nor could it be realistically achieved.

Acute iron toxicity, caused by the overdose of medicinal iron, is the leading cause of accidental poisoning in small children. As few as five to six high-potency tablets can provide enough iron to kill a child weighing 22 pounds. In adults, high intake of iron supplements can cause constipation, nausea, vomiting, and diarrhea, especially when the supplements are taken on an empty stomach.

Pica: ingestion of nonfood substances such as dirt, clay, or laundry starch.

Zinc

The small amount of zinc contained in the body (about 2 g) is found in almost all cells and is especially concentrated in the eyes, bones, muscles, and prostate gland. Zinc in tissues is not available to maintain serum levels when intake is inadequate, so a regular and sufficient intake is necessary.

Zinc is a component of DNA and RNA and is part of more than 100 enzymes involved in growth, metabolism, sexual maturation and reproduction, and the senses of taste and smell. Zinc plays important roles in immune system functioning and wound healing. Mean intake among American adults exceeds the RDA for zinc.

There is no single laboratory test that adequately measures zinc status, so zinc deficiency is not readily diagnosed. Risk factors for zinc deficiency include poor calorie intake, alcoholism, and malabsorption syndromes such as celiac disease, Crohn disease, and short bowel syndrome. Vegetarians are also at increased risk because zinc is only half as well absorbed from plants as it is from animal sources. Although overt zinc deficiency is not common in the United States, the effects of marginal intakes are poorly understood.

Iodine

Iodine is found in the muscles, the thyroid gland, the skin, the skeleton, endocrine tissues, and the bloodstream. It is an essential component of thyroxine (T_4) and triiodothyronine (T_3), the thyroid hormones responsible for regulating metabolic rate, body temperature, reproduction, growth, the synthesis of blood cells, and nerve and muscle function.

Most foods are naturally low in iodine. The iodine content of vegetables and grains varies with the soil content (Haldimann, Alt, Blanc, and Blondeau, 2005). Processed foods often contain salt that is not iodized (Dasgupta, Liu, and Dyke, 2008). Milk is naturally low in iodine but has become an important source of iodine in part because of the use of iodine chemicals to sanitize and disinfect udders, milking machines, and milk tanks. However, the iodine in dairy products from sanitizing agents is unintentional and usually not regulated (Perrine, Herrick, Serdula, and Sullivan, 2010). Likewise, some breads provide iodine due to the use of iodate dough conditioners. Seafood is a natural source of iodine due to iodine in seawater. The United States has generally been considered iodine sufficient since table salt began to be voluntarily iodized in 1924 (Perrine et al., 2010). Worldwide, iodine deficiency is a major problem and the leading cause of mental retardation (De Benoist, McLean, Andersson, and Rogers, 2008). Iodine deficiency disorders include goiter, hypothyroidism, cretinism, stillbirths, and delayed psychomotor and cognitive development (Zimmermann, Jooste, and Pandav, 2008). The effect of **goitrogens** on iodine balance is clinically insignificant except when iodine deficiency exists.

Goitrogens: thyroid antagonists found in cruciferous vegetables (e.g., cabbage, cauliflower, broccoli), soybeans, and sweet potatoes.

Selenium

Selenium is a component of a group of enzymes, called glutathione peroxidases, that function as antioxidants to disarm free radicals produced during normal oxygen metabolism. Selenium, as part of selenoproteins, regulates thyroid hormone actions; other functions are still being investigated, such as the potential role of selenium in preventing cardiovascular disease, neurodegenerative diseases, and certain cancers (Brenneisen, Steinbrenner, and Sies, 2005; Steinbrenner and Sies, 2009).

Although areas of the country with selenium-poor soil produce selenium-poor foods, mass transportation mitigates the effect on total selenium intake (IOM, 2000). Also, because selenium is associated with protein, some meats and seafood provide selenium. Although the average American adult consumes more than the RDA of selenium, many consumers habitually consume high amounts of selenium through supplements (Steinbrenner, Speckmann, Pinto, and Sies, 2011).

There is a narrow range between too little and too much selenium, and adverse effects can occur even when selenium intake is below levels considered toxic (Whanger, Vendeland, Park, and Xia, 1996). For instance, a surprising finding of the Nutritional Prevention of Cancer (NPC) trial was that participants who received selenium supplements over a 12-year period were more likely to develop type 2 diabetes than those who were given a placebo (Stranges et al., 2007). It is not known whether high serum selenium was a consequence or cause of type 2 diabetes.

Selenium deficiency is rare in the United States. It is most likely to occur secondary to severe gastrointestinal problems, such as Crohn disease, or from surgical removal of part of the stomach. People with acute severe illness who develop inflammation and widespread infection often have low blood levels of selenium.

Copper

Copper is distributed in muscles, liver, brain, bones, kidneys, and blood. Copper is a component of several enzymes involved in hemoglobin synthesis, collagen formation, wound healing, and maintenance of nerve fibers. Copper also helps cells to use iron and plays a role in energy metabolism.

Americans typically consume adequate amounts of copper. Excess zinc intake has the potential to induce copper deficiency by impairing its absorption, but copper deficiency is rare. Supplements, not food, may cause copper toxicity, as do some genetic disorders, such as Wilson disease.

Manganese

Mean manganese intake among American adults is well above the AI, and dietary deficiencies have not been noted. Manganese toxicity is a well-known occupational hazard for miners who inhale manganese dust over a prolonged period of time, leading to central nervous system abnormalities with symptoms similar to those of Parkinson disease. There is some evidence to suggest that high manganese intake from drinking water, which may be more bioavailable than manganese from food, also produces neuromotor deficits similar to Parkinson disease. The UL for adults is set at 11 mg/day, approximately four times the usual intake.

Fluoride

Cariogenic: cavity promoting.

Fluoride promotes the mineralization of developing tooth enamel prior to tooth eruption and the remineralization of surface enamel in erupted teeth. It concentrates in plaque and saliva to inhibit the process by which **cariogenic** bacteria metabolize carbohydrates to produce acids that cause tooth decay. Fluoridation of municipal water in the second half of the 20th century is credited with a major decline in the prevalence and severity of dental caries in the U.S. population.

Fluoridation of municipal water is endorsed by the National Institute of Dental Health, the Academy of Nutrition and Dietetics, the American Medical Association, the National Cancer Institute, and the Centers for Disease Control and Prevention (CDC). According to the CDC (2012), 73.9% of Americans had access to optimally fluoridated water in 2010. National health goals are to increase fluoridation to 79.6% or more of the U.S. population served by municipal water systems (CDC, 2012). It is estimated that for every $1 spent on fluoridation, $38 or more is saved in treatment costs. Studies show that water fluoridation reduces tooth decay by approximately 25% over a person's lifetime (CDC, 2012). Children under the age of 8 years are susceptible to mottled tooth enamel if they ingest several times more fluoride than the recommended amount during the time of tooth enamel formation. The swallowing of fluoridated toothpaste is to blame.

Chromium

Chromium enhances the action of the hormone insulin to help regulate blood glucose levels. A deficiency of chromium is characterized by high blood glucose and impaired insulin response.

Even though chromium is widespread in foods, many foods provide less than 1 to 2 μg per serving. Because existing databases lack information on chromium, few food intake studies utilizing few laboratories are available to estimate usual intake. However, it appears that average intake is adequate. Unrefined foods are higher in chromium than processed foods.

Molybdenum

Molybdenum plays a role in red blood cell synthesis and is a component of several enzymes. Average American intake falls within the recommended range. Dietary deficiencies and toxicities are unknown.

Other Trace Elements

Although definitive evidence is lacking, future research may reveal that other trace elements are essential for human nutrition. However, evidence is difficult to obtain, and quantifying human need is even more formidable. In addition, as with all trace minerals, the potential for toxicity exists. Consider the following:

- Nickel, silicon, vanadium, and boron have been demonstrated to have beneficial health effects in some animals and may someday be classified as essential for humans.
- Cobalt is an essential component of vitamin B_{12}, but it is not an essential nutrient and does not have an RDA.
- It is possible that minute amounts of cadmium, lithium, tin, and even arsenic are also essential to human life.

WATER AND MINERALS IN HEALTH PROMOTION

Water

One of the *Dietary Guidelines for Americans, 2010* selected messages for consumers is to drink water instead of sugary drinks (USDA, USDHHS, 2010). This corresponds to the recommendation to reduce the intake of food and beverages with added sugars. The American Heart Association recommends no more than 450 calories/week from sugar-sweetened beverages, or fewer than three 12-oz cans/week of sweetened beverages (Lloyd-Jones et al., 2010). Sugar-sweetened beverages are linked to poor diet quality, weight gain, obesity, and in adults, type 2 diabetes (Malik, Schulze, and Hu, 2006; Vartanian, Schwartz, and Brownell, 2007).

In both adults and children, soft drink consumption has increased over the last 30 years (Ogden, Kit, Carroll, and Park, 2011). As much as 50% of added sugars in a typical American diet may come from sugar-sweetened beverages (Johnson et al., 2009). Overall findings regarding sugar drink consumption between 2005 and 2008 indicate that

- Males consume 175 calories/day from sugar-sweetened drinks, and females consume 94 cal/day.
- The intake of sugar drinks peaks in the 12- to 19-year-old age group and then decreases with age.
- Approximately half of the population consumes sugar-sweetened drinks on any given day.
- Five percent of people on any given day consume at least 567 calories from sugar-sweetened drinks, the equivalent of more than four 12-oz cans of cola.

The Beverage Guidance Panel, a group of nutrition experts formed to provide guidance on the nutritional benefits and risks of various types of beverages, concurs that the current high intake of sweetened beverages contributes to an excess calorie intake and is a factor in the development of obesity (Popkin et al., 2006). Although naturally calorie-free plain water could be used to completely satisfy fluid needs, other beverages have value in that they may provide nutrients, phytochemicals, and interest to the diet. A sample beverage plan for a 2200-calorie diet where calories from beverages are limited to 10% or less of total calories is featured in Box 6.4.

Minerals

Because Americans on average consume fewer fruits, vegetables, whole grains, and milk and milk products than recommended, certain nutrients, including certain minerals, may be

Box 6.4   THE BEVERAGE GUIDANCE PANEL'S SUGGESTED PLAN

For a 2200-calorie diet with less than 10% of calories from beverages, drink approximately

- 6 glasses, or at least half of total fluid intake, of water. It is fine to meet fluid needs with only water.
- 3 to 4 cups of unsweetened tea and coffee, if desired. If not, substitute water.
- 2 glasses of low-fat milk
- 4 oz of 100% fruit juice
- If alcohol is consumed, limit intake to no more than one drink daily for women or 1 to 2 drinks daily for men.
- "Diet" beverages made with artificial sweeteners are not recommended but up to 1 to 2 glasses daily can be consumed (modified from the original recommendation to limit diet beverages to 32 oz or less daily).

Source: Popkin, B., Armstrong, L., Bray, G., et al. (2006). A new proposed guidance system for beverage consumption in the United States. *American Journal of Clinical Nutrition, 83,* 529–542.

consumed at levels low enough to be a public health concern (USDA, USDHHS, 2010). Specifically, the *Dietary Guidelines for Americans, 2010* makes recommendations for three minerals (USDA, USDHHS, 2010):

- Reduce daily sodium intake to less than 2300 mg and further reduce intake to 1500 mg among persons who are 51 years and older and those of any age who are African American or have hypertension, diabetes, or chronic kidney disease. The 1500-mg recommendation applies to about half of the U.S. population, including children and the majority of adults. The American Heart Association recommends all Americans limit their intake of sodium to 1500 mg/day (American Heart Association, 2012).
- Choose foods that provide more potassium and calcium.

Sodium and Potassium

Randomized controlled trials and epidemiologic studies show that a high sodium or low potassium intake increases blood pressure, which is a risk factor for coronary heart disease, stroke, congestive heart failure, and renal diseases (Cook et al., 2009; Strazzullo, D-Elia, Landala, and Cappuccio, 2009; Trials of Hypertension Prevention Collaborative Research Group, 1997). On average, blood pressure increases progressively and continuously over the continuum of sodium intake without an obvious threshold. Tips for reducing sodium intake appear in Box 6.5.

Because the Daily Value (DV) for sodium used on food labels predates the latest AI and UL set for sodium, those values do not reliably reflect a food's contribution to recommended (lower) sodium intake levels. The Daily Reference Value for sodium used on the "Nutrition Facts" label is 2400 mg, which exceeds the current UL set at 2300 mg. A food that supplies 50% of the DV for sodium in a serving actually provides 1200 mg, which is 100% of the current AI for adults age 71 years and older. Until the DV figure is updated, %DV is best used to compare the sodium content of similar products, not to estimate intake with the goal of consuming the AI. Descriptive terms on food labels do have legally defined meanings and can assist in food selection (Box 6.6).

Box 6.5   TIPS FOR LOWERING SODIUM INTAKE

- Avoid or limit convenience foods, such as boxed mixes, frozen dinners, and canned foods.
- Eat home-cooked meals more often.
- Eat more fresh or frozen vegetables.
- Compare labels to choose brands or varieties with the lowest amount of sodium.
- Use fresh veggies in place of pickles.
- Substitute low-sodium tuna and roasted chicken for deli meats.
- Replace sausages and hot dogs with fresh meats, such as rotisserie chicken.
- Use cheese sparingly.
- Choose nut butters with no sodium added.
- Cook rice and pasta without salt.
- Switch to pasta sauce without added salt or combine equal parts of no-salt-added tomato sauce with bottled pasta sauce.
- Choose cereals with no added salt, such as shredded wheat, puffed whole-grain cereal, and unsalted oatmeal.
- Use lower salt condiments, such as salt-free ketchup, Worcestershire sauce, vinegar, and low-sodium mayonnaise.
- Substitute homemade vinegar and oil dressing for bottled varieties.
- If you use canned vegetables, drain away liquid and rinse thoroughly.
- Limit salty snacks.
- Instead of salt, season food with spices, herbs, lemon, vinegar, or salt-free seasonings.

A high potassium intake may counter the effects of a high sodium intake, which may explain why Yang et al. (2011) observed a stronger association between cardiovascular disease and the ratio of sodium and potassium consumed than with either sodium or potassium intake alone. Likewise, the DASH (Dietary Approaches to Stop Hypertension) study showed that a diet rich in potassium, calcium, magnesium, and fiber combined with

Box 6.6   DESCRIPTORS OF SODIUM CONTENT

If the label says . . .	One serving contains . . .
Sodium free	Less than 5 mg
Very low sodium	Less than 35 mg
Low sodium	Less than 140 mg
Reduced or less sodium	At least 25% less sodium compared with a standard serving size of the traditional food
Light in sodium	50% less sodium than the traditional food (restricted to more than 40 calories per serving or more than 3 g fat per serving)
Salt free	Less than 5 mg
Unsalted or no added salt	No salt added during processing (this does not necessarily mean the food is sodium free)

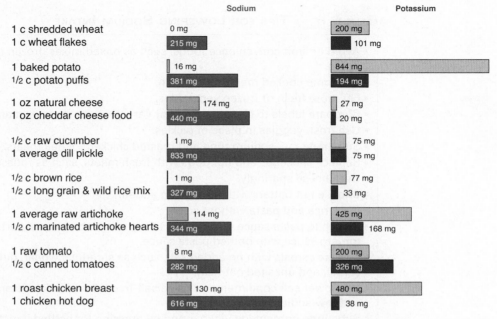

FIGURE 6.5 Effect of food processing on the sodium and potassium content of selected foods.

a reduced sodium intake lowers blood pressure in hypertensive and normotensive people (Obarzanek et al., 2001).

From a public health standpoint, increasing potassium intake could result in greater health benefits than simply restricting sodium (van Mierlo, Greyling, Zock, Kok, and Geleijnse, 2010). Food sources are recommended over supplements, and fruits and vegetables are preferred because potassium is better absorbed from them than from meat, milk, and cereal products. Substituting more wholesome or natural foods for processed foods increases potassium intake while lowering sodium. Figure 6.5 illustrates how food processing generally lowers potassium content and raises sodium content.

More Calcium

Calcium is best known for its importance in optimal bone health. Much research has been done on its role, either alone or with vitamin D, in preventing chronic disease. Moderate evidence shows that the intake of milk and milk products is linked to a lower risk of cardiovascular disease, type 2 diabetes, and lower blood pressure in adults (USDA, USDHHS, 2010). The majority of epidemiologic studies consistently show a decrease in the risk of colorectal cancer and adenomas at higher levels of intake of both calcium and vitamin D compared to low intakes (Zhang and Giovannucci, 2011). Observational and clinical studies also indicate that dairy calcium intake may play a role in weight regulation and obesity (Bush et al., 2010; Faghih, Abadi, Hedavati, and Kimiagar, 2011; Shahar et al., 2010).

Although Americans are urged to meet their RDA for calcium through food, 43% of adults take calcium supplements and the percentage rises to 70% among older women (IOM, 2011). Recently, questions have been raised about the safety of calcium supplements. For instance,

- An examination of cohort participants of the European Prospective Investigation into Cancer and Nutrition Study showed that calcium supplements may actually increase the risk of myocardial infarction (Kuanrong, Kaaks, Linseisen, and Rohrmann, 2012).

- Increased rates of cardiovascular events were reported in women allocated to calcium supplements in the Auckland Calcium Study, a 5-year randomized, placebo-controlled trial in healthy older women (Bolland et al., 2008).
- A meta-analysis of randomized, placebo-controlled trials of calcium supplements without vitamin D showed that calcium supplements increased the risk of myocardial infarction by 31% (Bolland et al., 2010).
- A reanalysis of data from the Women's Health Initiative Calcium/Vitamin D Supplementation Study found that calcium supplements, with or without vitamin D, modestly increase the risk of cardiovascular events, especially myocardial infarction, a finding that was obscured in the original study analysis by the widespread use of personal calcium supplements (Bolland, Grey, Avenell, Gamble, and Reid, 2011).

Generally, three daily servings of milk, yogurt, or cheese plus nondairy sources of calcium are needed to ensure an adequate calcium intake. Milk is a "nearly perfect" source because it contains vitamin D and lactose, which promote calcium absorption. People who are lactose intolerant can obtain calcium from yogurt; hard cheeses; and low-oxalate green vegetables, such as broccoli, bok choy, collard greens, and kale. Significant amounts of calcium can be found in calcium-fortified foods, such as fruit juices, tomato juice, and ready-to-eat breakfast cereals.

How Do You Respond?

Do zinc lozenges cure the common cold? Systematic review and meta-analysis of randomized, placebo-controlled trials show that oral zinc taken within 24 hours of the onset of common cold symptoms significantly reduces both the duration and severity of symptoms (Science, Johnstone, Roth, Guyatt, and Loeb, 2012; Singh and Das, 2011). Side effects were common, with bad taste and nausea reported most frequently. Prolonged high serum levels of zinc can interfere with copper metabolism; long-term effects of zinc used prophylactically are not known. Large high-quality studies are needed to determine optimal dose and formulation (Rao and Rowland, 2011).

Does chlorine in drinking water cause cancer? When organic matter is present in water, chlorine reacts with it to form a by-product called trihalomethane (THM). If THM forms, it is in such small quantities that it is not a cancer risk. The benefits of chlorine in preventing outbreaks of cholera, hepatitis, and other diseases far outweigh the negligible effects of THM.

What are chelated minerals? A chelated mineral is surrounded by an amino acid to protect it from other food components such as oxalates and phytates that can bind to the mineral and prevent it from being absorbed. Chelated minerals are probably not worth the added expense because chelated calcium is absorbed 5% to 10% better than ordinary calcium but costs about five times more.

Case Study

Bill is a 45-year-old bachelor who eats a grab-and-go breakfast, eats all of his lunches out, and has takeout or "something easy" for dinner. Bill's doctor is concerned that his blood pressure is progressively rising with every office visit and has advised him to "cut out the salt" to lower his sodium intake. Bill rarely uses salt from a salt shaker and

(continues on page 150)

CASE STUDY (continued)

is unsure what else he can do to lower his sodium intake. A typical day's intake is as follows:

Breakfast:	Black coffee Two jelly doughnuts
Midmorning snack:	Black coffee Cookies
Lunch:	Two fast-food tacos with tortilla chips and salsa or a 6-in cold cut submarine with potato chips Cola
Midafternoon snack:	Candy bar
Dinner:	If takeout, Chinese food or pizza If "something easy," boxed macaroni and cheese with a couple of hot dogs, canned soup with a cold cut sandwich, or frozen TV dinners
Dessert:	Instant pudding or ice cream or candy bars
Evening snacks:	Cereal and milk or potato chips and dip

- What foods did Bill eat yesterday that were high in sodium? What foods were relatively low in sodium? What would be better choices for him when eating out? How could he lower his sodium intake while still relying on "something easy" when he prepares food at home?
- Knowing that potassium may help blunt the effect of a high sodium intake on blood pressure, what foods would you recommend he add to his diet that would increase his potassium intake?
- In overweight people, weight loss helps lower high blood pressure. Bill is "a little heavy." What changes/substitutions would help him lose weight?

STUDY QUESTIONS

1. A healthy, young adult client asks how much water he should drink daily. Which of the following would be the nurse's best response?
   a. "The old adage is true: drink eight 8-oz glasses of water daily."
   b. "Drink to satisfy thirst and you will consume adequate fluid."
   c. "You can't overconsume water, so drink as much as you can spread out over the course of the day."
   d. "It is actually not necessary to drink water at all. It is equally healthy to meet your fluid requirement with sugar-free soft drinks."

2. When developing a teaching plan for a client who is lactose intolerant, which of the following foods would the nurse suggest as sources of calcium the client could tolerate?
   a. Cheddar cheese, bok choy, broccoli
   b. Spinach, beet greens, skim milk
   c. Poultry, meat, eggs
   d. Whole grains, nuts, and cocoa

3. The nurse knows her instructions about reading labels for sodium information have been effective when the client verbalizes
   a. "Foods labeled as 'no salt added' are sodium free."
   b. "The %DV on the 'Nutrition Facts' labels is based on the current adult AI of 1500 mg Na."
   c. "The best way to use the 'Nutrition Facts' label is to compare the sodium content or %DV of one brand or variety of a food to another."
   d. "Spaghetti sauce labeled 'reduced sodium' has less sodium in it than spaghetti sauce labeled as 'light in sodium.'"

4. Which of the following recommendations would be most effective at increasing potassium intake?
   a. Choose enriched grains in place of whole grains.
   b. Eat more fruits and vegetables.
   c. Eat more seafood and poultry in place of red meat.
   d. Because there are few good dietary sources of potassium, it is best obtained by taking potassium supplements.

5. A client asks why eating less sodium is important for healthy people. The nurse's best response is
   a. "Low-sodium diets tend to be low in fat and therefore may reduce the risk of heart disease."
   b. "Low-sodium diets are only effective at preventing high blood pressure, not lowering existing high blood pressure, so the time to implement a low-sodium diet is when you are healthy."
   c. "Blood pressure tends to go up as sodium intake rises—without an obvious threshold; lowering sodium regardless of how much you consume may help prevent or delay high blood pressure."
   d. "Low-sodium diets are inherently low in calories and help people lose weight, which can help prevent a variety of chronic diseases."

6. Which of the following recommendations would be most effective at helping a client maximize iron absorption?
   a. Drink orange juice when you eat iron-fortified breakfast cereal.
   b. Avoid drinking coffee when you eat red meat.
   c. Drink milk with all meals.
   d. Eat dried peas and beans in place of red meat.

7. A client says he never adds salt to any foods that his wife serves, so he believes he is consuming a low-sodium diet. Which of the following is the nurse's best response?
   a. "If you don't add salt to any of your foods, you are probably eating a low-sodium diet. Continue with that strategy."
   b. "Even though you aren't adding salt to food at the table, your wife is probably salting food as she cooks. She should stop doing that."
   c. "Lots of foods are naturally high in sodium, such as milk and meat; in addition to not using a salt shaker, you must also limit foods that are naturally high in sodium."
   d. "The major sources of sodium are processed and convenience foods. Limiting their intake makes the biggest impact on overall sodium intake."

8. What should you tell the client about taking mineral supplements?
   a. "Most Americans are deficient in minerals, so it is wise to take a multimineral supplement."
   b. "Like water-soluble vitamins, if you consume more minerals than your body needs, you will excrete them in the urine, so do not worry about taking in too much."
   c. "If you do not have a mineral deficiency, taking supplements can lead to a potentially excessive intake that can cause adverse health effects."
   d. "Mineral deficiencies do not exist in the United States, so you do not need to waste your money on them."

KEY CONCEPTS

- Because water is involved in almost every body function, is not stored, and is excreted daily, it is more vital to life than food.
- Under normal conditions, water intake equals water output to maintain water balance. In most healthy people, thirst is a reliable indicator of need.

■ The body's need for water is influenced by many variables, including activity, climate, and health. A general guideline is to consume 1.0 mL of fluid per calorie consumed, with a minimum of 1500 mL/day.

■ Minerals are inorganic substances that cannot be broken down and rearranged in the body.

■ Mineral toxicities are not likely to occur from diet alone. They are most often related to excessive use of mineral supplements, environmental exposure, or alterations in metabolism.

■ Depending on the mineral involved, the body can maintain mineral balance by altering the rate of absorption, altering the rate of excretion, or releasing minerals from storage when needed.

■ The absorption of many minerals is influenced by mineral–mineral interactions. Too much of one mineral may promote a deficiency of another mineral.

■ Sodium, potassium, and chloride are electrolytes because they carry electrical charges when they are dissolved in solution.

■ Macrominerals are needed in relatively large amounts and are found in the body in quantities greater than 5 g. Trace minerals are needed in very small amounts and are found in the body in amounts less than 5 g.

■ Approximately 75% of sodium consumed in the average American diet is from processed food. Virtually all Americans consume more than the UL for sodium.

■ The potassium content of the diet tends to decrease as the sodium content increases, largely because high-sodium processed foods tend to be low in potassium.

■ Many American adults consume less than the RDA for calcium, placing them at risk for osteoporosis and possibly hypertension. Milk and yogurt are the richest sources of calcium, and their vitamin D and lactose content promote its absorption.

■ Phosphorus is pervasive in foods and is also widely used in food additives to extend shelf life, enhance flavor, or improve quality characteristics. Americans consume more than they need.

■ Although most Americans consume less than the RDA for magnesium, overt deficiency symptoms are rare and occur only secondary to certain diseases such as protein malnutrition and alcoholism.

■ Trace minerals are not less important than major minerals; "trace" refers to the small amount normally found and needed in the body.

■ The typical American diet supplies only 6 to 7 mg of iron per 1000 calories, so menstruating females typically do not eat enough calories to meet their RDA of 18 mg. Iron deficiency anemia is one of the most common nutritional deficiencies in the world.

■ Americans generally consume adequate amounts of zinc. A regular intake is necessary because zinc in tissues cannot be released to maintain normal blood levels.

■ The natural iodine content of most foods is low. Iodized salt, dairy products, and breads provide added iodine. Processed foods are often made with salt that is not iodized. People living in the United States are generally considered to have sufficient iodine intake.

■ Selenium is a component of substances that act as antioxidants. It is being studied for its potential to decrease the risk of cardiovascular disease, neurodegenerative diseases, and certain cancers.

■ Fluoridated water has dramatically reduced the prevalence and severity of cavities in the U.S. population. Bottled water may not be fluoridated.

■ Americans are urged to reduce their intake of sodium because of its potential role in the development of hypertension. The UL established for sodium is lower than the DV used on the "Nutrition Facts" label.

■ A high potassium intake may blunt the effect of a high sodium intake. Americans are urged to increase their potassium intake by eating more fruits and vegetables. Meat, fish, whole grains, and legumes are also sources of potassium, but potassium is less well absorbed from them than the potassium in fruits and vegetables.

Check Your Knowledge Answer Key

1. **FALSE** Although many healthy people do not consume the eight 8-oz glasses of fluid recommended daily, the body is able to maintain homeostasis over a wide range of intakes.
2. **FALSE** Although the body rids itself of some excess minerals such as sodium and potassium through urinary excretion, homeostasis of other minerals is achieved by adjusting the rate of mineral absorption (e.g., iron, calcium).
3. **FALSE** Calcium is the most plentiful mineral in the body. For most Americans, sodium is the most abundant mineral in the diet.
4. **TRUE** An increase in sodium intake is associated with an increase in blood pressure. In addition, the dose-dependent rise in blood pressure is progressive, continuous, and appears to occur throughout the continuum of sodium intake without an obvious threshold.
5. **FALSE** People are urged to get their nutrients from food rather than supplements. Recent studies suggest calcium supplements, with or without vitamin D, may increase the risk of cardiovascular events.
6. **TRUE** Foods high in sodium tend to be low in potassium (e.g., processed foods like frozen entrees), and foods high in potassium tend to be low in sodium (e.g., fresh vegetables and whole grains).
7. **FALSE** The "major" and "trace" descriptions refer to the relative quantity of the mineral found in the body, not to its importance in maintaining health.
8. **TRUE** For most people, thirst is a reliable indicator of fluid needs. Exceptions are the elderly, children, and during hot weather or strenuous exercise.
9. **TRUE** Trace mineral balance is a function not only of the quantity of the element consumed but also of the presence of other trace minerals and dietary factors. For instance, nonheme iron absorption is impaired by tea but enhanced by orange juice.
10. **FALSE** A chronically low intake of calcium compromises the density and strength of bones but does not lead to hypocalcemia. Serum levels of calcium are maintained within normal range, regardless of calcium intake at the expense of calcium in bones.

Student Resources on thePoint

For additional learning materials, activate the code in the front of this book at
http://thePoint.lww.com/activate

Websites

Iron Overload Diseases Association at **www.ironoverload.org**
National Dairy Council at **www.nationaldairycouncil.org**
National Academy of Sciences, Institute of Medicine for Reference Dietary Intakes at **www.nap.edu**
National Institutes of Health: Facts about dietary supplements (including mineral supplements) at **http://dietary-supplements.info.nih.gov**
Nutrient sources at USDA National Nutrient Database for Standard Reference, Release 25, at **http://www.ars.usda.gov/Services/docs.htm?docid=22769**

References

American Heart Association. (2012). *Healthy diet goals.* Available at http://www.heart.org/HEARTORG/GettingHealthy/NutritionCenter/HealthyDietGoals/Healthy-Diet-Goals_UCM_310436_SubHomePage.jsp. Accessed on 9/28/12.

Baily, R., Fulgoni, V., Keast, D., & Dwyer, J. (2011). Dietary supplement use is associated with higher intakes of minerals from food sources. *American Journal of Clinical Nutrition, 94,* 1376–1381.

Bell, R., Draper, J., Tzeng, D., Shin, H. K., & Schmidt, G. R. (1977). Physiological responses of human adult to foods containing phosphate additives. *The Journal of Nutrition, 107,* 45–50.

Bolland, M., Avenell, A., Baron, J., Grey, A., MacLennan, G. S., Gamble, G. D., & Reid, I. R. (2010). Effect of calcium supplements on risk of myocardial infarction and cardiovascular events: Meta-analysis. *British Medical Journal, 341,* c3690.

Bolland, M., Barber, P., Doughty, R., Mason, B., Horne, A., Ames, R., . . . Reid, I. R. (2008). Vascular events in healthy older women receiving calcium supplementation: Randomized controlled trial. *British Medical Journal, 336,* 262–266.

Bolland, M., Grey, A., Avenell, A., Gamble, G. D., & Reid, I. R. (2011). Calcium supplements with or without vitamin D and risk of cardiovascular events: Reanalysis of the Women's Health Initiative limited access dataset and meta-analysis. *British Medical Journal, 342,* d2040.

Brenneisen, P., Steinbrenner, H., & Sies, H. (2005). Selenium, oxidative stress, and health aspects. *Molecular Aspects of Medicine, 26,* 256–267.

Bush, N., Alvarex, J., Choquett, S., Hunter, G. R., Oster, R. A., Darnell, B. E., & Gower, B. A. (2010). Dietary calcium intake is associated with less gain in intra-abdominal adipose tissue over 1 year. *Obesity, 18,* 2101–2104.

Bussemaker, E., Hillebrand, U., Hausberg, M., Pavenstädt, H., & Oberleithner, H. (2010). Pathogenesis of hypertension: Interactions among sodium, potassium, and aldosterone. *American Journal of Kidney Disease, 55,* 1111–1120.

Centers for Disease Control and Prevention. (2012). *Community water fluoridation.* Available at www.cdc.gov/fluoridation/benefits/background.htm. Accessed on 9/26/12.

Cook, N., Obarzanek, E., Cutler, J., Buring, J. E., Rexrode, K. M., Kumanyika, S. K., . . . Whelton, P. K. (2009). Trials of Hypertension Prevention Collaborative Research Group. Joint effects of sodium and potassium intake on subsequent cardiovascular disease: The Trials of Hypertension Prevention follow-up study. *Archives of Internal Medicine, 169,* 32–40.

Dasgupta, P., Liu, Y., & Dyke, J. (2008). Iodine nutrition: Iodine content of iodized salt in the United States. *Environmental Science and Technology, 42,* 1315–1323.

De Benoist, B., McLean, E., Andersson, M., & Rogers, L. (2008). Iodine deficiency in 2007: Global progress since 2003. *Food and Nutrition Bulletin, 29,* 195–202.

Faghih, S., Abadi, A., Hedavati, M., & Kimiagar, S. (2011). Comparison of the effects of cows' milk, fortified soy milk, and calcium supplement on weight and fat loss in premenopausal overweight and obese women. *Nutrition, Metabolism and Cardiovascular Diseases, 21,* 499–503.

Haldimann, M., Alt, A., Blanc, A., & Blondeau, K. (2005). Iodine content of food groups. *Journal of Food Composition and Analysis, 18,* 461–471.

Institute of Medicine. (2000). *Dietary Reference Intakes for vitamin C, vitamin E, selenium, and carotenoids.* Washington, DC: National Academy Press.

Institute of Medicine. (2001). *Dietary Reference Intakes for vitamin A, vitamin K, arsenic, boron, chromium, copper, iodine, iron, manganese, molybdenum, nickel, silicon, vanadium, and zinc.* Washington, DC: National Academy Press.

Institute of Medicine. (2005). *Dietary Reference Intakes for water, potassium, sodium, chloride, and sulfate.* Available at http://www.nap.edu/catalog.php?record_id=10925#. Accessed on 9/25/12.

Institute of Medicine. (2011). *Dietary Reference Intakes for calcium and vitamin D.* Available at http://www.nap.edu. Accessed on 2/17/12.

Johnson, R., Appel, L., Brands, M., Howard, B. V., Lefevre, M., Lustig, R. H., . . . Wylie-Rosett, J. (2009). Dietary sugars intake and cardiovascular health. A scientific statement from the American Heart Association. *Circulation, 120,* 1011–1020.

Kuanrong, L., Kaaks, R., Linseisen, J., & Rohrmann, S. (2012). Associations of dietary calcium intake and calcium supplementation with myocardial infarction and stroke risk and overall cardiovascular mortality in the Heidelberg cohort of the European Prospective Investigation into Cancer and Nutrition study (EPIC-Heidelberg). *Heart, 98,* 920–925.

Lloyd-Jones, D., Hong, Y., Labarthe, D., Mozaffarian, D., Appel, L. J., Van Horn, L., . . . Rosamond, W. D. (2010). Defining and setting national goals for cardiovascular health promotion and disease reduction: The American Heart Association's strategic impact goal through 2020 and beyond. *Circulation, 121,* 586–613.

MacFarquhar, J., Broussard, D., Melstrom, P., Hutchinson, R., Wolkin, A., Martin, C., . . . Jones, T. F. (2010). Acute selenium toxicity associated with a dietary supplement. *Archives of Internal Medicine, 170,* 256–261.

Malik, V., Schulze, M., & Hu, F. (2006). Intake of sugar-sweetened beverages and weight gain: A systematic review. *American Journal of Clinical Nutrition, 84,* 274–288.

Obarzanek, E., Sacks, F., Vollmer, W., Bray, G. A., Miller, E. R., III, Lin, P. H., . . . Proschan, M. A. (2001). Effects on blood lipids of a blood pressure-lowering diet: The Dietary Approaches to Stop Hypertension (DASH) Trial. *American Journal of Clinical Nutrition, 74*, 80–89.

Office of Dietary Supplements, National Institutes of Health. (2009). *Magnesium.* Available at http://ods.od.nih.gov/factsheets/magnesium.asp. Accessed on 9/25/12.

Ogden, C., Kit, B., Carroll, M., & Park, S. (2011). *Consumption of sugar drinks in the United States, 2005–2008* (NCHS Data Brief, no. 71). Available at http://www.cdc.gov/nchs/data/databriefs/db71.pdf. Accessed on 1/22/13.

Perrine, C., Herrick, K., Serdula, M., & Sullivan, K. (2010). Some subgroups of reproductive age women in the United States may be at risk for iodine deficiency. *Journal of Nutrition, 140*, 1489–1494.

Popkin, B., Armstrong, L., Bray, G., Caballero, B., Frei, B., & Willett, W. C. (2006). A new proposed guidance system for beverage consumption in the United States. *American Journal of Clinical Nutrition, 83*, 529–542.

Rao, G., & Rowland, K. (2011). Zinc for the common cold—Not if, but when. *Journal of Family Practice, 60*, 669–671.

Science, M., Johnstone, J., Roth, D., Guyatt, G., & Loeb, M. (2012). Zinc for the treatment of the common cold: A systematic review and meta-analysis of randomized controlled trials. *Canadian Medical Association Journal, 184*, E551–E561.

Shahar, D., Schwarzfuchs, D., Fraser, D., Vardi, H., Thiery, J., Fiedler, G. M., . . . Shai, I. (2010). Dairy calcium intake, serum vitamin D, and successful weight loss. *American Journal of Clinical Nutrition, 92*, 1017–1022.

Singh, M., & Das, R. (2011). Zinc for the common cold. *Cochrane Database System Review, 2*, CD001365.

Steinbrenner, H., & Sies, H. (2009). Protection against reactive oxygen species by selenoproteins. *Biochimica et Biophysica Acta, 1970*, 1478–1485.

Steinbrenner, H., Speckmann, B., Pinto, A., & Sies, H. (2011). High selenium intake and increased diabetes risk: Experimental evidence for interplay between selenium and carbohydrate metabolism. *Journal of Clinical Biochemistry and Nutrition, 48*, 40–45.

Stranges, S., Marshall, J., Natarajan, R., Donahue, R. P., Trevisan, M., Combs, G. F., . . . Reid, M. E. (2007). Effects of long-term selenium supplementation on the incidence of type 2 diabetes: A randomized trial. *Annals of Internal Medicine, 147*, 217–223.

Strazzullo, P., D-Elia, L., Landala, N., & Cappuccio, F. (2009). Salt intake, stroke, and cardiovascular disease: Meta-analysis of prospective studies. *British Medical Journal, 339*, b4567.

Trials of Hypertension Prevention Collaborative Research Group. (1997). Effects of weight loss and sodium reduction intervention on blood pressure and hypertension incidence in overweight people with high-normal blood pressure: The Trials of Hypertension Prevention, phase II. *Archives of Internal Medicine, 157*, 657–667.

Tussing-Humphreys, L., & Braunschweig, C. (2011). Anemia in postmenopausal women: Dietary inadequacy of nondietary factors? *Journal of American Dietetic Association, 111*, 528–531.

U.S. Department of Agriculture, Agricultural Research Service. (2010). *Nutrient intakes from food: Mean amounts consumed per individual, by gender and age. What We Eat in American, NHANES 2007–2008.* Available at www.ars.usda.gov/ba/bhnrc/fsrg. Accessed on 6/9/12.

U.S. Department of Agriculture, U.S. Department of Health and Human Services. (2010). *Dietary guidelines for Americans, 2010* (7th ed.). Available at www.health.gov/dietaryguidelines. Accessed on 9/24/12.

Valtin, H. (2002). "Drink at least eight glasses of water a day." Really? Is there scientific evidence for "8 × 8"? *American Journal of Physiology. Regulatory, Integrative and Comparative Physiology, 283*, R993–R1004.

van Mierlo, L., Greyling, A., Zock, P., Kok, F. J., & Geleijnse, J. M. (2010). Suboptimal potassium intake and potential impact on population blood pressure. *Archives of Internal Medicine, 170*, 1501–1502.

Vartanian, L., Schwartz, M., & Brownell, K. (2007). Effects of soft drink consumption on nutrition and health: A systematic review and meta-analysis. *American Journal of Public Health, 97*, 667–675.

Whanger, P., Vendeland, S., Park, Y., & Xia, Y. (1996). Metabolism of subtoxic levels of selenium in animals and humans. *Annals of Clinical and Laboratory Science, 26*, 99–113.

World Health Organization. (2012). *Micronutrient deficiencies. Iron deficiency anaemia.* Available at www.who.int/nutrition/topics/ida/en/index.html. Accessed on 9/26/12.

Yang, Q., Liu, T., Kuklina, E., Flanders, W. D., Hong, Y., Gillespie, C., . . . Hu, F. B. (2011). Sodium and potassium intake and mortality among US adults. Prospective data from the Third National Health and Nutrition Examination Survey. *Archives of Internal Medicine, 171*, 1183–1191.

Zhang, X., & Giovannucci, E. (2011). Calcium, vitamin D and colorectal cancer chemoprevention. *Best Practice and Research. Clinical Gastroenterology, 25*, 485–494.

Zimmermann, M., Jooste, P., & Pandav, C. (2008). Iodine-deficiency disorders. *The Lancet, 372*, 1251–1262.

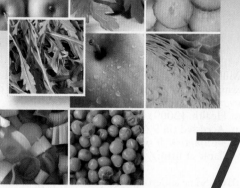

7 Energy Balance

TRUE FALSE

☐ ☐ **1** A food that is high in "energy" is high in calories.

☐ ☐ **2** A pound of body fat is equivalent to 3500 calories.

☐ ☐ **3** People shaped like "apples" are at greater health risk than people shaped like "pears."

☐ ☐ **4** The formulas to calculate body mass index (BMI) are different for men and women.

☐ ☐ **5** Calorie-dense foods provide a relatively high amount of calories with low levels of vitamins, minerals, and other beneficial substances.

☐ ☐ **6** The majority of calories expended daily by most Americans are spent on basal needs.

☐ ☐ **7** Building muscle speeds metabolic rate.

☐ ☐ **8** To reap health benefits, you must participate in continuous activity for at least 30 minutes.

☐ ☐ **9** Sitting too much is a health risk even when physical activity goals are met.

☐ ☐ **10** An effective strategy for limiting calorie intake is to limit food and beverages high in added sugar and solid fat.

LEARNING OBJECTIVES

Upon completion of this chapter, you will be able to

1 Estimate an individual's total calorie requirements.
2 Determine an individual's BMI.
3 Evaluate weight status based on BMI.
4 Assess a person's waist circumference.
5 Give examples of the healthiest ways to reduce calorie intake.
6 Evaluate a person's usual activity level based on Dietary Guidelines recommendations.

Calorie: unit by which energy is measured; the amount of heat needed to raise the temperature of 1 kg of water by 1°C. Technically, calorie is actually kilocalorie or kcal.

Technically, a **calorie** is the amount of energy required to raise the temperature of 1 kg of water by 1°C. In nutrition, calories are the measure of the amount of energy in a food or used by the body to fuel activity. Energy balance is a function of calorie intake versus calorie output (Fig. 7.1).

This chapter addresses the dynamics of energy balance and how total calorie requirements are estimated. Methods to determine healthy body weight and standards for evaluating

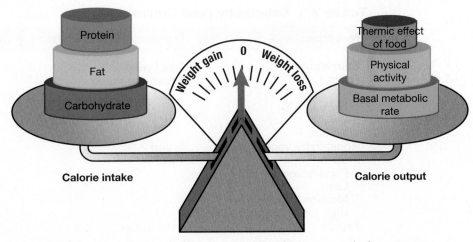

■ FIGURE 7.1   Energy balance: calorie intake versus calorie output.

body weight are presented. Energy in health promotion focuses on the *Dietary Guidelines for Americans, 2010* (DGA) recommendations for weight management and physical activity (PA).

ENERGY INTAKE

Calories come from carbohydrates, protein, fat, and alcohol. The total number of calories in a food or diet can be estimated by multiplying total grams of these nutrients by the appropriate calories per gram—namely, 4 cal/g for carbohydrates and protein, 9 cal/g for fat, and 7 cal/g for alcohol.

In practice, "counting calories" is an imprecise and painstaking process dependent on knowing accurate portion sizes of all foods consumed and the exact nutritional composition of each item, neither of which conditions is easily met. Even when all food consumed is measured, the nutrient values available in food composition references represent *average* not *actual* nutrition content based on analysis of a number of food samples.

A less accurate but easier way to estimate calorie intake is to estimate or count the number of servings from each food group a person consumes. Multiply the number of servings by the average amount of calories in a serving and then add the calories from each group to get an approximation of the total calories consumed. Be aware that representative foods within each of the Exchange Lists for Diabetics food groups are generally free of added fat or sugar (Table 7.1). For instance, items like onion rings, brownies, and sugar-sweetened cereals are not part of those food groups. As with "counting calories," the accuracy of "counting servings" depends on the quality of foods consumed and accuracy of portion size estimation.

ENERGY EXPENDITURE

The body uses energy for involuntary activities and purposeful PA. The total of these expenditures represents the number of calories a person uses in a day.

Table 7.1 Calories by Food Groups

Food Group	Representative Serving Size	Average Calories per Serving
Starch/grains	1 oz bread	80
Fruits	1 medium piece	60
Milk	1 cup	
Skim or 1%		100
2%		120
Whole		160
Nonstarchy vegetables	½ cup	25
Protein foods	1 oz	
Plant-based protein		Varies
Lean		45
Medium fat		75
High fat		100
Fat/oils	1 tsp butter	45

Source: American Diabetes Association, American Dietetic Association. (2008). *Choose your foods: Exchange lists for diabetes.* Alexandria, VA: The American Diabetes Association.

Basal Metabolism

Basal Metabolic Rate (BMR) or Basal Energy Expenditure (BEE): the amount of calories expended in a 24-hour period to fuel the involuntary activities of the body at rest and after a 12-hour fast.

Resting Metabolic Rate (RMR) or Resting Energy Expenditure (REE): the amount of calories expended in a 24-hour period to fuel the involuntary activities of the body at rest. RMR does not adhere to the criterion of a 12-hour fast, so it is slightly higher than BEE because it includes energy spent on digesting, absorbing, and metabolizing food.

Basal metabolism is the amount of calories required to fuel the involuntary activities of the body at rest after a 12-hour fast. These involuntary activities include maintaining body temperature and muscle tone, producing and releasing secretions, propelling the gastrointestinal (GI) tract, inflating the lungs, and beating the heart. For most people, the **basal metabolic rate (BMR)** or **basal energy expenditure (BEE)** accounts for approximately 60% to 70% of total calories expended. The less active a person is, the greater is the proportion of calories used for BEE. The term "BEE" is often used interchangeably with **resting metabolic rate (RMR)** or **resting energy expenditure (REE)** even though they are slightly different measures.

One imprecise, rule-of-thumb guideline for estimating BMR is to multiply healthy weight (in pounds) by 10 for women and 11 for men. For example, a 130-pound woman expends approximately 1300 cal/day on BMR (130 lb × 10 cal/lb = 1300 calories). When actual weight exceeds healthy weight, an "adjusted" weight of halfway between healthy and actual can be used. For instance, if healthy weight is 130 lb, but actual weight is 170 lb, 150 lb would be the "adjusted" weight for estimating basal calories. Methods used to determine BMR and total calorie requirements in the clinical setting are discussed in Chapter 16.

A drawback of using a rule-of-thumb method for determining BMR is that it is based only on weight; it does not account for other variables that affect metabolic rate, such as body composition. Lean tissue (muscle mass) contributes to a higher metabolic rate than fat tissue. Therefore, people with more muscle mass have higher metabolic rates than do people with proportionately more fat tissue. This explains why men, who have a greater proportion of muscle, have higher metabolic rates than women, who have a greater proportion of fat. Conversely, the loss of lean tissue that usually occurs with aging beginning sometime around age 30 years is one reason why calorie requirements decrease as people get older. However, strength training exercise can lead to significant gains in muscle strength and size—and thus increase BMR—even among frail, institutionalized 90-year-old men and women (Fiatarone et al., 1990). Other factors that affect BMR appear in Table 7.2.

Table 7.2 Factors That Affect BMR

Variables	Effect on Metabolism
Age	Loss of lean body mass with age lowers BMR.
Growth	The formation of new tissue, as seen in children and during pregnancy, increases BMR.
Stresses	Stresses, such as infection and many diseases, raise BMR.
Thyroid hormones: tetraiodothyronine (thyroxine, or T_4) and triiodothyronine (T_3)	An oversecretion of thyroid hormones (hyperthyroidism) speeds up BMR; undersecretion of thyroid hormones (hypothyroidism) lowers BMR. The change may be as great as 50%.
Fever	BMR increases 7% for each degree Fahrenheit above 98.6.
Height	When considering two people of the same gender who weigh the same, the taller one has a higher BMR than the shorter one because of a larger surface area.
Extreme environmental temperatures	Very hot and very cold environmental temperatures increase the BMR because the body expends more energy to regulate its own temperature.
Starvation, fasting, and malnutrition	Part of the decline in BMR that occurs with these conditions is attributed to the loss of lean body tissue. Hormonal changes may contribute to the decrease in metabolic rate.
Weight loss from calorie deficits	With smaller body mass, less energy is required to fuel metabolism.
Smoking	Nicotine increases BMR.
Caffeine	Increases BMR
Certain drugs, such as barbiturates, narcotics, and muscle relaxants	Decrease BMR
Sleep, paralysis	Decrease BMR

Physical Activity

Physical activity (PA), or voluntary muscular activity, accounts for approximately 30% of total calories used, although it may be as low as 20% in sedentary people and as high as 50% in people who are very active. The actual amount of energy expended on PA depends on the intensity and duration of the activity and the weight of the person performing the activity. The more intense and longer the activity, the greater is the amount of calories burned. Heavier people, who have more weight to move, use more energy than lighter people to perform the same activity.

Although it is possible to get a reasonable estimate of total calories expended in a day by keeping a thorough record of all activity for a 24-hour period, it is a tedious process. An easier rule-of-thumb method for estimating daily calories expended on PA is to calculate the percentage increase above BMR on the basis of estimated intensity of usual daily activities.

Thermic Effect of Food

Thermic Effect of Food: an estimation of the amount of energy required to digest, absorb, transport, metabolize, and store nutrients.

The **thermic effect of food** is another category of energy expenditure that represents the "cost" of processing food. In a normal mixed diet, it is estimated to be about 10% of the total calorie intake. For instance, people who consume 1800 cal/day use about 180 calories to process their food. The actual thermic effect of food varies with the composition of food eaten, the frequency of eating, and the size of meals consumed. Although it represents an actual and legitimate use of calories, the thermic effect of food in practice is often disregarded when calorie requirements are estimated because it constitutes such a small amount of energy and is imprecisely estimated.

Estimating Total Energy Expenditure

Total calorie needs can be imprecisely estimated by using predictive equations, of which more than 200 have been published. The following are different approaches for estimating calorie needs; all yield estimates, not precise measurements.

- Add the results of the rule-of-thumb methods described earlier for estimating BMR and calories spent on activity (Box 7.1).
- Use a simple formula of calories per kilogram of body weight, such as 25 cal/kg to 30 cal/kg, which is often used for nonobese adults. This formula is adjusted upward or downward based on the client's age, weight, or activity level.
- Use a standard reference that lists estimated daily calorie needs based on gender, age, and activity. Table 7.3 lists estimated daily calorie needs.

Box 7.1 ESTIMATING TOTAL ENERGY EXPENDITURE

1. Estimate basal metabolic rate (BMR)

Multiply your healthy weight (in pounds) by 10 for women or 11 for men. If you are overweight, multiply by the average weight within your healthy weight range (see Chapter 14).

_____ (weight in pounds) × _____ = _____ calories for BMR

2. Estimate total calories according to usual activity level

Choose the category that describes your usual activities and then multiply BMR by the appropriate percentage.

Sedentary: mostly sitting, driving, sleeping, standing, reading, typing, and other low-intensity activities	20
Light activity: light exercise such as walking not more than 2 hours/day	30
Moderate activity: moderate exercise such as heavy housework, gardening, and very little sitting	40
High activity: active in physical sports or a labor-intensive occupation such as construction work	50

3. Add BMR calories and physical activity calories

_____ calories for BMR + _____ calories spent on activity = _____ calories spent on involuntary and physical activity

4. Add estimate of thermic effect of food

_____ calories spent on involuntary and voluntary activity + 10% for processing food = _____ total calories expended daily

Table 7.3 Estimated Calorie Needs per Day by Age, Gender, and Physical Activity Level*

Age	Activity Level for Males			Age	Activity Level for Females[‡]		
	Sedentary[†]	Moderately Active[†]	Active[†]		Sedentary[†]	Moderately Active[†]	Active[†]
2	1000	1000	1000	2	1000	1000	1000
3	1000	1400	1400	3	1000	1200	1400
4	1200	1400	1600	4	1200	1400	1400
5	1200	1400	1600	5	1200	1400	1600
6	1400	1600	1800	6	1200	1400	1600
7	1400	1600	1800	7	1200	1600	1800
8	1400	1600	2000	8	1400	1600	1800
9	1600	1800	2000	9	1400	1600	1800
10	1600	1800	2200	10	1400	1800	2000
11	1800	2000	2200	11	1600	1800	2000
12	1800	2200	2400	12	1600	2000	2200
13	2000	2200	2600	13	1600	2000	2200
14	2000	2400	2800	14	1800	2000	2400
15	2200	2600	3000	15	1800	2000	2400
16	2400	2800	3200	16	1800	2000	2400
17	2400	2800	3200	17	1800	2000	2400
18	2400	2800	3200	18	1800	2000	2400
19–20	2600	2800	3000	19–20	2000	2200	2400
21–25	2400	2800	3000	21–25	2000	2200	2400
26–30	2400	2600	3000	26–30	1800	2000	2400
31–35	2400	2600	3000	31–35	1800	2000	2200
36–40	2400	2600	2800	36–40	1800	2000	2200
41–45	2200	2600	2800	41–45	1800	2000	2200
46–50	2200	2400	2800	46–50	1800	2000	2200
51–55	2200	2400	2800	51–55	1600	1800	2200
56–60	2200	2400	2600	56–60	1600	1800	2200
61–65	2000	2400	2600	61–65	1600	1800	2000
66–70	2000	2200	2600	66–70	1600	1800	2000
71–75	2000	2200	2600	71–75	1600	1800	2000
76 and up	2000	2200	2400	76 and up	1600	1800	2000

Note: Values depict amounts of calories needed to maintain calorie balance for various gender and age groups at three different levels of physical activity. The estimates are rounded to the nearest 200 calories. An individual's calorie needs may be higher or lower than these average estimates.

*Based on estimated energy requirements (EER) equations, using reference heights (average) and reference weights (healthy) for each age–gender group. For children and adolescents, reference height and weight vary. For adults, the reference man is 5 ft 10 in tall and weighs 154 pounds. The reference woman is 5 ft 4 in tall and weighs 126 pounds. EER equations are from the Institute of Medicine. (2002). *Dietary Reference Intakes for energy, carbohydrate, fiber, fat, fatty acids, cholesterol, protein, and amino acids.* Washington, DC: The National Academies Press.

[†]Sedentary means a lifestyle that includes only the light physical activity associated with typical day-to-day life. Moderately active means a lifestyle that includes physical activity equivalent to walking about 1.5 to 3 miles per day at 3 to 4 miles per hour, in addition to the light physical activity associated with typical day-to-day life. Active means a lifestyle that includes physical activity equivalent to walking more than 3 miles per day at 3 to 4 miles per hour, in addition to the light physical activity associated with typical day-to-day life.

[‡]Estimates for females do not include women who are pregnant or breastfeeding.

Source: Britten, P., Marcoe, K., Yamini, S., & Davis, C. (2006). Development of food intake patterns for the MyPyramid Food Guidance System. *Journal of Nutrition Education and Behavior, 38*(Suppl. 6), S78–S92.

From: U.S. Department of Agriculture, U.S. Department of Health and Human Services. (2010). *Dietary guidelines for Americans, 2010* (7th ed.). Available at www.health.gov/dietaryguidelines. Accessed on 2/24/11.

EVALUATING WEIGHT STATUS

From a health perspective, "healthy" or "desirable" weight is that which is statistically correlated to good health. But the relationship between body weight and good health is more complicated than simply the number on the scale. The amount of body *fat* a person has and where a person's weight is distributed also influence health risks, as does the presence of certain diseases or conditions, such as type 2 diabetes and cardiovascular disease. Table 7.4 summarizes the standards for evaluating ideal body weight, body mass index, and waist circumference. These values are relatively arbitrary because risk exists on a continuum without absolute cutoffs.

Ideal Body Weight

Ideal Body Weight: the formula given here is a universally used standard in clinical practice to quickly estimate a person's reasonable weight based on height, even though this and all other methods are not absolute.

The Hamwi method is a quick and easy way to compute **"ideal" body weight** (IBW) based on an adult's height and gender. The formula is as follows:

For women: Allow 100 pounds for the first 5 ft of height
Add 5 pounds for each additional inch of height

For men: Allow 106 pounds for the first 5 ft of height
Add 6 pounds for each additional inch of height.

Using this formula, a 5 ft 6 in tall women would have an "ideal" weight of 130 pounds and a man of the same height would have an "ideal" weight of 142 pounds. IBW can be adjusted upward or downward by 10% based on estimation of a person's frame size. Likewise, for people who are less than 5 ft tall, 2½ pounds are subtracted for each inch under 5 ft. Although this formula is simple to use, it does not take into account body composition or distribution of body fat, both of which impact health risk.

Body Mass Index

In the clinical setting, body mass index (BMI) has replaced traditional height–weight calculations of "ideal" or "desirable" body weight. In 2003, the U.S. Preventive Services Task Force (USPSTF) concluded that BMI is an acceptable measure for identifying adults

Table 7.4 Evaluating Weight

Standard	Interpretation
Percentage of "ideal" body weight (% IBW)	≤69% severe malnutrition 70%–79% moderate malnutrition 80%–89% mild malnutrition 90%–110% within normal range 110%–119% overweight ≥120% obese ≥200% morbidly obese
Body mass index (BMI)	≤18.5 may ↑ health risk 18.5–24.9 healthy weight 25–29.9 overweight 30–34.9 obesity class 1 35–39.9 obesity class 2 ≥40 obesity class 3

with excess weight (USPSTF, 2003). Although the USPSTF recently updated the 2003 statement on screening for obesity and overweight in adults, screening tests were not part of its review (Moyer, 2012).

The formula to calculate BMI is weight in kilograms divided by height in meters squared or weight in pounds divided by height in inches squared multiplied by 703. Nomograms and tables that plot height and weight to determine BMI eliminate complicated mathematical calculations (Table 7.5).

Despite its widespread use as a screening tool, BMI is not without controversy. For instance, the BMI levels that define overweight and obesity are somewhat arbitrary because the relationship between increasing weight and risk of disease is continuous. Also, BMI does not take body composition into account; a lean athlete may have well-developed muscle mass and little fat tissue, yet if his BMI is high, he would fall under the designation of overweight or obese. Conversely, an elderly person may have a normal BMI and be deemed "healthy" despite a high amount of body fat masked by a low percentage of muscle mass. Last, ethnic differences exist in the relationship between BMI and health risks. For instance, because of genetic differences in body composition, the health risks of obesity occur at a BMI lower than 30 for Asian Americans and higher than 30 for Black Americans.

Waist Circumference

Recent evidence indicates that waist circumference may be an acceptable alternative to BMI measurement in some subpopulations (Moyer, 2012). In fact, the location of excess body fat may be a more important and reliable indicator of disease risk than the degree of total body fatness. Storing a disproportionate amount of total body fat in the abdomen increases risks for type 2 diabetes and cardiovascular disease. Generally, men and postmenopausal women tend to store excess fat in the upper body, particularly in the abdominal area, whereas premenopausal women tend to store excess fat in the lower body, particularly in the hips and thighs. Regardless of gender, people with a high distribution of abdominal fat (i.e., "apples") have a greater relative health risk than people with excess fat in the hips and thighs (i.e., "pears") (Fig. 7.2). The current waist circumference recognized as abdominal obesity in the United States is 40 in or more for men and 35 in or more for women (Alberti et al., 2009). As with BMI, ethnic groups differ in regard to where risk begins in relation to waist circumference.

ENERGY BALANCE IN HEALTH PROMOTION

The state of energy balance is the relationship between the amount of calories consumed and the amount of calories expended. As illustrated in Figure 7.3, when calorie intake and output are approximately the same over time, body weight is stable. A "positive" energy balance occurs when calorie intake exceeds calorie output, whether the imbalance is caused by overeating, low activity, or both (Fig. 7.4). Over time, the calories consumed in excess of need contribute to weight gain. Because a pound of body fat is equivalent to 3500 calories, an "extra" 500 cal/day for a whole week can result in a 1-pound weight gain. Conversely, a "negative" calorie balance occurs when calorie output exceeds intake, whether the imbalance is from decreasing calorie intake, increasing PA, or (preferably) both (Fig. 7.5).

In 2009–2010, 68.8% of Americans 20 years of age and older were overweight or obese, and 35.7% of American adults were obese (National Center for Health Statistics, 2012). Excess weight, the outcome of a positive energy balance, also increases the risk of cardiovascular disease, hypertension, type 2 diabetes, and certain cancers (U.S.

Table 7.5 Body Mass Index

	Normal							Overweight						Obese			
BMI	19	20	21	22	23	24	25	26	27	28	29	30	31	32	33	34	35
Height (inches)								**Body Weight (pounds)**									
58	91	96	100	105	110	115	119	124	129	134	138	143	148	153	158	162	167
59	94	99	104	109	114	119	124	128	133	138	143	148	153	158	163	168	173
60	97	102	107	112	118	123	128	133	138	143	148	153	158	163	168	174	179
61	100	106	111	116	122	127	132	137	143	148	153	158	164	169	174	180	185
62	104	109	115	120	126	131	136	142	147	153	158	164	169	175	180	186	191
63	107	113	118	124	130	135	141	146	152	158	163	169	175	180	186	191	197
64	110	116	122	128	134	140	145	151	157	163	169	174	180	186	192	197	204
65	114	120	126	132	138	144	150	156	162	168	174	180	186	192	198	204	210
66	118	124	130	136	142	148	155	161	167	173	179	186	192	198	204	210	216
67	121	127	134	140	146	153	159	166	172	178	185	191	198	204	211	217	223
68	125	131	138	144	151	158	164	171	177	184	190	197	203	210	216	223	230
69	128	135	142	149	155	162	169	176	182	189	196	203	209	216	223	230	236
70	132	139	146	153	160	167	174	181	188	195	202	209	216	222	229	236	243
71	136	143	150	157	165	172	179	186	193	200	208	215	222	229	236	243	250
72	140	147	154	162	169	177	184	191	199	206	213	221	228	235	242	250	258
73	144	151	159	166	174	182	189	197	204	212	219	227	235	242	250	257	265
74	148	155	163	171	179	186	194	202	210	218	225	233	241	249	256	264	272
75	152	160	168	176	184	192	200	208	216	224	232	240	248	256	264	272	279
76	156	164	172	180	189	197	205	213	221	230	238	246	254	263	271	279	287

Source: Adapted from U.S. Department of Health and Human Services. (1998). *Clinical guidelines on the identification, evaluation, and treatment of overweight and obesity in adults: The evidence report.* Rockville, MD: U.S. Department of Health and Human Services.

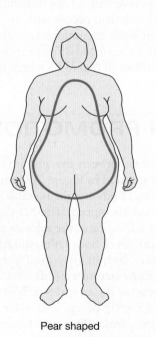

Pear shaped

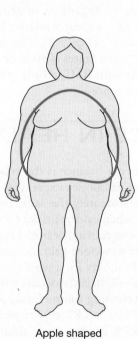

Apple shaped

■ **FIGURE 7.2** Pear shape versus apple shape.

Extreme Obesity																		
36	37	38	39	40	41	42	43	44	45	46	47	48	49	50	51	52	53	54

Body Weight (pounds)

172	177	181	186	191	196	201	205	210	215	220	224	229	234	239	244	248	253	258
178	183	188	193	198	203	208	212	217	222	227	232	237	242	247	252	257	262	267
184	189	194	199	204	209	215	220	225	230	235	240	245	250	255	261	266	271	276
190	195	201	206	211	217	222	227	232	238	243	248	254	259	264	269	275	280	285
196	202	207	213	218	224	229	235	240	246	251	256	262	267	273	278	284	289	295
203	208	214	220	225	231	237	242	248	254	259	265	270	278	282	287	293	299	304
209	215	221	227	232	238	244	250	256	262	267	273	279	285	291	296	302	308	314
216	222	228	234	240	246	252	258	264	270	276	282	288	294	300	306	312	318	324
223	229	235	241	247	253	260	266	272	278	284	291	297	303	309	315	322	328	334
230	236	242	249	255	261	268	274	280	287	293	299	306	312	319	325	331	338	344
236	243	249	256	262	269	276	282	289	295	302	308	315	322	328	335	341	348	354
243	250	257	263	270	277	284	291	297	304	311	318	324	331	338	345	351	358	365
250	257	264	271	278	285	292	299	306	313	320	327	334	341	348	355	362	369	376
257	265	272	279	286	293	301	308	315	322	329	338	343	351	358	365	372	379	386
265	272	279	287	294	302	309	316	324	331	338	346	353	361	368	375	383	390	397
272	280	288	295	302	310	318	325	333	340	348	355	363	371	378	386	393	401	408
280	287	295	303	311	319	326	334	342	350	358	365	373	381	389	396	404	412	420
287	295	303	311	319	327	335	343	351	359	367	375	383	391	399	407	415	423	431
295	304	312	320	328	336	344	353	361	369	377	385	394	402	410	418	426	435	443

Department of Agriculture [USDA], U.S. Department of Health and Human Services [USDHHS], 2010).

Poor food choices and physical inactivity contribute to the current state of energy imbalance in the United States. For instance, MyPlate recommends Americans limit their intake of solid fats and added sugars to no more than 15% of total calories; yet on average,

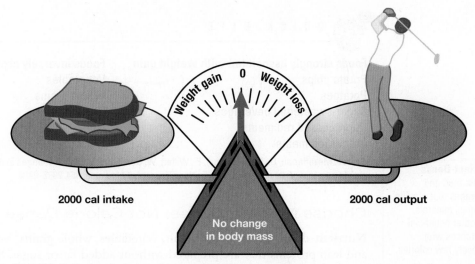

2000 cal intake   2000 cal output

No change
in body mass

■ FIGURE 7.3   A state of energy balance: calorie intake is equal to calorie output.

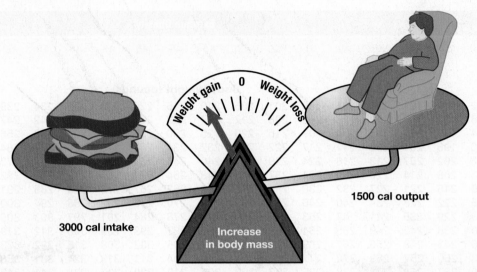

■ FIGURE 7.4   A positive energy balance: calorie intake is greater than calorie output.

Americans consume approximately 35% of their total calories in the form of empty calories (ChooseMyPlate.gov). Likewise, fewer than 5% of adults participate in 30 minutes of PA each day (USDA, USDHHS, 2010).

Food Choices

The *Dietary Guidelines for Americans, 2010* contain two main interrelated concepts: maintain calorie balance over time to achieve and sustain a healthy weight and focus on consuming nutrient-dense foods and beverages (USDA, USDHHS, 2010). Key recommendations that pertain to calorie balance and weight management are listed in Box 7.2.

Some lifestyle strategies to attain and maintain healthy weight are discussed in the following section. As a clinical issue, the management of overweight and obesity, including therapeutic diet approaches, is presented in Chapter 14.

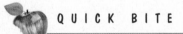 **Q U I C K   B I T E**

Foods strongly associated with weight gain	Foods inversely associated with weight gain
Potato chips	Vegetables
Potatoes	Whole grains
Sugar-sweetened beverages	Fruits
Unprocessed red meats	Nuts
Processed meats	Yogurt

Source: Mozaffarian, D., Hao, T., Rimm, E., Willett, W. C., & Hu, F. B. (2011). Changes in diet and lifestyle and long-term weight gain in women and men. *New England Journal of Medicine, 364*, 2392–2404.

Nutrient-Dense Items: food and beverages that provide vitamins, minerals, and other beneficial substances with relatively few calories.

Choose Nutrient-Dense, Not Calorie-Dense Items

Nutrient-dense items include fruit, vegetables, whole grains, legumes, nuts, nonfat milk, and lean proteins that are prepared without added fat or sugar. Substituting these healthy

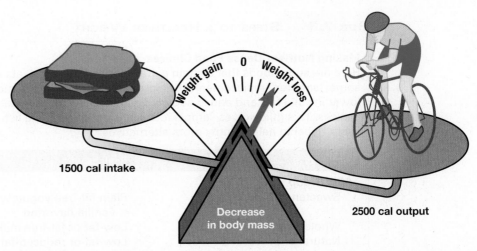

■ FIGURE 7.5   A negative energy balance: calorie intake is less than calorie output.

Calorie-Dense Items: food and beverages that provide relatively high calories per amounts of vitamins, minerals, and other beneficial substances.

choices for **calorie-dense items**, such as regular soft drinks, most desserts, fried foods, full-fat dairy products, high-fat meat, alcohol, and most fast foods, lowers calorie intake while increasing nutrient intake (Box 7.3). Strategies that may make healthy eating easier include eating out less often, bringing healthy snacks from home instead of relying on vending machine options, and stocking the pantry and refrigerator with only healthy items.

Note that the emphasis is on healthy and wholesome choices, not commercially prepared "junk" foods that have been modified to be "fat free" or "sugar free." Those labels may give the impression that the food is also "calorie free," but that is not necessarily true. Fat-free milk is a good choice because milk is a fundamentally healthy food made healthier by the elimination of fat. In contrast, fat-free cookies are still cookies—"treats" made with sugar and refined flour—not an inherently healthy food. In both cases, these fat-free foods still contain calories from protein and carbohydrates.

Eat Only to Relieve Hunger

Eating should not be used as a diversion from boredom, loneliness, anxiety, or stress, nor should it be used in response to external cues, such as the time of day or commercial advertising. Likewise, eating only to the point of satisfaction, and not until feeling "stuffed," by focusing on internal cues for satiety, helps control calorie intake. Mindful eating practices

---

BOX 7.2   *DIETARY GUIDELINES FOR AMERICANS, 2010 KEY RECOMMENDATIONS TO BALANCE CALORIES TO MANAGE WEIGHT*

- Prevent and/or reduce overweight and obesity through improved eating and physical activity behaviors.
- Control total calorie intake to manage body weight. For people who are overweight or obese, this will mean consuming fewer calories from foods and beverages.
- Increase physical activity and reduce time spent in sedentary behaviors.
- Maintain appropriate calorie balance during each stage of life—childhood, adolescence, adulthood, pregnancy and breastfeeding, and older age.

Box 7.3   Steps to a Healthier Weight

Making Nutrient-Dense Food Choices
Here are some foods that contain extra calories from solid fats and added sugars and some "smarter" replacements. Choices on the right side are more nutrient dense—lower in solid fats and added sugars. Try these new ideas instead of your usual choices. This guide gives sample ideas; it is not a complete list. Use the "Nutrition Facts" label to help identify more alternatives.

Instead of ...	Replace with ...
Milk Group	
Sweetened fruit yogurt	Plain fat-free yogurt with fresh fruit or vanilla flavoring
Whole milk	Low-fat or fat-free milk
Natural or processed cheese	Low-fat or reduced-fat cheese
Protein Foods	
Beef (chuck, rib, brisket)	Beef (loin, round), fat trimmed off
Chicken with skin	Chicken without skin
Lunch meats (such as bologna)	Low-fat lunch meats (95%–97% fat free)
Hot dogs (regular)	Hot dogs (lower fat)
Bacon or sausage	Canadian bacon or lean ham
Refried beans	Cooked or canned kidney or pinto beans
Grain Group	
Granola	Reduced-fat granola
Sweetened cereals	Unsweetened cereals with cut-up fruit
Pasta with cheese sauce	Pasta with vegetables (primavera)
Pasta with white sauce (alfredo)	Pasta with red sauce (marinara)
Croissants or pastries	Toast or bread (try whole-grain types)
Fruit Group	
Apple or berry pie	Fresh apple or berries
Sweetened applesauce	Unsweetened applesauce
Canned fruit packed in syrup	Canned fruit packed in juice or "lite" syrup
Vegetable Group	
Deep-fried French fries	Oven-baked French fries
Baked potato with cheese sauce	Baked potato with salsa
Fried vegetables	Steamed or roasted vegetables
Solid Fats	
Cream cheese	Light or fat-free cream cheese
Sour cream	Plain low-fat or fat-free yogurt
Regular margarine or butter	Light-spread margarines, diet margarine
Added Sugars	
Sugar-sweetened soft drinks	Seltzer mixed with 100% fruit juice
Sweetened tea or drinks	Unsweetened tea or water
Syrup on pancakes or French toast	Unsweetened applesauce or berries as a topping
Candy, cookies, cake, or pastry	Fresh or dried fruit
Sugar in recipes	Experiment with reducing amount and adding spices (cinnamon, nutmeg, etc.)

Source: ChooseMyPlate.gov. U.S. Department of Agriculture.

include eating slowly and not doing other things while eating, such as watching television, driving, or talking on the telephone.

Maintain a Consistent Eating Pattern

Avoiding periods of hunger may help avoid bingeing; people become less discriminating in their food choices when they are "starving." Breakfast is important for children and adults; observational studies show an inverse relationship between the frequency of eating breakfast and the risk for obesity and other chronic diseases such as type 2 diabetes (Song, Chun, Obayashi, Cho, and Chung, 2005; Wyatt et al., 2002).

Right Portion Sizes

Portion sizes have grown over the last 20 years (Table 7.6). For instance,

- The number of "large-sized" food packages sold in grocery stores increased 10-fold between 1970 and 2000 (Young and Nestle, 2003).
- Jumbo-sized portions in restaurants are consistently 250% larger than regular portions (Wansink and Ittersum, 2007).
- The average dinner plate used in the home has increased from approximately 10 in in diameter to approximately 12 in in diameter (Wansink, 2006). A study by Pratt, Croager, and Rosenberg (2012) showed that a small increase in the size of dishware can lead to a substantial increase in calories available for consumption.

Over time, the effects of larger portion sizes distort peoples' perception of how much food is "normal" or necessary to create a feeling of fullness and alter their ability to monitor how much food they have consumed, resulting in an increase in the amount of food consumed in a single eating occasion (Wansink and Ittersum, 2007). "Portion distortion" appears to be a widespread problem not linked to income, education, hunger, or body

Table 7.6 Portion Distortion: A Comparison Between Portion Sizes 20 Years Ago and Today

	20 Years Ago	Today
Bagel	3 in diameter 140 calories	6 in diameter 350 calories
Blueberry muffin	1.5 oz 210 calories	5 oz 500 calories
Chicken Caesar salad	1½ cups 390 calories	3 cups 790 calories
Coffee	8 oz with milk and sugar 45 calories	16 oz with milk, sugar, and syrup 350 calories
French fries	2.4 oz 210 calories	6.9 oz 610 calories
Soda	6.5 oz 85 calories	20 oz 250 calories
Spaghetti with meatballs	1 cup pasta with sauce and 3 meatballs 500 calories	2 cups pasta with sauce and 3 large meatballs 1025 calories

Source: U.S. Department of Health and Human Services, National Heart Lung and Blood Institute, National Institutes of Health. (2004). *Portion distortion.* Available at hp2010.nhlbihin.net/portion/index.htm. Accessed on 10/5/12.

weight (Wansink and Ittersum, 2007). Even overconsumption of healthy food can lead to a positive calorie balance and weight gain over time.

According to Wansink and Ittersum (2007), telling people to remind themselves not to overeat is not the answer; changing the environment that led to large portion sizes is easier. Strategies to make food less accessible and less visible include

- Switching to smaller plates, bowls, and glasses
- Buying smaller packages of food at the grocery store; forgo the jumbo size
- Buying prepackaged, portion-controlled items, such as 100-calorie packs
- Storing food out of sight
- Ordering smaller portions at restaurants
- Filling a doggie bag before beginning to eat

Activity Choices: Move More, Sit Less

The *2008 Physical Activity Guidelines for Americans* (USDHHS, 2008) urge all adults to avoid inactivity (Table 7.7). Although any exercise is better than none, the benefits of

Table 7.7 **2008 Physical Activity Guidelines for Americans Summary**

Key Guidelines for Adults

- All adults should avoid inactivity. Some physical activity is better than none, and adults who participate in any amount of physical activity gain some health benefits.
- For substantial health benefits, adults should do at least 150 minutes (2 hours and 30 minutes) a week of moderate-intensity or 75 minutes (1 hour and 15 minutes) a week of vigorous-intensity aerobic physical activity, or an equivalent combination of moderate- and vigorous-intensity aerobic activity. Aerobic activity should be performed in episodes of at least 10 minutes, and preferably, it should be spread throughout the week.
- For additional and more extensive health benefits, adults should increase their aerobic physical activity to 300 minutes (5 hours) a week of moderate-intensity or 150 minutes a week of vigorous-intensity aerobic physical activity, or an equivalent combination of moderate- and vigorous-intensity activity. Additional health benefits are gained by engaging in physical activity beyond this amount.
- Adults should also do muscle-strengthening activities that are moderate or high intensity and involve all major muscle groups on 2 or more days a week, as these activities provide additional health benefits.

Key Guidelines for Older Adults

The Key Guidelines for Adults also apply to older adults. In addition, the following guidelines are just for older adults:

- When older adults cannot do 150 minutes of moderate-intensity aerobic activity a week because of chronic conditions, they should be as physically active as their abilities and conditions allow.
- Older adults should do exercises that maintain or improve balance if they are at risk of falling.
- Older adults should determine their level of effort for physical activity relative to their level of fitness.
- Older adults with chronic conditions should understand whether and how their conditions affect their ability to do regular physical activity safely.

Source: U.S. Department of Health and Human Services. (2008). *Physical activity guidelines for Americans.* Available at http://www.health.gov/paguidelines/guidelines/summary.aspx. Accessed on 10/4/12.

increasing activity are dose dependent and occur along a continuum. A minimum of 2 hours and 30 minutes per week of moderate-intensity aerobic activity is recommended to gain substantial health benefits. For more extensive health benefits, 5 hours per week of moderate-intensity aerobic activity are suggested. Additional benefits are obtained with even higher amounts of aerobic activity. Tips for increasing activity appear in Box 7.4. Exercising with the support of others helps maintain motivation (Fig. 7.6).

In addition to regular aerobic exercises, muscle-strengthening activities that involve all major muscle groups are recommended on 2 or more days a week. Muscle-strengthening activities, which include strength training, resistance training, and strength and endurance exercises, build muscle, which helps to raise metabolic rate and increase the likelihood of weight loss and body fat loss. Changes in body composition—more muscle, less fat—are positive outcomes of muscle-strengthening activities that are not reflected on the scale, as are improved bone density and decreased risk of osteoporosis.

Independent of the time spent exercising, observational epidemiologic studies show that the more time spent being sedentary, the greater the risk of weight gain (Mozaffarian, Hao, Rimm, Willett, and Hu, 2011), obesity (Hu, Li, Colditz, Willett, and Manson, 2003), and other chronic diseases, such as type 2 diabetes (Grontved and Hu, 2011) and cardiovascular disease (Wijndaele et al., 2011). Experimental studies show that prolonged sitting suppresses lipase and insulin activity in muscles, leading to metabolic abnormalities (Bergouignan, Rudwill, Simon, and Blanc, 2011). Clearly, too much sitting is a health risk and is not the same as too little exercise. Strategies to reduce sedentary activity include limiting television viewing and replacing television time with more physically active pursuits.

BOX 7.4   TIPS FOR INCREASING PHYSICAL ACTIVITY

- **Find something enjoyable.** The best chance of success comes from choosing a physical activity (PA) that is enjoyable to the individual. The best activity or exercise is one that is performed, not just contemplated.
- **Use the buddy system.** Committing to an exercise program or increased PA with a friend makes the activity less of a chore and helps to sustain motivation.
- **Spread activity over the entire day if desired.** This recommendation is particularly important for people who "don't have time to exercise." Many people find it easier to fit three 10-minute activity periods into a busy lifestyle than to find 30 uninterrupted minutes to dedicate to activity.
- **Start slowly and gradually increase activity.** For people who have been inactive, it is prudent to start with only a few minutes of daily activity, such as walking, and gradually increase the frequency, duration, and then intensity. People with existing health problems such as diabetes, heart disease, and hypertension should consult a physician before beginning a PA program, as should all men older than 40 years and all women older than 50 years.
- **Move more.** Just moving more can make a cumulative difference in activity. Take the stairs instead of the elevator, park at the far end of the parking lot, walk around while talking on the portable phone, walk instead of driving short distances, play golf without a golf cart or caddy, or fidget.
- **Keep an activity log.** Just as people tend to underestimate the amount of food they eat, people usually overestimate the amount of PA they perform. Documenting the type and duration of activity can help to track progress.

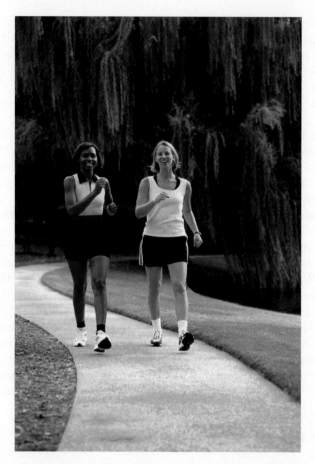

■ **FIGURE 7.6** Women power walking. Enlisting the support of a "buddy" helps sustain motivation.

How Do You Respond?

Do calories eaten at night promote weight gain? What determines whether or not calories are stored as fat is not when they are eaten but in what quantity. Food eaten in the evening is not more calorically dense than it is during the day, but mindless snacking in the evening, if it causes calorie intake to exceed calorie expenditure, can lead to weight gain over time.

Which diet is best for losing weight—a low-carb diet or a low-fat diet? *Any diet that creates a calorie deficit leads to weight loss over time.* What ultimately determines weight loss is the amount of calories consumed compared to the amount of calories expended, not what macronutrient the calories are from. In other words, if a 1500-calorie intake will promote weight loss, it does not matter if these calories come from French fries and cola or carrots and kidney beans. From a health standpoint, the recommended distribution of calories is 45% to 55% carbohydrate, 15% to 35% protein, and 20% to 35% fat (National Academy of Sciences, Institute of Medicine, 2005).

Case Study

Tonya is 5 ft 3 in tall, weighs 151 pounds, and is 38 years old. Her waist circumference is 37 in. As a receptionist for a law firm and mother of two socially active children, her life is busy but sedentary. She simply does not have the time or energy to stay with an exercise program after working all day and caring for her children. She would like to lose about 20 pounds but knows "dieting" doesn't work for her—all the diets she has tried in the past have left her hungry and feeling deprived. Losing weight has taken on greater importance since her doctor told her that both her blood pressure and glucose level are at "borderline" high levels.

- What is her BMI? Assess her weight based on BMI.
- Estimate her total calorie requirements using the rule-of-thumb method of calculating BMR and adding calories for a sedentary lifestyle. How does it compare to the level of calories recommended in Table 7.3 for a woman of her age and sedentary lifestyle? Which calorie level do you think is most accurate? Why?
- How many calories would she need to eat to lose 1 pound of weight per week if her activity level stays the same? Two pounds per week? Is a 2-pound weight loss per week a reasonable goal?
- To help her avoid feeling hungry while eating fewer calories, what foods would you recommend she consume more of? She knows she should drink fewer soft drinks. What advice would you give her to help her do that?

STUDY QUESTIONS

1. For most Americans, the largest percentage of their total calories expended daily is from
   a. Physical activity
   b. Thermal effect of food
   c. Basal energy expenditure
   d. Sitting

2. The nurse knows her instructions about portion control have been effective when the client verbalizes she will
   a. Prepare a doggie bag after she feels she is full enough while eating out.
   b. Use a smaller dinner plate.
   c. Be careful not to overfill her cereal bowl when she serves herself from the large, family-sized box.
   d. Remind herself not to overeat.

3. A client asks how she can speed up her metabolism. The best response is
   a. "You can't. Metabolic rate is genetically determined."
   b. "Ask your doctor to check your thyroid hormone levels. Taking thyroid hormone will stimulate metabolism."
   c. "Include resistance training in your exercise program because adding muscle tissue will increase metabolic rate."
   d. "Eat fewer calories because that will stimulate metabolic rate."

4. How much weight will a person lose in a week if he eats 500 fewer calories/day than he needs and increases his exercise expenditure by 500 calories/day?
   a. 1 pound/week
   b. 2 pounds/week
   c. 3 pounds/week
   d. There isn't enough information provided to estimate weekly weight loss.

5. Using the rule-of-thumb formula, how many calories/day would a healthy-weight adult who weighs 70 kg need?
   a. 2350 to 2800 calories
   b. 2100 to 2350 calories
   c. 1750 to 2100 calories
   d. 1400 to 1750 calories

6. Waist circumference is an indicator of
   a. Percentage of body fat
   b. Abdominal fat content
   c. The ratio of body fat to muscle mass
   d. Body mass index

7. Which of the following substitutions results in a healthier choice?
   a. Beef loin instead of beef rib
   b. Refried beans instead of cooked or canned pinto beans
   c. Natural cheese instead of low-fat cheese
   d. Baked potato with cheese sauce instead of baked potato with salsa

8. A BMI of 26 is classified as
   a. Normal
   b. Overweight
   c. Class 1 obesity
   d. Class 2 obesity

KEY CONCEPTS

■ Calories are a measure of energy. The body obtains calories from carbohydrates, protein, fat, and alcohol.

■ Basal metabolism refers to the calories used to conduct the involuntary activities of the body, such as beating the heart and inflating the lungs. For most Americans, basal metabolism accounts for approximately 60% to 70% of total daily calories used.

■ The sum of calories spent on basal metabolism and physical activity (PA) represent a person's total calorie expenditure.

■ The thermic effect of food is the cost of digesting, absorbing, and metabolizing food. At about 10% of total calories consumed, it is a small part of total energy requirements and is often not factored into the total energy equation.

■ MyPlate calorie levels are based on gender, age, and activity. Sedentary women need approximately 1600 to 2000 cal/day, and sedentary men need 2000 to 2600 cal/day.

■ Desirable weight is defined as weight for height that is statistically correlated to good health. Ideal body weight, BMI, and waist circumference may be used to assess risk related to overweight and obesity.

■ BMI may be the best method of evaluating weight status, but it does not account for how weight is distributed. Overweight is defined as a BMI of 25 to 29.9; obesity is defined as a BMI of 30 or higher.

■ Waist circumference is a tool to assess for abdominal fatness. "Apples" (people with upper body obesity) have more health risks than "pears" (people with lower body obesity).

■ The *Dietary Guidelines for Americans, 2010* urge Americans to control calorie intake to manage weight, increase PA, and reduce time spent in sedentary behaviors.

- Healthy food choices involve eating less of items that are high in added sugar and fat and more of nutrient-dense foods like fruits, vegetables, whole grains, nonfat dairy products, and lean protein.
- Portion sizes have grown over the last two decades, and people often overestimate how much food they really need. Portion control is facilitated by eating less at restaurants, using smaller dinner plates, and buying prepackaged, portion-controlled foods.
- The vast majority of Americans do not get the recommended amount of PA. The benefits of PA are dose dependent.
- Exercise leads to only modest weight loss if calories are not also restricted. In the long term, exercise promotes weight loss by promoting fat loss and preventing loss of muscle, which contributes to metabolic rate.

Check Your Knowledge Answer Key

1. **TRUE** Calorie is a unit of measure pertaining to energy in foods. Thus, a food that is high in "energy" is high in calories.

2. **TRUE** One pound of body fat is equivalent to 3500 calories. In theory, to lose 1 pound of weight per week, a daily deficit of 500 calories for 7 days is necessary, whether from eating less, doing more, or both.

3. **TRUE** People of either gender with a high distribution of abdominal fat ("apples") have a greater health risk than people with excess fat in the hips and thighs ("pears").

4. **FALSE** The formulas to calculate BMI are used for either men or women.

5. **TRUE** Calorie-dense foods have relatively high levels of calories for the amount of nutrients they provide.

6. **TRUE** On average, basal metabolism accounts for 60% to 70% of total calories expended in a day. Active people use a smaller percentage of total calories on BMR.

7. **TRUE** Building muscle speeds metabolic rate because lean tissue is metabolically active compared with fat tissue, which is relatively inert and requires few calories to exist.

8. **FALSE** Activity does not need to be sustained for any given duration to provide health benefits. Snippets of activity accumulated over the entire day can provide the same health benefits as one exercise session of the same total length of time.

9. **TRUE** The best exercise is one the individual sticks with. Exercise prescriptions are not one-size-fits-all.

10. **TRUE** Sitting too much, even if physical activity goals are met, is a health risk.

Student Resources on thePoint

For additional learning materials, activate the code in the front of this book at
http://thePoint.lww.com/activate

Websites

American College of Sports Medicine at **www.acsm.org**
American Council on Exercise at **www.acefitness.org**
Calculate your own BEE at **http://www-users.med.cornell.edu/~spon/picu/calc/beecalc.htm**
National Institute of Diabetes and Digestive and Kidney Diseases, Physical Activity and Weight
    Control at **www.niddk.nih.gov/health/nutrit/pubs/physact.htm**
President's Council on Physical Fitness and Sports at **www.fitness.gov**

References

Alberti, K., Eckel, R., Grundy, S., Zimmet, P. Z., Cleeman, J. I., Donato, K. A., . . . Smith, S. C., Jr. (2009). Harmonizing the metabolic syndrome. A joint interim statement of the International Diabetes Federation Task Force on Epidemiology and Prevention; National Heart, Lung, and Blood Institute: American Heart Association; World Heart Federation; International Atherosclerosis Society; and International Association for the Study of Obesity. *Circulation, 120,* 1640–1645.

Bergouignan, A., Rudwill, F., Simon, C., & Blanc, S. (2011). Physical inactivity as the culprit of metabolic inflexibility: Evidence from bedrest studies. *Journal of Applied Physiology, 111,* 1201–1210.

Fiatarone, M., Marks, E., Ryan, N., Meredith, C. N., Lipsitz, L. A., & Evans, W. J. (1990). High-intensity strength training in nonagenarians. Effects on skeletal muscle. *Journal of the American Medical Association, 263,* 3029–3034.

Grontved, A., & Hu, F. (2011). Television viewing and risk of type 2 diabetes, cardiovascular disease, and all-cause mortality: A meta-analysis. *Journal of the American Medical Association, 305,* 2448–2455.

Hu, R., Li, T., Colditz, G., Willett, W. C., & Manson, J. E. (2003). Television watching and other sedentary behaviors in relation to risk of obesity and type 2 diabetes mellitus in women. *Journal of the American Medical Association, 289,* 1785–1791.

Moyer, V. (2012). Screening for and management of obesity in adults: US Preventive Services Task Force recommendation statement. *Annals of Internal Medicine, 157,* 373–378.

Mozaffarian, D., Hao, T., Rimm, E., Willett, W. C., & Hu, F. B. (2011). Changes in diet and life-style and long-term weight gain in women and med. *New England Journal of Medicine, 364,* 2392–2404.

National Academy of Sciences, Institute of Medicine. (2005). *Dietary Reference Intakes for energy, carbohydrate, fiber, fat, fatty acids, cholesterol, protein, and amino acids.* Washington, DC: The National Academies Press.

National Center for Health Statistics. (2012). *Health, United States, 2011: With special feature on socioeconomic status and health.* Hyattsville, MD: National Center for Health Statistics.

Pratt, I., Croager, E. & Rosenberg, M. (2012). The mathematical relationship between dishware size and portion size. *Appetite, 58,* 299–302.

Song, W., Chun, O., Obayashi, S., Cho, S., & Chung, C. E. (2005). Is consumption of breakfast associated with body mass index in US adults. *Journal of the American Dietetic Association, 105,* 1373–1382.

U.S. Department of Agriculture, U.S. Department of Health and Human Services. (2010). *Dietary guidelines for Americans, 2010* (7th ed.). Available at www.health.gov/dietaryguidelines. Accessed on 10/8/12.

U.S. Department of Health and Human Services. (2008). *Physical activity guidelines for Americans.* Washington, DC. Available at www.health.gov/paguidelines. Accessed 10/8/12.

U.S. Preventive Services Task Force. (2003). Screening for obesity in adults: Recommendations and rational. *Annals of Internal Medicine, 139,* 930–932.

Wansink, B. (2006). *Mindless eating: Why we eat more than we think.* New York, NY: Bantam Dell.

Wansink, B., & Ittersum, K. (2007). Portion size me: Downsizing our consumption norms. *Journal of the American Dietetic Association, 107,* 1103–1106.

Wijndaele, K., Brage, S., Besson, H., Khaw, K. T., Sharp, S. J., Luben, R., . . . Ekelund, U. (2011). Television viewing and incident cardiovascular disease: Prospective associations and mediation analysis. In the EPIC Norfolk study. *PLoS One, 6,* e20058.

Wyatt, H., Grunwald, G., Mosca, C., Klem, M. L., Wing, R. R., & Hill, J. O. (2002). Long-term weight loss and breakfast in subjects in the National Weight Control Registry. *Obesity Research, 10,* 78–82.

Young, L., & Nestle, M. (2003). Expanding portion sizes in the US marketplace: Implications for nutritional counseling. *Journal of the American Dietetic Association, 103,* 231–234.

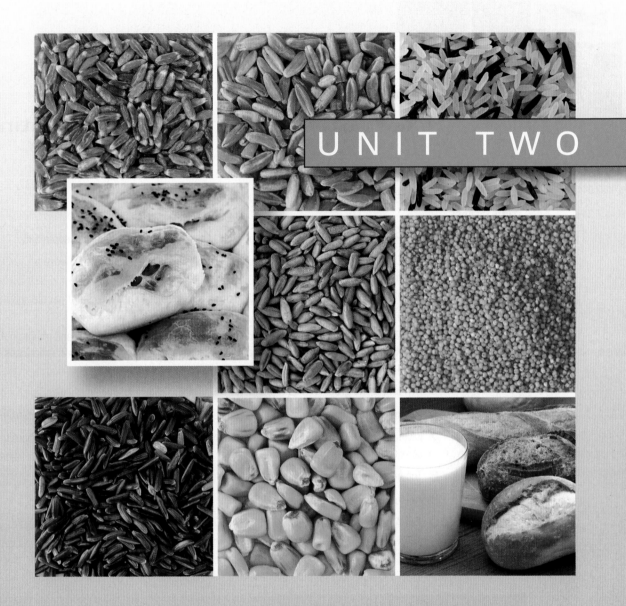

Nutrition in Health Promotion

8 Guidelines for Healthy Eating

LEARNING OBJECTIVES

Upon completion of this chapter, you will be able to

1 Discuss the overall objectives of Healthy People 2020 in the area of nutrition and overweight.
2 Compare Recommended Dietary Allowance (RDA) and Adequate Intake (AI).
3 Summarize the *Dietary Guidelines for Americans, 2010*.
4 Design a day's intake for your own MyPlate that illustrates variety and moderation.
5 Evaluate an individual's intake according to the appropriate MyPlate plan.
6 Give examples of foods with solid fats or added sugars.
7 Compare nutrition recommendations from the American Heart Association, the American Cancer Society, and the American Institute for Cancer Research.

A healthy diet provides enough of all essential nutrients to avoid deficiencies but not excessive amounts that may increase the risk of nutrient toxicities or chronic diseases. Today, nutrient deficiency diseases are rare in the United States except among the poor, elderly, alcoholics, fad dieters, and hospitalized patients. Conversely, 4 of the 10 leading causes of death in the United States are associated with dietary excesses—namely, heart disease, cancer, stroke, and diabetes (Murphy, Xu, and Kochanek, 2012). Many other health problems, such as obesity, hypertension, and hypercholesterolemia, are related, at least in part, to dietary excesses. Healthy eating and regular exercise are essential for reducing the risk of chronic disease (U.S. Department of Agriculture [USDA], U.S. Department of Health and Human Services [USDHHS], 2010).

QUICK BITE

The 10 leading causes of death in the United States in 2010 (in descending order)

1. Heart disease
2. Cancer
3. Chronic lower respiratory diseases
4. Cerebrovascular diseases
5. Accidents
6. Alzheimer disease
7. Diabetes
8. Nephritis, nephrotic syndrome, and nephrosis
9. Influenza and pneumonia
10. Suicide

Source: Murphy, Xu, & Kochanek. (2012). Deaths: Preliminary data for 2010. *National Vital Statistics Report, 60*(4). Available at http://www.cdc.gov/nchs/data/nvsr60/nvsr60_04.pdf

OVERVIEW

Dietary Reference Intakes (DRIs): a set of four nutrient-based reference values used to plan and evaluate diets.

This chapter focuses on recommended nutrient intake values and recommended eating patterns. Topics include the **Dietary Reference Intakes (DRIs)**, Healthy People 2020, the Dietary Guidelines for Americans, MyPlate, and intake recommendations from leading health agencies.

NUTRIENT REFERENCE VALUES

Recommended Dietary Allowances (RDAs): the average daily dietary intake level sufficient to meet the nutrient requirement of 97% to 98% of healthy individuals in a particular life stage and gender group.

Historically, the **Recommended Dietary Allowances (RDAs)** in the United States and the Recommended Nutrient Intakes in Canada established recommended levels of nutrients set at a level to protect people from nutrient-deficiency diseases. The old RDAs have been replaced with a new set of standards, the DRIs, which incorporate an expanded focus of reducing the risk of chronic diseases associated with dietary excesses.

Dietary Reference Intakes

In the early 1990s, Canadian scientists and the Food and Nutrition Board of the Institute of Medicine embarked on a comprehensive, multiyear project to update and expand nutrient intake recommendations. The outcome has been a series of in-depth reports featuring a new set of references called DRIs that cover vitamins, minerals, the energy nutrients, cholesterol, fiber, electrolytes, and water.

The DRIs is a group name that includes four separate reference values that are based on the concepts of probability and risk (Otten, Hellwig, and Meyers, 2006). They include

- Updated RDAs
- Estimated Average Requirement (EAR)
- Adequate Intake (AI)
- Tolerable Upper Intake Level (UL)

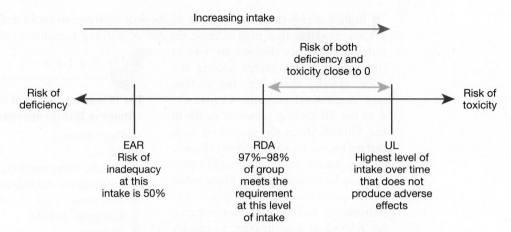

■ **FIGURE 8.1** Representation of DRI along a continuum of intake.

Each of these reference values has a specific purpose and represents a different level of intake (Fig. 8.1). Nutrients have either an RDA or an AI; not all nutrients have an established UL (Table 8.1). Each reference value is viewed as an average daily intake over time, at least 1 week for most nutrients. Summary tables of the DRIs appear in Appendices 1, 2, and 3. Additional reference values include Acceptable Macronutrient Distribution Ranges (AMDRs) and an Estimated Energy Requirement (EER).

DRIs are used by scientists and nutritionists who work in research or academic settings and by dietitians who plan menus for specific populations, such as elderly feeding programs, schools, prisons, hospitals, nursing homes, and military feeding programs. They are also used to assess the adequacy of an individual's intake by comparing estimated intake with estimated requirements. Keep in mind that obtaining a reliable estimate of a person's actual intake is difficult due to reporting errors, flaws in estimating portion sizes, and day-to-day variation in food intake. Unless a person has participated in a nutrient requirement study, it is impossible to quantify exact nutrient requirements for an individual. Because consumers eat food and not nutrients, the DRIs are not suited to teaching people how to make healthy choices.

Recommended Dietary Allowances

The RDAs represent the average daily recommended intake to meet the nutrient requirements of 97% to 98% of healthy individuals by life stage and gender. The recommendations are based on specific criteria indicators for estimating requirements, such as plasma and serum nutrient concentrations, and are set high enough to account for daily variations in intake. When estimating the nutritional needs of people with health disorders, health professionals use the RDAs as a starting point and adjust them according to the individual's need.

Estimated Average Requirement

Estimated Average Requirement (EAR): the nutrient intake estimated to meet the requirement of half of the healthy individuals in a particular life stage and gender group.

Estimated Average Requirement (EAR) values are used to determine RDA values; they are not used as a stand-alone reference. The EAR is the amount of a nutrient that is estimated to meet the requirement of half of healthy people in a lifestyle or gender group. "Average" actually means *median*. By definition, the EAR exceeds the requirements of half of the group and falls below the requirements of the other half. The EAR is not based solely on the prevention of nutrient deficiencies but includes consideration for reducing the risk of chronic disease and takes into account the bioavailability of the nutrient—that is, how its absorption is impacted by other food components.

Table 8.1 Standards Applied to Each Nutrient for People Age 1 Year and Older

Nutrient	RDA	AI	UL*
Total water		✓	
Macronutrients			
Carbohydrate	✓		
Fiber		✓	
Linoleic acid		✓	
Alpha-linolenic acid		✓	
Protein	✓		
Fat-soluble vitamins			
Vitamin A	✓		✓
Vitamin D	✓		✓
Vitamin E	✓		✓
Vitamin K		✓	
Water-soluble vitamins			
Thiamin	✓		
Riboflavin	✓		
Niacin	✓		✓
Vitamin B_6	✓		✓
Folate	✓		✓
Vitamin B_{12}	✓		
Pantothenic acid		✓	
Biotin		✓	
Choline		✓	✓
Vitamin C	✓		✓
Elements			
Calcium	✓		
Chromium		✓	
Copper	✓		✓
Fluoride		✓	✓
Iodine	✓		✓
Iron	✓		✓
Magnesium	✓		✓
Manganese		✓	✓
Molybdenum	✓		✓
Phosphorus	✓		✓
Selenium	✓		✓
Zinc	✓		✓
Potassium		✓	
Sodium		✓	✓
Chloride		✓	✓

*A UL has also been established for boron and nickel even though neither nutrient has an RDA or AI.

Adequate Intake

Adequate Intake (AI): an intake level thought to meet or exceed the requirement of almost all members of a life stage and gender group. An AI is set when there are insufficient data to define an RDA.

An **Adequate Intake (AI)** is set when an RDA cannot be determined due to lack of sufficient data on requirements. It is a recommended average daily intake level thought to meet or exceed the needs of virtually all members of a life stage or gender group based on observed or experimentally determined estimates of nutrient intake by groups of healthy people. The primary purpose of the AI is as a goal for the nutrient intake of individuals. This is similar to the use of the RDA except that the RDA is expected to meet the needs of almost all healthy people, while in the case of an AI, it is not known what percentage of people are covered.

Tolerable Upper Intake Level

Tolerable Upper Intake Level (UL): the highest average daily intake level of a nutrient likely to pose no danger to most individuals in the group.

The **Tolerable Upper Intake Level (UL)** is the highest level of average daily nutrient intake that is likely to pose no risk of adverse health effects to almost all individuals in the general population. It is not intended to be a recommended level of intake; there is no benefit in consuming amounts greater than the RDA or AI.

Acceptable Macronutrient Distribution Ranges

Acceptable Macronutrient Distribution Ranges (AMDRs): an intake range as a percentage of total calories for energy nutrients.

The **Acceptable Macronutrient Distribution Ranges (AMDRs)** are broad ranges for each energy nutrient, expressed as a percentage of total calories consumed. These ranges are associated with reduced risk of chronic disease and are such that an adequate intake of all nutrients can be obtained. Over time, intakes above or below this range may increase the risk of chronic disease or deficiency, respectively. The AMDRs for adults are as follows:

	% Total Calories Consumed
Carbohydrate	45–65
Protein	10–35
Fat	20–35
Linoleic acid (*n*-6)	5–10
Alpha-linolenic acid (*n*-3)	0.6–1.2

Estimated Energy Requirements (EERs): level of calorie intake estimated to maintain weight in normal-weight individuals based on age, gender, height, weight, and activity.

Estimated Energy Requirements

Similar to the EAR, the EERs are defined as the dietary energy intake predicted to maintain energy balance in healthy, normal-weight individuals of a defined age, gender, weight, height, and level of physical activity consistent with good health. Exceeding the EER may produce weight gain. See Chapter 7 for more on determining energy needs.

HEALTHY EATING GUIDELINES

Many government and health agencies issue healthy eating guidelines based on a food group approach to eating. For instance, Healthy People 2020 is a public health initiative that includes benchmarks for nutrition and weight. In practice, the most prominent tools to assist Americans in making wise food choices are the Dietary Guidelines for Americans and its companion tool, MyPlate. The American Heart Association, the American Cancer Society, and the American Institute for Cancer Research have also issued dietary recommendations to help Americans choose diets aimed at reducing the risk of chronic diseases.

Healthy People 2020

Under the jurisdiction of the USDHHS, Healthy People is a program that focuses on improving the health of all Americans and eliminating health disparities. Updated every 10 years after its inception 30 years ago, Healthy People sets public health goals and objectives and monitors the nation's progress toward meeting those objectives.

The newest edition, Healthy People 2020, has approximately 1200 objectives organized into 42 focus areas ranging from cancer and diabetes to substance abuse and immunizations. At the time of its launch in December 2010, 911 objectives were measurable with baseline data and established targets (USDHHS, 2010). The overall objectives under nutrition and weight status are listed in Box 8.1. Healthy People 2020 states that Americans who eat a healthful diet

- Eat a variety of nutrient-dense foods within and across food groups, especially whole grains, fruits, vegetables, low-fat or fat-free milk and milk products, and lean proteins.
- Limit the intake of saturated fat, trans fat, cholesterol, added sugars, sodium, and alcohol.
- Balance calorie intake with calorie needs.

Box 8.1   HEALTHY PEOPLE 2020: SUMMARY OF NUTRITION AND WEIGHT STATUS OBJECTIVES

Goal: Promote health and reduce chronic disease risk through consumption of healthful diets and achievement and maintenance of healthy body weights.

Healthier Food Access

1. Increase the number of States with nutrition standards for foods and beverages provided to preschool-aged children in child care.
2. Increase the proportion of schools that offer nutritious foods and beverages outside of school meals.
3. Increase the number of States that have state-level policies that incentivize food retail outlets to provide foods that are encouraged by the Dietary Guidelines.
4. (Developmental) Increase the proportion of Americans who have access to a food retail outlet that sells a variety of foods that are encouraged by the *Dietary Guidelines for Americans*.

Healthcare and Worksite Settings

5. Increase the proportion of primary care physicians who regularly measure the body mass index of their patients.
6. Increase the proportion of physician office visits that include counseling or education related to nutrition or weight.
7. (Developmental) Increase the proportion of worksites that offer nutrition or weight management classes or counseling.

Weight Status

8. Increase the proportion of adults who are at a healthy weight.

9. Reduce the proportion of adults who are obese.
10. Reduce the proportion of children and adolescents who are considered obese.
11. (Developmental) Prevent inappropriate weight gain in youth and adults.

Food Insecurity

12. Eliminate very low food security among children.
13. Reduce household food insecurity and in doing so reduce hunger.

Food and Nutrient Consumption

14. Increase the contribution of fruits to the diets of the population aged 2 years and older.
15. Increase the variety and contribution of vegetables to the diets of the population aged 2 years and older.
16. Increase the contribution of whole grains to the diets of the population aged 2 years and older.
17. Reduce consumption of calories from solid fats and added sugars in the population aged 2 years and older.
18. Reduce consumption of saturated fat in the population aged 2 years and older.
19. Reduce consumption of sodium in the population aged 2 years and older.
20. Increase consumption of calcium in the population aged 2 years and older.

Iron Deficiency

21. Reduce iron deficiency among young children and females of childbearing age.
22. Reduce iron deficiency among pregnant females.

Source: Healthy People 2020. Available at http://www.healthypeople.gov/2020/topicsobjectives2020/objectiveslist.aspx?topicId=29

Dietary Guidelines for Americans

The Dietary Guidelines for Americans, published jointly every 5 years by the USDHHS and the USDA, serves as the federal policy on nutrition, dictating how education, communication, and food assistance programs are conducted by the government. They are evidence-based recommendations designed to help people attain and maintain a healthy weight, reduce the risk of chronic disease, and promote overall health for Americans age 2 years and older. Unlike previous editions, the 2010 version is intended not just for "healthy" people but also for people at increased risk of chronic disease. This is in response to the current epidemic of overweight and obesity in all ages and segments of American society.

The Dietary Guidelines comprise 23 key recommendations with 6 additional recommendations for specific population groups (Box 8.2). An underlying principle is that nutrient needs should be primarily met by eating food. The major themes are to maintain calorie balance to achieve and maintain healthy weight and to focus on eating nutrient-dense food

---

Box 8.2   *DIETARY GUIDELINES FOR AMERICANS, 2010 RECOMMENDATIONS*

Key Recommendations

Balancing Calories to Manage Weight
Prevent and/or reduce overweight and obesity through improved eating and physical activity.
Control total calorie intake to manage body weight. For people who are overweight or obese, this will mean consuming fewer calories from foods and beverages.
Increase physical activity and reduce time spent in sedentary behaviors.
Maintain appropriate calorie balance during each stage of life—childhood, adolescence, adulthood, pregnancy and breastfeeding, and older age.

Foods and Food Components to Reduce
Reduce daily sodium intake to less than 2300 mg and further reduce intake to 1500 mg among persons who are age 51 years and older and those of any age who are African American or have hypertension, diabetes, or chronic kidney disease. The 1500-mg recommendation applies to about half of the U.S. population, including children and the majority of adults.
Consume less than 10% of calories from saturated fatty acids by replacing them with monounsaturated and polyunsaturated fatty acids.
Consume less than 300 mg/day of dietary cholesterol.
Keep trans fatty acid consumption as low as possible by limiting foods that contain synthetic sources of trans fats, such as partially hydrogenated oils, and by limiting other solid fats.
Reduce the intake of calories from solid fats and added sugars.
Limit the consumption of foods that contain refined grains, especially refined grain foods that contain solid fats, added sugars, and sodium.
If alcohol is consumed, it should be consumed in moderation—up to one drink per day for women and two drinks per day for men—and only by adults of legal drinking age.*

Foods and Nutrients to Increase
Individuals should meet the following recommendations as part of a healthy eating pattern while staying within their calorie needs:

Increase vegetable and fruit intake.
Eat a variety of vegetables, especially dark green and red and orange vegetables and beans and peas.

Box 8.2	*DIETARY GUIDELINES FOR AMERICANS, 2010* RECOMMENDATIONS (continued)

Consume at least half of all grains as whole grains. Increase whole-grain intake by replacing refined grains with whole grains.

Increase intake of fat-free or low-fat milk and milk products, such as milk, yogurt, cheese, or fortified soy beverages.[†]

Choose a variety of protein foods, which include seafood, lean meat and poultry, eggs, beans and peas, soy products, and unsalted nuts and seeds.

Increase the amount and variety of seafood consumed by choosing seafood in place of some meat and poultry.

Replace protein foods that are higher in solid fats with choices that are lower in solid fats and calories and/or are sources of oils.

Use oils to replace solid fats where possible.

Choose foods that provide more potassium, dietary fiber, calcium, and vitamin D, which are nutrients of concern in American diets. These foods include vegetables, fruits, whole grains, and milk and milk products.

Recommendations for Specific Population Groups

Women Capable of Becoming Pregnant[‡]

Choose foods that supply heme iron, which is more readily absorbed by the body, additional iron sources, and enhancers of iron absorption, such as vitamin C–rich foods.

Consume 400 μg/day of synthetic folic acid (from fortified foods and/or supplements) in addition to food forms of folate from a varied diet.[§]

Women Who Are Pregnant or Breastfeeding[‡]

Consume 8 to 12 oz of seafood per week from a variety of seafood types.

Because of its high methyl mercury content, limit white (albacore) tuna to 6 oz per week, and do not eat the following four types of fish: tilefish, shark, swordfish, and king mackerel.

If pregnant, take an iron supplement, as recommended by an obstetrician or other health-care provider.

Individuals Ages 50 Years and Older

Consume foods fortified with vitamin B_{12}, such as fortified cereals, or dietary supplements.

Building Healthy Eating Patterns

Select an eating pattern that meets nutrient needs over time at an appropriate calorie level.

Account for all foods and beverages consumed and assess how they fit within a total healthy eating pattern.

Follow food safety recommendations when preparing and eating foods to reduce the risk of foodborne illnesses.

*See Chapter 3 in the *Dietary Guidelines for Americans, 2010*, Foods and Food Components to Reduce, for additional recommendations on alcohol consumption and specific population groups. There are many circumstances when people should not drink alcohol.

[†]Fortified soy beverages have been marketed as "soymilk," a product name consumers could see in supermarkets and consumer materials. However, U.S. Food and Drug Administration's (FDA) regulations do not contain provisions for the use of the term soymilk. Therefore, in this document, the term "fortified soy beverage" includes products that may be marketed as soymilk.

[‡]Includes adolescent girls.

[§]"Folic acid" is the synthetic form of the nutrient, whereas "folate" is the form found naturally in foods.

Source: Adapted from U.S. Department of Agriculture, U.S. Department of Health and Human Services. (2010). *Dietary guidelines for Americans, 2010* (7th ed.). Available at http://www.cnpp.usda.gov/Publications/DietaryGuidelines/2010/PolicyDoc/Chapter4.pdf. Accessed on 1/22/13.

and beverages. In the *Dietary Guidelines for Americans, 2010*, the basic messages for consumers are as follows:

- Enjoy your food, but eat less.
- Avoid oversized portions.
- Make half your plate fruits and vegetables.
- Make at least half your grains whole grains.
- Switch to fat-free or low-fat (1%) milk.
- Compare sodium in foods, such as soup, bread, and frozen meals, and choose foods with lower amounts of sodium.
- Drink water instead of sugary drinks.

MyPlate

In early 2011, MyPlate replaced MyPyramid as the new graphic by which the Dietary Guidelines for Americans are translated into food choices for healthy individuals older than 2 years. It features a place setting with half of the dinner plate devoted to fruits and vegetables, ¼ to protein foods, and ¼ to grains; dairy accompanies the plate (Fig. 8.2) (USDA, Center for Nutrition Policy and Promotion, 2011). Consistent with the Dietary Guidelines, it is based on the philosophy that nutrient needs, to the greatest extent possible, should be met through food, not supplements. As a total diet approach, it covers all aspects of the diet, from calories and fat to particular types of vegetable subgroups and whole grains.

MyPlate includes an interactive online guidance system. Visitors to the website www.choosemyplate.gov enter their age, gender, weight, height, and physical activity level to see the Daily Food Plan most appropriate for their estimated calorie needs. There are food patterns for 12 different calorie levels ranging from 1000 to 3200 calories that increase in increments of 200 calories (Table 8.2). This individualization of food intake patterns reflects not only the broad range of calorie needs across the population but also the increasing attention paid to obesity as a major health problem.

Figure 8.3 illustrates the format used to convey basic MyPlate plan recommendations. The pdf version of a MyPlate plan features the recommended daily amounts from each group and additional basic information, as illustrated in the 2000-calorie MyPlate Daily Food Plan in Figure 8.4.

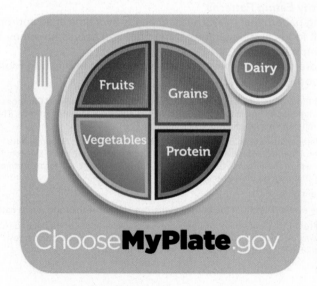

■ FIGURE 8.2 MyPlate. (USDA, Center for Nutrition Policy and Promotion. [2011]. Available at www.choosemyplate.gov)

Table 8.2 USDA Food Patterns

For each food group or subgroup,[a] recommended average daily intake amounts[b] at all calorie levels. Recommended intakes from vegetable and protein foods subgroups are per week. For more information and tools for application, go to MyPlate.gov.

Calorie Level of Pattern[c]	1000	1200	1400	1600	1800	2000	2200	2400	2600	2800	3000	3200
Fruits	1 c	1 c	1½ c	1½ c	1½ c	2 c	2 c	2 c	2 c	2½ c	2½ c	2½ c
Vegetables[d]	1 c	1½ c	1½ c	2 c	2½ c	2½ c	3 c	3 c	3½ c	3½ c	4 c	4 c
Dark-green vegetables	½ c/wk	1 c/wk	1 c/wk	1½ c/wk	1½ c/wk	1½ c/wk	2 c/wk	2 c/wk	2½ c/wk	2½ c/wk	2½ c/wk	2½ c/wk
Red and orange vegetables	2½ c/wk	3 c/wk	3 c/wk	4 c/wk	5½ c/wk	5½ c/wk	6 c/wk	6 c/wk	7 c/wk	7 c/wk	7½ c/wk	7½ c/wk
Beans and peas (legumes)	½ c/wk	½ c/wk	½ c/wk	1 c/wk	1½ c/wk	1½ c/wk	2 c/wk	2 c/wk	2½ c/wk	2½ c/wk	3 c/wk	3 c/wk
Starchy vegetables	2 c/wk	3½ c/wk	3½ c/wk	4 c/wk	5 c/wk	5 c/wk	6 c/wk	6 c/wk	7 c/wk	7 c/wk	8 c/wk	8 c/wk
Other vegetables	1½ c/wk	2½ c/wk	2½ c/wk	3½ c/wk	4 c/wk	4 c/wk	5 c/wk	5 c/wk	5½ c/wk	5½ c/wk	7 c/wk	7 c/wk
Grains[e]	3 oz-eq	4 oz-eq	5 oz-eq	5 oz-eq	6 oz-eq	6 oz-eq	7 oz-eq	8 oz-eq	9 oz-eq	10 oz-eq	10 oz-eq	10 oz-eq
Whole grains	1½ oz-eq	2 oz-eq	2½ oz-eq	3 oz-eq	3 oz-eq	3 oz-eq	3½ oz-eq	4 oz-eq	4½ oz-eq	5 oz-eq	5 oz-eq	5 oz-eq
Enriched grains	1½ oz-eq	2 oz-eq	2½ oz-eq	2 oz-eq	3 oz-eq	3 oz-eq	3½ oz-eq	4 oz-eq	4½ oz-eq	5 oz-eq	5 oz-eq	5 oz-eq
Protein foods[d]	2 oz-eq	3 oz-eq	4 oz-eq	5 oz-eq	5 oz-eq	5½ oz-eq	6 oz-eq	6½ oz-eq	6½ oz-eq	7 oz-eq	7 oz-eq	7 oz-eq
Seafood	3 oz/wk	5 oz/wk	6 oz/wk	8 oz/wk	8 oz/wk	8 oz/wk	9 oz/wk	10 oz/wk	10 oz/wk	11 oz/wk	11 oz/wk	11 oz/wk
Meat, poultry, eggs	10 oz/wk	14 oz/wk	19 oz/wk	24 oz/wk	24 oz/wk	26 oz/wk	29 oz/wk	31 oz/wk	31 oz/wk	34 oz/wk	34 oz/wk	34 oz/wk
Nuts, seeds, soy products	1 oz/wk	2 oz/wk	3 oz/wk	4 oz/wk	4 oz/wk	4 oz/wk	4 oz/wk	5 oz/wk	5 oz/wk	5 oz/wk	5 oz/wk	5 oz/wk
Dairy[f]	2 c	2½ c	2½ c	3 c	3 c	3 c	3 c	3 c	3 c	3 c	3 c	3 c
Oils[g]	15 g	17 g	17 g	22 g	24 g	27 g	29 g	31 g	34 g	36 g	44 g	51 g
Maximum SoFAS[h] limit, calories (% of calories)	137 (14%)	121 (10%)	121 (9%)	121 (8%)	161 (9%)	258 (13%)	266 (12%)	330 (14%)	362 (14%)	395 (14%)	459 (15%)	596 (19%)

[a] All foods are assumed to be in nutrient-dense forms, lean or low-fat and prepared without added fats, sugars, or salt. Solid fats and added sugars may be included up to the daily maximum limit identified in the table. Food items in each group and subgroup are

Fruits All fresh, frozen, canned, and dried fruits and fruit juices: for example, oranges and orange juice, apples and apple juice, bananas, grapes, melons, berries, raisins.

Vegetables

Dark-green vegetables   All fresh, frozen, and canned dark-green leafy vegetables and broccoli, cooked or raw: for example, broccoli; spinach; romaine; collard, turnip, and mustard greens.

Red and orange vegetables   All fresh, frozen, and canned red and orange vegetables, cooked or raw: for example, tomatoes, red peppers, carrots, sweet potatoes, winter squash, and pumpkin.

(continues on page 188)

Table 8.2 USDA Food Patterns (continued)

Beans and peas (legumes)	All cooked beans and peas: for example, kidney beans, lentils, chickpeas, and pinto beans. Does not include green beans or green peas. (See additional comment under protein foods group.)
Starchy vegetables	All fresh, frozen, and canned starchy vegetables: for example, white potatoes, corn, green peas.
Other vegetables	All fresh, frozen, and canned other vegetables, cooked or raw: for example, iceberg lettuce, green beans, and onions.
Grains	
Whole grains	All whole-grain products and whole grains used as ingredients: for example, whole wheat bread, whole-grain cereals and crackers, oatmeal, and brown rice.
Enriched grains	All enriched refined-grain products and enriched refined grains used as ingredients: for example, white breads, enriched grain cereals and crackers, enriched pasta, white rice.
Protein foods	All meat, poultry, seafood, eggs, nuts, seeds, and processed soy products. Meat and poultry should be lean or low-fat and nuts should be unsalted. Beans and peas are considered part of this group as well as the vegetable group but should be counted in one group only.
Dairy	All milks, including lactose-free and lactose-reduced products and fortified soy beverages, yogurts, frozen yogurts, dairy desserts, and cheeses. Most choices should be fat-free or low-fat. Cream, sour cream, and cream cheese are not included due to their low calcium content.

[b]Food group amounts are shown in cup (c) or ounce-equivalents (oz-eq). Oils are shown in grams (g). Quantity equivalents for each food group are

- Grains, 1 ounce-equivalent is: 1 one-ounce slice bread; 1 ounce uncooked pasta or rice; ½ cup cooked rice, pasta, or cereal; 1 tortilla (6" diameter); 1 pancake (5" diameter); 1 ounce ready-to-eat cereal (about 1 cup cereal flakes).
- Vegetables and fruits, 1 cup equivalent is: 1 cup raw or cooked vegetable or fruit; ½ cup dried vegetable or fruit; 1 cup vegetable or fruit juice; 2 cups leafy salad greens.
- Protein foods, 1 ounce-equivalent is: 1 ounce lean meat, poultry, seafood; 1 egg; 1 tbsp peanut butter; ½ ounce nuts or seeds. Also, ¼ cup cooked beans or peas may also be counted as 1 ounce-equivalent.
- Dairy, 1 cup equivalent is: 1 cup milk, fortified soy beverage, or yogurt; 1½ ounces natural cheese (e.g., cheddar); 2 ounces of processed cheese (e.g., American).

[c]See Appendix 6 for estimated calorie needs per day by age, gender, and physical activity level. Food intake patterns at 1000, 1200, and 1400 calories meet the nutritional needs of children ages 2 to 8 years. Patterns from 1600 to 3200 calories meet the nutritional needs of children ages 9 years and older and adults. If a child ages 4 to 8 years needs more calories and, therefore, is following a pattern at 1600 calories or more, the recommended amount from the dairy group can be 2½ cups per day. Children ages 9 years and older and adults should not use the 1000, 1200, or 1400 calorie patterns.

[d]Vegetable and protein foods subgroup amounts are shown in this table as weekly amounts, because it would be difficult for consumers to select foods from all subgroups daily.

[e]Whole-grain subgroup amounts shown in this table are minimums. More whole grains up to all of the grains recommended may be selected, with offsetting decreases in the amounts of enriched refined grains.

[f]The amount of dairy foods in the 1200 and 1400 calorie patterns have increased to reflect new RDAs for calcium that are higher than previous recommendations for children ages 4 to 8 years.

[g]Oils and soft margarines include vegetable, nut, and fish oils and soft vegetable oil table spreads that have no trans fats.

[h]SoFAS are calories from solid fats and added sugars. The limit for SoFAS is the remaining amount of calories in each food group in each food pattern after selecting the specified amounts in each food group in nutrient-dense forms (forms that are fat-free or low-fat and with no added sugars). The number of SoFAS is lower in the 1200, 1400, and 1600 calorie patterns than in the 1000 calorie pattern. The nutrient goals for the 1200 to 1600 calorie patterns are higher and require that more calories be used for nutrient-dense foods from the food groups.

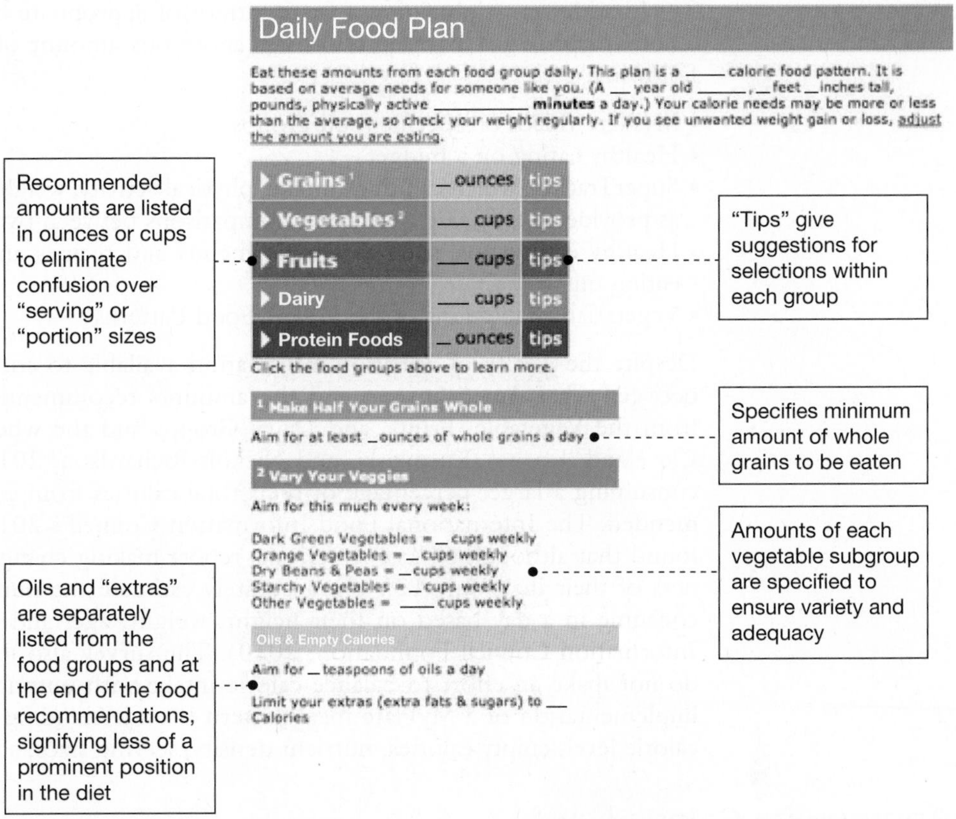

Daily Food Plan

Eat these amounts from each food group daily. This plan is a _____ calorie food pattern. It is based on average needs for someone like you. (A __ year old _____, __ feet __inches tall, pounds, physically active _____ minutes a day.) Your calorie needs may be more or less than the average, so check your weight regularly. If you see unwanted weight gain or loss, adjust the amount you are eating.

Recommended amounts are listed in ounces or cups to eliminate confusion over "serving" or "portion" sizes

▶ Grains¹	_ ounces	tips
▶ Vegetables²	_ cups	tips
▶ Fruits	_ cups	tips
▶ Dairy	_ cups	tips
▶ Protein Foods	_ ounces	tips

Click the food groups above to learn more.

"Tips" give suggestions for selections within each group

¹ Make Half Your Grains Whole

Aim for at least _ ounces of whole grains a day ●

Specifies minimum amount of whole grains to be eaten

² Vary Your Veggies

Aim for this much every week:

Dark Green Vegetables = _ cups weekly
Orange Vegetables = _ cups weekly
Dry Beans & Peas = _ cups weekly
Starchy Vegetables = _ cups weekly
Other Vegetables = _____ cups weekly

Amounts of each vegetable subgroup are specified to ensure variety and adequacy

Oils & Empty Calories

Aim for _ teaspoons of oils a day

Limit your extras (extra fats & sugars) to _ Calories

Oils and "extras" are separately listed from the food groups and at the end of the food recommendations, signifying less of a prominent position in the diet

■ FIGURE 8.3
Format of ChooseMyPlate .gov. (USDA, Center for Nutrition Policy and Promotion. [2011]. Available at www .choosemyplate.gov)

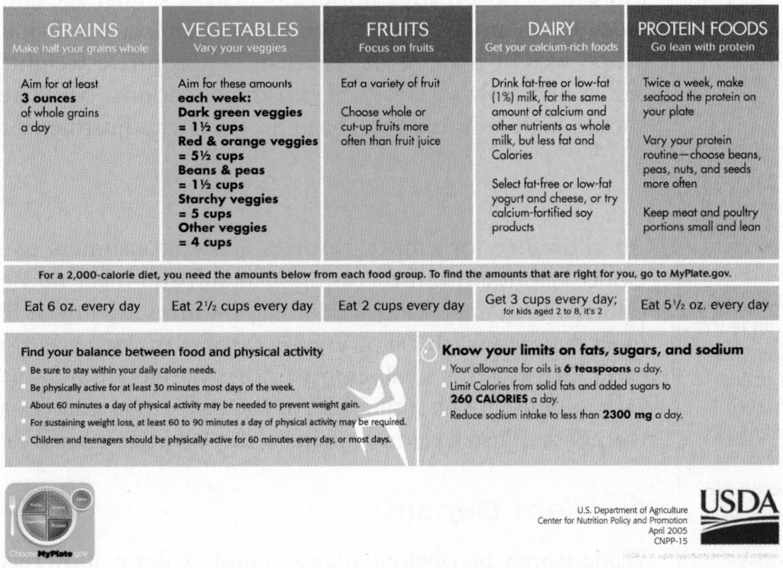

GRAINS Make half your grains whole	VEGETABLES Vary your veggies	FRUITS Focus on fruits	DAIRY Get your calcium-rich foods	PROTEIN FOODS Go lean with protein
Aim for at least **3 ounces** of whole grains a day	Aim for these amounts **each week: Dark green veggies = 1½ cups Red & orange veggies = 5½ cups Beans & peas = 1½ cups Starchy veggies = 5 cups Other veggies = 4 cups**	Eat a variety of fruit Choose whole or cut-up fruits more often than fruit juice	Drink fat-free or low-fat (1%) milk, for the same amount of calcium and other nutrients as whole milk, but less fat and Calories Select fat-free or low-fat yogurt and cheese, or try calcium-fortified soy products	Twice a week, make seafood the protein on your plate Vary your protein routine—choose beans, peas, nuts, and seeds more often Keep meat and poultry portions small and lean

For a 2,000-calorie diet, you need the amounts below from each food group. To find the amounts that are right for you, go to MyPlate.gov.

| Eat 6 oz. every day | Eat 2½ cups every day | Eat 2 cups every day | Get 3 cups every day; for kids aged 2 to 8, it's 2 | Eat 5½ oz. every day |

Find your balance between food and physical activity
- Be sure to stay within your daily calorie needs.
- Be physically active for at least 30 minutes most days of the week.
- About 60 minutes a day of physical activity may be needed to prevent weight gain.
- For sustaining weight loss, at least 60 to 90 minutes a day of physical activity may be required.
- Children and teenagers should be physically active for 60 minutes every day, or most days.

Know your limits on fats, sugars, and sodium
- Your allowance for oils is **6 teaspoons** a day.
- Limit Calories from solid fats and added sugars to **260 CALORIES** a day.
- Reduce sodium intake to less than **2300 mg** a day.

U.S. Department of Agriculture
Center for Nutrition Policy and Promotion
April 2005
CNPP-15

USDA

■ FIGURE 8.4   PDF version of MyPlate's 2000-Calorie Daily Food Plan. (USDA, Center for Nutrition Policy and Promotion. [2011]. Available at www.choosemyplate.gov)

In addition to obtaining a food pattern of appropriate calorie level, visitors to www .choosemyplate.gov have access to an enormous amount of information, including the following:

- MyPlate videos on specific food groups
- Healthy eating on a budget
- SuperTracker, which can track intake, physical activity, weight, and nutrition goals, as well as provide side-by-side nutritional comparisons between two different items
- Healthy eating tips, such as sample menus and recipes and how to eat healthy when eating out
- Vegetarian adaptations of the USDA Food Patterns

Despite the wealth of nutrition information available to consumers, there is a large gap between what Americans eat and the amounts recommended in the Daily Food Plans from the Vegetable, Fruits, and Dairy Groups and the whole-grain subgroup (Britten, Cleveland, Koegel, Kuczynski, and Nickols-Richardson, 2012). Likewise, Americans are consuming a larger percentage of their total calories from empty calories than is recommended. The International Food Information Council's 2010 Food and Healthy Survey found that although 64% of Americans report making changes to improve the healthfulness of their diet, only 12% can accurately estimate the number of calories they should consume in a day based on their height, weight, age, and activity (International Food Information Council Foundation, 2010). The survey also found that 58% of Americans do not make an effort to balance calorie intake with output. Fundamental to successful implementation of a MyPlate meal pattern is understanding the concepts of appropriate calorie level, empty calories, nutrient density, serving sizes, and variety.

Appropriate Calorie Level

The specific Daily Food Plan calorie level recommended for an individual is actually an estimate of how many calories a person of similar age and average height and weight needs to maintain an appropriate weight, not an exact individual requirement. If an individual's actual weight is more or less than "appropriate weight," weight change may occur as a result of following MyPlate recommendations. MyPlate makes a disclaimer that weight should be monitored to determine whether adjustments to calorie intake need to be made.

Empty Calories

Empty Calories: items with solid fats and/or added sugars that provide calories with few or no nutrients. Sometimes all the calories in an item are empty, such as in regular soft drinks. Sometimes only some of the total calories are considered empty, such as the calories from added sugar in sweetened yogurt.

An allowance for **empty calories** allows consumers to incorporate small amounts of or empty calories into their eating plan and still meet nutrient needs without exceeding total calorie constraints. Empty calorie allowances are low at 8% to 19% of total calories, and for most Americans, the allowance is toward the lower end of this range (Table 8.3) (Britten et al., 2012). This small empty calorie budget allows for only small amounts of alcohol or calorie-dense items *if* the bulk of the day's food choices are of nutrient-dense foods. More than 35% of usual calorie intake in the United States is from empty calories.

Nutrient Density

While it may be obvious that an empty calorie allowance can be used for "extras" to the meal plan, such as a glass of wine or can of cola, consumers may not realize that empty calories may be "eaten up" by choosing foods within the existing plan that are high in fat or added sugar. At each calorie level, the recommendations for the amount of food to consume are based on nutrient-dense representative foods within each group, such as the

Table 8.3 Empty Calorie Budgets

Age and Gender	Estimated Limit for Empty Calories for Those Who Are Not Physically Active	
	Total Daily Calorie Needs*	Daily Limit for Empty Calories
Children 2–3 yr	1000	140[†]
Children 4–8 yr	1200–1400	120
Girls 9–13 yr	1600	120
Boys 9–13 yr	1800	160
Girls 14–18 yr	1800	160
Boys 14–18 yr	2200	270
Females 19–30 yr	2000	260
Males 19–30 yr	2400	330
Females 31–50 yr	1800	160
Males 31–50 yr	2200	270
Females 51+ yr	1600	120
Males 51+ yr	2000	260

*These amounts are appropriate for individuals who get less than 30 minutes of moderate physical activity most days. Those who are more active need more total calories and have a higher limit for empty calories. To find your personal total calorie needs and empty calories limit, enter your information into "My Daily Food Plan."

[†]The limit for empty calories is higher for children 2 and 3 years old than it is for some older children, because younger children have lower nutrient needs and smaller recommended intakes from the basic food groups.

Healthiest Foods: subjectively defined as foods that provide the most nutrients with the least amount of extraneous calories from fat or added sugar.

very leanest cuts of meat trimmed of all visible fat. To the extent possible, they are without added sugars or sodium (Britten et al., 2012). If more calorically dense food choices are made, such as choosing whole milk instead of fat-free milk, the difference in calories is considered part of the empty calorie allowance, which is small. Selecting the **healthiest food** choices from each food group is vital for achieving appropriate calorie and nutrient recommendations.

Portion Sizes

Just as the quality of foods chosen influences total calorie intake, so does the quantity of foods eaten. Previously, MyPyramid recommended the number of servings from each group, which is not the same as the number of portions. For instance, a serving of pasta is ½ cup but a usual portion may be 3 cups at a restaurant. MyPlate has eliminated quantity confusion by specifying total amounts per day, such as 6 oz of grains and 2½ cups of vegetables. Instead of counting the number of portions eaten per day, consumers are now faced with the challenge of estimating how many servings their portion sizes are. Using common objects is an excellent way to convey the concept of normal **serving sizes**. Strategies to downsize **portion sizes** include using smaller dinnerware at home and using a tall slender glass instead of a short wide one.

QUICK BITE

This amount . . .	Looks like . . .
3 oz of meat	a deck of cards
2 tbsp of peanut butter	a ping-pong ball
1 oz of cheese	4 dice
½ cup of nuts	a level adult handful
½ cup cooked pasta, rice, or cereal	a scoop of ice cream
1 medium-sized piece of fruit	a baseball

Serving Size: the amount of food "officially" recommended.

Portion Size: the amount of food usually consumed.

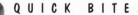

QUICK BITE

A comparison between 1-oz grain equivalent *serving* and a typical American *portion*

	Amount that qualifies as 1-oz grain equivalent	Common portion
Bread	1 slice	2 slices
Pancakes	1 (4½ in diameter)	3 (4½ in diameter)
Popcorn	3 cups, popped	12 cups, popped
Rice or pasta	½ cup cooked	1 cup cooked
Tortillas	1 small (6 in)	1 large (12 in)

Source: www.ChooseMyPlate.gov

Variety

Following a varied diet helps ensure that the more than 40 known essential nutrients are consumed in adequate amounts based on the rationale that some nutrients, such as iron, calcium, vitamin C, and vitamin A, are concentrated in a few foods. For instance, choosing a variety of vegetables, such as carrots, broccoli, tomatoes, and garbanzo beans, helps ensure adequate nutrient intake because each has a different nutrient profile. Conversely, choosing a variety of refined grains (e.g., white bread, white pasta, hamburger bun) does little to ensure nutritional adequacy, because although they are each different foods, their nutrient profile is remarkably similar. Likewise, eating a variety of foods from fat-dense food groups (e.g., protein food group and fat group) may contribute to a higher total calorie intake. A study conducted on people who have successfully maintained significant weight loss found their diets had very low variety in all food groups, especially groups with higher fat density (Raynor, Jeffery, Phelan, Hill, and Wing, 2005).

Recommendations from Health Agencies

Many health agencies publish guidelines or recommendations for healthy eating including the American Heart Association (Lichtenstein et al., 2006), the American Cancer Society (Kushi et al., 2012), and the American Institute for Cancer Research (World Cancer Research Fund, American Institute for Cancer Research, 2007) (Table 8.4). The recommendations are similar to each other and to the Dietary Guidelines for Americans. They urge Americans to become more physically active, choose more nutrient-dense foods, and limit alcohol intake.

Guidelines and Graphics in Other Countries

Cultural differences in communicating symbolism and other cultural norms influence the shape of food guides in other countries. Similar to MyPlate, a circle or dinner plate with each section depicting relative proportion to the total diet is used by many countries, including the United Kingdom (Fig. 8.5), Germany, and Mexico. Korea and China use a pagoda shape, and Canada uses a rainbow shape (Fig. 8.6). Despite the differences in the shape of the graphics, the core recommendations are consistently similar: eat plenty of grains, vegetables, and fruit; limit fat, saturated fat, and sugars; eat a variety of foods; and eat to balance intake with activity.

Table 8.4 Comparison of Nutrition and Lifestyle Recommendations from the American Heart Association, the American Cancer Society, and the American Institute for Cancer Research

Criteria	Our 2006 Diet and Lifestyle Recommendations by the American Heart Association*	American Cancer Society Guidelines for Nutrition and Physical Activity for Cancer Prevention[†]	American Institute for Cancer Research Diet and Guidelines for Cancer Prevention[‡]
Weight/ calorie balance	Use up at least as many calories as you take in.	▪ Achieve and maintain healthy weight throughout life. ▪ Be as lean as possible throughout life without being underweight. ▪ Avoid excessive weight gain throughout the life cycle.	Be as lean as possible without becoming underweight.
Physical activity	Aim for at least 30 minutes of moderate physical activity on most days of the week or—best of all—at least 30 minutes every day.	▪ Engage in regular physical activity and limit the intake of high-calorie food and beverages. ▪ Adopt a physically active lifestyle. ▪ Adults: get at least 150 minutes or more of moderate-intensity or 75 minutes of vigorous-intensity activity, or an equivalent combination, spread throughout the week.	Be physically active for at least 30 minutes each day.
Food	▪ Eat a variety of nutritious foods from all the food groups. ▪ Eating a variety of fruits and vegetables may help you control your weight and your blood pressure. ▪ Unrefined whole-grain foods contain fiber that can help lower your blood cholesterol and help you feel full, which may help you manage your weight. ▪ Eat fish at least twice a week. ▪ Eat less of the nutrient-poor foods. ▪ Choose lean meats and poultry without skin and prepare them without added saturated and trans fat. ▪ Select fat-free, 1%, and low-fat dairy products. ▪ Cut back on foods containing partially hydrogenated vegetable oils to reduce trans fat in your diet. ▪ Cut back on foods high in dietary cholesterol. Aim to eat less than 300 mg of cholesterol each day. ▪ Cut back on beverages and foods with added sugars. ▪ Choose and prepare foods with little or no salt. Aim to eat less than 2300 mg of sodium per day.	▪ Eat a variety of healthy foods, with an emphasis on plant sources. ▪ Choose foods and beverages in amounts that help you achieve and maintain a healthy weight. ▪ Limit consumption of processed and red meats. ▪ Eat at least 2½ cups of vegetables and fruits each day. ▪ Choose whole grains instead of refined grains.	▪ Eat more of a variety of vegetables, fruits, whole grains, and legumes such as beans. ▪ Don't use supplements to protect against cancer. ▪ Limit consumption of red meats (such as beef, pork, and lamb) and avoid processed meats. ▪ Limit consumption of energy-dense foods (particularly processed foods high in added sugar, low in fiber, or high in fat). ▪ Avoid sugary drinks. ▪ Limit consumption of salty foods and foods processed with salt (sodium).

(continues on page 194)

Table 8.4 Comparison of Nutrition and Lifestyle Recommendations from the American Heart Association, the American Cancer Society, and the American Institute for Cancer Research (continued)

Criteria	Our 2006 Diet and Lifestyle Recommendations by the American Heart Association*	American Cancer Society Guidelines for Nutrition and Physical Activity for Cancer Prevention[†]	American Institute for Cancer Research Diet and Guidelines for Cancer Prevention[‡]
Alcohol	If you drink alcohol, drink in moderation. That means 1 drink per day for women and 2 drinks per day for men.	If you drink alcoholic beverages, limit consumption. Drink no more than 1 drink per day for women or 2 drinks per day for men.	If consumed at all, limit daily alcoholic drinks to 2 for men and 1 for women.
Tobacco	Don't smoke tobacco, and stay away from tobacco smoke.	Stay away from tobacco.	Do not use, smoke, or chew tobacco.

Sources: *Lichtenstein, A., Appel, L., Brands, M., Carnethon, M., Daniels, S., Franch, H. A., . . . Wylie-Rosett, J. (2006). Diet and lifestyle recommendations. Revision 2006. A scientific statement from the American Heart Association Nutrition Committee. *Circulation, 114,* 82–96.

[†]Kushi, L., Doyle, C., McCullough, M., Rock, C. L., Demark-Wahnefried, W., Bandera, E. V., . . . Gansler, T. (2012). American Cancer Society guidelines on nutrition and physical activity for cancer prevention. Reducing the risk of cancer with healthy food choices and physical activity. *CA: A Cancer Journal for Clinicians, 62,* 30–67.

[‡]World Cancer Research Fund, American Institute for Cancer Research. (2007). *Food, nutrition, physical activity and the prevention of cancer: A global perspective.* Washington, DC: American Institute for Cancer Research.

The eatwell plate

Use the eatwell plate to help you get the balance right. It shows how much of what you eat should come from each food group.

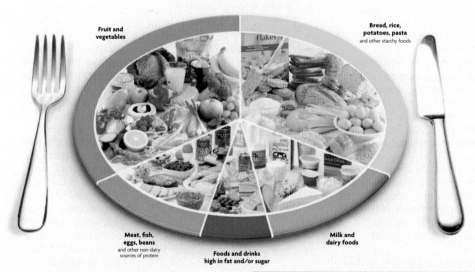

So, try to eat:
- plenty of fruit and vegetables
- plenty of bread, rice, potatoes, pasta, and other starchy foods—choose whole grain varieties whenever you can
- some milk and dairy foods
- some meat, fish, eggs, beans, and other nondairy sources of protein
- just a small amount of foods and drinks high in fat and/or sugar

8 TIPS FOR EATING WELL
1. Base your meals on starchy foods
2. Eat lots of fruit and vegetables
3. Eat more fish
4. Cut down on saturated fat and sugar
5. Try to eat less salt—no more than 6 g/day
6. Get active and try to be a healthy weight
7. Drink plenty of water
8. Don't skip breakfast

■ **FIGURE 8.5** Great Britain's food guide: The Balance of Good Health Food Standards Agency (United Kingdom).

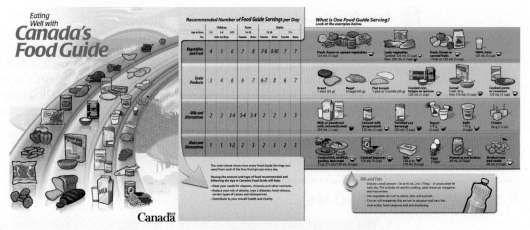

■ **FIGURE 8.6**   Canada's Food Guide to Healthy Eating. (© Her Majesty the Queen in Right of Canada, represented by the Minister of Healthy Canada, 2007.)

How Do You Respond?

Which foods are "good"? Which foods are "bad"? Instead of thinking of individual foods as good or bad, consider how a food fits within the context of the total intake. For instance, broccoli is among the best plant foods available, yet if someone ate only broccoli all day long, it would not be "good" because it does not supply adequate amounts of all essential nutrients for health. What matters is how often a particular food is eaten, what size the portion is, *why* a particular food is eaten (e.g., by choice or from mindless eating), and overall calorie balance. If most of a person's intake is of healthful foods, small amounts of less-than-healthful choices can fit into the diet without wreaking great havoc as long as total calorie intake is appropriate. The keys to fitting in less-than-healthful foods are to eat them *infrequently, in small amounts, and by conscious decision.*

How can I eat healthy if I don't like whole wheat bread? Just as there are no good or bad foods, there is not one particular food you must eat to be healthy, nor is there one particular food you must never eat to be healthy. Instead of whole wheat bread, consider whole wheat bagels or tortillas made with whole wheat flour for sandwiches and wraps. "Low-calorie" breads are another alternative; although they lack the phytochemicals, vitamins, and minerals of whole wheat bread, they do provide generous amounts of fiber added in place of some starch. Besides whole wheat bread, other sources of insoluble fiber include bran and whole-grain cereals and dried peas and beans.

Case Study

Andrew wants to eat healthier and went online to learn about MyPlate. He came away overwhelmed at all the information and was turned off by reading about ounces and cups—concepts that are unfamiliar to him. He is clearly interested in changing his food habits but is stuck on the idea that that isn't possible unless he weighs and measures his food. He is wondering if eating healthier is worth the trouble.

- How would you encourage him to approach the goal of eating healthier? What information would you gather about his usual intake? His willingness to change? How would you use MyPlate to help him make better choices without overwhelming him?

(continues on page 196)

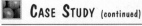

CASE STUDY (continued)

- Andrew's doctor told him he is not meeting his RDA for vitamin C based on what Andrew told him about his eating habits. Andrew is worried that he will develop scurvy. Can you assume that he is at risk for scurvy if he isn't consuming the RDA for vitamin C? Why may the doctor's assessment be flawed? How can you determine if Andrew isn't consuming enough vitamin C? What would you tell Andrew to calm his fears?

STUDY QUESTIONS

1. The greatest percentage of calories in the diet should come from
   a. Carbohydrates
   b. Protein
   c. Fat
   d. Either carbohydrate or protein

2. The Dietary Guidelines for Americans recommend Americans increase their intake of
   a. Refined grains
   b. Beef, pork, and chicken
   c. Fat-free or low-fat milk
   d. Calories from solid fats

3. "Moderate" alcohol consumption is
   a. Three to four drinks per week for women, six to eight drinks per week for men
   b. Up to one drink per day for both men and women
   c. Up to one drink per day for women, up to two drinks per day for men
   d. Up to two drinks per day for women, up to three drinks per day for men

4. The nurse knows her instructions about grain equivalents have been understood when the client verbalizes that one grain equivalent is equal to
   a. One slice of bread
   b. Two cups of ready-to-eat cereal
   c. One cup of cooked pasta
   d. One cup of cooked rice

5. A client states that there is no way he can eat all the vegetables recommended in his MyPlate plan. Which of the following would be the nurse's best response?
   a. "If you can't eat all the vegetables, make up for the difference by eating more fruit."
   b. "Be sure you take a daily multivitamin to provide the nutrients that may be missing from your diet."
   c. "Set a goal of eating larger quantities of the vegetable servings you currently eat and gradually increase the servings and variety as you become more skillful in adding vegetables to your diet."
   d. "No one can. The recommendations are only a guide. Just eat what you can."

6. The nurse knows her instructions about portion sizes have been effective when the client verbalizes that ½ cup cooked cereal looks like
   a. A scoop of ice cream
   b. An adult handful
   c. A ping-pong ball
   d. A softball

7. Which of the following items contains empty calories?
   a. Whole milk
   b. Whole wheat bread
   c. Orange juice
   d. Steamed broccoli

8. According to the Dietary Guidelines, a "nutrient of concern" that may be deficient in a typical American diet is
   a. Protein
   b. Potassium
   c. Vitamin C
   d. Zinc

KEY CONCEPTS

- A healthy diet provides optimal amounts of all essential nutrients to prevent deficiency symptoms and not excessive amounts that may cause nutrient toxicities or increase the risk of chronic diseases such as heart disease, cancer, stroke, and diabetes.
- DRIs are a set of reference values: the new RDAs, EARs, AIs, and ULs. Individual nutrients do not have each of these reference values; a nutrient has an EAR plus either an RDA or an AI. ULs are not established for all nutrients.
- The DRIs are primarily for professional use because they deal with quantities of nutrients as opposed to amounts of food.
- The RDAs are amounts of essential nutrients considered adequate to meet the nutritional needs of 97% to 98% of healthy people in a gender or life stage group. The AIs are similar to the RDA, but it is not known what percentage of people are meeting nutritional needs by consuming the AI.
- UL is the highest intake of a nutrient over time that does not pose a risk. There is no benefit to consuming amounts between the RDA and UL of a nutrient.
- Healthy People 2020 is a comprehensive blueprint for monitoring the nation's progress toward becoming healthier. It states a healthful diet contains a variety of nutrient-dense foods; is limited in saturated fat, trans fat, cholesterol, added sugar, sodium, and alcohol; and has a calorie level that is in balance with calorie need.
- The Dietary Guidelines for Americans are intended to help the public choose diets that promote health, reduce the risk of chronic disease, and help them attain and maintain healthy weight. They are revised every 5 years.
- The major messages conveyed by the Dietary Guidelines for Americans relate to balancing calories to achieve healthy weight and focus on eating nutrient-dense food and beverages. Recommendations include healthy eating patterns and foods/food components that should be limited.
- MyPlate is the newest generation of graphic to illustrate the Dietary Guidelines for Americans. MyPlate meal plans are available in 12 different calorie levels for individualization based on a person's age, gender, and level of activity.
- Consumers need to understand that it may be necessary to monitor their weight because MyPlate calorie recommendations are population-based estimates, not individual requirements.
- Empty calorie allowances are small, and if not strictly adhered to, total calorie intake will exceed recommended levels.
- Portion control is vital to staying within calorie restraints. Consumers may benefit from learning to estimate portion sizes using common household items.

■ Because a "healthy" diet not only limits excess calories but also provides adequate amounts of all essential nutrients, wise food choices are necessary, including eating a variety of foods within the vegetable and fruit groups.

■ Circles, a rainbow, a pagoda, and a plate are used as food graphics in other countries. Worldwide, food guides consistently recommend a high intake of whole grains, fruits, and vegetables.

■ The American Heart Association, the American Cancer Society, and the American Institute for Cancer Research each recommend a plant-based diet to reduce the risk of chronic disease.

Check Your Knowledge Answer Key

1. **FALSE** The RDAs are intended for healthy people and also people at risk of chronic disease.

2. **FALSE** The DRIs are most often used by dietitians to plan and evaluate menus and by researchers studying nutrition. Because they focus on nutrients, not foods, they are of limited value in teaching people how to choose healthy diets.

3. **FALSE** The Tolerable Upper Intake Level is the highest intake of a nutrient that does not produce any adverse effects. There is no advantage in consuming amounts greater than the RDA.

4. **TRUE** The Dietary Guidelines for Americans are intended to help people attain and maintain a healthy weight, reduce the risk of chronic disease, and promote wellness in Americans 2 years of age and older.

5. **TRUE** MyPlate, like its predecessor, is the graphic designed to illustrate the Dietary Guidelines for Americans.

6. **TRUE** MyPlate is actually a group of 12 different Daily Food Plans so that dietary advice can be personalized for a person's gender, age, height, weight, and activity patterns.

7. **FALSE** MyPlate specifies how many cups or ounces a person should consume from each group instead of using the vague term "servings."

8. **TRUE** Too much variety can contribute to overeating, depending on how variety is achieved. Variety in fruit and vegetables has a positive impact on the nutritional adequacy of the diet without promoting excessive calorie intake. Conversely, variety in snacks, entrees, and high-carbohydrate foods may contribute to overeating. Isn't it generally harder to limit food intake at a buffet than a traditional restaurant?

9. **TRUE** Discretionary calories can be "extras," but extra may not translate to extra food if selections within the food plan are not ones that are lowest in fat and added sugars. Discretionary calories may be used to choose higher calorie foods within the existing plan instead of adding extra food.

10. **TRUE** Both the American Cancer Society and American Heart Association recommend a plant-based diet to reduce the risk of chronic disease.

Student Resources on thePoint

For additional learning materials, activate the code in the front of this book at
http://thePoint.lww.com/activate

Websites

American Cancer Society at **www.cancer.org**
American Heart Association at **www.americanheart.org**
American Institute for Cancer Research at **www.aicr.org**
Dietary Guidelines for Americans at **www.health.gov/dietaryguidelines**
Dietary Reference Intakes from the National Academy Press are found at **www.nap.edu**
Healthy People 2010 at **www.healthypeople.gov**
International Dietary Guidelines, under Topics A-Z available at **www.nal.usda.gov/fnic**
MyPlate at **www.choosemyplate.gov**

References

Britten, P., Cleveland, L., Koegel, K., Kuczynski, K. J., & Nickols-Richardson, S. M. (2012). Updated US Department of Agriculture Food Patterns meet goals of the 2010 Dietary Guidelines. *Journal of the Academy of Nutrition and Dietetics, 112*, 1648–1655.

International Food Information Council Foundation. (2010). *2010 food and health survey: Consumer attitudes toward food safety, nutrition & health*. Available at www.foodinsight.org/Content/3651/2010FinalFullReport.pdf. Accessed on 10/11/12.

Kushi, L., Doyle, C., McCullough, M., Rock, C. L., Demark-Wahnefried, W., Bandera, E. V., . . . Gansler, T. (2012). American Cancer Society guidelines on nutrition and physical activity for cancer prevention. Reducing the risk of cancer with healthy food choices and physical activity. *CA: A Cancer Journal for Clinicians, 62*, 30–67.

Lichtenstein, A., Appel, L., Brands, M., Carnethon, M., Daniels, S., Franch, H. A., . . . Wylie-Rosett, J. (2006). Diet and lifestyle recommendations. Revision 2006. A scientific statement from the American Heart Association Nutrition Committee. *Circulation, 114*, 82–96.

Murphy, S., Xu, J., & Kochanek, K. (2012). Deaths: Preliminary data for 2010. *National Vital Statistics Report, 60*(4). Available at www.cdc.gov/nchs/data/nvsr/nvsr60/nvsr60_04.pdf. Accessed on 10/9/12.

Otten, J., Hellwig, J., & Meyers, L. (Eds.). (2006). *Dietary reference intakes. The essential guide to nutrient requirements*. Washington, DC: National Academy Press.

Raynor, H., Jeffery, R., Phelan, S., Hill, J. O., & Wing, R. R. (2005). Amount of food group variety consumed in the diet and long-term weight loss maintenance. *Obesity Research, 13*, 883–890.

U.S. Department of Agriculture, Center for Nutrition Policy and Promotion. (2011). *MyPlate*. Available at www.choosemyplate.gov. Accessed on 10/11/12.

U.S. Department of Agriculture, U.S. Department of Health and Human Services. (2010). *Dietary guidelines for Americans, 2010* (7th ed.). Available at www.health.gov/dietaryguidelines. Accessed on 2/24/11.

U.S. Department of Health and Human Services. (2010). *HHS announces the nation's new health promotion and disease prevention agenda*. Available at http://www.healthypeople.gov/2020/about/DefaultPressRelease.pdf. Accessed on 10/9/12.

World Cancer Research Fund, American Institute for Cancer Research. (2007). *Food, nutrition, physical activity, and the prevention of cancer: A global perspective*. Washington DC: American Institute for Cancer Research.

9 Consumer Issues

TRUE FALSE

☐ ☐ **1** Most Americans believe food and nutrition play a role in maintaining or improving health.

☐ ☐ **2** The serving sizes listed on the "Nutrition Facts" label are based on amounts typically eaten.

☐ ☐ **3** The Percent Daily Value listed on the "Nutrition Facts" label is based on a 2000-calorie diet.

☐ ☐ **4** Structure/function claims that appear on food labels are accurate and reliable.

☐ ☐ **5** Supplement manufacturers must prove that their products are safe and effective before they can be marketed.

☐ ☐ **6** Supplement manufacturers must list potential side effects on the label.

☐ ☐ **7** Organically grown foods are better for you than their conventionally raised counterparts.

☐ ☐ **8** Bacteria cause the majority of foodborne illnesses.

☐ ☐ **9** Genetically modified food is to be used with caution.

☐ ☐ **10** Irradiated food may contain small amounts of radioactive substances.

LEARNING OBJECTIVES

Upon completion of this chapter, you will be able to

1 Analyze a nutrition or health claim for credibility.

2 Evaluate a "Nutrition Facts" label to make better food choices.

3 Compare how the regulation and marketing of dietary supplements differ from regulation and marketing of drugs.

4 Advise clients of questions to consider before using a supplement.

5 Implement practices to help retain the nutritional value of food.

6 Discuss functional foods.

7 Interpret labeling on organic products.

8 Teach clients about the four simple steps to keep food safe.

9 Debate whether genetically modified food is safe.

10 Explain the reason why some foods are irradiated.

Functional Foods: commonly (not legally) defined as foods that provide health benefits beyond basic nutrition.

Food Irradiation: treatment of food with approved levels of ionizing radiation for a prescribed period of time and a controlled dose to destroy bacteria and parasites that would otherwise cause foodborne illness.

The proliferation of cyberspace information—and misinformation—gives millions of Americans ready access to nutritional concepts. Advances in food technology have brought us **functional foods**, bioengineering, and **food irradiation** as well as new questions about food safety and optimal nutrition. The ever-evolving science of nutrition has progressed from three square meals a day and a well-rounded diet to MyPlate. This is an era that presents old and new challenges for health professionals.

This chapter explores what consumers believe about food and nutrition and where they get their information. A variety of consumer issues are explored, including food labels, dietary supplements, retaining the nutrient content of food, functional food, organic foods, foodborne illnesses, biotechnology, and irradiation.

CONSUMER INFORMATION AND MISINFORMATION

In a recent survey, 60% or more of Americans either somewhat or strongly believed that food and beverages can provide a wide array of specific health benefits (International Food Information Council [IFIC] Foundation, 2008). Over the last two decades, the perceived role of food has shifted from simply a means to prevent deficiency diseases to a tool for preventing chronic health problems and delaying aging. According to the American Dietetic Association (ADA, 2009), this food as medicine paradigm is fueled by several factors, including

- Consumer interest in managing their own health
- Increases in older and ethnic subpopulations
- Escalating health-care costs
- A highly competitive food market with small profit margins
- Technologic advances, such as biotechnology
- Changes in food regulations
- Evidence-based science that links diet to a reduced risk of chronic disease

QUICK BITE

When asked to identify their top two to three sources of information about nutrition and health, consumers cited the following:

News media	71%
Internet	52%
Medical sources	36%
Friends/family	18%
Labels on products	5%
Diet and health books	3%
Researchers and scientists	4%

Source: International Food Information Council Foundation. (2007). *2005 Consumer attitudes toward functional foods/foods for health. Executive summary.* Available at www.foodinsight.org/Content/6/IFICExecSumAINGLE_vF2.pdf. Accessed on 10/15/12.

More than two-thirds of Americans surveyed agreed that reading or hearing about the relationship between food and health is of interest to them, but 45% stated that food and health information is confusing and conflicting (IFIC Foundation, 2008). Consumers grow skeptical when what seems like fact today is considered fiction tomorrow.

Media

Nearly three-fourths of Americans identify the news media, especially the Internet (52%) and television news (27%), as their top source of health and nutrition information (IFIC Foundation, 2007). However, only 24% rate the media as a believable source (IFIC

Box 9.1 JUDGING RELIABILITY OF NUTRITION "NEWS"

Who is promoting the message? Anyone who stands to benefit economically by promoting a food, supplement, or diet is not likely to be an objective resource.

What is the message? Generally, if it sounds too good to be true, it usually is.

When was the study conducted, the results published, or the website updated? Even seemingly legitimate information can become quickly outdated.

Where was the study conducted? Was the site a reputable research institution or an impressive-sounding but unknown facility? Internet addresses ending in .edu (educational institutions), .org (organizations), or .gov (government agencies) are more credible than those ending in .com (commercial), whose main objective may be to sell a product.

Why was the article written—to further the reader's awareness and knowledge or to sell or promote a product? Question objectivity when the author or site has a financial interest.

Foundation, 2007). Consumers are right to be skeptical: "breaking news" may be little more than "spin" (a favorable slant) or incomplete coverage of preliminary results from scientific studies, which are often discounted later as more research is completed. The distinction between correlation and causation may be blurred, and inappropriate conclusions may be made from study results. Features or articles that fail to identify how much or little of a food should be eaten, how often it should be eaten, or to whom the advice applies do not give consumers enough information to appropriately judge what the study means to them personally. Other types of media inaccuracy include generalizing a study to a broader population than was actually studied and overstating the size of the effect. And although the information available on the Internet is vast, there are no regulatory safeguards in place to ensure that the information is accurate. Junk science coexists with legitimate data. It is the responsibility of each individual consumer to evaluate the reliability of information (Box 9.1).

Combating Misinformation

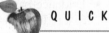

QUICK BITE

Red flags or "buzz words" signaling that a health or nutrient claim may be fraudulent include the following:

Breakthrough
Easy
Enzymatic process
Discovered in Europe
New
Mysterious
Quick
Secret
Absolutely safe
Miraculous cure
Ancient formula
All natural
Exclusive formula
Scientifically proven

Determining whether information is valid and reliable may be easier than persuading a client that he or she has been a victim of hype. Many people assume that anything that appears in print form (e.g., in a book, magazine, or newspaper) is accurate, and not everyone recognizes the shortcomings of the World Wide Web. If clients' beliefs are unsupported but harmless, you may risk alienating them for no reason by trying to convince them they're misinformed. Determine how much of an emotional investment the client has in believing the misinformation. Be aware that casual or judgmental dismissal of misinformation can cause clients to become defensive and distrustful;

clients may conclude that you are not as up-to-date as they are about nutrition, and they may reject you as a credible reference.

Food Labels

Sixty-two percent of Americans polled said that food labels influence to "great extent" or "moderately" their decision to try a food or food component (IFIC Foundation, 2007). Information provided on a label includes Nutrition Facts and an ingredient list; nutrient content claims, health claims, and structure/function claims may also be found.

Nutrition Facts

The Nutrition Facts label gives consumers "facts" they need to know to make informed decisions as they shop for food. Figure 9.1 lists facts about the Nutrition Facts label.

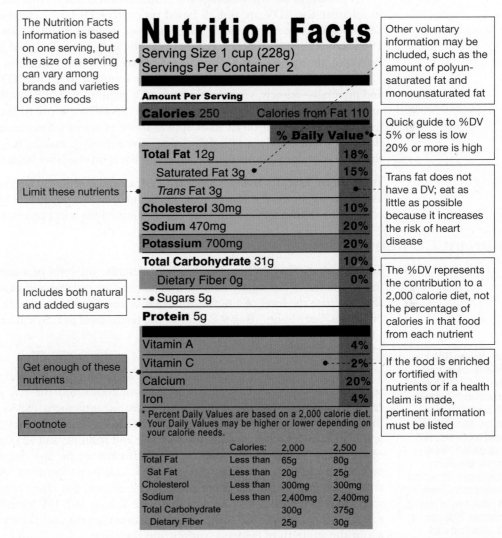

■ FIGURE 9.1   Nutrition facts label. (*Source:* U.S. Food and Drug Administration)

Everything Hinges on Portion Size. All information that appears on the Nutrition Facts label is specific for the portion size listed. So if the actual portion size eaten differs from that listed, all the "facts" are incorrect. Because different varieties of a food differ in weight, there may be slight differences in the serving size among different manufacturers. For instance, the serving size of Barbara's Bakery Puffins cereal is ¾ cup, 30 g; Kellogg's Special K is 1 cup, 31 g; and Kellogg's Rice Krispies is 1¼ cup, 33 g. Food label serving sizes may also differ from size equivalents used in MyPlate.

Percent Daily Value (%DV): the percentage of how much of a particular nutrient or fiber a person should consume based on a 2000-calorie diet.

Percent Daily Value May Not Be Accurate for an Individual. The **Percent Daily Value (%DV)** stated on the label may underestimate or overestimate the contribution to an individual's diet, depending on how many calories the individual actually needs. For nutrients whose amounts are based on a percentage of total calories (e.g., carbohydrates, fiber, fat, saturated fat), the %DV is calculated on the basis of a 2000-calorie diet. For people who need fewer than 2000 calories daily, such as most women and elderly men, the %DV listed on the label actually underestimates the contribution a serving makes to the total needed daily. For young active men who need more than 2000 cal/day, the %DV overestimates actual contribution.

A wrinkle in the usefulness of the Nutrition Facts label is that the nutrient amounts used to calculate the %DV are not all based on current Dietary Reference Intakes (DRIs). The %DVs for vitamin A, vitamin D, calcium, iron, vitamin E, folate, and zinc are based on the 1968 Recommended Dietary Allowances. Similarly, the value used for sodium is 2400 mg, even though the new Adequate Intake (AI) set for sodium intake in adults is 1500 mg.

Another caveat is that manufacturers are required to list the %DV of only four vitamins and minerals—namely, vitamin A, vitamin C, calcium, and iron—unless the food is enriched or fortified with others. However, a manufacturer may choose to list other nutrients, which may make one brand of an item appear more nutritious than another. For instance, one brand of yogurt boasts a 10% daily value of vitamin B_{12}, making it look superior to another that also contains vitamin B_{12} but does not list it on the label because it is not required.

Ingredient List. Ingredients are listed in descending order by weight. The further down the list an item appears, the less of that ingredient is in the product. This information gives the consumer a relative idea of how much of each ingredient is in a product but not the proportion.

Nutrient Content Claims

Terms such as "low," "free," and "high" describe the level of a nutrient or substance in a food. The terms are legally defined and so they are reliable and valid. Nutrient claims may also compare the level of a nutrient to that of comparable food with terms such as "more," "reduced," or "light." Box 9.2 defines the terms used in nutrient claims.

Health Claims

Daily Values (DVs): are reference values established by the FDA for use on food labels. For some nutrients (e.g., sodium), they are amounts that should not be exceeded; for others (e.g., fiber), they are amounts to strive toward. For nutrient intakes that are based on the percentage of calories consumed, 2000 calories is the standard used.

The U.S. Food and Drug Administration (FDA) has approved certain health claims about the relationship between specific nutrients or foods and the risk of a disease or health-related condition that meet significant scientific agreement (SSA) (Box 9.3). Items that make one of these claims also meet other requirements: (1) they do not exceed specific levels for total fat, saturated fat, cholesterol, and sodium; and (2) they contain at least 10% of the **Daily Values (DVs)** (before supplementation) for any one or all of the following: protein, dietary fiber, vitamin A, vitamin C, calcium, and iron. Additional health claim criteria are specific for the claim made. For instance, the claim regarding calcium and osteoporosis is only allowed on foods that have at least 20% DV for calcium. These claims are referred to as *unqualified* health claims because they do not require a qualifying statement about the strength of evidence supporting the claim.

Box 9.2   DEFINITIONS OF TERMS USED IN NUTRIENT CLAIMS

Free means the product contains virtually none of that nutrient. "Free" can refer to calories, sugar, sodium, salt, fat, saturated fat, and cholesterol.

Low means there is a small enough amount of a nutrient that the product can be used frequently without concern about exceeding dietary recommendations. Low sodium, low calorie, low fat, low saturated fat, and low cholesterol are all defined as to the amount allowed per serving. For instance, to be labeled low cholesterol, a product must have no more than 20 mg cholesterol per serving.

Very low refers to sodium only. The product cannot have more than 35 mg sodium per serving.

Reduced or less means the product has at least a 25% reduction in a nutrient compared to the regular product.

Light or lite means the product has fewer calories than a comparable product or 50% of the fat found in a comparable product.

Good source means the product provides 10% to 19% of the daily value for a nutrient.

High, rich in, or excellent source means the product has at least 20% of the daily value for a nutrient.

More means the product has at least 10% more of a desirable nutrient than does a comparable product.

Lean refers to meat or poultry products with less than 10 g fat, less than 4 g saturated fat, and less than 95 mg cholesterol per standardized serving and per 100 g.

Extra lean refers to meat or poultry products with less than 5 g fat, less than 2 g saturated fat, and less than 95 mg cholesterol per standardized serving and per 100 g.

The FDA allows certain qualified health claims when the relationship between food, a food component, and a supplement is not strong enough to meet SSA or published authoritative standards. Specific FDA-approved labeling language must be used for qualified health claims, and companies must petition the FDA for prior written permission to make a qualified health claim. The weakest claim is as follows: "Very limited and preliminary scientific research suggests [health claim]. The FDA concludes that there is little scientific evidence supporting this claim." Examples of qualified health claims are listed in Box 9.4.

Structure/Function Claims

Structure/function claims offer the possibility that a food may improve or support body function, which is a fine distinction from the approved health claims that relate a food or nutrient to a disease. An example of a disease claim needing approval is "suppresses appetite to treat obesity," whereas a function claim that does not need approval is "suppresses appetite to aid weight loss." These structure claims had previously been used primarily by supplement manufacturers with the disclaimer that "These statements have not been evaluated by the FDA. This product is not intended to diagnose, treat, cure or prevent any disease." Structure/function claims are now appearing on food labels and do not require a disclaimer. Unlike health claims that can only appear on foods that meet other nutritional criteria (e.g., they cannot be high in fat, cholesterol, sodium), structure/function claims can appear on "junk" foods. Structure/function claims do not require FDA approval, so there may be no evidence to support the claim. See Box 9.5 for structure/function claims that do not need prior approval.

Box 9.3	UNQUALIFIED HEALTH CLAIMS BASED ON SIGNIFICANT SCIENTIFIC AGREEMENT

Cancer Risk
- Dietary fat
- Fruits and vegetables
- Fiber-containing grain products
- Whole-grain foods and certain cancers

Coronary Heart Disease Risk
- Saturated fat and cholesterol
- Fruits, vegetables, and grain products that contain fiber, particularly soluble fiber
- Plant sterol/stanol esters
- Soluble fiber, such as that found in whole oats and psyllium seed husk
- Soy protein
- Whole-grain foods
- Phytosterols

Decreased Risk of Dental Caries
- Sugar alcohols

Hypertension Risk
- Sodium
- Potassium (also decreased risk of stroke)

Neural Tube Defect Risk
- Folate

Osteoporosis Risk
- Calcium
- Calcium and vitamin D

Box 9.4	SELECTED QUALIFIED HEALTH CLAIMS

Cancer Risk
- Green tea
- Selenium
- Antioxidant vitamins
- Tomatoes and/or tomato sauce (prostate, ovarian, gastric, and pancreatic cancers)

Cardiovascular Disease Risk
- Nuts
- Walnuts
- Monounsaturated fatty acids from olive oil
- Omega-3 fatty acids
- B vitamins
- Unsaturated fatty acids from canola oil
- Corn oil

Hypertension Risk (and Pregnancy-Induced Hypertension and Preeclampsia)
- Calcium

Box 9.5	STRUCTURE/FUNCTION CLAIMS THAT DO NOT NEED APPROVAL

Improves memory
Improves strength
Improves digestion
Boosts stamina
For common symptoms of premenstrual syndrome (PMS)
For hot flashes
Helps you relax
Helps enhance muscle tone or size
Relieves stress
Helps promote urinary tract health
Maintains intestinal flora
For hair loss associated with aging
Prevents wrinkles
For relief of muscle pain after exercise
To treat or prevent nocturnal leg muscle cramps
Helps maintain normal cholesterol levels
Provides relief of occasional constipation
Supports the immune system

Future Directions

Over the last decade, many food manufacturers and retailers have added a variety of nutrition symbols and rating systems to the front of food packages to show how nutritious they are. For instance, PepsiCo Smart Spot and the American Heart Association Heart Check utilize a single symbol to provide summary information about the nutrient content of a product. The Whole Grain Council's Whole Grain Stamp is an example of a front-of-package symbol used to indicate the presence of a food group or ingredient. Although intended to simplify choices for consumers, these front-of-package labels may actually increase confusion (Institute of Medicine [IOM], 2011).

The IOM formed a committee, with the Centers for Disease Control and Prevention, the FDA, and the Center for Nutrition Policy and Promotion in the U.S. Department of Agriculture as cosponsors, to study the issue of front-of-package nutrition rating systems. The committee concluded that it is time for a fundamental shift from simply providing nutrition information to also providing guidance on making healthier food choices (IOM, 2011). It describes a successful symbol system as one that

- Is simple, not requiring sophisticated nutrition knowledge
- Provides guidance rather than specific facts
- Uses a scaled or ranking system
- Features readily remembered names or identifiable symbols

Such a system would complement the Nutrition Facts label, not replace it. Weeks before the IOM committee report was issued, the Grocery Manufacturers Association and Food Marketing Institute unveiled Facts Up Front, a voluntary front-of-package labeling initiative that features an icon with four nutrients: calories, saturated fat, sodium, and sugar (Fig. 9.2) (Grocery Manufacturers Association, 2010). Participating food and beverage companies have the option to add up to two nutrients that have positive health benefits—namely, potassium, fiber, protein, vitamin A, vitamin C, vitamin D, calcium, and iron. Smaller packages may limit the icon to just calories. The icon began appearing in the marketplace in late 2011.

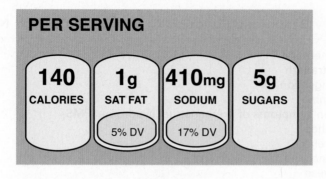

PER SERVING

140 CALORIES   **1g** SAT FAT   **410mg** SODIUM   **5g** SUGARS

5% DV   17% DV

■ **FIGURE 9.2**   Facts Up Front

Although the icon does not provide the guidance the IOM report recommended, the FDA has issued its support of Facts Up Front labeling but stopped short of endorsing the program (Scott-Thomas, 2012). The FDA intends to assess whether the system is applied in a way that promotes public health and is useful to consumers.

CONSUMER-RELATED CONCERNS

Poor diet is clearly associated with several major causes of morbidity and mortality, including cardiovascular disease, hypertension, type 2 diabetes, obesity, and certain types of cancer (ADA, 2009). As knowledge of nutrition in health and disease continues to grow, consumers interested in self-directed care will increasingly look to diet-related strategies to ensure health and wellness (ADA, 2009). Some of those strategies may include using dietary supplements, retaining the nutritional value of foods, choosing functional foods, and opting for organic foods. Other issues covered include foodborne illness, biotechnology, and irradiation.

Dietary Supplements

Herbs: plants or parts of plants used to alleviate health problems or promote wellness.

The term dietary supplement is a group name for products that contain one or more dietary ingredients including vitamins, minerals, **herbs** or other botanicals, amino acids, and other substances. They are intended to *add to* (supplement) the diets of some people, not to replace a healthy diet. Supplements are taken by mouth as a capsule, tablet, lozenge, liquid, or tea. Labeling laws require the front label to state that the product is a dietary supplement. Figure 9.3 depicts a supplement label.

More than half of American adults take a dietary supplement (Gahche et al., 2011), collectively spending about $28.1 billion per year (Nutrition Business Journal, 2011). Although multivitamins/multiminerals are the most commonly used dietary supplements, approximately 18% of total U.S. supplement sales in 2010 were for herbs and botanicals (Nutrition Business Journal, 2011). The top 10 selling herbal dietary supplements in food, drug, and mass marketing retail channels in the United States are summarized in Table 9.1.

Whereas the functions and requirements of vitamins and minerals are fairly well understood, scientific research is lacking for many herbal products. Many people mistakenly believe "natural" is synonymous with "safe." They assume that herbs must be harmless because they come from flowers, leaves, and seeds. In truth, herbs are not guaranteed to be safe or effective.

In June 2007, the FDA announced a final rule establishing current good manufacturing practice requirements (CGMPs) for dietary supplements. For the first time, identity,

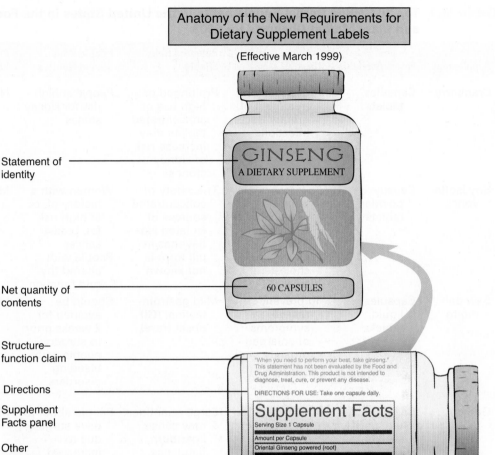

Anatomy of the New Requirements for
Dietary Supplement Labels

(Effective March 1999)

Statement of identity

Net quantity of contents

Structure–function claim

Directions

Supplement Facts panel

Other ingredients in descending order of predominance and by common name or proprietary blend.

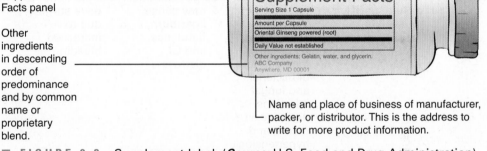

GINSENG
A DIETARY SUPPLEMENT

60 CAPSULES

"When you need to perform your best, take ginseng." This statement has not been evaluated by the Food and Drug Administration. This product is not intended to diagnose, treat, cure, or prevent any disease.

DIRECTIONS FOR USE: Take one capsule daily.

Supplement Facts

Serving Size 1 Capsule

Amount per Capsule

Oriental Ginseng powered (root)

Daily Value not established

Other ingredients: Gelatin, water, and glycerin.
ABC Company
Anywhere, MD 00001

Name and place of business of manufacturer, packer, or distributor. This is the address to write for more product information.

■ FIGURE 9.3   Supplement label. (**Source:** U.S. Food and Drug Administration)

purity, quality, and composition of dietary supplements were required to be accurately reflected on the label. The final rule is a significant step in protecting consumers by ensuring supplements that

- Are free of contaminants or impurities such as natural toxins, bacteria, pesticides, glass, lead, or other substances
- Contain the stated amount of a dietary ingredient
- Are properly packaged
- Are made from ingredients that were properly handled

In addition, the final rule requires that manufacturers report all serious dietary supplement adverse events to the FDA. Still, there are major differences between how supplements and drugs are regulated and marketed.

Table 9.1 Top 10 Selling Herbal Supplements in the United States in the Food, Drug, and Mass Market Channels for 2009

Supplement	Forms Available	Uses	Potential Side Effects	People Who Should Not Use	Potential Herb–Drug Interactions
Cranberry	Capsules, tablets	Prevention and treatment of urinary tract infections	Prolonged or high use of concentrated tablets may increase risk of kidney stones	People at high risk for kidney stones	No reported adverse interactions
Soy isoflavones	Capsules, powder, tablets	To lessen symptoms of menopause such as hot flashes, to lower serum cholesterol levels	The safety of concentrated sources of isolated isoflavones in pill form is not known	Women with a history of, or at high risk for, breast cancer People with altered thyroid function	May reduce the absorption of thyroid medications when taken concurrently
Saw palmetto	Capsules, liquid, tablets	To prevent or relieve symptoms of enlarged prostate	Mild gastrointestinal (GI) upset (rare)	Should be avoided for 2 weeks prior to surgery; people with bleeding disorders	May increase bleeding time when taken with anticoagulants, aspirin, supplements of vitamin E or ginkgo; may interfere with hormone and contraceptive drug therapies
Garlic	Capsules, liquid, powder, tablets	To lower cholesterol and/or triglyceride levels; may be useful in the treatment of bacterial and fungal infections, digestive ailments, and hypertension	Large quantities may cause heartburn, flatulence, and GI distress	People about to have surgery, due to increased bleeding	May increase bleeding time when taken with other blood-thinning supplements or anticoagulants; may decrease effectiveness of cyclosporine, some calcium channel blockers, chemotherapeutic agents, antifungals, glucocorticoids, and others; may interfere with the effectiveness of oral contraceptives; avoid if used with nonnucleoside reverse transcriptase inhibitor antiretroviral drugs
Echinacea	Capsules, liquid, tablets; also sold in herbal teas and throat lozenges	To prevent or treat colds and the flu	Minor GI upset, increased urination, allergic reactions (especially in people allergic to grass pollens)	People with autoimmune diseases such as multiple sclerosis, lupus Not recommended to be used for >8 successive weeks	May decrease effectiveness of immune-suppressing drugs, such as cyclosporine, azathioprine, prednisone, and other corticosteroids

Table 9.1 **Top 10 Selling Herbal Supplements in the United States in the Food, Drug, and Mass Market Channels for 2009** (continued)

Supplement	Forms Available	Uses	Potential Side Effects	People Who Should Not Use	Potential Herb–Drug Interactions
Ginkgo biloba	Capsules, infusions, liquid, tablets	To improve memory, to treat peripheral vascular disease	Mild headache, GI upset, constipation, allergic skin reactions Consumption of ginkgo seeds can be fatal	Should be avoided at least 36 hours prior to surgery; people with bleeding disorders or diabetes	Anticoagulants, aspirin, vitamin E or garlic supplements, trazodone, fluoxetine (Prozac), antidiabetics, thiazide diuretics
Milk thistle	Capsules, tablets, soft gels, liquid, tincture	To treat alcoholic liver cirrhosis, to reduce the risk of cancers of the prostate and skin	Minimal occurrence of side effects that include GI upset and skin rash	None known	May increase clearance of glucuronidated drugs, such as select statin medications, acetaminophen, diazepam, digoxin, morphine
St. John's wort	Capsules, liquid, tea, tablets, powders	To treat depression, anxiety, seasonal affective disorder, sleep disorders	Dry mouth, dizziness, GI symptoms, increased sensitivity to sunlight, fatigue	People sensitive to sunlight or using ultraviolet treatment People with bipolar disorder; people scheduled for surgery; may increase dementia in people with Alzheimer disease	Do not use with antidepressant medications; may decrease the effectiveness of oral contraceptives, theophylline, digoxin, and numerous other drugs for epilepsy, heart disease, immunosuppression, and psychosis
Ginseng	Capsules, gel caps, tablets, tea	To improve mental alertness or increase energy As an aphrodisiac or stress reliever	Generally not associated with adverse side effects	People with untreated hypertension Women with a history of breast cancer	May increase bleeding time when taken with other blood-thinning supplements or medications; when used with caffeine, may stimulate hypertension; may interfere with corticosteroids, digoxin, diabetes medications, and estrogen therapy
Black cohosh	Capsules, liquid, tablets, teas	Relief of menopausal symptoms, premenstrual syndrome, dysmenorrhea	GI upset, headaches, dizziness, weight gain, cramping, feeling of heaviness in the legs	Women with a history of breast cancer or at risk of breast cancer (an animal study showed black cohosh promoted cancer metastasis)	May increase the risk of liver damage in people taking potentially hepatotoxic drugs or supplements

Sources: Cavaliere, C., Rea, P., Lynch, M., & Blumenthal, M. (2010). *Herbal supplement sales rise in all channels in 2009*. Available at http://cms.herbalgram.org/herbalgram/issue86/article3530.html. Accessed on 10/16/12; and Fragakis, A., & Thomson, C. (2007). *The health professional's guide to popular dietary supplements* (3rd ed.). Chicago, IL: The American Dietetic Association.

Supplement Regulation

In their medicinal sense, herbs are technically unapproved drugs; approximately 30% of drugs used today originated from plants (e.g., paclitaxel, aspirin, digoxin). In the United States, dietary supplements are regulated by the FDA as *foods,* which means they do not have to meet the same standards as drugs and over-the-counter medications. Supplements differ greatly from conventional drugs in how they are marketed and regulated.

Safety and Effectiveness Are Not Proven. Before a drug can be marketed, the FDA must authorize its use based on the results of clinical studies performed to determine safety, effectiveness, possible interactions with other substances, and appropriate doses. In contrast, the regulations regarding dietary supplements are lax. Supplement ingredients sold in the United States before October 15, 1994, are assumed to be safe and so do not require FDA review for safety before they are marketed. Dietary supplement manufacturers that want to market a **new dietary ingredient** must submit information to the FDA that supports their conclusion that *reasonable* evidence exists that the product is safe for human consumption. Manufacturers do not have to *prove* to the FDA that dietary supplements are safe or effective; however, they are not supposed to market unsafe or ineffective products.

Once a product is marketed, the responsibility lies with the FDA to prove danger rather than with the manufacturer to prove safety. They do this through adverse event monitoring and research. When the FDA determines that a supplement is unsafe, it issues a consumer advisory discouraging its use. Only one supplement, ephedra, has actually been banned by the FDA in an unprecedented move that resulted from a 7-year review of tens of thousands of public comments and peer-reviewed scientific literature on the safety of ephedra. Despite the ban, consumers are still able to buy ephedra.

Strength Is Not Standardized. Dietary supplements are not required to be standardized in the United States. In fact, there is no legal definition of **standardization** as it applies to supplements, so the concentration of active compounds in different batches of supposedly identical plant material can vary greatly. The difference in concentration may be related to several factors such as the variety of plant used and the part of the plant used (e.g., the stems or leaves).

Dosages Are Not Standardized. Recommended dosages vary among manufacturers because there is no premarket testing to determine optimum dosage or maximum safe dosage. Other than the manufacturers' responsibility to ensure safety, there are no regulations that limit a "serving size" of any supplement.

Claims on Packaging Do Not Require FDA Approval. Although dietary supplements cannot claim to be used for the diagnosis, treatment, cure, or prevention of disease, they can be labeled with statements explaining their purported effect on the structure or function of the human body (e.g., "alleviates fatigue") or their role in promoting well-being (e.g., "improves mood"). These statements do not require FDA approval, but the label must include the following disclaimer: "This statement has not been evaluated by the FDA. This product is not intended to diagnose, treat, cure, or prevent any disease."

Warnings Are Not Required. Unlike drugs, supplements are not required to carry warning labels about potential side effects, adverse effects, or supplement–drug interactions. There are also no advisories about who should not use the product.

Supplements Are Self-Prescribed. A major concern with self-medication is that consumers may misdiagnose their condition or forsake effective conventional medical care to treat themselves "naturally." Another problem with self-medicating is that patients may not inform their physicians about their use of herbs, so side effects and herb–drug interactions go undiagnosed and unreported.

New Dietary Ingredient: supplement ingredient not marketed in the United States before October 15, 1994.

Standardization: a manufacturing process that ensures product consistency from batch to batch.

Advice for Supplement Users

Clients who choose to use supplements should

- Ask critical questions beforehand, such as whether there is any scientific evidence to support the use of the product or if there are any potential adverse side effects associated with its use.
- Check with the FDA website for consumer advisories on supplements to avoid.
- Discuss supplement use with the physician.
- Take only single supplement products and keep the dose small to prevent and manage adverse side effects and supplement–drug interactions.
- Take supplements at different times from prescribed medications to help reduce the potential for supplement–drug interactions.
- Discontinue supplements immediately if adverse side effects or supplement–drug interactions occur.
- Avoid herbs and other botanical supplements if they are pregnant or lactating women or children under the age of 6 years.

Retaining the Nutrient Content of Food

Even when it is carefully planned, an eating plan may not provide optimal amounts of all nutrients if the food has been improperly stored or overly processed. Food generally begins to lose its nutrients the moment harvesting or processing begins; the more done to a food before it is eaten, the greater the loss of naturally present nutrients. Heat, light, air, soaking in water, mechanical injury, dry storage, and acidic or alkaline food processing ingredients can hasten nutrient losses. Vitamins, minerals, and fibers are particularly vulnerable to the effects of food processing. Tips to retain the nutrient value of foods are featured in Box 9.6.

Box 9.6   TIPS FOR RETAINING THE NUTRIENT VALUE OF FOODS

- Don't buy produce that is damaged or wilted or that has been improperly stored. Produce picked when fully ripe is higher in nutrients than produce picked when green.
- Refrigerate most fruits and vegetables immediately to slow enzyme activity and retain nutrients. Keep produce in the refrigerator crisper or in moisture-proof bags.
- Wash, don't soak, produce to avoid leaching nutrients.
- Avoid peeling and paring vegetables before cooking because a valuable layer of nutrients is stored directly beneath the skin. If necessary, scrape or pare as thin a layer as possible.
- Avoid cutting produce into small pieces: the more surface area exposed, the greater the nutrient loss.
- Prepare vegetables as close to serving time as possible to avoid excessive exposure to light and air. Don't thaw frozen vegetables before cooking.
- Eat some fruits and vegetables raw.
- Cook produce in as little water as possible to avoid leaching vitamins. Stir fry, steam, microwave, or pressure cook vegetables to retain nutrients. If water is used in cooking, save it and use it as stock for soups, gravies, or sauces.
- Shorten cooking time as much as possible. Cook vegetables to the tender crunchy, rather than to the mushy, stage of doneness; cover the pan to retain heat; and preheat the pan or water before adding foods to speed heating time.
- Cook only as many vegetables as are needed at a time because reheating causes considerable loss of vitamins.

Functional Foods

Functional foods are one of the fastest growing segments of the food industry. The term has no legal meaning in the United States; it is currently a marketing, not regulatory, term. It generally applies to foods or food components that provide health benefits beyond basic nutrition. Functional foods may be natural (Table 9.2) or manufactured.

Manufactured functional foods are a blend of food and pharmacy ("phoods") in which food has one or more functional ingredients added, such as vitamins, minerals,

Table 9.2 Natural Functional Foods

Food	Active Ingredient	Potential Health Benefits
Blueberries	Anthocyanins	May reduce the risk of Alzheimer disease through anti-inflammatory and antioxidant properties
Soy foods	Soy protein	Lower total and low-density lipoprotein (LDL) cholesterol, may inhibit tumor growth
Oats	Soluble fiber (beta-glucan)	Lower total and LDL cholesterol
Fatty fish	Omega-3 fatty acids	Lower triglycerides, lower heart disease, lower cardiac deaths, and lower fatal and nonfatal heart attacks
Purple grape juice or red wine	Resveratrol	Decrease platelet aggregation
Cranberry juice	Proanthocyanidins	Reduces bacteriuria
Green tea	Catechins	Reduces the risk of certain cancers, such as breast and prostate
Tomatoes and tomato products	Lycopene	Reduce the risk of prostate, ovarian, gastric, and pancreatic cancer
Yogurt and fermented dairy products	Probiotics	Promote gastrointestinal health
Nuts	Monounsaturated fatty acids and vitamin E	Reduce the risk of cardiovascular disease
Citrus fruits	Flavanones	Neutralize free radicals; promote cellular antioxidant defenses
Cruciferous vegetables (e.g., broccoli, cauliflower, cabbage)	Sulforaphane	Reduce the risk of certain types of cancer
Garlic, onions, leeks, scallions	Sulfur compounds	Lower total and LDL cholesterol; may promote healthy immune function
Orange, red, and dark green fruits and vegetables	Beta-carotene	Neutralize free radicals, which may damage cells; may inhibit cancer growth
Spinach, kale, collard greens	Lutein	Lower risk of age-related macular degeneration

Sources: American Dietetic Association. (2009). Position of the American Dietetic Association: Functional foods. *Journal of the American Dietetic Association, 109,* 735–746; International Food Information Council Foundation. (2009). *Functional foods fact sheet: Antioxidants.* Available at www.foodinsight.org/Resources/Detail.aspx?topic=Functional_Foods_Fact_Sheet_Antioxidants. Accessed on 10/23/12. American Institute for Cancer Research. (2012). Phytochemicals: The cancer fighters in the foods we eat. Available at http://preventcancer.aicr.org/site/PageServer?pagename=elements_phytochemicals. Accessed on 10/23/12.

phytochemicals, or herbs. New functional foods with unique combinations of ingredients are being introduced in the marketplace faster than science can provide information on their safety. Like supplements, once functional foods are marketed, adverse effects are brought to light only if consumers alert the FDA to suspected problems.

As scientific evidence mounts in the role of specific nutrients or food substances in preventing chronic diseases such as heart disease, cancer, diabetes, hypertension, and osteoporosis, it is likely that more foods will be considered functional and the supply of manufactured functional foods will expand exponentially. It is the position of the ADA that functional foods have a potentially beneficial effect on health when consumed as part of a varied diet on a regular basis (ADA, 2009). Functional foods should be viewed as an option in the continuum of good nutrition, not as a "magic bullet" to cure all dietary ills.

Organically Grown Foods

Organic: in a chemical sense, organic means carbon containing. Generally, organic refers to living organisms; as such, all foods are technically organic.

Sales of **organic** food and beverages in the United States have grown from $1 billion in 1990 to $26.7 billion in 2010 (Organic Trade Association, 2011). Although fruits and vegetables are the top-selling organic products, dairy, beverages, packaged and prepared foods, and bread and grains comprised 63% of total organic sales in 2008 (Dimitri and Oberholtzer, 2009). Consumers have the impression that organic vegetables and fruits are safer, more nutritious, and healthier—ideas promoted by the organic food industry, its advocates, food marketers, and even some physicians and scientists (Tarver, 2012).

Organic foods are grown without synthetic fertilizers and pesticides. Instead, "natural" products, such as manure, compost, and other organic wastes, are used to fertilize crops, and chemicals that occur naturally in the environment, such as sulfur, nicotine, and copper, may be used as pesticides. Insects that do not harm a particular crop may be used to control other insects known to cause crop damage. Crop rotation, tillage, and cover crops are used to manage soil. Food irradiation, sewage sludge, and bioengineered plants cannot be used.

Organically Grown or Organically Produced: foods produced with little or no synthetic fertilizers or pesticides (e.g., plants) and no antibiotics or hormones (e.g., livestock).

Regulations are also in place for raising organically grown livestock. **Organically produced** feed must be used for a specified period of time toward the end of gestation; animals may be given vitamin and mineral supplements, but the use of growth hormones and antibiotics is prohibited; and animals treated with medication cannot be sold as organic.

The U.S. Department of Agriculture (USDA) ensures that the production, processing, and certification of **organically grown** foods adhere to strict national standards and that organic labeling meets criteria that define the four official organic categories (Fig. 9.4). Most consumers assume that produce sold at local farmers' markets is grown locally and is organic, but neither is necessarily true.

Organic food is usually more expensive because of higher production costs, greater losses, and smaller yields. For instance, a gallon of organic milk typically costs twice as much as a gallon of store brand or name brand milk. However, not all organic foods are appreciably more expensive than their conventional counterparts, such as oranges, grapes, and bread.

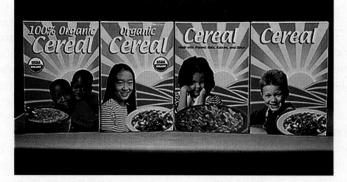

■ FIGURE 9.4   Sample cereal boxes showing four labeling categories for organic labeling. From left: cereal with 100% organic ingredients; cereal with 95% to 100% organic ingredients; cereal made with at least 70% organic ingredients; and cereal with less than 70% organic ingredients. (*Source:* U.S. Department of Agriculture website)

Are organically produced foods more nutritious or safer than their conventionally raised counterparts? A recent review of 17 human studies and 223 evaluations of nutrient and contamination levels in a wide range of foods revealed a lack of strong evidence in the literature that organic foods are significantly more nutritious than conventional foods. However, the review also found that eating organic foods may lower exposures to pesticide residues and antibiotic-resistant bacteria (Smith-Spangler et al., 2012). Among the findings are the following:

- The only nutrient higher in organic produce than conventional produce was phosphorus, a nutrient typically not lacking in American diets. Weak evidence suggests that organic produce may have higher levels of phenols, a class of phytochemicals, and that organic milk and chicken have more omega-3 fatty acids than their conventional counterparts.
- Eating organic produce in place of conventional produce may reduce pesticide exposure by 30%, but both types of produce generally have pesticide levels well below established tolerance levels set by the Environmental Protection Agency. What is not known is whether chronic ingestion of pesticides at low levels over years or decades is a health risk (Schardt, 2007).
- Organic and conventional produce and livestock were at equal risk of being contaminated; *Salmonella* and *Campylobacter* bacteria were common in both organic and conventional animal products. However, organic chicken and pork were less likely to be contaminated with antibiotic-resistant bacteria.

To help consumers reduce their exposure to pesticides, the Environmental Working Group (EWG) compiles an annual list of the "Dirty Dozen" and the "Clean 15," which identify fruits and vegetables with the most and least levels of pesticides, respectively (EWG, 2012) (Table 9.3). However, their methodology and interpretation of residue findings have been called into question in a recent study by Winter and Katz (2011). They found that that exposure to detected pesticides on the "Dirty Dozen" posed negligible risks to consumers and that replacing the "Dirty Dozen" with organically grown varieties did not result in any appreciable reduction of consumer risk. For instance, in 75% of the pesticide/ food combinations studied, they found consumer exposure estimates more than 1 million times *lower* than doses given to laboratory animals continuously over their lifetimes that do not show adverse effects (Winter, 2011). Despite the controversy regarding the risks of pesticide residues in food, both sides agree that the benefits of eating a diet rich in fruits and vegetables outweigh any potential risks of pesticide exposure (EWG, 2012).

Table 9.3 Dirty Dozen and the Clean 15

Ranking is based on the
▪ Percentage of samples with detectable pesticides ▪ Percentage of samples with two or more pesticides ▪ Average number of pesticides found on a sample ▪ Average concentration of all pesticides found ▪ Maximum number of pesticides found on a single sample ▪ Total number of pesticides found

The Dirty Dozen	Clean 15
1. Apples	1. Onions
2. Celery	2. Sweet corn
3. Sweet bell peppers	3. Pineapples
4. Peaches	4. Avocado
5. Strawberries	5. Cabbage
6. Nectarines (imported)	6. Sweet peas
7. Grapes	7. Asparagus
8. Spinach	8. Mangoes
9. Lettuce	9. Eggplant
10. Cucumbers	10. Kiwi
11. Blueberries (domestic)	11. Cantaloupe (domestic)
12. Potatoes	12. Sweet potatoes
Plus green beans and kale/greens	13. Grapefruit
because they may contain pesticide	14. Watermelon
residues of special concern	15. Mushrooms

Source: Environmental Working Group Food News. (2012). *EWG's 2010 shopper's guide to pesticides in produce.* Available at www.ewg.org/foodnews/summary/. Accessed on 10/17/12.

Whether produce is grown organically or conventionally, thoroughly rinsing all fruits and vegetables under running water and discarding the outer leaves, where appropriate, are vital to reduce exposure to natural dangers such as bacteria and man-made risks such as chemical residues.

FOOD SAFETY CONCERNS

Food safety concerns include preventing foodborne illnesses that can occur from improperly handled or stored food. Other current issues of food safety include biotechnology and irradiation.

Foodborne Illness

Foodborne Illness: an illness transmitted to humans via food.

The Centers for Disease Control and Prevention (CDC) estimates that every year, approximately 48 million Americans experience a **foodborne illness**, resulting in 128,000 hospitalizations and 3000 deaths (CDC, 2011). Eight known pathogens account for the vast majority of those estimates (Fig. 9.5, Table 9.4). Although more than half of foodborne illnesses are caused by viruses, the majority of deaths are attributed to bacteria (Scallan et al., 2011).

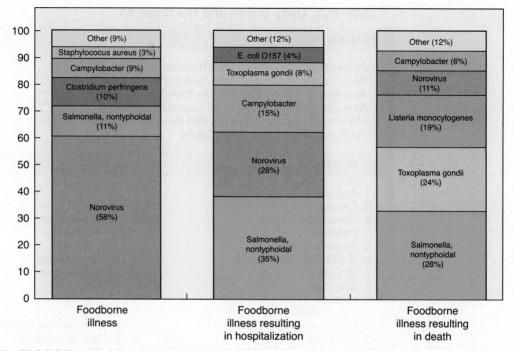

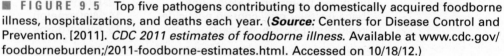

■ **FIGURE 9.5**   Top five pathogens contributing to domestically acquired foodborne illness, hospitalizations, and deaths each year. (**Source:** Centers for Disease Control and Prevention. [2011]. *CDC 2011 estimates of foodborne illness.* Available at www.cdc.gov/foodborneburden;/2011-foodborne-estimates.html. Accessed on 10/18/12.)

The microorganisms that cause foodborne illness are found widely in nature and are transmitted to people from within food (e.g., meat and fish), from on food (e.g., eggshell or vegetables), from unsafe water, or from human or animal feces. Foods most often associated with foodborne illness are the following:

- Raw or undercooked foods of animal origin, such as meat, poultry, eggs, shellfish, and unpasteurized milk
- Raw fruits and vegetables, which can be contaminated with animal feces in manure or water used to wash them
- Raw sprouts, which are grown under conditions that are ideal for promoting the growth of microbes
- Unpasteurized fruit juice
- Any uncooked food that was handled by someone who is ill

The most common symptoms of foodborne illness may be mistaken for the flu—diarrhea, nausea, vomiting, fever, abdominal pain, and headaches. Most cases are self-limiting and run their course within a few days. Symptoms that warrant medical attention include bloody diarrhea (possible *Escherichia coli* 0157:H7 infection), a stiff neck with severe headache and fever (possible meningitis related to *Listeria*), excessive diarrhea or vomiting (possible life-threatening dehydration), and any symptoms that persist for more than 3 days. Infants, pregnant women, the elderly, and people with compromised immune systems (e.g., people with AIDS or cancer, organ transplant recipients, people taking corticosteroids) are particularly vulnerable to the effects of foodborne illness.

The major cause of foodborne illnesses is unsanitary food handling. To reduce the risk of contamination, proper personal hygiene and handwashing must be practiced by all food handlers. Steps must be taken to prevent cross-contamination between raw and cooked

Table 9.4 Top Pathogens Contributing to Domestically Acquired Foodborne Illnesses, Hospitalizations, and Death in the United States

Pathogen	Type of Pathogen	Common Food Vehicles	Onset	Symptoms	Other
Norovirus (food poisoning; viral gastro-enteritis)	Virus	Fruits, vegetables, meat, and salads prepared or handled by infected person; oysters from contaminated water	24–48 hours	Explosive and projectile vomiting, watery diarrhea, cramps, headache, mild fever, muscle aches	Environmentally hardy; also transferred from person to person and from contact with surfaces. Very contagious. Severe illness is rare.
Salmonella species (salmonellosis)	Bacteria	Raw and undercooked eggs, poultry, meats, milk and dairy products; fresh produce, including raw sprouts (alfalfa, bean); shrimp; sauces; and salad dressings	6–72 hours	Nausea, vomiting, cramps, fever, diarrhea, headache. Arthritic symptoms may occur 3–4 weeks after onset of acute symptoms.	Can be fatal. Incidence is increasing in the United States.
Campylobacter jejuni (campylobacter enteritis)	Bacteria	Unpasteurized milk and cheeses made from it; undercooked poultry, raw beef, unchlorinated water	2–5 days	Gastroenteritis; diarrhea, fever, abdominal cramps, vomiting	Small percentage develops severe complications, such as bacteremia, meningitis, hepatitis, pancreatitis, and Guillain-Barré syndrome.
Clostridium perfringens (perfringens food poisoning)	Bacteria	Meat, poultry, stuffing, gravy, and cooked foods held or stored at inappropriate temperature	16 hours	Intense abdominal cramps, diarrhea, headache, the chills	The "cafeteria germ," associated with steam table foods not kept hot enough. Illness usually over within 24 hours
Escherichia coli (*E. coli* 0157-H7; hemorrhagic colitis, hemolytic-uremic syndrome)	Bacteria	Undercooked beef, especially ground beef; raw milk; unpasteurized fruit juice and cider; alfalfa and radish sprouts; plant foods fertilized with raw manure or irrigated with contaminated water	2–5 days	Severe abdominal cramps and diarrhea. Hemorrhagic colitis may lead to hemolytic-uremic syndrome (severe anemia and renal failure)	

(continues on page 220)

Table 9.4 Top Pathogens Contributing to Domestically Acquired Foodborne Illnesses, Hospitalizations, and Death in the United States (continued)

Pathogen	Type of Pathogen	Common Food Vehicles	Onset	Symptoms	Other
Listeria mono- cytogenes (listeriosis)	Bacteria	Raw milk, deli-type salads, processed meats, soft cheese, under- cooked poultry, ice cream, raw vegetables, raw and cooked poultry	2 days to 3 weeks; severe form may have in- cubation period of 3 days to 3 months	Healthy people may have no or mild symptoms. Sudden fever, headache, back- ache, occasional abdominal pain, and diarrhea Septicemia and meningitis may lead to death. One-third of con- firmed cases in pregnant women may end in spontaneous abortion or still- birth; infants born alive may have bacteremia and meningitis.	This bacterium thrives in cold temperatures and appears to be able to sur- vive short-term pasteurization. Mortality from lis- teric meningitis may be as high as 70%.
Staphylococcus aureus (staphylo- coccal food poisoning)	Bacteria	Meat and meat products; custard- or cream-filled baked goods, sandwich fillings; poultry and egg products; salad made of egg, tuna, chicken, potato, and macaroni	1–7 hours	Severe nausea, vomiting, diar- rhea, abdominal cramps	Of healthy people, 50% are carriers. Most frequently found in the nose, throat, on skin and hair, and in infected boils, pimples, cuts, and burns. Frequently transmit- ted to foods by human carriers
Toxoplasma gondii	Parasite	Raw or undercooked meats (e.g., pork, lamb, wild game), untreated water from rivers or ponds; contact with cat, rat, ro- dent, or bird feces (e.g., handling cats, cleaning cat litter box, gardening); shell- fish, raw or under- cooked clams and oysters	1–3 weeks	Swollen glands, fever, muscle aches CNS disorders, such as mental retardation and visual impair- ments, in children	Especially danger- ous to pregnant women; may cause stillbirth, miscarriage; can pass to fetus More than 60 mil- lion Americans may be infected with *T. gondii* but are asymp- tomatic because the immune sys- tem prevents ill- ness caused by the parasite.

Source: U.S. Food and Drug Administration. (2012). *The bad bug book. Foodborne pathogenic microorganisms and natural toxins hand- book* (2nd ed.). Available at http://www.fda.gov/downloads/Food/FoodSafety/FoodborneIllness/FoodborneIllnessFoodbornePathogensNatural Toxins/BadBugBook/UCM297627.pdf. Accessed on 10/23/12.

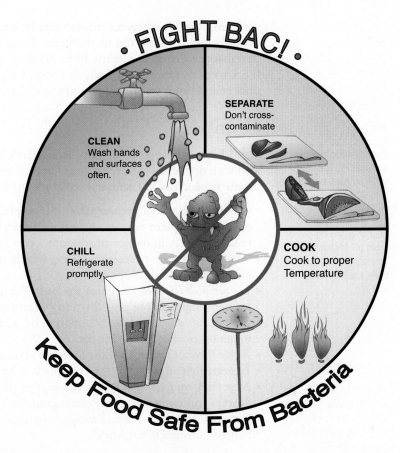

FIGURE 9.6   Fight BAC! infographic.
(**Source:** Partnership for Food Safety
Education)

foods and through food handlers. Because heat kills most bacteria, thorough cooking of meat and fish is vital, as is pasteurization of all milk products. Adequate refrigeration inhibits the growth of bacteria. Figure 9.6 depicts the four simple steps to keep food safe, promoted by the Fight BAC! (as in bacteria) campaign of the Partnership for Food Safety Education. See the Partnership for Food Safety Education website for additional food safety tips.

Mad Cow Disease (Bovine Spongiform Encephalopathy)

Mad cow disease is the common name for bovine spongiform encephalopathy (BSE), a slowly progressive, degenerative, fatal disease affecting the central nervous system of adult cattle. Although the exact cause is unknown, BSE is believed to be caused by prions, an infectious form of a type of protein. BSE was first reported in 1986 in the United Kingdom and is believed to have originated when scrapie-infected sheep meat and bone meal were fed to cattle (scrapie is the sheep version of BSE). Evidence suggests the disease proliferated when BSE-contaminated cattle protein was fed to calves. Unlike bacteria, prions are resistant to heat and so are not destroyed by cooking. Eating BSE-infected beef products is believed to cause a variant form of Creutzfeldt–Jakob disease (vCJD), which is the human version of BSE.

Measures to Prevent Mad Cow Disease

Although the FDA and other federal agencies have had regulatory measures in place since 1989 to prevent BSE from entering the U.S. food supply, the first case of BSE in the United States was identified in December 2003. Fortunately, the animal's organs infected with prions never entered the food supply, and the rest of the meat from that cow was successfully recalled from the marketplace. Since then, the USDA has enacted additional rules to enhance safeguards against BSE. To date, a total of four cases of BSE have occurred in the United States, none of which reached the food supply. Research is ongoing to better understand prion transmission and the diseases it causes.

Food Biotechnology

Food Biotechnology:
a process that involves taking a gene with a desirable trait from one plant and inserting it into another with the goal of changing one or more of its characteristics; also called genetically engineered food.

Food biotechnology combines plant science with genetics to improve food. Genes associated with desirable characteristics are moved from one plant to another—a quicker and more precise version of old-fashioned crossbreeding. The positive results are numerous and varied:

- *Healthier crops and greater yields.* Some plants are genetically modified to increase their resistance to plant viruses and other diseases; this means they can be raised using fewer pesticides to help reduce production costs and environmental residues.
- *Greater resistance to severe weather,* which reduces crop losses and increases year-round availability of fresh crops.
- *Longer shelf life and increased freshness.* Plants can be made to ripen more slowly, staying fresher longer—a big plus for transportation.
- *Higher nutritional value.* Plants can be genetically modified to contain more vitamins, minerals, or protein, or less fat.
- *Better flavor.* Genetic modification has produced sweeter melons and sweeter strawberries.
- *Improved characteristics.* An example is celery without strings.
- *New food varieties through crossbreeding.* Broccoflower (a blend of broccoli and cauliflower) and tangelos (a tangerine–grapefruit hybrid) are examples.
- *Potential to alleviate world hunger.* Stronger crops with enhanced nutritional value may benefit consumers worldwide.

In the United States, more than 165 million acres of biotech crops were planted in 2010 (Biotechnology Industry Organization, 2011). Eighty-six percent of all the corn and 93% of all soybeans in the United States are grown using biotechnology. Ingredients made from these top crops, such as soybean oil, corn oil, and corn syrup, are pervasive in processed foods available in U.S. grocery stores (from cereals and frozen pizza to hot dogs and soft drinks). Other leading biotech crops include cotton, soybeans, canola, squash, papaya, alfalfa, and sugar beet (Biotechnology Industry Organization, 2011). In addition to permeating the food supply, biotechnology has created new diagnostic tests, therapies, and vaccines, beginning with FDA approval of recombinant human insulin in 1982 (Biotechnology Industry Organization, 2011).

Numerous national and worldwide agencies, including the U.S. National Academies of Science, the World Health Organization, the American Medical Association, International Food Technologists, and the Academy of Nutrition and Dietetics, have taken the position that biotech products are as safe as similar crops that have undergone traditional or organic breeding. Still, opponents to biotechnology cite concern over the risk of allergic reactions based on the idea that a protein from a food identified as a major allergen (e.g., milk, soybeans, eggs) could be incorporated into a food that typically does not cause an allergic reaction, leaving susceptible consumers vulnerable to an allergic reaction. However, the FDA requires scientific evidence that genetically modified products do not contain protein from any of the high-allergy foods. Because the FDA asserts that genetically modified foods do not pose a health or safety risk, mandatory labeling is not required unless the food contains new allergens, has a modified nutritional profile, or represents a new plant. Despite the relative consensus among the scientific community that it is safe, biotechnology has not been used long enough to know whether long-term complications may develop. People who do not want to consume genetically engineered foods can avoid these products by using organically produced foods.

Food Irradiation

To many consumers, the term irradiated food conjures up visions of radioactive fallout. In truth, irradiation is a safe and effective technology that can prevent many foodborne illnesses by reducing or eliminating pathogens, controlling insects, or killing parasites. Irradiation also reduces food losses from infestation, contamination, and spoilage (University of Wisconsin Food Irradiation Education Group, 2012).

Irradiation does not use heat and thus is sometimes referred to as "cold pasteurization." Bacteria, mold, fungi, and insects are destroyed as the food is exposed to radiant energy, including gamma rays, electron beams, and x-rays. A small amount of new compounds are formed that are similar to the changes seen in food as it is cooked, pasteurized, frozen, or otherwise prepared. Except for a slight decrease in thiamin, the nutrient content is essentially unchanged. Because irradiation kills any living cells that may be contained in the food, such as in seeds or potatoes, shelf life may be prolonged. For instance, irradiated potatoes do not sprout during storage. However, irradiation does not hide spoilage or eliminate the need for safe food handling; irradiated food can still become contaminated through cross-contamination.

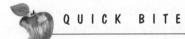

QUICK BITE

Foods allowed to be irradiated in the United States include

Wheat and wheat flour to control mold
White potatoes to inhibit sprouting
Pork to kill trichina parasites
Fresh produce to control insects
Iceberg lettuce and spinach to kill bacteria
Many spices and dry vegetable seasonings for sterilization
Fresh red meat and poultry to reduce bacterial pathogens

Irradiation is the most extensively studied food-processing technique available in the world and is used by 37 countries on more than 40 foods (USDA, Food Safety and Inspection Service, 2012). More than a half million tons of food are irradiated throughout the world every year (University of Wisconsin Food Irradiation Education Group, 2012). The FDA first approved the use of radiation in 1963 and is responsible for establishing the maximum radiation dose allowed on foods. Federal law requires irradiated food to be labeled with the international symbol, the radura (Fig. 9.7), and state "Treated with irradiation" or "Treated by irradiation." Research on irradiation as a part of an overall system of ensuring food safety is ongoing.

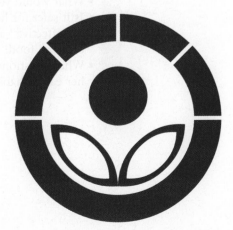

■ **FIGURE 9.7**   Radura: international symbol for irradiation.

HOW DO YOU RESPOND?

Does the word "sugars" on the Nutrition Facts label just indicate added sugar? Sugars on the label refer to both added and natural sugars, which is why plain milk lists 12 g of sugar—all of it is naturally occurring lactose.

Can you prevent foodborne illness by washing produce? While washing produce—even varieties that you peel—is recommended, it cannot guarantee food safety. For instance, it is difficult to remove sticky bacteria from leafy greens like spinach. Even "triple" washed or thoroughly washed ready-to-eat bags of spinach, lettuce, and mixed greens may be contaminated with bacteria, because the cleaning process using chlorinated water kills only 90% to 95% of microbes when performed correctly. And with other produce, such as melon, mango, or apple, if bacteria have migrated to the inside of the fruit, such as traveling through the apple core to the interior, washing will not remove it. Safe food handling at home is important but cannot guarantee safety.

CASE STUDY

Maria is 52 years old, has a normal body mass index (BMI), and does not have any health problems. She prides herself on being "into" holistic treatments and goes to the doctor only when her attempts to treat herself fail. She occasionally takes one aspirin a day because she has heard that it can prevent heart attacks. She tries to eat a healthy diet and uses supplements to give her added protection against chronic diseases, especially heart disease, which runs in her family. Currently, she takes ginkgo biloba to prevent memory loss, garlic to prevent heart disease, and fish oil supplements to keep her blood thin. She routinely drinks omega-3–fortified orange juice and organic milk. She attributes the bruises on her legs to being clumsy. She is thinking about adding vitamin E to her regimen because she heard it may also lower the risk of heart disease. To save money, she is thinking about discontinuing her use of garlic pills and fish oil supplements and instead eating more garlic and fish in her diet.

- What are the dangers of her present regimen? What may be responsible for the bruising she is experiencing?
- What would you tell Maria about the use of supplements in general? About the types and combination of supplements she is currently using? What specific changes would you suggest she make?
- What would you tell her about using omega-3–fortified milk and juice?
- Is it safer for her to eat more garlic and fish instead of taking them as supplements? Is it as "effective" as taking them as supplements? Could she "overdose" on garlic and fish oil from food?
- What questions would you ask about her diet to see if there are any improvements in her eating habits she could make to reduce the risk of heart disease?

STUDY QUESTIONS

1. Which statement indicates that the client needs further instruction about reading nutrition labels?
   a. "The %DV is the contribution of a serving of a food to a 2000-calorie diet."
   b. "The %DV represents the percentage of calories in that food from each nutrient."
   c. "The amount of sugar on the label includes both natural and added sugars."
   d. "The serving size listed on the label can vary among brands and varieties of the same food."

2. The client asks if a tea that claims to "improve memory" really works. Which of the following would be the nurse's best response?
   a. "If the tea claims to improve memory, it has been tested and proven effective at improving memory."
   b. "Claims on food labels are not regulated by law and cannot be trusted."
   c. "Function claims like 'improve memory' can be used on labels without supporting proof that they are accurate."
   d. "That type of claim is illegal and should not appear on any food label."

3. Which statement about supplements is accurate?
   a. "All supplements must be tested for safety and effectiveness before they can be marketed."
   b. "Supplement dosages are standardized."
   c. "Proper handling of supplement ingredients is required by law."
   d. "Warnings about potential side effects or interactions must be stated on the packaging."

4. Which supplement should be used with caution by people taking anticoagulants?
   a. Echinacea
   b. St. John's wort
   c. Cranberry
   d. Garlic

5. A client asks how she can minimize her risk of foodborne illness. Which of the following should the nurse include in the response as the best way to reduce the risk? Select all that apply.
   a. "Wash your hands before and after handling food."
   b. "Rely on organically grown foods as much as possible."
   c. "Cook foods thoroughly."
   d. "Avoid cross-contamination by using separate surfaces for meats and foods that will be eaten raw."

6. The best response to a client's question about whether organic food is worth the extra cost is
   a. "Is there anything more important to spend money on than your health?"
   b. "There is no difference in pesticide levels and nutritional value of organically grown foods compared to conventional foods."
   c. "Buying organic foods is an individual decision; some may have more nutritional value than their conventional counterparts, and they do have lower pesticide levels."
   d. "It is worth it to buy organic produce but not organic products."

7. Which of the following practices helps preserve the nutritional value of produce?
   a. Refrigerating vegetables in the crisper
   b. Adding baking soda to the water when steaming vegetables
   c. Cutting vegetables into small pieces before boiling to hasten the cooking time
   d. Thawing frozen vegetables prior to cooking

8. A client asks how she can avoid buying foods that are genetically engineered. The nurse's best response is
   a. "Foods labeled as 'organic' cannot be genetically engineered."
   b. "There is no way to avoid genetically engineered foods."
   c. "Buy foods that have the radura symbol on them; they cannot be genetically engineered."
   d. "Genetically engineered food must have that fact stated on the front label where consumers can clearly see it."

KEY CONCEPTS

- The field of nutrition is rapidly changing and growing. New challenges in nutrition stem from advances in food technology, the explosion of information available on the World Wide Web, and the concept of food as medicine.
- The majority of Americans surveyed believe that food and beverages can supply specific health benefits (IFIC Foundation, 2008). They also are interested in hearing about the role of nutrition in health but are often confused by food and health information.
- To judge the validity and reliability of nutrition "news," ask who, what, when, where, and why. Beware of claims that sound too good to be true, quick fixes, and recommendations that are intended to help sell a product.
- Nutrition misinformation is everywhere and can be difficult to refute in a client who is convinced that what he or she knows is accurate.
- The Nutrition Facts label is intended to provide consumers with reliable and useful information to help avoid nutritional excesses such as fat, saturated fat, cholesterol, and sodium.
- The %DV listed on food labels for fat, saturated fat, carbohydrate, and dietary fiber is based on a 2000-calorie diet. The %DV for these nutrients underestimates the contribution in diets containing fewer than 2000 calories.
- Ingredients are listed in order of descending weight.
- Unqualified health claims on food labels are based on significant scientific agreement and include statements such as "calcium may help prevent osteoporosis" and "low sodium may help prevent high blood pressure."
- Qualified health claims are supported by scientific evidence but do not meet the standard for significant scientific agreement. Examples of qualified health claims include the role of nuts in reducing cardiovascular disease risk and the role of green tea in reducing cancer risk.
- Structure/function claims, such as "improves mood," "relieves stress," and "for hot flashes," can be used without FDA approval and do not have to carry a disclaimer.
- A dietary supplement is a product (other than tobacco) intended to supplement the diet and that contains one or more of the following: vitamins, minerals, herbs or other botanicals, amino acids, or any combination of these ingredients.
- Dietary supplements are regulated by the FDA like food; proof of their safety and effectiveness is not required before marketing. When a dietary supplement is deemed to be unsafe by the FDA, consumer advisories are issued and the manufacturer is requested, not ordered, to stop selling the product. As such, harmful supplements may remain on the market.
- People choosing to use supplements should first check with the FDA for consumer advisories and consult with their physicians. Many supplements can render certain drugs ineffective or potentiate the effectiveness of drugs.

- Pregnant and lactating women and children under the age of 6 years should not use dietary supplements.
- To help retain their nutrient value, plants should be purchased fresh, stored properly, and cooked for a minimum amount of time in a minimum amount of water.
- Functional foods contain substances that appear to enhance health beyond their basic nutritional value. Incorporating more natural functional foods into the diet is prudent; the use of manufactured functional foods may pose risks.
- There is a lack of strong evidence in the literature that organically grown foods are nutritionally superior to their conventionally grown counterparts. Because of production costs, higher losses, and lower yields, they are generally more expensive than other foods. However, organic produce consistently has lower levels of pesticides, and organic meats are less likely to be contaminated with antibiotic-resistant bacteria.
- The majority of foodborne illnesses are caused by norovirus; the majority of foodborne illness–related deaths are attributed to bacteria. Other causes of foodborne illness are parasites, molds, and unknown causes.
- The foods most commonly causing foodborne illness are those that are eaten raw or undercooked, such as fresh fruits and vegetables, raw meat and shellfish, undercooked poultry and eggs, and unpasteurized milk and fruit juices. Improper food handling, such as inadequate cooking and poor personal hygiene, is the major cause of foodborne illness.
- Food biotechnology uses genetic modification to improve the characteristics of a food. Biotechnology has created plant foods that are more resistant to disease, stay fresher longer, have higher nutritional value, or are more resistant to severe weather. The FDA considers biotechnology safe.
- Irradiation is used to reduce or eliminate pathogens that can cause foodborne illness. The food remains uncooked and completely free of any radiation residues. Strict regulations and ongoing research protect consumers from potential risks regarding irradiation.

Check Your Knowledge Answer Key

1. **TRUE** Most Americans believe food and nutrition are important for good health but may be confused by nutrition and health messages.

2. **TRUE** The serving sizes used on the Nutrition Facts label are based on amounts typically eaten. However, they may not represent what an *individual* consumes.

3. **TRUE** The %DVs for fat, saturated fat, carbohydrate, and fiber listed on the Nutrition Facts label are based on a 2000-calorie diet. The values are not accurate percentages for anyone who eats more or less than 2000 cal/day. The %DV for other nutrients, such as cholesterol and sodium, are based on Daily Reference Values that are constant for all people over the age of 4 years regardless of total calorie intake.

4. **FALSE** Structure/function claims are not regulated by the FDA; their use does not require prior approval nor is a disclaimer necessary.

5. **FALSE** Supplement manufacturers do not have to prove safety or effectiveness before marketing a product, although they are not supposed to sell dangerous or ineffective products.

6. **FALSE** Warning labels about potential side effects or supplement–drug interactions are not required, nor is a statement regarding who should *not* use the product such as pregnant and lactating women, children under 6 years of age, or people with certain chronic illnesses.

7. **FALSE** While some organically grown foods may have higher nutritional profiles than their conventionally grown counterparts, it is not known whether the difference is significant in terms of overall intake. Likewise, organically grown produce does have fewer pesticides than conventionally grown fruits and vegetables, but the health implications are not clear.

8. **FALSE** Norovirus is responsible for an estimated 58% of all foodborne illnesses.

9. **FALSE** Genetically modified foods are not labeled as such unless the food contains new allergens, has a modified nutritional profile, or represents a new plant.

10. **FALSE** Irradiated food is completely free of radiation residues.

Student Resources on thePoint

For additional learning materials, activate the code in the front of this book at
http://thePoint.lww.com/activate

Websites

Reliable nutrition information

Academy of Nutrition and Dietetics at **www.eatright.org**
American Cancer Society at **www.cancer.org**
American Diabetes Association at **www.diabetes.org**
Cancer Net, National Cancer Institute, National Institutes of Health at **www.nci.nih.gov**
Case Western Reserve consumer health information at **www.netwellness.org**
Center for Science in the Public Interest at **www.cspinet.org**
Government site for nutrition at **www.nutrition.gov**
Health on the Net Foundation at **www.hon.ch**
International Food Information Council at **www.ific.org**
Mayo Clinic at **www.mayohealth.org**
National Council Against Health Fraud, Inc. at **www.ncahf.org**
National Heart, Lung, and Blood Institute, National Institutes of Health at **www.nhlbi.nih.gov**
Office of Disease Prevention and Health Promotion, U.S. Department of Health and Human Services at **www.odphp.osophs.dhhs.gov**
PubMed, National Library of Medicine at **www.ncbi.nlm.nih.gov/Pubmed/**
U.S. Department of Agriculture Food and Nutrition Information Center at **www.nal.usda.gov/fnic**
U.S. Department of Health and Human Services Healthfinder at **www.healthfinder.gov**
U.S. Food and Drug Administration Center for Food Safety and Applied Nutrition at **www.fda.gov/AboutFDA/CentersOffices/OfficeofFoods/CFSAN/default.htm**
World Health Organization at **www.who.int**

Supplement information

Office of Dietary Supplements (ODS) of the National Institutes of Health at **http://ods.od.nih.gov/**
The International Bibliographic Information on Dietary Supplements (IBIDS) NIH Office of Dietary Supplements at **http://ods.od.nih.gov/Health_Information/IBIDS.aspx**
The National Center for Complementary and Alternative Medicine Clearinghouse provides information on complementary and alternative medication at **www.nccam.nih.gov**
U.S. Food and Drug Administration Center for Food Safety and Applied Nutrition at **www.fda.gov/AboutFDA/CentersOffices/OfficeofFoods/CFSAN/default.htm**.
Check out "Tips for the Savvy Supplement User: Making Informed Decisions and Evaluating Information."
U.S. Pharmacopeia at **www.usp.org**

Food safety

International Food Information Council at **www.ific.org**
Partnership for Food Safety Education at **www.fightbac.org**
U.S. Food and Drug Administration at **www.fda.gov**

References

American Dietetic Association. (2009). Position of the American Dietetic Association: Functional foods. *Journal of the American Dietetic Association, 109*, 735–746.

Biotechnology Industry Organization. (2011). *Food crops derived from agricultural biotechnology. Frequently asked questions about food labeling and safety.* Available at www.bio.org/articles/food-crops-derived-agricultural-biotechnology. Accessed on 10/18/12.

Centers for Disease Control and Prevention. (2011). *CDC 2011 estimates of foodborne illness: Findings.* Available at www.cdc.gov/foodborneburden/2011-foodborne-estimates.html. Accessed on 10/18/12.

Dimitri, C., & Oberholtzer, L. (2009). *Marketing US organic foods. Recent trends from farms to consumers* (USDA, ERS, Economic Information Bulletin Number 28). Available at www.ers.usda.gov/publications/eib58_1_.pdf. Accessed on 10/19/12.

Environmental Working Group. (2012). *EWS's 2012 shopper's guide to pesticides in produce.* Available at www.ewg.org/foodnews/summary. Accessed on 10/17/12.

Gahche, J., Bailey, R., Burt, V., Hughes, J., Yetley, E., Dwyer, J., . . . Sempos, C. (2011). *Dietary supplement use among US adults has increased since NHANES III (1988–1994)* (NCHS Data Brief No. 61) Hyattsville, MD: National Center for Health Statistic.

Grocery Manufacturers Association. (2010). *Facts Up Front front-of-pack labeling initiative.* Available at www.gmaonline.org/issues-policy/health-nutrition/facts-up-front-front-of-pack-labeling-initiative. Accessed on 10/19/12.

Institute of Medicine. (2011). *Front-of-package nutrition rating systems and symbols. Promoting healthier choices.* Available at http://www.iom.edu/~/media/Files/Report%20Files/2011/Front-of-Package-Nutrition-Rating-Systems-and-Symbols-Promoting-Healthier-Choices/frontofpackagereportbrieffornap.pdf. Accessed on 10/16/12.

International Food Information Council Foundation. (2007). *2007 consumer attitudes toward functional foods/food for health.* Available at www.foodinsight.org/Content/6/IFICExecSumSINGLE_vF2.pdf. Accessed on 10/15/12.

International Food Information Council Foundation. (2008). *2008 food and health survey. Consumer attitudes toward food, nutrition and health. A trended survey.* Available at www.foodinsight.org/Content/6/IFICFdn2008FoodandHealthSurvey.pdf. Accessed on 10/16/12.

Nutrition Business Journal. (2011). *NBJ's supplement business report.* Available at http://newhope360.com/site-files/newhope360.com/files/uploads/2011/10/TOCEXECSUMM110930.supp%20report%20FINAL-2.pdf. Accessed on 10/19/12.

Organic Trade Association. (2011). *Industry statistics and projected growth.* Available at www.ota.com/organic/mt/business.html. Accessed on 10/16/12.

Scallan, E., Hoekstra, R., Angulo, F., Tauxe, R. V., Widdowson, M., Roy S. L., . . . Griffin, P. M. (2011). Foodborne illness acquired in the United States—Major pathogens. *Emerging Infectious Diseases.* Available at www.nc.cdc.gov/eid/article/17/1/p1-1101_article.htm. Accessed on 10/18/12.

Schardt, D. (2007). Organic food. Worth the price? *Nutrition Action Health Letter, 34*(1), 3–8.

Scott-Thomas, C. (2012). *FDA offers support in industry roll-out of Facts Up Front labeling.* Available at http://www.foodnavigator-usa.com/content/view/print/616127. Accessed on 10/16/12.

Smith-Spangler, C., Brandeau, M., Hunter, G., Bavinger, J. C., Pearson, M., Eschbach, P. J., . . . Bravata, D. M. (2012). Are organic foods safer or healthier than conventional alternatives? *Annals of Internal Medicine, 157*, 348–366.

Tarver, T. (2012). Is the pathway to health organic? *Food Technology, 66*, 27–33.

U.S. Department of Agriculture, Food Safety and Inspection Service. (2012). *Irradiation and food safety. Answers to frequently asked questions.* Available at www.fsis.usda.gov/Fact_Sheet?Irradiation_and_Food_Safety/index.asp. Accessed on 10/19/12.

University of Wisconsin Food Irradiation Education Group. (2012). *The facts about food irradiation.* Available at http://uw-food-irradiation.engr.wisc.edu/Facts.html. Accessed on 10/19/12.

Winter, C. (2011). *Expert perspective: Eat your fruits and veggies and don't fear the "dirty" rhetoric.* Available at http://www.foodinsight.org/Newsletter/Detail.aspx?topic=Expert_Perspective_Eat_Your_Fruits_and_Veggies_and_Don_t_Fear_the_Dirty_Rhetoric. Accessed on 10/19/12.

Winter, C., & Katz, J. (2011). Dietary exposure to pesticide residues from commodities alleged to contain the highest contamination levels. *Journal of Toxicology, 2011*, 589674.

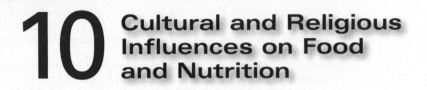

10 Cultural and Religious Influences on Food and Nutrition

LEARNING OBJECTIVES

Upon completion of this chapter, you will be able to

1 Debate the value of using convenience foods to prepare home-cooked meals.
2 Select the healthiest choices from a restaurant menu.
3 Give examples of how culture influences food choices.
4 Explain the general ways in which people's food choices change as they become acculturated to a new area.
5 Contrast American cultural values with those of traditional cultures.
6 Assess a person's dietary acculturation.
7 Summarize dietary laws followed by major world religions.

Culture: encompasses the total way of life of a particular population or community at a given time.

The nutritional requirements among people of similar age and gender are essentially the same throughout the world, yet an infinite variety of food and food combinations can satisfy those requirements. How a person chooses to satisfy nutritional requirements is influenced by many variables, including culture, socioeconomic status, personal factors, and religion.

This chapter discusses what America eats and the impact of **culture** on food choices. Traditional food practices of major cultural subgroups in the United States are presented, as are religious food practices.

AMERICAN CUISINE

Foodway: an all-encompassing term that refers to all aspects of food including what is edible, the role of certain foods in the diet, how food is prepared, the use of foods, the number and timing of daily meals, how food is eaten, and health beliefs related to food.

American cuisine is a rich and complex melting pot of foods and cooking methods that have been adapted and adopted from cuisines brought to the United States by immigrants. Early settlers from northern and southern Europe came with their own established **foodway** that changed in response to what was available in the New World. Native Americans made significant contributions to American cuisine by introducing items such as corn, squash, beans, cranberries, and maple syrup. Later, West African slaves brought okra, watermelon, black-eyed peas, and taro and influenced the regional cuisine in the southeastern United States with fried, boiled, and roasted dishes made with pork and pork fat. Likewise, American Southwest cuisine was shaped by flavors and ingredients brought across the border by Mexican Indians and Spanish settlers.

QUICK BITE

Examples of convenience items with a positive impact on nutrition

Fresh fruits and vegetables from the salad bar
Washed spinach
Prewashed and cut vegetables
Bagged salad mixes
Frozen vegetables
Fresh sushi
Whole-grain rolls from the bakery section
Prepared hummus
Fully cooked roasted chickens
Lean delicatessen meats

In the early 1850s, the first wave of Chinese immigrants came to the United States to join the gold rush. They brought stir-fry, a novel cooking method, and new foods such as egg rolls, fried rice, and spare ribs. The first wave of Italian immigrants arrived around 1880, and although they were unable to replicate their native foods, they utilized the available ingredients to create Americanized versions of lasagna, manicotti, veal parmigiana, and meatballs. Today, Italian food is mainstream American fare.

The influx of immigrants continued, and cuisines from around the globe melded. Today, it is difficult to determine which foods are truly American and which are an adaptation from other cultures. Swiss steak, Russian dressing, and chili con carne are American inventions. And although ethnic restaurants and ethnic foods sections in grocery stores offer distinct fare, cross-cultural food creations, such as Tex-Mex wontons and tofu lasagna, reaffirm the ongoing melting pot nature of American cuisine.

Although a "typical American diet" is difficult to define, Box 10.1 offers a snapshot view of what and how America eats. Driven by expediency and ease, convenience foods and restaurant-sourced meals (either eat in or takeout) are a driving force in current food trends.

Convenience Foods

Convenience Food: broadly defined as any product that saves time in food preparation, ranging from bagged fresh salad mixes to frozen packaged complete meals.

Convenience foods range from convenient ingredients used to make home-cooked meals to complete, heat-and-serve meals. According to an online Harris poll conducted in 2010, 75% of people who prepare meals at home either very often or occasionally use pre-prepared

Box 10.1   A SNAPSHOT VIEW OF WHAT AND HOW AMERICA EATS

- More than 80% eat at home more than three times a week.
- More than 45% take at least 30 minutes to make dinner.
- 53% eat a vegetarian dinner entrée at home once or twice a week.
- 48% name vegetables as a favorite side dish.
- 51% eat out at least once a week.
- The most frequently named favorite cuisine when eating out was American at 19%.
- 42% sometimes take calorie counts on the menu into account when ordering at a restaurant; 35% rarely or never do.

Source: *What America Eats 2012: A survey.* Available at http://www.epicurious.com/articlesguides/everydaycooking/family/whatamericaeats. Accessed on 10/24/12.

and/or frozen ingredients and kitchen appliances such as microwaves and toaster ovens to speed both cooking and clean up (Corso, 2010). Generally, the more convenient the meal is, the greater the impact all around on time, budget, and nutritional value. When time is short, frozen complete or nearly complete meals or boxed "helper" type entrées earn their designation as "convenient." They generally cost more than "from-scratch" items and lack that "homemade" taste but are less expensive than takeout and are easy and quick to prepare. And variety abounds, from typical American fare, such as meatloaf and pot roast, to vegetarian, Mexican, Chinese, Southwestern, and Italian cuisines. On the downside, these products tend to be high in sodium and relatively low in fiber and provide little to no fruit, vegetables, and whole grains. The 1- to 2-cup portion sizes listed on the label may leave many people hungry. With a little planning and effort, they can be part of a healthy diet. See Box 10.2 for tips on balancing convenience with nutrition.

Box 10.2   TIPS FOR BALANCING CONVENIENCE WITH NUTRITION

Read the label to comparison shop. Calories, fat, saturated fat, and sodium can vary greatly among different brands of similar items. A rule-of-thumb guideline is to limit sodium to less than 800 mg and fat to no more than 10 to 13 g in a meal that provides 300 to 400 calories.

Look for "healthy" on the label. The government allows "healthy" on the label of meals or entrées that limit sodium to 140 mg/100 g of food. And "healthy" foods must also provide 3 g or less of total fat or 1 g of saturated fat per 100 g of food. They are a better choice than the products not labeled "healthy" yet may still lack adequate fiber.

Add additional ingredients to "stretch" the meal. For instance, adding a bag of frozen vegetables, a can of tomatoes, or a can of garbanzo or black beans provides nutrients and increases volume.

Add healthy side dishes. A convenience "meal" that provides 300 to 400 calories may leave many people hungry. Adding quick and easy side dishes, such as bagged salad mixes, raw vegetables, whole-grain rolls, an instant cup of soup, or piece of fresh fruit, can greatly increase nutritional and satiety values.

Adjust the seasoning when possible. Some frozen meal solutions contain a separate seasoning packet; using half satisfies taste while cutting sodium.

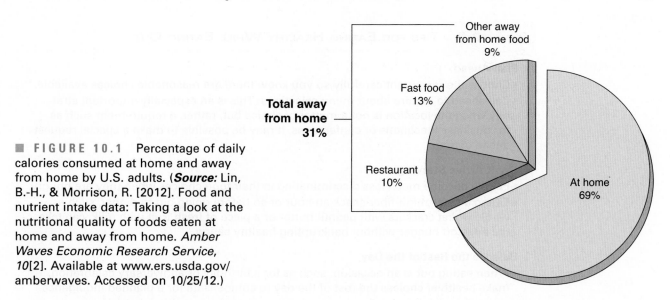

■ **FIGURE 10.1**   Percentage of daily calories consumed at home and away from home by U.S. adults. (**Source:** Lin, B.-H., & Morrison, R. [2012]. Food and nutrient intake data: Taking a look at the nutritional quality of foods eaten at home and away from home. *Amber Waves Economic Research Service, 10*[2]. Available at www.ers.usda.gov/amberwaves. Accessed on 10/25/12.)

Restaurant-Sourced Meals

According to a recent online poll by Mandala Research, the average American eats 4.8 restaurant meals per week, which includes both dining in and carrying out (LivingSocial, 2011). On average, Americans spend 42% of their food budget on food away from home (FAFH) (Todd, Mancino, and Lin, 2010). Fast food contributes the greatest percentage of calories of FAFH (Fig. 10.1).

Although eating out may be easy and quick, diet quality generally suffers. A study by Todd et al. (2010) found that for the average adult, eating one meal of FAFH increases daily calorie intake by 134 calories. In addition, FAFH decreases the number of servings of fruit, vegetables, whole grains, and dairy per 1000 calories consumed; moreover, fiber, calcium, and iron intakes decline. Conversely, FAFH increases sodium per 1000 calories and the percentage of calories from saturated fat, solid fat, alcohol, and added sugar. Because eating out has evolved from a special treat to a regular event, planning and menu savvy are needed to ensure that eating out is consistent with, not contradictory to, eating healthy. Tips for eating healthy while eating out appear in Box 10.3. "Best bet" choices from various ethnic restaurants are listed in Box 10.4.

THE IMPACT OF CULTURE

QUICK BITE

Culture

- Has an inherent value system that defines what is "normal"
- Is learned, not instinctive
- Is passed from generation to generation
- Has an unconscious influence on its members
- Resists change but is not static

Culture has a profound and unconscious effect on food choices. Yet, within all cultures, individuals or groups of individuals may behave differently from the socially standardized foodway because of age, gender, state of health, household structure, or socioeconomic status. Race, ethnicity, and geographic region are often inaccurately assumed to be synonymous

Box 10.3 TIPS FOR EATING HEALTHY WHILE EATING OUT

Plan Ahead
- Choose the restaurant carefully so you know there are reasonable choices available.
- Call ahead to inquire about menu selections. This is an especially important strategy when the location is not a matter of choice but, rather, a requirement such as for business luncheons or conferences. It may be possible to make a special request ahead of time.

Don't Arrive Starving
- People become much less discriminating in their food choices when they are hungry.
- Eating a small, high-fiber snack an hour or so before going out to dinner, such as whole wheat crackers with peanut butter or a piece of fresh fruit with milk, can take the edge off hunger without bankrupting healthy eating.

Balance the Rest of the Day
- When eating out *is* an occasion, such as for a birthday or anniversary celebration, make healthier choices the rest of the day to compensate for a planned indulgence.

Practice Portion Control
- Order the smallest size meat available.
- Create a doggie bag *before eating*; if you wait until the end of the meal, there may not be any left.
- Order regular size, not biggie size or super size.
- Order a la carte. Is a value meal a "better value" if it undermines your attempt to eat healthily?
- Order a half portion, when available.
- Order two (carefully chosen) appetizers in place of an entrée, or order an appetizer and split an entrée with a companion.

Know the Terminology
"Fatty" words to watch out for include

- Buttered
- Battered
- Breaded
- Deep fried
- Au gratin
- Creamy
- Crispy

- Alfredo
- Bisque
- Hollandaise
- Parmigiana
- Béarnaise
- En croute

- Escalloped
- French fried
- Pan fried
- Rich
- Sautéed
- With gravy, with mayonnaise, with cheese

Less fatty terms are: baked, braised, broiled, cooked in its own juice, grilled, lightly sautéed, poached, roasted, steamed.

Beware of Hidden Fats, Such as
- High-fat meats
- Nuts
- Cream and full-fat milk
- Full-fat salad dressings and mayonnaise

Make Special Requests
- Order sauces and gravies "on the side" to control portions.
- Ask that lower fat items be substituted for high-fat items (e.g., a baked potato instead of French fries).
- Request an alternate cooking method (e.g., broiled instead of fried).

Box 10.4	Best Bet Choices from Fast-Food and Ethnic Restaurants

Fast Foods
English muffins or bagels with spreads on the side
Butter, margarine, or syrups on the side—not added to food
Baked potato—plain or with reduced-fat or fat-free dressings or salsa
Pretzels or baked chips
Regular, small, or junior sizes
Ketchup, mustard, relish, BBQ sauce, and fresh vegetables as toppings
Grilled chicken sandwiches without "special sauce"
Veggie burger
Small roast beef on roll
Fruit 'n yogurt parfait
Lean, 6-in subs on whole-grain rolls
Side salads with reduced-fat or fat-free dressings
Salads with grilled chicken
Low-fat or nonfat milk
Fresh fruit
Specialty coffees with skim milk

Salad Bars
Dark, leafy greens
Plain raw vegetables
Chickpeas, kidney beans, peas
Low-fat cottage cheese
Hard-cooked egg
Fresh fruit
Lean ham, turkey
Reduced-fat or fat-free dressings

Pizza
Thin crust
Vegetables: onions, spinach, tomatoes, broccoli, mushrooms, peppers
Lean meats: Canadian bacon, ham, grilled chicken, shrimp, crab meat
Half-cheese pizza
Salad as a side dish

Buffet
Survey the buffet before beginning.
Use a small plate.
Pile food no thicker than a deck of cards.
Practice the "plate method": one-quarter meat, three-quarters plants.

Mexican
Sauces: salsa, mole, picante, enchilada, pico de gallo
Guacamole and sour cream on the side
Black bean soup, gazpacho
Soft, nonfried tortillas as in bean burritos or enchiladas
Refried beans (without lard)
Arroz con pollo (chicken with rice)
Grilled meat, fish, or chicken
Steamed vegetables
Soft-shell chicken or veggie tacos

(continues on page 236)

Box 10.4   BEST BET CHOICES FROM FAST-FOOD AND ETHNIC RESTAURANTS (continued)

A la carte or half entrée
Fajitas: chicken, seafood, vegetable, beef
Flan (usually a small portion)

Chinese
Hot-and-sour soup, wonton soup
Chicken chow mein
Chicken or beef chop suey
Szechuan dishes
Shrimp with garlic sauce
Stir-fried and teriyaki dishes
Noodles: lo mein, chow fun, Singapore noodles
Steamed rice instead of fried
Steamed spring rolls
Tofu
Steamed dumplings and other dim sum instead of egg rolls
Fortune cookies
Use chopsticks
No MSG

Italian
Minestrone
Garden salad; vinegar and oil dressing
Breadsticks, bruschetta, Italian bread
Sauces: red clam, marinara, wine, cacciatore, fra diavolo, marsala
Shrimp, veal, chicken without breading
Choose vegetables for a side dish instead of pasta or potatoes.
Limit "unlimited" bread or breadsticks.
Italian ice or fruit

Indian
Raw vegetable salads, Mulligatawny soup (lentil soup)
Tandoori meats
Condiments: fruits and vegetable chutneys, raita (cucumber and yogurt sauce)
Lentil and chickpea curries
Chicken and vegetables
Chicken rice pilaf
Basmati rice
Naan (bread baked in tandoori oven)
Dal

Japanese
Boiled green soybeans, miso soup, bean soups
Sushi—cooked varieties include imitation crab, cooked shrimp, scrambled egg
Most combinations of grilled meats or seafood
Teriyaki chicken or seafood
Steamed rice, rice noodles
Green tea

Box 10.4	BEST BET CHOICES FROM FAST-FOOD AND ETHNIC RESTAURANTS (continued)

Greek
Lentil soup
Greek salad, tabouli
Chicken, lamb, pork souvlaki salad or sandwich
Shish kebabs
Pita bread

Make a meal of appetizers: baba ghanoush (smoked eggplant), hummus (mashed chickpeas), dolma (stuffed grape leaves), and tabouli (cracked wheat salad). Olive oil is often poured on the baba ghanoush, hummus, and other foods, so ask for it on the side.

with culture. This misconception leads to stereotypic grouping, such as assuming that all Jews adhere to orthodox food laws or that all Southerners eat sausage, biscuits, and gravy. **Subgroups** within a culture display a unique range of cultural characteristics that affect food intake and nutritional status. What is edible, the role of food, how food is prepared, the symbolic use of food, and when and how food is eaten are among the many characteristics defined by culture.

Subgroups: a unique cultural group that coexists within a dominant culture.

Culture Defines What Is Edible

Edible: foods that are part of an individual's diet.

Inedible: foods that are usually poisonous or taboo.

Culture determines what is **edible** and what is **inedible**. To be labeled a food, an item must be readily available, safe, and nutritious enough to support reproduction. However, cultures do not define as edible all sources of nutrients that meet those criteria. For instance, in the United States, horsemeat, insects, and dog meat are not considered food, even though they meet the food criteria. Culture overrides flavor in determining what is offensive or unacceptable. For example, you may like a food (e.g., rattlesnake) until you know what it is; this reflects disliking the *idea* of the food rather than the actual food itself. An unconscious food selection decision process appears in Figure 10.2.

The Role of Certain Foods in the Diet

Every culture has a ranking for its foods that is influenced by cost and availability. Major food categories include core foods, secondary foods, and peripheral, or occasional, foods.

Core Foods

Core Foods: the important and consistently eaten foods that form the foundation of the diet; they are the dietary staples.

Core foods provide a significant source of calories and are regularly included in the diet, usually on a daily basis. Core foods are typically complex carbohydrates, such as cereal grains (rice, wheat, millet, corn), starchy tubers (potatoes, yams, taro, cassava), and starchy vegetables (plantain or green bananas). In much of the world, high-fat, energy-dense diets have replaced traditional diets high in complex carbohydrates (Caprio et al., 2008).

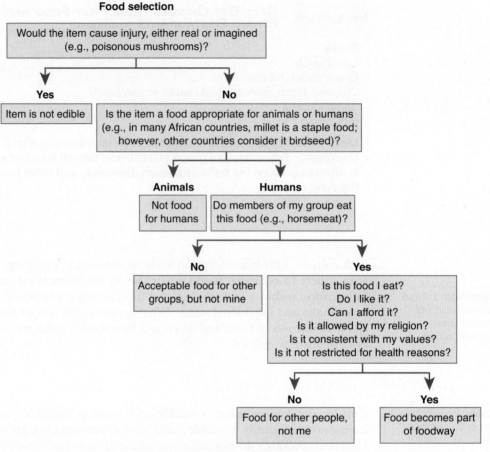

FIGURE 10.2 Food selection decision making.

Secondary Foods

Secondary Foods: foods that are widespread in the diet but not eaten consistently.

Foods widely consumed, but not on a daily basis, are considered **secondary foods**, such as vegetables, legumes, nuts, fish, eggs, and meats. Secondary foods used by a culture vary with availability. For instance, the types of legumes used in Chinese culture include mung beans and soybeans, whereas those used in Latin American culture include black beans and pinto beans.

Peripheral Foods

Peripheral, or Occasional, Foods: foods that are infrequently consumed.

Peripheral, or occasional, foods, eaten sporadically, are typically based on an individual's preferences, not cultural norms. They may be foods that are reserved for special occasions, not readily available, or not generally well tolerated, as is the case with milk among Asian Americans.

How Food Is Prepared

Traditional methods of preparation vary between and within cultural groups. For instance, vegetables often are stir-fried in Asian cultures but boiled in Hispanic cultures. Traditional seasonings also vary among cultures and may be the distinguishing feature between one

Table 10.1 Examples of Seasonings Used by Various Cultures

Cultural Group	Distinguishing Flavors
Asian Indian	Garam masala (curry blend of coriander, cumin, fenugreek, turmeric, black pepper, cayenne, cloves, cardamom, and chili peppers), mint, saffron, mustard, fennel, cinnamon
Brazilian (Bahia)	Chili peppers, dried shrimp, ginger root, palm oil
Chinese	Soy sauce, rice wine, ginger root
French	Butter, cream, wine, bouquet garni (tarragon, thyme, bay leaf)
German	Sour cream, vinegar, dill, mustard, black pepper
Greek	Lemon, onions, garlic, oregano, olive oil
Italian	Tomato, garlic, basil, oregano, olive oil
Japanese	Soy sauce, sugar, rice wine vinegar
Korean	Soy sauce, garlic, ginger root, black pepper, scallions, chili peppers, sesame seeds or oil
Mexican	Tomatoes, onions, chili peppers, cumin
Puerto Rican	Sofrito (seasoning sauce of tomatoes, onions, garlic, bell peppers, cilantro, capers, pimento, annatto seeds, and lard)
Thai	Fermented fish sauce, coconut milk, chili peppers, garlic, ginger root, lemon grass, tamarind

Source: Kittler, P., Sucher, K., & Nahikian-Nelms, M. (2012). *Food and culture* (6th ed.). Belmont, CA: Wadsworth Cengage Learning.

culture's foods and another's (Table 10.1). The choice of seasonings varies among geographic regions and between seasons, based on availability. With home-prepared meals, seasonings are adjusted to suit the family's preferences.

Symbolic Use of Foods

Each culture has food customs and bestows symbolism on certain foods. Custom determines what foods are served as meals versus snacks and what foods are considered feminine versus masculine. Symbolically, food can be used to express love, to reward or punish, to display piety, to express moral sentiments, to demonstrate belongingness to a group, or to proclaim the separateness of a group. On a personal level, food may be used inappropriately to relieve anxiety, reduce stress, ease loneliness, or to substitute for sex. Culture also determines which foods are used in celebration and which provide comfort. People who move to other cultures may retain their own cultural comfort foods as a link with the past.

When and How Food Is Eaten

All cultures eat at least once a day. Some may eat five or more meals each day. Dinner may start at 6 p.m. in Australia or 7 to 9 p.m. in Kenya. A Lebanese custom is to arrive anytime when invited for dinner, even as early as 9 or 10 a.m. Food may be eaten with chopsticks, a knife and fork, or fingers. In the United States, bad manners in eating may be associated with animal behavior, as in "He eats like a pig," "She chews like a cow," or "Don't wolf down your food."

Cultural Values

Cultural values define desirable and undesirable personal and public behavior and social interaction. Understanding the client's cultural values and their impact on health and food choices facilitates cross-cultural nutrition care. Table 10.2 highlights the contrast between selected American cultural values and values of more traditional cultures.

Health Beliefs

Each culture has a unique point of view on life, health, and illness, and the meaning of each in society (Kittler, Sucher, and Nahikian-Nelms, 2012). Almost all cultures define certain foods that promote wellness, cure disease, or impart medicinal properties. For instance, hot oregano tea seasoned with salt is used to treat an upset stomach in Vietnamese culture. Some cultures define foods that create equilibrium within the body and soul (Kittler et al., 2012).

Culture also shapes body image. In the United States, "you can never be too thin," and thinness, particularly in women, is equated with beauty and status. Overweight and obesity may be viewed as a character flaw. Conversely, thinness has historically been a risk factor for poor health or associated with poverty. In many cultures today, including those of some

Table 10.2 A Contrast of Cultural Values

American Values	Traditional Values	Potential Considerations of Traditional Values
Personal control	Fate	
Individuals believe they have personal control over their future.	Individuals may accept what happens to them as out of their control.	Clients may not consider themselves active participants in their own healing but rather recipients.
Individualism	Group welfare	
Interests of the individual have preference over the interests of the group.	The group is valued over the individual; decisions may be made by the group, not the individual.	Involve family in planning. Emphasize the good of the entire family rather than individual benefits.
Time dominates	Human interaction dominates	
"Being on time" and "not wasting time" are virtues.	Personal interaction is more important than time management.	Expediency and efficiency may be counter-productive. Pause while talking. Avoid interruptions.
Informality	Formality	
Informality is viewed as a sign of friendliness.	Informality may be equated with disrespect.	Use a formal tone, especially with older people.
Directness	Indirectness	
Honest, open communication is considered effective communication.	Straightforwardness may be rude or too personal.	It may be appropriate to avoid eye contact. Talking in the third person, such as "someone who wants to eat less sodium may choose fresh vegetables over canned" is valued over "you should. . . ." Asking questions may be considered disrespectful; ask questions judiciously.

Africans, Mexicans, American Indians, and Caribbean Islanders, being overweight is a sign of health, beauty, and prosperity (Kittler et al., 2012). To some people, "healthy eating" is synonymous with eating large quantities of food rather than making more nutritious food choices.

Dietary Acculturation

Dietary Acculturation: the process that occurs as members of a minority group adopt the eating patterns and food choices of the host country.

Acculturation: the process that occurs as people who move to a different cultural area adopt the beliefs, values, attitudes, and behaviors of the dominant culture; not limited to immigrants but affects anyone (to varying degrees) who moves from one community to another.

Dietary acculturation occurs when eating patterns of immigrants change to resemble those of the host country. In the United States, **acculturation** is linked to increased risk of chronic disease and obesity; however, its effect on diet quality is inconsistent (Sofianou, Fung, and Tucker, 2011). For instance, a study by Batis, Hernandez-Barrera, Barquera, Rivera, and Popkin (2011) found that dietary acculturation in Mexican Americans leads to positive changes, such as higher intakes of low-fat meat and fish, high-fiber bread, and low-fat milk, but also to negative effects, such as higher intakes of saturated fat, sugar, dessert, salty snacks, pizza, and French fries. Likewise, studies show that acculturation in Asian Americans causes an increase in the intake of grains, dairy products, fruits, and vegetables but also of fat and sweets (Lv and Carson, 2004; Satia et al., 2001). Clearly, acculturation is a highly complex, dynamic, multidimensional process that is impacted by a variety of personal, cultural, and environmental factors (Satia, 2009). Associations of acculturation with diet are often inconsistent and do not fit an expected pattern (Satia, 2009).

Generally, food habits are one of the last behaviors people change through acculturation, possibly because eating is done in the privacy of the home, not in full view of the majority culture. Usually, first-generation Americans adhere more closely to cultural food patterns and have at least one native meal daily (Brown, 2005). They may cling to traditional foods to affirm their cultural identity. Second-generation Americans do not have the direct native connection and may follow cultural patterns only on holidays and at family gatherings, or they may give up ethnic foods but retain traditional methods of preparation. Children tend to adopt new ways quickly as they learn from other children at school. Points to keep in mind regarding dietary acculturation appear in Box 10.5.

Box 10.5   POINTS TO CONSIDER REGARDING DIETARY ACCULTURATION

- Generally with acculturation, the intake of sweets and fats increases, neither of which has a positive effect on health.
- Because dietary acculturation is most likely to change food choices for breakfast and lunch rather than dinner, focus on promoting healthy "American" food choices for those meals.
- Portion control is a better option than advising someone to eliminate an important native food from their diet. Lower fat or lower sodium options, when available, may also be an acceptable option for the client. While giving up soy sauce may not be an option for a Chinese American, using a reduced-sodium version may be doable.
- It is essential to determine how often a food is consumed in order to determine the potential impact of that food. For instance, lard is unimportant in the context of the total diet if it is used in cooking only on special occasions.
- Don't assume the client knows what American foods are considered healthy.
- Suggest fruits and vegetables that are similar in texture to those that are familiar but unavailable to the client.

Interrelated changes in food choices that occur as part of acculturation are as follows:

- *New foods are added to the diet.* Status, economics, information, taste, and exposure are some of the reasons why new foods are added to the diet. Eating "American" food may symbolize status and make people feel more connected to their new culture. Frequently, new foods are added because they are relatively inexpensive and widely available.
- *Some traditional foods are replaced by new foods.* This often occurs because traditional foods may be difficult to find, are too expensive, or have lengthy preparation times. For many ethnic groups who move to the United States, breakfast and lunch are most likely to be composed of convenient American foods, whereas traditional foods are retained for the major dinner meal, which has greater emotional significance.
- *Some traditional foods are rejected.* To become more like their peers, children and adolescents are more likely than older adults to reject traditional foods. Traditional foods may also be rejected because of an increased awareness of the role of nutrition in the development of chronic diseases. For instance, one reason why Indians who have resided in the United States for a relatively long period tend to eat significantly less ghee (clarified butter served with rice or spread on Indian breads) may be that they are trying to decrease their intake of saturated fat.

Understanding Acculturation

It is important to understand acculturation so that interventions to promote healthy food choices can be tailored to be culturally and individually appropriate. Ideally, clients will retain healthy traditional food practices, adopt healthy new food behaviors, and avoid forming less healthy American dietary habits. While first-generation citizens usually need help choosing American replacements for their native foods, second-generation citizens may need help selecting healthy American foods.

To be effective in encouraging clients to make healthier food choices, health-care professionals must possess specific knowledge about food habits, preferences, and practices among the cultural and ethnic groups they see in their practice (Goody and Drago, 2009). Questions that may aid in the understanding of food habits include the following:

- What traditional foods do you eat daily?
- What are your favorite foods?
- What foods do you eat on holidays or special occasions?
- What traditional foods do you no longer eat?
- What new foods do you eat? Remember that new immigrants may not know the name of American foods.
- What prompted you to eat these new foods?
- Do you regularly eat new foods?
- What foods do you eat to keep you healthy?
- What natural herbs or home remedies do you use?
- What foods do you avoid to prevent illness?
- Do you balance some foods with other foods?
- Are there foods you will not eat? Is it because of personal preference, cultural norms, or religious mandate?
- Do you have enough food to eat each day?
- For hospitalized clients: Are there any special customs or religious practices you want performed before or after a meal?

Suggestions for conducting effective cross-cultural nutrition counseling are listed in Box 10.6.

Box 10.6	SUGGESTIONS FOR CONDUCTING EFFECTIVE CROSS-CULTURAL NUTRITION COUNSELING

- Establish rapport; respect cultural differences.
- Be knowledgeable about cultural food habits and health beliefs.
- Be attuned to cultural and individual variations.
- Use culturally appropriate verbal and nonverbal communication.
- Determine the primary written and spoken language used in the client's home.
- Use trained interpreters when necessary.
- Determine whether the client prefers direct or indirect communication.
- Pare down information to only what the client needs to know.
- Emphasize the positive food practices of traditional health beliefs and food customs.
- Provide written material only after determining reading ability.
- Communicate consistent messages.

TRADITIONAL DIETS OF SELECTED CULTURAL SUBGROUPS IN THE UNITED STATES

The U.S. Census Bureau (2008) projects that by the year 2050, about 54% of the U.S. population will consist of minority groups. The nutritional implication of this shift in cultural predominance is that cultural competence will become increasingly important to nursing care. Nutrition information that is technically correct but culturally inappropriate does not produce behavior change. Cultural competence facilitates nutrition care consistent with the individual's attitudes, beliefs, and values.

The U.S. Office of Management and Budget established seven sociopolitical categories, which include five racial categories (Whites, African Americans, Asian Americans, Native Americans, and Native Hawaiians and other Pacific Islanders) and two ethnic categories (Hispanic or Latino and Not Hispanic or Latino) (Office of Management and Budget, 1997). Each of these categories has multiple, diverse subgroups. For instance, the category of Native Americans comprises more than 575 federally recognized tribes and more than 300 other tribes, each with their own language and culture (Kagawa-Singer, Dadia, Yu, and Surbone, 2010). In addition, multiracial individuals represent a growing population.

Three major cultural subgroups in the United States are highlighted in the following sections. Their leading causes of death appear in Table 10.3. Although generalizations can be made about traditional eating practices and dietary changes related to acculturation, actual food choices vary greatly within a subgroup on the basis of national, regional, ethnic, and individual differences.

African Americans

The majority of African Americans can trace their ancestors to West Africa, although some have immigrated from the Caribbean, Central America, and East African countries. Because most are many generations away from their original homeland, much of their native heritage has been assimilated, lost, or modified.

Traditional Food Practices

"Soul food" describes traditional southern African American foods and cooking techniques that evolved from West African, slave, and postabolition cuisine. Many soul food customs

Table 10.3 Leading Causes of Death of Selected Groups in the United States

Cause of Death Rank	African Americans	Hispanic or Latino Americans	Asian Americans	White Americans
1	Heart disease	Cancer	Cancer	Heart disease
2	Cancer	Heart disease	Heart disease	Cancer
3	Stroke	Unintentional injuries	Stroke	Chronic lower respiratory disease
4	Unintentional injuries	Stroke	Unintentional injuries	Stroke
5	Diabetes	Diabetes	Diabetes	Unintentional injuries
6	Nephritis, nephrotic syndrome, and nephrosis	Chronic liver disease and cirrhosis	Influenza and pneumonia	Alzheimer disease
7	Chronic lower respiratory disease	Chronic lower respiratory diseases	Chronic lower respiratory disease	Diabetes
8	Homicide	Influenza and pneumonia	Suicide	Influenza and pneumonia
9	Septicemia	Homicide	Nephritis, nephrotic syndrome, and nephrosis	Nephritis, nephrotic syndrome, and nephrosis
10	HIV/AIDS	Nephritis, nephrotic syndrome, and nephrosis	Alzheimer disease	Suicide

Source: Centers for Disease Control and Prevention, Office of Minority Health and Health Disparities. Available at www.cdc.gov/omhd/populations/definitions.htm. Accessed on 10/29/12.

and practices are shared by white Americans in the southern United States, particularly those of lower socioeconomic status or living in rural areas (Kulkarni, 2004).

Traditional soul foods tend to be high in fat, cholesterol, and sodium and low in protective nutrients, such as potassium (fruits and vegetables), fiber (whole grains and vegetables), and calcium (milk, cheese, and yogurt). Corn and corn products (grits and cornmeal) are the primary grain. Meats are often breaded and fried. A variety of beef and pork cuts are consumed, as are poultry, oxtail, tripe, and tongue. Table 10.4 highlights traditional soul foods and the impact of acculturation on food choices.

Although soul food has become a symbol of African American identity and African heritage, today African Americans' food habits usually reflect their current socioeconomic status, geographic location, and work schedule more than their African or southern heritage (Kittler et al., 2012). Soul food may be reserved for special occasions and holidays.

Health Beliefs

The health beliefs and practices of some African Americans are a blend of traditional African concepts as well as those encountered through early contact with both Native Americans and Whites (Kittler et al., 2012). Some African Americans believe that ill health is due to bad luck or fate. Home remedies and natural therapies may be frequently used.

Table 10.4 Traditional Soul Foods and the Effects of Acculturation

Food Group	Foods Commonly Consumed	Effects of Acculturation
Grains	Rice, grits, cornbread, biscuits, muffins, dry and cooked cereals, macaroni	Substitution of commercially made bread for homemade biscuits
Vegetables	Green leafy vegetables (collard, mustard, turnip, and dandelion greens), kale, spinach, and pokeweed are collectively known as "greens" Corn, sweet and white potatoes	Vegetable intake remains low and is based on availability; greens remain popular.
Fruit	Apples, bananas, berries, peaches, and watermelon, eaten based on availability	Fruit intake remains low and is based on availability.
Milk	Whole milk (commonly referred to as "sweet milk") and buttermilk	Greater consumption of milk, at least among blacks living in urban areas
Meat and Beans	A variety of beef, pork, poultry, and fish; oxtail, tripe, tongue Dried beans (pinto, navy, lima, butter, kidney); fresh or dried peas (black-eyed, field, green, crowder, butter); beans with pork; succotash (corn with lima beans)	Packaged and luncheon meats are popular; intake of fatty meats, such as sausage and bacon, is high.
Fats	Butter, lard, bacon, fatback, salt pork, meat drippings, vegetable shortening	
Beverages	Coffee, fruit drinks, fruit wine, soft drinks, tea	

Source: Kittler, P., Sucher, K., & Nahikian-Nelms, M. (2012). *Food and culture* (6th ed.). Belmont, CA: Wadsworth Cengage Learning.

Nutrition-Related Health Problems

African Americans score just slightly below the national population average on the Healthy Eating Index (HEI), a tool developed by the U.S. Department of Agriculture (USDA) Center for Nutrition Policy and Promotion that measures dietary factors, such as the intake of total fat, saturated fat, cholesterol, and sodium as well as dietary variety (Ervin, 2011). In a study among patients with one or more chronic diseases, Blacks were 92% more likely than Whites to have low diet quality (Chen, Cheskin, Shi, and Wang, 2011). In general, African Americans

- Are less likely than Whites to meet the USDA guidelines and have the lowest fruit and vegetable intake among U.S. racial/ethnic groups (Casagrande, Wang, Anerson, and Gary, 2007) (Fig. 10.3). They also have higher intakes of fat and cholesterol compared to Whites (Chen et al., 2011). Fat intake is related to a high meat intake, the popularity of frying, and high intake of fast foods.
- Have a high prevalence of obesity. According to 2009–2010 data, the prevalence of obesity (body mass index [BMI] ≥30) among adult Black American men is 38.8%; among Black women, the prevalence is 58.5% (Centers for Disease Control and Prevention, 2012). Studies have shown that, in general, African Americans accept or are comfortable with larger body sizes (Boyington et al., 2008) and may also feel less guilty about overeating (Satia, 2009).
- Have double the rate of death from heart disease and stroke compared with Whites (OMH, 2012a). African Americans are 60% more likely to have a cerebrovascular accident than their White counterparts (OMH, 2012a).

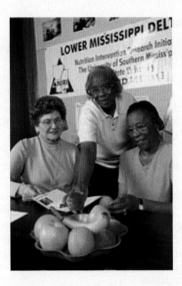

■ **FIGURE 10.3** In general, African Americans should increase their intake of fruits and vegetables (USDA).

- Have a significantly higher prevalence of hypertension (42%) than Whites (29.1%) (Fryar, Hirsch, Eberhardt, Yoon, and Wright, 2010). African Americans are also more likely to develop complications related to hypertension, such as heart disease, stroke, and end-stage renal disease.
- Have a higher prevalence of diabetes (14.5%) than Whites (8.3%) (Fryar et al., 2010).
- Have an infant mortality rate that is 2.3 times higher than Whites (OMH, 2012a).

Mexican Americans

The OMH describes Hispanics or Latinos as people of Cuban, Mexican, Puerto Rican, South or Central American, or other Spanish culture or origin regardless of race (OMH, 2012c). They are a diverse group differing in native language, customs, history, and foodways. According to 2011 U.S. Census Bureau population estimates, approximately 52 million Hispanics are living in the Unites States, which represents 16.7% of the American population (OMH, 2012c). Mexicans are the largest subgroup at 63% of the Hispanic American population.

Traditional Food Practices

The traditional Mexican diet, influenced by Spanish and Native American cultures, is generally a low-fat, high-fiber diet rich in complex carbohydrates and vegetable proteins, with an emphasis on corn, corn products, beans, and rice. Tortillas are a staple and may be consumed at every meal. Pork, goat, and poultry are the most used animal proteins; they are usually served ground or chopped as part of a mixed dish. Vegetables are also rarely served separately; they are incorporated into soups, rice, pasta, and tortilla-based dishes. Milk is not widely used, and lactose intolerance is common. Table 10.5 highlights traditional Mexican food practices and the impact of acculturation.

Health Beliefs

Traditional health beliefs are a blend of European folk medicine introduced from Spain and Native American rituals. Health is viewed as a gift from God, and illness is caused by outside forces unless it is punishment from God for sin (Kittler et al., 2012). Illness is inevitable and to be endured. Certain foods may be considered "cold" or "hot" for healing purposes. Prayer is appropriate for all illnesses, and lighting of candles on behalf of a sick person is common (Kittler et al., 2012).

Table 10.5 Traditional Mexican Foods and the Effects of Acculturation

Food Group	Foods Commonly Consumed	Effects of Acculturation
Grains	Corn, rice	Rice eaten as part of a mixed dish with vegetables decreases; intake of plain rice increases. Flour tortillas are used more often than corn tortillas. Intake of white bread and sweetened cereals increases.
Vegetables	Cactus, calabaza criolla (green pumpkin), chili peppers, corn, jicama, lettuce, onions, peas, plantains, potatoes, squash, tomatillos, tomatoes, yams, yucca	Intake of most vegetables decreases.
Fruit	Avocados, bananas, carambola, cherimoya, coconut, passion fruit, guava, lemons, limes, mangoes, melon, oranges, papaya, pineapple, strawberries	Intake of bananas, apples, oranges, orange juice, and cantaloupe remains relatively constant.
Milk	Goat and cow's milk (whole is preferred), evaporated milk, café con leche, hot chocolate, cheese	Milk intake increases related to its use with a new food, such as ready-to-eat breakfast cereal; whole milk is replaced with low-fat or nonfat milk.
Meat and beans	Beef, goat, pork, chicken, turkey, shrimp, eggs Legumes: black beans, chickpeas, kidney beans, pinto beans	Red meat intake increases. Legume intake falls. Intake of traditional meat and vegetable preparations declines drastically.
Fats	Butter, lard, Mexican cream	Butter, margarine, and salad dressing intake increases related to introduction of cooked vegetables and salads.
Beverages	Fruit-based beverage	Severe decline in fruit-based beverage consumption; increased use of highly sweetened drinks (e.g., Kool-Aid, soft drinks) and caffeinated beverages Alcohol intake increases.

Source: Kittler, P., Sucher, K., & Nahikian-Nelms, M. (2012). *Food and culture* (6th ed.). Belmont, CA: Wadsworth Cengage Learning.

Nutrition-Related Health Problems

Mexican Americans have the highest HEI scores of all ethnic groups, especially regarding fruit and vegetable intake (Ervin, 2011). However, acculturation generally *decreases* the quality of the diet. Studies on Mexico-born Americans show that the intake of fiber, fruit, legumes, and vegetables decreases with duration of residence in the United States, whereas consumption of processed foods, refined carbohydrates, and added sugars increases (Sofianou et al., 2011). Acculturation also changes food consumption behaviors, such as increases in eating out, eating at fast-food outlets, and eating salty snacks, which contribute to higher fat and sodium intakes (Ayala, Baquero, and Klinger, 2008). In general, Hispanic/Mexican Americans have

- A high prevalence of overweight and obesity. Based on statistics for 2007–2010, the prevalence of obesity is 36.3% among Mexican males and 44.6% among Mexican females, with obesity defined as a BMI of 30 or higher (OMH, 2012c). For overweight (BMI ≥25), the prevalence is 81.3% among Mexican males and 78.0% among Mexican females (OMH, 2012c). Compared to Whites, the concept of ideal weight may be higher for Mexican Americans.
- A higher prevalence of type 2 diabetes (15.3% among Mexican Americans) than either African Americans (14.6%) or Whites (8.3%) (Fryar et al., 2010). In 2008, Hispanics

were 1.5 times more likely than Whites to die from diabetes and 1.6 times more likely to be treated for end-stage renal disease related to diabetes (OMH, 2012c).

- A lower risk of dying from a stroke and lower rates of hypertension and hypercholesterolemia than Whites (OMH, 2012c). Although heart disease is the leading cause of death, Hispanics are less likely to have coronary heart disease and are less likely to die from heart disease than Whites. Hispanics also generally have lower rates of cancer.

Chinese Americans

The term "Asian Americans" encompasses a diverse population originating from at least 37 different ethnic groups; Pacific Islander includes about 25 nationalities (Kagawa-Singer et al., 2010). Chinese, alone or in any combination, is the largest Asian American subgroup in the United States (Hoeffel, Rastogi, Kim, and Shahid, 2012). Two dietary commonalities exist between these diverse cultures: (1) emphasis on rice and vegetables with relatively little meat and (2) cooking techniques that include meticulous attention to preparing ingredients before cooking. Chinese food practices and health and nutrition status are described in the following section.

Traditional Food Practices

Traditional Chinese foods and the effect of acculturation are highlighted in Table 10.6. Grains are the foundation of the traditional diet—predominately rice in southern China and wheat, in the form of noodles, dumplings, pancakes, and steamed bread, in northern China. A variety of vegetables are used extensively; other foods commonly consumed include sea vegetables, nuts, seeds, beans, soy foods, vegetable and nut oils, herbs and spices, tea, wine, and beer. A variety of animal proteins are consumed; the use of fish and seafood depends on availability. Most Chinese food is cooked; the exception is fresh fruit, which is eaten infrequently. Few dairy products are consumed because lactose intolerance is common. Calcium is provided by

Table 10.6 Traditional Chinese Foods and the Effects of Acculturation

Food Group	Foods Commonly Consumed	Effects of Acculturation
Grains	Rice, wheat, buckwheat, corn, millet, sorghum	Rice remains a staple, but the intake of wheat bread and cereals increases.
Vegetables	Amaranth, asparagus, bamboo shoots, bean sprouts, bitter melon, cassava, cauliflower, celery, bok choy, Napa cabbage, chili peppers, Chinese broccoli, Chinese long beans, eggplant, flat beans, garlic, lily root, dried and fresh mushrooms, okra, onions, seaweed, spinach, taro	Raw vegetable and salad intake increases. Traditional vegetables are replaced by more commonly available ones.
Fruit	Apples, bananas, coconut, dates, figs, kumquats, lime, litchi, mango, oranges, passion fruit, pineapple, pomegranates, tangerines, watermelon	Intake of temperate fruits increases (e.g., apples, grapes, pears, peaches).
Milk	Cow's milk, buffalo milk	Milk, ice cream, and cheese intake increases.
Meat and beans	Almost all sources of protein are eaten.	Intake of meat and ethnic dishes increases.
Fats	Butter, lard, corn oil, peanut oil, sesame oil, soybean oil, suet	Fat intake increases as fast-food intake increases.
Beverages	Tea (southern China), soup (northern China), wine, beer	

Source: Kittler, P., Sucher, K., & Nahikian-Nelms, M. (2012). *Food and culture* (6th ed.). Belmont, CA: Wadsworth Cengage Learning.

tofu, small fish (bones are eaten), and soups made with bones that have been partially dissolved by vinegar in making stock. Sodium intake is generally assumed to be high because of traditional food preservation methods (salting and drying) and condiments (e.g., soy sauce).

Health Beliefs

Asian cultures believe that health and illness are related to the balance between yin and yang forces in the body. Yin represents female, cold, and darkness; yang represents male, hot, and light. Digested foods turn into air that is either yin or yang. Diseases caused by yin forces are treated with yang foods, and diseases caused by yang forces are treated with yin foods. Pregnancy is considered a yang or "hot" condition, so women following traditional practices during pregnancy eat yin foods such as most fruits and vegetables, seaweed, cold drinks, juices, and rice water. Yang foods include chicken, meat, pig's feet, meat broth, nuts, fried food, coffee, and spices. The hot–cold theory of foods and illness also exists in Puerto Rico and Mexico, but the food designations are not universal within or across cultures.

Nutrition-Related Health Problems

The traditional Chinese diet is low in fat and dairy products and high in complex carbohydrates and sodium (Kittler et al., 2012). With Americanization, the diet becomes higher in fat, protein, sugar, and cholesterol. In general,

- Asian American women have the highest life expectancy of all ethnic groups in the United States (OMH, 2012b). Life expectancy varies among Asian subgroups: Filipino women, 81.5 years; Japanese women, 84.5 years; and Chinese women, 86.1 years.
- The prevalence of obesity is low at 11.6% for Asians age 18 years and older (OMH, 2012b). However, Filipino adults are 70% more likely to be obese compared to the overall Asian population.
- Asians Americans have the same rate of diabetes as Whites (OMH, 2012b).
- The leading cause of death among Asian Americans is cancer. Asian/Pacific Islander men are 40% less likely to have prostate cancer than White men, but they are twice as likely to have stomach cancer. Asian/Pacific Islander women are 20% less likely to have breast cancer than White women but are almost three times as likely to have stomach cancer (OMH, 2012b).

FOOD AND RELIGION

Kosher: a word commonly used to identify Jewish dietary laws that define "clean" foods, "unclean" foods, how food animals must be slaughtered, how foods must be prepared, and when foods may be consumed (e.g., the timing between eating milk products and meat products).

Religion tends to have a greater impact on food habits than nationality or culture does (e.g., Orthodox Jews follow **kosher** dietary laws regardless of their national origin). However, religious food practices vary significantly even among denominations of the same faith. National variations also exist. How closely an individual follows dietary laws is based on his or her degree of orthodoxy. An overview of religious food practices follows. Table 10.7 outlines major features of various religious dietary laws.

Christianity

The three primary branches of Christianity are Roman Catholicism, Eastern Orthodox Christianity, and Protestantism. Dietary practices vary from none to explicit.

- Roman Catholics do not eat meat on Ash Wednesday or on Fridays of Lent. Food and beverages are avoided for 1 hour before communion is taken. Devout Catholics observe several fast days during the year.
- Eastern Orthodox Christians observe numerous feast and fast days throughout the year.

Table 10.7 **Summary of Dietary Laws of Selected Religions**

	Orthodox Judaism	Islam	Hinduism	Buddhism
Meat	Cannot be eaten with dairy products		Beef is prohibited	Avoided by the most devout
Pork and pork products	Prohibited	Prohibited	Avoided by the most devout	Avoided by the most devout
Lacto-ovo vegetarianism			Encouraged	Practiced by many
Seafood	Only fish with fins and scales are allowed		Restricted	Avoided by the most devout
Alcohol		Prohibited	Avoided by the most devout	
Coffee/tea		Strongly discouraged		
Ritual slaughter of animals	Yes	Yes		
Moderation		Practiced		Practiced
Partial or total fasting	Practiced	Practiced	Practiced	Practiced

Sources: ElGindy, G. (2005). *Cultural competence. Understanding Buddhist patient's dietary needs.* Available at MinorityNurse.com. Accessed on 11/1/12; ElGindy, G. (2005). *Cultural competence. Hindu dietary practices: Feeding the body, mind and soul.* Available at MinorityNurse.com. Accessed on 11/1/12; and ElGindy, G. (2005). *Cultural competence. Meeting Jewish and Muslim patients' dietary needs.* Available at MinorityNurse.com. Accessed on 11/1/12.

The only denominations in the Protestant faith with dietary laws are the Mormons (Church of Jesus Christ of Latter-Day Saints) and Seventh-Day Adventists.

- Mormons do not use coffee, tea, alcohol, or tobacco. Followers are encouraged to limit meats and consume mostly grains. Some Mormons fast 1 day a month.
- Most Seventh-Day Adventists are lacto-ovo vegetarians; those who do eat meat avoid pork. Overeating is avoided, and coffee, tea, and alcohol are prohibited. An interval of 5 to 6 hours between meals is recommended with no snacking between meals. Water is consumed before and after meals. Strong seasonings, such as pepper and mustard, are avoided.

Judaism

In the United States, there are three main Jewish denominations: Orthodox, Conservative, and Reform. Hasidic Jews are a sect within the Orthodox. These groups differ in their interpretation of the precepts of Judaism. Orthodox Jews believe that the laws are the direct commandments of God, so they adhere strictly to dietary laws. Reform Jews follow the moral law but may selectively follow other laws; for instance, they may not follow any religious dietary laws. Conservative Jews fall between the other two groups in their beliefs and adherence to the laws. They may follow the Jewish dietary laws at home but take a more liberal attitude on social occasions. Because Jews have diverse backgrounds and nationalities, their food practices vary widely.

Because dietary laws are rigid, Orthodox Jews rarely eat outside the home except at homes or restaurants with kosher kitchens. Milk and dairy products are used widely but cannot be consumed at the same meal with meat or poultry. Dairy products are not allowed within 1 to 6 hours after eating meat or poultry, depending on the individual's ethnic

Pareve: dairy-free.

tradition. Meat and poultry cannot be eaten for 30 minutes after dairy products have been consumed. Margarine labeled **pareve**, nondairy creamers, and oils may be used with meats. Fruits, vegetables, plain grains, pastas, plain legumes, and eggs are considered kosher and can be eaten with either dairy or meat products.

Food preparation is prohibited on the Sabbath. Religious holidays are celebrated with certain foods. For example, only unleavened bread is eaten during Passover, and a 24-hour fast is observed on Yom Kippur.

Islam

Halal: Islamic dietary laws.

Haram: foods that are prohibited.

Muslims eat as a matter of faith and for good health. Basic guidance concerning food laws is revealed in the Quran (the divine book) from Allah (the Creator) to Muhammad (the Prophet). For Muslims, health and food are considered acts of worship for which Allah must be thanked (ElGindy, 2005b). There are 11 generally accepted rules pertaining to **halal** (permitted) and **haram** (prohibited) foods. Islam also stresses certain hygienic practices, such as washing hands before and after eating and frequent teeth cleaning.

Hinduism

Ahimsa: nonviolence as applicable to foods.

A love of nature and desire to live a simple natural life are the basis of Hinduism (ElGindy, 2005a). A number of health beliefs and dietary practices stem from the idea of living in harmony with nature and having mercy and respect for all of God's creations. Generally, Hindus avoid all foods that are believed to inhibit physical and spiritual development. Eating meat is not explicitly prohibited, but many Hindus are vegetarian because they adhere to the concept of **ahimsa**.

Another influential concept is that of purity. Some foods, such as dairy products (e.g., milk, yogurt, ghee [clarified butter]), are considered to enhance spiritual purity. When prepared together, pure foods can improve the purity of unpure foods. Some foods, such as beef or alcohol, are innately polluted and can never be made pure.

Jainism, a branch of Hinduism, also promotes the nonviolent doctrine of ahimsa. Devout Jains are complete vegetarians and may avoid blood-colored foods (e.g., tomatoes) and root vegetables (because harvesting them may cause the death of insects).

Buddhism

The Buddhist code of morality is set forth in the Five Moral Precepts, which are to not (1) kill or harm living things; (2) steal; (3) engage in sexual misconduct; (4) lie; and (5) consume intoxicants, such as alcohol, tobacco, or mind-altering drugs. Believing that thoughtful food decisions can contribute to spiritual enlightenment, a Buddhist asks himself these questions (ElGindy, 2005c):

- What food is this? This question evaluates the origin of the food and how it reached the individual.
- Where does it come from? This question considers the amount of work necessary to grow the food, prepare it, cook it, and bring it to the table.
- Why am I eating it? This question reflects on whether the individual deserves or is worthy of the food.
- When should I eat and benefit from this food? This question is based on the idea that food is a necessity and a healing agent and people are subjected to illness without food.
- How should I eat it? This question considers the premise that food is only received and eaten for the purpose of realizing the proper way to reach enlightenment.

In the Buddhist faith, life revolves around nature with its two opposing energy systems of yin and yang (ElGindy, 2005c). Examples of these opposing energy systems are heat/cold, light/darkness, good/evil, and sickness/health. Illnesses may result from an imbalance of yin and yang. Most Buddhists subscribe to the concept of ahimsa (not killing or harming), so many are lacto-ovo vegetarians. Some eat fish; some avoid only beef. Buddhist dietary practices vary widely depending on the sect and country. Buddhist monks avoid eating solid food after the noon hour.

How Do You Respond?

Is all fast food bad? No, not all fast foods are "bad." "Bad" is a relative term that depends on how often and how much. But even when "healthy" selections are made, such as a grilled chicken sandwich or a plain baked potato, fast-food meals tend to be low in fiber, fruit, vegetables, and milk/dairy products. While an occasional fast-food meal will not jeopardize someone's nutritional status, a steady diet of it can be detrimental for what it provides (too much fat, calories, and sodium) and for what it lacks.

Case Study

Elizabet moved to the Midwest at the age of 26 years from her native country, Iceland, where she ate seafood almost every evening for dinner. She ate fruit and vegetables daily, but the variety was limited. In her new home, she complains that good seafood is hard to find—that it is not as fresh as it is at home, it tastes different, and it is more expensive. She also misses the dark brown and black breads she is accustomed to; she is willing to try American breads but is unsure what variety is "good." American fast food is well known to her, but she does not want to rely on that to satisfy her need for familiar foods. She wants to eat foods that are healthy, tasty, and affordable.

- What questions would you ask Elizabet before coming up with suggestions about foods she could try?
- What would you say to her about her frustration with the seafood available locally? What suggestions would you make to her?
- What would you tell her about healthy breads? What fruits would you recommend as healthy, tasty, and affordable? What vegetables?

STUDY QUESTIONS

1. Which of the following items would be the healthiest choice from a Mexican restaurant?
    a. Cheese quesadillas
    b. Arroz con pollo
    c. Taco salad
    d. Guacamole with taco chips

2. A descriptive word that indicates a low-fat cooking technique is
    a. Au gratin
    b. Breaded
    c. Roasted
    d. Battered

3. A first-generation Chinese American has been advised to consume less sodium. What native food would the nurse ask about to get an idea of how much sodium he consumes?
   a. Soybeans
   b. Soy sauce
   c. Wonton
   d. Bok choy

4. A negative impact of acculturation on Mexican American food choices is often a decrease in fiber intake related to a decrease in the intake of (select all that apply)
   a. Legumes
   b. Whole-grain cereals
   c. Whole wheat bread
   d. Vegetables
   e. Fruit

5. What are the nutritional characteristics of a traditional soul food diet? Select all that apply.
   a. High in fat
   b. High in sodium
   c. High in fiber
   d. High in cholesterol
   e. Low in calcium

6. Which of the following is a healthy traditional food practice of Chinese Americans that should be encouraged?
   a. None; an American diet is healthier
   b. High intake of milk and dairy products
   c. Frequent use of fresh fruit
   d. Extensive use of vegetables in mixed dishes

7. When developing a teaching plan for an overweight woman from Mexico, which approach would be best?
   a. Tell the client she will feel better if she loses some of the extra weight she is carrying around.
   b. Encourage more "nutritious" food choices.
   c. Advise the client that "healthy eating" will help her shed inches.
   d. Provide a low-calorie diet and encourage her to eat low-calorie American foods, such as artificially sweetened soda and low-fat ice cream.

8. Muslims are prohibited from consuming
   a. Alcohol
   b. Eggs
   c. Beef
   d. Shellfish

KEY CONCEPTS

- American cuisine has evolved from a melting pot of food, flavors, and cooking techniques contributed by immigrants over the course of U.S. history. It continues to undergo change.
- Convenience foods range from pre-prepared ingredients to use to make a home-cooked meal (e.g., fresh cut vegetables and bagged salad) to complete, heat-and-serve meals. Convenience "meals" tend to be high in sodium and low in fiber, fruit, vegetables, and whole grains. Portion sizes are smaller than most people normally consume.
- The average American eats out approximately five times a week. Fast-food restaurants are the most popular choice for food away from home. Fast-food "value" meals are high in calories, fat, and sodium, in part because the portion sizes are large.

■ Suggestions to help control portion sizes while eating out include ordering two appetizers as a meal, splitting an entrée with a companion, ordering a "child"-sized meal, or creating a doggie bag before beginning to eat.

■ Culture defines what is edible; how food is handled, prepared, and consumed; what foods are appropriate for particular groups within the culture; the meaning of food and eating; attitudes toward body size; and the relationship between food and health. Yet, food habits vary considerably among individuals and families within a cultural group based on personal factors, socioeconomic factors, and religious factors.

■ Core foods are an indispensable part of the diet and consist of grains or starchy vegetables. Secondary foods are nutrient rich and add variety and ethnic identity to meals. Occasional or peripheral foods are used infrequently.

■ Cultural values identify behavior that is desirable and define how people should interact within society. American values are often very different from values of other cultures. Understanding a client's cultural values facilitates communication.

■ Culture defines body image and desirable weight. In the United States, thinness is valued, particularly for women. In some other cultures, thinness is equated with poverty; heavier weight is considered desirable and a sign of prosperity.

■ Dietary acculturation occurs as people who move to a new area change their food habits to some degree. New foods are added to their diet or substituted for traditional foods, and some traditional foods are rejected. Availability and cost influence food choices.

■ Acculturation can have a negative or positive effect on nutrition and health. Generally, as immigrants adopt the "typical American diet," their intake of fat, sugar, and calories goes up, and their intake of fiber, fruits, vegetables, and vegetable protein goes down. New Americans should be encouraged to retain the healthy eating practices of their native diet.

■ Generalizations can be made about traditional eating practices of subcultures within the United States. However, an individual's food choices deviate from these based on personal preferences, socioeconomic status, and degree of acculturation.

■ Traditional soul food is high in fat, cholesterol, and sodium and low in fiber, fruit, vegetables, and calcium. Socioeconomic factors, geographic area, and work schedules have a greater impact on the intake of African Americans than does the traditional soul food diet.

■ African Americans have a higher prevalence of overweight/obesity, hypertension, and type 2 diabetes than Whites. Morbidity and mortality for mothers and infants are also higher. The leading cause of death for African Americans is heart disease.

■ Mexican Americans have a higher prevalence of overweight/obesity and type 2 diabetes than Whites. Compared to Whites, they are less likely to die from a stroke and have lower rates of hypertension. The leading cause of death is heart disease.

■ Asian women have the longest life expectancy of all ethnic groups in the United States. The prevalence of overweight/obesity among Asian Americans is lower than in Whites. Cancer is the leading cause of death.

■ Religion tends to have a greater impact on food habits than nationality or culture. People are more likely to eat ethnic food from a different culture than they are to eat food that is prohibited by the mandates of their religion.

Check Your Knowledge Answer Key

1. **TRUE** Religion tends to have a greater impact on food choices than culture does.

2. **FALSE** Race, ethnicity, and geographic region are often inaccurately assumed to be synonymous with culture. This misconception leads to stereotyping.

3. **TRUE** Core foods tend to be complex carbohydrates, such as cereal grains, starchy tubers, and starchy vegetables. These core foods are the indispensable foundation of the diet and provide significant calories.

4. **TRUE** Both Hinduism and Buddhism promote vegetarianism.

5. **FALSE** The hot–cold theory of health and diet refers to Asian cultures' belief that health and illness are related to the balance between yin and yang forces in the body. Yin represents female, cold, and darkness; yang represents male, hot, and light.

6. **TRUE** Usually, first-generation Americans adhere more closely to cultural food patterns to preserve their ethnic identity compared with subsequent generations.

7. **TRUE** For many ethnic groups who move to the United States, breakfast and lunch are most likely to be composed of convenient American foods, while traditional foods are retained for the major dinner meal, which has greater emotional significance.

8. **TRUE** Eating food prepared away from home tends to increase a person's intake of calories, sodium, added sugar, and saturated and solid fat.

9. **FALSE** Dietary acculturation can lead to positive or negative changes in food choices. For instance, Mexican Americans dramatically reduce their intake of lard and Mexican cream through the process of acculturation, which is a positive change. However, substituting sweetened drinks (e.g., Kool-Aid and soft drinks) for the traditional beverage made from fruit has a negative impact on nutritional intake.

10. **FALSE** Although restaurant portions tend to be much larger than the standard serving size, the same is not true for convenience foods. The portion sizes listed on the label of convenience meals tend to be much smaller than what Americans typically consume in a meal.

Student Resources on thePoint

For additional learning materials, activate the code in the front of this book at
http://thePoint.lww.com/activate

Websites

Cultural/Ethnic Food Guide Pyramids, USDA National Agricultural Library at **http://fnic.nal
.usda.gov/dietary-guidance/myplatefood-pyramid-resources/ethniccultural-food-pyramids**
Ethnic medicine information including nutrition information: Harborview Medical Center,
University of Washington at **www.ethnomed.org**
Office of Minority Health at **http://minorityhealth.hhs.gov/**
Oldways Preservation & Exchange Trust at **www.oldwayspt.org**
Website for information on fast food and eating out: Center for Science in the Public Interest at
www.cspinet.org

References

Ayala, G., Baquero, B., & Klinger, S. (2008). A systemic review of the relationship between acculturation and diet among Latinos in the United States: Implications for future research. *Journal of the American Dietetic Association, 108,* 1330–1344.

Batis, C., Hernandez-Barrera, L., Barquera, S. Rivera, J. A., & Popkin, B. M. (2011). Food acculturation drives dietary differences among Mexicans, Mexican Americans, and Non-Hispanic whites. *Journal of Nutrition, 141,* 1898–1906.

Boyington, J., Carter-Edwards, L., Piehl, M., Hutson, J., Langdon, D., & McManus, S. (2008). Cultural attitudes toward weight, diet, and physical activity among overweight African American girls. *Preventing Chronic Disease, 5,* A36.

Brown, D. (2005). Dietary challenges of new Americans. *Journal of the American Dietetic Association, 105,* 1704–1706.

Caprio, S., Daniels, S., Drewnowski, A., Kaufman, F. R., Palinkas, L. A., Rosenbloom, A. L., & Schwimmer, J. B. (2008). Influence of race, ethnicity, and culture on childhood obesity: Implications for prevention and treatment. A consensus statement of Shaping America's Health and the Obesity Society. *Diabetes Care, 31,* 2211–2221.

Casagrande, S., Wang, Y., Anerson, C., & Gary, T. (2007). Have Americans increased their fruit and vegetable intake? The trends between 1988 and 2002. *American Journal of Preventive Medicine, 32,* 257–263.

Centers for Disease Control and Prevention. (2012). QuickStats: Prevalence of obesity among adults ages ≥ 20 years, by race/ethnicity and sex—National Health and Nutrition Examination Survey, United States, 2009–2010. *Morbidity and Mortality Weekly Report, 61,* 130.

Chen, X., Cheskin, L., Shi, L., & Wang, Y. (2011). Americans with diet-related chronic diseases report higher diet quality than those without these diseases. *Journal of Nutrition, 141,* 1543–1551.

Corso, R. (2010). *Three in ten Americans love to cook, while one in five do not enjoy it or don't cook.* Available at www.harrisinterctive.com/NewsRoom?HarrisPolls/tabid447/mid/1508/articled/444/ctl/ReadCustom%20Default/Default.aspx. Accessed on 10/26/12.

ElGindy, G. (2005a). *Cultural competence Q & A: Hindu dietary practices: Feeding the body, mind and soul.* Available at www.minoritynurse.com/features/health/10-25-05b.html. Accessed on 2/6/08.

ElGindy, G. (2005b). *Cultural competence Q & A: Meeting Jewish and Muslim patients' dietary needs.* Available at www.minoritynurse.com/features/health/03-01-05f.html. Accessed on 2/6/08.

ElGindy, G. (2005c). *Cultural competence Q & A: Understanding Buddhist patients' dietary needs.* Available at www.minoritynurse.com/features/health/05-03-05a.html. Accessed on 2/6/08.

Ervin, B. (2011). Healthy Eating Index—2005 total and component scores for adults aged 20 and over: National Health and Nutrition Examination Survey, 2003–2004. *National Health Statistics Reports, Number 44,* December 13, 2011.

Fryar, C., Hirsch, R., Eberhardt, M., Yoon, S. S., & Wright, J. D. (2010). *NCHS Data Brief. Hypertension, high serum total cholesterol, and diabetes: Racial and ethnic prevalence differences in US adults, 1999–2006.* Available at www.cdc.gov/nchs/data/databriefs/db36.htm. Accessed on 10/30/12.

Goody, C., & Drago, L. (2009). Using cultural competence constructs to understand food practices and provide diabetes care and education. *Diabetes Spectrum, 22,* 43–47.

Hoeffel, E., Rastogi, S., Kim, M., & Shahid, H. (2012). *The Asian population: 2010. 2010 Census Brief.* Available at www.census.gov//rpod/cen2010/briefs/c2010br-11.pdf. Accessed on 10/30/12.

Kagawa-Singer, M., Dadia, A., Yu, M., & Surbone, A. (2010). Cancer, culture, and health disparities. Time to chart a new course? *CA: A Cancer Journal for Clinicians, 60,* 12–39.

Kittler, P., Sucher, K., & Nahikian-Nelms, M. (2012). *Food and culture* (6th ed.). Belmont, CA: Wadsworth Cengage Learning

Kulkarni, K. (2004). Food, culture, and diabetes in the United States. *Clinical Diabetes, 22,* 190–192.

LivingSocial. (2011). *Reservation nation? Despite recession, Americans eat whopping 250 restaurant meals per year, says LivingSocial dining survey.* Available at http://corporate.livingsocial.com/september. Accessed on 10/26/12.

Lv, N., & Carson, D. (2004). Dietary pattern change and acculturation of Chinese Americans in Pennsylvania. *Journal of the American Dietetic Association, 104,* 771–778.

Office of Management and Budget. (1997). *Revisions to the standards for the classification of federal data on race and ethnicity. Federal Register Notice 10/30/97.* Available at www.whitehouse.gov/omb/fedreg_1997standards/. Accessed on 10/31/12.

Office of Minority Health. (2012a). *African American profile.* Available at http://minorityhealth.hhs.gov/templates/browse.aspx?lvl=3&lvlid=23. Accessed on 10/29/12.

Office of Minority Health. (2012b). *Asian American/Pacific Islander profile.* Available at http://minorityhealth.hhs.gov/templates/browse.aspx?lvl=3&lvlid=29. Accessed on 10/29/12.

Office of Minority Health. (2012c). *Hispanic/Latino profile.* Available at http://minorityhealth.hhs.gov/templates/browse.aspx?lvl=3&lvlid=31. Accessed on 10/29/12.

Satia, J. (2009). Diet-related disparities: Understanding the problem and accelerating solutions. *Journal of the American Dietetic Association, 109,* 610–615.

Satia, J., Patterson, R., Kristal, A., Hislop, T. G., Yasui, Y., & Taylor, V. M. (2001). Development of scales to measure dietary acculturation among Chinese-Americans and Chinese-Canadians. *Journal of the American Dietetic Association, 101,* 548–553.

Sofianou, A., Fung, T., & Tucker, K. (2011). Differences in diet pattern adherence by nativity and duration of US residence in the Mexican-American Population. *Journal of the American Dietetic Association, 111,* 1563–1569.

Todd, J., Mancino, L., & Lin, B. *The impact of food away from home on adult diet quality (Feb 1, 2010)* (USDA-ERS Economic Research Report Paper No. 90). Available at http://ssrn.com/abstract=1557129. Accessed on 10/30/12.

U.S. Census Bureau. (2008). *An older and more diverse nation by mid-century.* Available at www.census.gov/newsroom/releases-archives/population/cb08-123.html#. Accessed on 10/31/12.

11 Healthy Eating for Healthy Babies

CHECK YOUR KNOWLEDGE

TRUE	FALSE		
☐	☐	**1**	Adequate weight gain during pregnancy ensures delivery of a normal-weight baby.
☐	☐	**2**	Obese women should not gain weight during pregnancy.
☐	☐	**3**	An important source of folic acid is ready-to-eat breakfast cereals.
☐	☐	**4**	Both inadequate and excessive maternal weight gain during pregnancy are associated with overweight or obesity in the offspring later in life.
☐	☐	**5**	To get enough calcium during pregnancy, women need to double their usual intake of milk.
☐	☐	**6**	Pregnant and lactating women are advised to eliminate fish and seafood from their diets to avoid mercury contamination.
☐	☐	**7**	Calorie needs do not increase during pregnancy until the second trimester.
☐	☐	**8**	Lactation increases calorie requirements more than pregnancy does.
☐	☐	**9**	An inadequate maternal intake of nutrients decreases the quantity of breast milk produced, not the quality.
☐	☐	**10**	Thirst is a good indicator for the need for fluid in most lactating women.

LEARNING OBJECTIVES

Upon completion of this chapter, you will be able to

1 Evaluate a woman's pattern and amount of weight gain during pregnancy based on her prepregnancy body mass index (BMI).

2 Assess a woman's intake of folic acid for adequacy in the preconception period and during pregnancy.

3 Assess whether a woman may benefit from a multivitamin and mineral supplement during pregnancy.

4 Plan a day's intake for a pregnant woman based on her MyPlate food intake pattern.

5 Give examples of nutrition interventions used for nausea, constipation, and heartburn during pregnancy.

6 Compare nutrition guidelines for healthy eating during pregnancy with the guidelines for lactation.

7 Identify risk factors for poor nutritional status during pregnancy.

8 List benefits of breastfeeding for mother and infant.

257

Although an optimal diet before and during pregnancy cannot *guarantee* a successful outcome of pregnancy, it can improve the chance of a healthy newborn baby, a healthy mom, and a healthy future for both. A woman who is well nourished and within her healthy weight range prior to conception provides an environment conducive to normal fetal growth and development during the critical first trimester of pregnancy. During pregnancy, the fetus cannot meet its genetic potential for development if the supply of energy and nutrients is inadequate. Conversely, excessive weight gain during pregnancy is strongly associated with maternal and fetal complications (Yogev and Catalano, 2009). An optimal diet provides enough, but not too many, calories and nutrients to optimize maternal and fetal health.

This chapter discusses dietary guidelines for women before, during, and after pregnancy. Weight gain recommendations, common problems of pregnancy, and nutrition interventions for maternal health conditions are presented.

PREPREGNANCY NUTRITION

Ideally, women enter pregnancy optimally nourished and at a healthy body weight. Dietary Guidelines key recommendations for women who are capable of becoming pregnant, as well as those who are pregnant or breastfeeding, appear in Box 11.1 Specific prepregnancy concerns, including healthy eating, various nutrients, and body weight, are discussed below.

Healthy Eating

The basic principles of healthy eating that apply to healthy people are also appropriate before, during, and after pregnancy: eat plenty of fruits and vegetables of various kinds and colors; whole-grain bread and cereals; lean protein foods; low-fat or fat-free milk and dairy products; and healthy fats in moderation. As with the general public, sodium, solid fats, added sugars, and refined grains should be limited.

Folic Acid

Folic Acid: synthetic form of folate found in multivitamins, fortified breakfast cereals, and enriched grain products.

Neural Tube Defect: a serious central nervous system birth defect, such as anencephaly (absence of a brain) and spina bifida (incomplete closure of the spinal cord and its bony encasement).

Folate: natural form of the B vitamin involved in the synthesis of DNA; only one-half is available to the body as synthetic folic acid.

The Institute of Medicine (IOM, 1998), Centers for Disease Control and Prevention (CDC, 2012c), *Dietary Guidelines for Americans, 2010* (U.S. Department of Agriculture [USDA], U.S. Department of Health and Human Services [USDHHS], 2010), and March of Dimes (MOD, 2012) are among the many experts who recommend that synthetic **folic acid** be consumed prior to conception to prevent **neural tube defects.** Because neural tube defects originate in the first month of pregnancy before a woman may even know she is pregnant, all women of childbearing age who are capable of becoming pregnant are urged to consume 400 µg of synthetic folic acid every day from fortified food or supplements in addition to consuming natural **folate** in a varied diet. Synthetic folic acid is recommended because it is better absorbed and has greater availability than natural folate in foods.

> ### QUICK BITE
>
> **Sources of folic acid**
> 100% fortified ready-to-eat breakfast cereals
> White bread, rolls, pasta, and crackers (In the United States and Canada, enriched flour is required to be fortified with folic acid.)
>
> **Sources of naturally occurring folate**
> Leafy green vegetables, such as spinach
> Citrus fruits
> Dried peas and beans, such as lentils, soybeans, pinto beans

| Box 11.1 | 2010 DIETARY GUIDELINES KEY RECOMMENDATIONS FOR WOMEN WHO ARE CAPABLE OF BECOMING PREGNANT, PREGNANT, OR BREASTFEEDING |

Women of Childbearing Age Who May Become Pregnant

- Choose foods that supply heme iron, which is more readily absorbed by the body, additional iron sources, and enhancers of iron absorption such as vitamin C–rich foods.
- Consume 400 micrograms (μg) per day of synthetic folic acid (from fortified foods and/or supplements) in addition to food forms of folate from a varied diet.
- Achieve and maintain a healthy weight before becoming pregnant. This may reduce the risk of complications during pregnancy, increase the chances of a healthy infant birth weight, and improve the long-term health of both mother and infant.
- Do not drink alcohol because alcohol can cause negative behavioral or neurologic consequences in the offspring when consumed during pregnancy, especially during the first few months. A safe level of alcohol intake during pregnancy has not been established.

Women Who Are Pregnant or Breastfeeding (Including Adolescent Girls)

- Consume 8 to 12 oz of seafood per week from a variety of seafood types.
- Due to their high methylmercury content, limit white (albacore) tuna to 6 oz per week and do not eat the following four types of fish: tilefish, shark, swordfish, and king mackerel.
- If pregnant, take an iron supplement, as recommended by an obstetrician or other health-care provider.
- If pregnant, consume 600 μg/day of dietary folate equivalents from all sources (natural and synthetic).
- Pregnant women are encouraged to gain weight within the 2009 Institute of Medicine (IOM) gestational weight gain guidelines (Table 11.1). Maternal weight gain during pregnancy outside the recommended range is associated with increased risks for maternal and child health.
- Pregnant women are advised to not drink alcohol because a safe level of intake has not been established. If breastfeeding women choose to drink, they should wait until the infant is at least 3 months of age and consume only one drink, waiting at least 4 hours before breastfeeding.

Source: U.S. Department of Agriculture, U.S. Department of Health and Human Services. (2010). *Dietary guidelines for Americans, 2010* (7th ed.). Available at www.health.gov/dietaryguidelines. Accessed on 2/24/11.

Heme Iron

The CDC recommends that all women who are capable of becoming pregnant be counseled to choose foods that provide heme iron, or other sources of iron in the diet, and nonheme iron absorption enhancers, such as vitamin C (CDC, 2012c). Iron deficiency screening is recommended so that anemia can be treated prior to conception.

Other Nutrients of Concern

Other nutrients of concern in women who are capable of becoming pregnant include (CDC, 2012c)

- Calcium. Women should be counseled about the importance of consuming calcium in an adequate amount; calcium supplements may be an option if calcium intake is inadequate.

- Essential fatty acids, particularly the essential omega-3 fatty acids. Seafood recommendations are to consume 8 to 12 oz of a variety of seafood per week and not more than 6 oz of canned albacore tuna weekly.
- Iodine. An iodine deficiency during pregnancy can cause neurologic damage from fetal hypothyroidism; population studies correlate iodine deficiency with impaired cognitive development in the fetus and in children (Ziesel, 2009). Women should be advised to consume the recommended amount of iodine before, during, and after pregnancy. Iodized salt is an acceptable source.
- Dietary supplements. Screening should identify all supplements used, including vitamins, minerals, herbs, weight loss products, and home remedies so that safety and efficacy can be discussed.

Healthy Weight

Healthy Weight: BMI of 18.5 to 24.9.

Approximately one in five American women begin pregnancy overweight and one in six enter pregnancy as obese (Andres, Shankar, and Badger, 2012). Obesity during pregnancy is associated with gestational diabetes, gestational hypertension, preeclampsia, birth defects, cesarean delivery, fetal macrosomia, perinatal deaths, postpartum anemia, and childhood obesity (American Dietetic Association [ADA], 2008). Infants of overweight mothers have greater body fat mass in the early neonatal period compared to infants born to lean women (Andres et al., 2012). Achieving **healthy weight** prior to conception is beneficial to mother and infant.

All women with a body mass index (BMI) of 18.5 or lower or 25 or higher should be counseled about the risks of unhealthy weight to maternal health and future pregnancies, including the risk of infertility. Clinical care recommendations are based on BMI (CDC, 2012b).

- Women who are overweight (BMI 25–29.9) should be treated for overweight when two or more risk factors are present or when waist circumference is high. Treatment should focus on producing moderate weight loss through nutrition and physical activity.
- Women who are obese (BMI ≥30) should be treated to produce substantial weight loss over a prolonged period; comorbidities should be considered when determining treatment options.
- Women who are underweight (BMI ≤18.5) should be evaluated for eating disorders and distorted body image.

NUTRITION AND LIFESTYLE DURING PREGNANCY

Low Birth Weight (LBW): a baby weighing less than 2500 g or 5.5 pounds.

The first prenatal visit should identify clients who present with a high-risk pregnancy (Box 11.2). A high-risk pregnancy is likely to produce a **low birth weight (LBW)** infant; LBW infants are more likely to experience complications during delivery and have a higher risk of physical and mental defects. Monitoring continues throughout pregnancy to identify high-risk criteria that may develop during gestation, such as excessive or inadequate weight gain or the development of gestational diabetes.

Many women are motivated during pregnancy to adopt healthy lifestyle changes, which have the potential to make a long-lasting impact on the health of mother and infant.

| **Box 11.2** | **FACTORS ASSOCIATED WITH HIGH-RISK PREGNANCIES** |

Age
Teens (especially 15 years or younger) and women 35 years or older

Anthropometric Data
Prepregnancy BMI of less than 18.5 or greater than 25
Inadequate or excessive weight gain during pregnancy

Dietary Data
Nutrient deficiencies or excesses
Disordered eating
Use of a therapeutic diet
Use of alcohol, tobacco, or drugs

Medical–Psychosocial Data
Chronic preexisting medical problems such as diabetes, heart disease, pulmonary
    disease, renal disease, maternal phenylketonuria
Development of gestational disorders, such as gestational diabetes and gestational
    hypertension
Poor obstetric history (low birth weight, stillbirth, abortion, fetal anomalies), high
    parity, multiparity.
Repetitive pregnancies at short intervals (younger than 18 months)
Low socioeconomic status, lack of family support, low level of education, problems
    with food availability

Pregnant women, like all Americans, are urged to follow a healthy eating pattern while staying within their calorie needs (USDA, USDHHS, 2010). This means they should

- Eat a variety of nutrient-dense food and beverages among the basic food groups.
- Be sure to include enough vegetables, fruits, whole grains, and milk and milk products because these foods provide nutrients of concern in the typical American diet—namely, potassium, fiber, calcium, and vitamin D.
- Limit their intake of saturated fat, trans fats, cholesterol, added sugars, and salt.
- Follow food safety guidelines to reduce the risk of foodborne illness.

Additional Dietary Guidelines recommendations for pregnant women appear in Box 11.1. Specific considerations are presented in the following section.

Amount of Weight Gain

Current weight gain recommendations for pregnancy are based on prepregnancy BMI (see Table 11.1). Recommended weight gain is 25 to 35 pounds in women of normal weight, 28 to 40 pounds for underweight women, 15 to 25 pounds for overweight women, and 11 to 20 pounds for women who are obese at the time of conception (National Research Council [NRC], 2009). Women pregnant with twins need to gain somewhat more weight than that recommended for single births but not double the amounts.

Among the IOM's key findings are that (1) women should enter pregnancy with a normal BMI to reduce the risks of adverse pregnancy outcomes associated with excess prepregnancy weight, and (2) although record numbers of American women have BMI values of 35, there is insufficient data available to issue specific weight gain recommendations for

Table 11.1 Recommended Weight Gain Ranges Based on Maternal Prepregnancy BMI

BMI	Prepregnancy BMI Status	Total Weight Gain (pounds)	Rate of Weekly Weight Gain in Second and Third Trimester (mean range in pounds per week)*
Less than 18.5	Underweight	28–40	1 (1–1.3)
18.5–24.9	Normal weight	25–35	1 (0.8–1)
25–29.9	Overweight	15–25	0.6 (0.5–0.7)
30 or greater	Obese (all classes)	11–20	0.5 (0.4–0.6)

*Calculations assume 1.1- to 4.4-pound weight gain in the first trimester.

Source: National Research Council. (2009). *Weight gain during pregnancy: Reexamining the guidelines.* Washington, DC: The National Academies Press.

this population (NRC, 2009). The report emphasizes the need for increased nutrition and exercise counseling to help women attain a normal BMI.

Excessive weight gain in pregnancy is common and most marked in women who are overweight or obese prior to pregnancy (Crozier et al., 2010). Excess weight increases the risk of gestational diabetes, gestational hypertension, preeclampsia, cesarean deliveries, complications during delivery, and postpartum weight retention (Ricciotti, 2008). Weight gain during pregnancy has been shown to independently predict long-term weight gain and obesity in women (Mamun et al., 2010). For the infant, excessive maternal weight gain increases the risk of hypoglycemia, large for gestational age, a low Apgar score, seizures, and polycythemia (ADA, 2008). Short-term and long-term studies show that offspring born to women who gained more than the recommended amount of weight during pregnancy are more likely to become overweight (Wrotniak, Shults, Butts, and Stettler, 2008). Unfortunately, there are no evidence-based recommendations on the most appropriate dietary and/or physical activity interventions to use to control excessive maternal weight gain (Crozier et al., 2010).

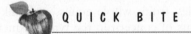

QUICK BITE

Weight gain distribution in normal pregnancy (pounds)

Birth weight of baby	7.5
Placenta	1.5
Increase in maternal blood volume	4
Increase in maternal fluid volume	4
Increase in uterus	2
Increase in breast tissue	2
Amniotic fluid	2
Maternal fat tissue	7
Total	30

In contrast, inadequate weight gain during pregnancy increases the risk of an LBW infant. LBW infants have a high incidence of postnatal complications and mortality. LBW is also associated with an increased risk of cardiovascular disease, hypertension, type 2 diabetes, dyslipidemia, and obesity later in life (Barker and Osmond, 1986; Godfrey and Barker, 2001). All women should receive guidelines on an appropriate rate and amount of weight gain based on their prepregnancy BMI (Josefson, 2011). Ongoing monitoring and counseling are appropriate during and after pregnancy to help avoid postpartum weight retention.

Weight Gain Pattern

Assuming a 1.1- to 4.4-pound weight gain in the first trimester of pregnancy, normal-weight women are urged to gain approximately 1 pound per week during the second and third trimesters; recommended amounts of weekly gain for underweight, overweight, and obese women are slightly different (see Table 11.1) (NRC, 2009). Although slightly higher or lower rates of weight gain can be considered normal, obvious or persistent deviations warrant further investigation.

Calorie Requirements

According to Dietary Reference Intakes (DRIs), pregnant women do not need any additional calories until the second trimester. Even then, the increase is surprisingly small: an extra 340 cal/day is recommended during the second trimester and an additional 452 cal/day in the third (IOM, 2005). Most pregnant women need a total of 2200 to 2900 cal/day (ADA, 2008). Throughout pregnancy, adequacy of calorie intake is measured by adequacy of weight gain.

Figure 11.1 illustrates sample MyPlate Daily Food Plan for a pregnant woman who normally requires 2000 cal/day. A 2000-calorie meal plan is shown for the first trimester, a 2400-calorie plan for the second trimester, and a 2600-calorie plan for the third trimester. The total calories in each of these plans slightly exceeds the actual estimated increase required (e.g., 2340 calories during the second trimester, 2452 calories in the third trimester) because these are general food group plans, not exact formulas. From the beginning to end of pregnancy, the *increase* in food recommended daily is

- 3 oz of grains
- 1 cup of vegetables
- 1 oz of protein foods
- 2 tsp oils

Daily Food Plan

	GRAINS Make half your grains whole	VEGETABLES Vary your veggies	FRUITS Focus on fruits	DAIRY Get your calcium-rich foods	PROTEIN FOODS Go lean with protein	OILS
1st Trimester Based on a 2000 calorie pattern*	6 ounces a day Aim for at least 3 ounces of whole grains a day	2 1/2 cups a day Aim for this much weekly: Dark green veggies - 3 cups Orange veggies - 2 cups Dry beans & peas - 3 cups Starchy veggie - 3 cups Other veggies - 6 1/2 cups	2 cups a day Eat a variety of fruit Go easy on fruit juices	3 cups a day Go low-fat or fat-free when you choose milk, yogurt or cheese	5 1/2 ounces a day Choose low-fat or lean meats and poultry. Vary your protein routine – choose more fish, beans, peas, nuts, and seeds	6 tsp a day
2nd Trimester Based on a 2400 calorie pattern*	8 ounces a day Aim for at least 3 1/2 ounces of whole grains a day	3 cups a day Aim for this much weekly: Dark green veggies - 3 cups Orange veggies - 2 cups Dry beans & peas - 3 cups Starchy veggie - 6 cups Other veggies - 7 cups	2 cups a day Eat a variety of fruit Go easy on fruit juices	3 cups a day Go low-fat or fat-free when you choose milk, yogurt or cheese	6 1/2 ounces a day Choose low-fat or lean meats and poultry. Vary your protein routine – choose more fish, beans, peas, nuts, and seeds	7 tsp a day
3rd Trimester Based on a 2600 calorie pattern*	9 ounces a day Aim for at least 4 ounces of whole grains a day	3 1/2 cups a day Aim for this much weekly: Dark green veggies - 3 cups Orange veggies - 2 cups Dry beans & peas - 3 cups Starchy veggie - 6 cups Other veggies - 7 cups	2 cups a day Eat a variety of fruit Go easy on fruit juices	3 cups a day Go low-fat or fat-free when you choose milk, yogurt or cheese	6 1/2 ounces a day Choose low-fat or lean meats and poultry. Vary your protein routine – choose more fish, beans, peas, nuts, and seeds	8 tsp a day

*These are only estimates of your needs. Check with your health care provider to make sure you are gaining weight appropriately.

The calories and amounts of food you need change with each trimester of pregnancy. Your plan may show different amounts of food for different months, to meet your changing nutritional needs. Changing the amount of calories you eat each trimester also helps you gain weight at the correct rate.

Know your limits on fats, sugars, and sodium

Total calories	Extras Limit extras (solid fats and sugars) to this much:
2000 calories	258 calories or less/day
2400 calories	330 calories or less/day
2600 calories	362 calories or less/day

FIGURE 11.1 Sample MyPlate Daily Food Plans for each trimester of pregnancy. (*Source:* U.S. Department of Agriculture, Center for Nutrition Policy and Promotion. [2011]. Available at www.choosemyplate.gov)

Table 11.2   Selected Nutritional Needs for Women (Aged 19–30 Years) During Pregnancy and Lactation

Nutrient	Nonpregnant Women	Pregnancy	Lactation
Calories	Individualized	1st tri: +0 2nd tri: +340 3rd tri: +450	1st 6 months: +330 2nd 6 months: +400
Protein (g)	46	71	71
Vitamin A (μg)	700	770	1300
Vitamin C (mg)	75	85	120
Vitamin D (IU)	600	600	600
Vitamin E (mg)	15	15	19
Vitamin K (μg)*	90*	90*	90*
Thiamin (mg)	1.1	1.4	1.4
Riboflavin (mg)	1.1	1.4	1.6
Niacin (mg)	14	18	17
Vitamin B_6 (mg)	1.3	1.9	2.0
Folate (μg)	400	600	500
Vitamin B_{12} (μg)	2.4	2.6	2.8
Calcium (mg)	1000	1000	1000
Iron (mg)	18	27	9
Magnesium (mg)	310	350	310
Selenium (μg)	55	60	70
Zinc (mg)	8	11	12

Recommended Dietary Allowances are in **boldface**; Adequate Intakes (AIs) appear in roman type followed by an asterisk (*).

tri, trimester.

Nutrient Requirements

Although most nutrient requirements increase during pregnancy (Table 11.2),

- Nutrient needs are not constant throughout the course of pregnancy. Nutrient needs generally change little during the first trimester (folic acid is an exception) and are at their highest during the last trimester.
- Nutrient needs do not increase proportionately. For instance, the need for iron increases by 50% during pregnancy, yet the requirement for vitamin B_{12} increases by only about 10%.
- Actual requirements during pregnancy vary among individuals and are influenced by previous nutritional status and health history including chronic illnesses, multiple pregnancies, and closely spaced pregnancies.
- The requirement for one nutrient may be altered by the intake of another. For instance, women who do not meet their calorie requirements need higher amounts of protein.
- Most women who are at low nutritional risk can meet their nutrient needs throughout pregnancy from food alone (ADA, 2008). Exceptions are discussed in the following section.

Folic Acid

Dietary Folate Equivalents (DFE): a measure of total folate available that accounts for the lower availability of natural folate in food compared to synthetic folic acid used in fortified foods and supplements. Total DFE = micrograms of food folate + 1.7 × micrograms of synthetic folic acid.

Folic acid has a vital role in DNA synthesis and thus is essential for the synthesis of new cells and transmission of inherited characteristics. It is recommended that pregnant women increase their intake of **dietary folate equivalents (DFE)** to 600 μg daily throughout pregnancy. A daily supplement ensures an adequate intake.

Iron

The DRI for iron increases by 50% during pregnancy to support the increase in maternal blood volume and to provide iron for fetal liver storage, which sustains the infant for the first 4 to 6 months of life. Even with careful selections, women are not likely to consume adequate amounts of iron during pregnancy from food alone. Infants born to women who have iron deficiency anemia have an increased risk of LBW and possibly preterm delivery and perinatal mortality (ADA, 2008). It is recommended that pregnant women take an iron supplement of 27 mg of iron daily; women who are anemic may need 60 mg of iron daily until the anemia resolves (ADA, 2008).

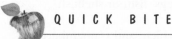

QUICK BITE

Good sources of iron*
Heme iron
  Lean red meat, poultry, fish
Nonheme iron
  100% iron-fortified ready-to-eat cereals
  Dried peas and beans, such as soybeans,
    lentils, lima beans

Baked potato with skin
Dried fruit

*Heme iron is well absorbed and not influenced by the presence of other dietary factors. Nonheme iron absorption is enhanced when eaten at the same time as foods high in vitamin C, such as citrus fruits or juices, tomato products, red peppers, cantaloupe, or strawberries.

Other Nutrient Supplements

A multivitamin and mineral supplement is recommended for pregnant women who (ADA, 2008)

- Have iron deficiency anemia
- Consume a poor-quality diet
- Do not consume enough foods from animal sources
- Smoke or abuse alcohol or drugs
- Are carrying two or more fetuses
- Have HIV, especially if access to antiretroviral treatment is limited

Specific supplements that may be needed based on individual circumstances are as follows:

- Complete vegans who are pregnant or breastfeeding should take supplements of vitamin B_{12} if a reliable dietary source is not consumed. Reliable sources are vegan foods fortified with vitamin B_{12}, such as yeast extracts, vegetable stock, veggie burgers, textured vegetable protein, soymilk, vegetable and sunflower margarines, and ready-to-eat breakfast cereals. All other nutrient needs can be met through a well-planned lacto-ovo vegetarian or vegan diet.
- Women who do not consume adequate vitamin D or have insufficient sunlight exposure should consume supplemental vitamin D to reduce the risk of low serum calcium in the infant and abnormal neonatal bone metabolism (ADA, 2008). Amounts greater than the Recommended Dietary Allowances (RDAs) do not appear to provide added benefits.

Fetal Alcohol Syndrome (FAS): a condition characterized by varying degrees of physical and mental growth failure and birth defects caused by maternal intake of alcohol.

Teratogen: anything that causes abnormal fetal development and birth defects.

Alcohol

Alcohol use during pregnancy can cause physical and neurodevelopmental problems, such as mental retardation, learning disabilities, and **fetal alcohol syndrome**. Alcohol does its damage by dehydrating fetal cells, leaving them dead or functionless, or by causing secondary nutrient deficiencies. Because alcohol is a potent **teratogen** and a "safe" level of consumption is not known, women are advised to completely avoid alcohol before and during pregnancy.

Avoiding Foodborne Illness

Foodborne risks are more dangerous for pregnant women than for most other adults. During pregnancy, listeriosis, caused by the bacterium *Listeria monocytogenes,* may cause only mild, flu-like illness in the mother but may lead to miscarriage, stillbirth, premature delivery, or neonatal infection (Ricciotti, 2008). Pregnant women are 20 times more likely to get listeriosis than other healthy adults, and approximately one-third of all listeriosis cases occur during pregnancy. To reduce the risk of listeriosis, pregnant women should *not* consume the following foods:

- Unpasteurized milk or products made with it
- Raw or undercooked meat, poultry, eggs, fish, or shellfish
- Refrigerated pâtés or meat spreads
- Certain soft cheeses such as feta, Brie, bleu, and Camembert
- Leftover foods and ready-to-eat foods, including hot dogs and deli meats, unless heated until steaming hot

Healthy people infected by the parasite *Toxoplasma gondii* may be asymptomatic or may have flu-like symptoms. During pregnancy, the consequences are more serious: if transmitted from mother to fetus in the first trimester, toxoplasmosis can cause mental retardation, blindness, and epilepsy. Eating raw meat is the cause of approximately half of toxoplasmosis infections (Ricciotti, 2008). Pregnant women should be instructed on how to prevent transmission of the parasite, including

- Cook meat thoroughly.
- Peel or wash fresh fruits and vegetables before eating.
- Avoid cross-contamination in the kitchen by cleaning surfaces and utensils exposed to raw food.
- Avoid changing cat litter (cats pass an environmentally resistant form of the organism in their feces).

Pica

Pica: purposeful ingestion of nonfood substances such as dirt, clay, starch, and ice.

Some women experience **pica**, the craving for and ingestion of nonfood items. The most commonly consumed items are earth, such as soil, clay, or baked clay (geophagy); raw starch (amylophagy); and ice (pagophagy). Geophagy occurs most often. Although pica can be found in all regions of the United States, it is more commonly reported among socioeconomically disadvantaged women living in rural and immigrant communities and in women of African heritage (Corbett, Ryan, and Weinrich, 2003). It is not known what causes pica, although cultural beliefs, hunger, and medicinal purpose may be factors (Njiru, Elchalal, and Paltiel, 2011). There is no evidence that micronutrient deficiencies cause a physiologic craving; iron deficiency was thought to be a risk factor for pica, but it may be a consequence (Njiru et al., 2011). Eating clay or soil may displace the intake of iron-rich foods from the diet and may interfere with iron absorption. An increased risk of premature birth, spontaneous abortion, and permanent neurocognitive and neurodevelopmental impairments can occur from exposure to metals in soil and clay, such as lead, arsenic, mercury, and cadmium (Kim and Nelson, 2012).

Caffeine

A high caffeine intake is associated with LBW but not with birth defects (ADA, 2008) or preterm birth (Maslova, Bhattacharya, Lin, and Michels, 2010). The ADA recommends pregnant women limit their intake of caffeine to 300 mg/day or less (Table 11.3).

Table 11.3 Caffeine Content of Selected Beverages and Foods

Item	Average Caffeine Content (mg)
8 oz coffee, generic brewed	133 (range 102–200)
16 oz coffee, generic brewed	266
16 oz Starbucks brewed coffee (Grande)	320
8 oz coffee, generic instant	93 (range 27–173)
8 oz coffee, generic decaffeinated	5 (range 3–12)
8 oz brewed tea	53 (range 40–120)
16 oz Snapple, lemon (and diet version)	42
12 oz Pepsi	38
12 oz Coca-Cola Classic	35
7-Up, Sprite	0
8.3 oz Red Bull	80
8 oz Ben & Jerry's coffee-flavored ice cream	68
1 stick Jolt caffeinated gum	33
1.55 oz Hershey's chocolate bar	9
1 Hershey Kiss	1
8 oz hot cocoa	9 (range 3–13)

Source: Center for Science in the Public Interest. (2012). *Caffeine content of food and drugs.* Available at http://www.cspinet.org/new/cafchart.htm. Accessed on 11/12/12.

Nonnutritive Sweeteners

The use of nonnutritive sweeteners during pregnancy has been studied extensively. Acesulfame potassium (Sunette, Sweet One), aspartame (NutraSweet, Spoonful, Equal), saccharin (Sweet 'N Low), and sucralose (Splenda) are all deemed to be safe during pregnancy when consumed at levels within the U.S. Food and Drug Administration (FDA) Acceptable Daily Intake (ADI) guidelines (ADA, 2008). The exception is that women with phenylketonuria (PKU) should not use aspartame because it is made from phenylalanine. However, a recent large, prospective cohort study found that high intakes (>1 serving/day) of both nonnutritive sweeteners and sugar-sweetened beverages are associated with an increased risk of preterm delivery (Englund-Ogge et al., 2012).

Herbal Supplements

Because little is known about the safety and efficacy of herbal supplements during pregnancy, it is recommended that they not be used during pregnancy and lactation. Herbal products, including herbal teas, are technically unapproved drugs; most drugs cross the placental barrier to some degree, exposing the fetus to potentially teratogenic effects. Unlike approved drugs, little animal or human testing has been done to determine if herbs can cause birth defects or potentially harm mothers and infants.

Fish

The FDA has issued advisories regarding fish and shellfish consumption during pregnancy due to the risk of methylmercury contamination (FDA, 2004). Mercury occurs naturally in the environment, including waterways. Bacteria in the water convert mercury to methylmercury, which is absorbed by fish low on the food chain and becomes concentrated in larger, longer living predatory fish at the top of the food chain. Nearly all fish contain trace amounts of mercury; it accumulates in humans primarily by eating fish.

Mercury can be toxic, particularly to developing brains in fetuses and young children. Mercury poisoning in a fetus can result in learning delays in walking or talking to more severe problems such as cerebral palsy, seizures, and mental retardation. To reduce the risk of methylmercury poisoning, women who are pregnant or lactating are advised to (FDA, 2004; USDA, USDHHS, 2010)

- Not eat shark, swordfish, king mackerel, and tilefish.
- Eat 8 to 12 oz of seafood per week from a variety of fish and shellfish that are lower in mercury, such as shrimp, salmon, pollock, catfish, and canned light tuna.
- Limit albacore ("white") tuna to 6 oz per week.
- Check local advisories about the safety of fish from local waters. If no advice is available, eat up to 6 oz per week of fish from local waters, but don't consume any other fish that week.

Even though fish and seafood are healthful sources of omega-3 fatty acids, which are essential for optimal fetal neurodevelopment, the conflicting message that fish is potentially toxic causes many women to avoid eating fish (Bloomingdale et al., 2010). Pregnant women may be more likely to consume fish if given advice on how much and what kinds of seafood are safe.

Physical Activity

Healthy pregnant women who do not have medical or obstetric complications are urged to follow the advice for all healthy adults: get at least 30 minutes of moderate exercise on most days of the week (American College of Obstetricians and Gynecologists, 2009). Safe exercise should be encouraged, with attention paid to fall risk and avoiding supine positions during the second and third trimesters (Fig. 11.2). Exercise may play a role in preventing and managing gestational diabetes (American College of Obstetricians and Gynecologists, 2009).

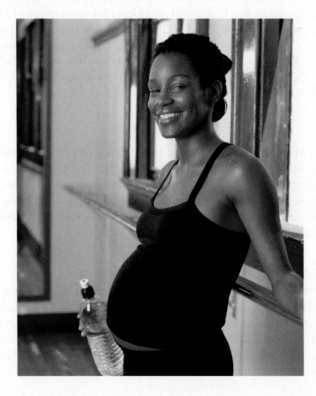

■ **FIGURE 11.2** Pregnant women are urged to get at least 30 minutes of moderate, safe exercise daily throughout their pregnancies.

Table 11.4 Common Complaints Associated with Pregnancy

Complaint	Possible Causes	Nutrition Interventions
Nausea and vomiting (common during the first trimester)	Hypoglycemia, decreased gastric motility, relaxation of the cardiac sphincter, anxiety	Eat easily digested carbohydrate foods (e.g., dry crackers, melba toast, dry cereal, hard candy) before getting out of bed in the morning. Eat frequent, small snacks of dry carbohydrates (e.g., crackers, hard candy) to prevent drop in glucose. Eat small frequent meals. Avoid liquids with meals. Limit high-fat foods because they delay gastric emptying. Eliminate individual intolerances and foods with a strong odor.
Constipation	Relaxation of gastrointestinal (GI) muscle tone and motility related to increased progesterone levels Increasing pressure on the GI tract by the fetus Decrease in physical activity Inadequate fiber and fluid intake Use of iron supplements	Increase fiber intake, especially intake of whole-grain breads and cereals. Look for breads that provide at least 2 g fiber/slice and cereals with at least 5 g fiber/serving. Drink at least eight 8-oz glasses of liquid daily. Try hot water with lemon or prune juice upon waking to help stimulate peristalsis. Participate in regular exercise.
Heartburn	Decrease in GI motility Relaxation of the cardiac sphincter Pressure of the uterus on the stomach	Eat small, frequent meals and eliminate liquids immediately before and after meals to avoid gastric distention. Avoid coffee, high-fat foods, and spices. Eliminate individual intolerances. Avoid lying down or bending over after eating.

Maternal Health

Common complaints associated with pregnancy, such as nausea, heartburn, and constipation, may be prevented or alleviated by nutrition interventions (Table 11.4). More serious health conditions in the mother, whether preexisting or gestational, can greatly impact the course of pregnancy and infant health. Diabetes mellitus, gestational hypertension, and maternal PKU are discussed in the following sections.

Diabetes Mellitus

Preexisting diabetes increases the risk of congenital malformations (ADA, 2008). Gestational diabetes, which appears in the latter half (after 24 weeks) of pregnancy, increases the risk of macrosomia and can make delivery difficult, increasing the risk of infant shoulder dislocation and cesarean delivery. Although symptoms of gestational diabetes disappear after delivery, women who have had gestational diabetes, especially those who continue to have impaired glucose tolerance in the postpartum period, are at high risk for type 2 diabetes

Box 11.3   Nutritional Management of Diabetes During Pregnancy

- The goals of diet are to achieve weight gain within the recommended range, keep blood glucose levels within the goal range, and avoid ketosis.
- Total calories required are determined on an individual basis based on an individual's goals.
- Carbohydrates are controlled, but a minimum of 175 g are needed daily.
- Clinical measures such as blood glucose levels and ketones determine how carbohydrates are distributed during the day.
- Glucose control may be improved by allowing fewer carbohydrates at breakfast and more at other meals.
- Exercise is encouraged if there are no medical or obstetrical complications.

Source: American Dietetic Association. (2008). Position of the American Dietetic Association: Nutrition and lifestyle for healthy pregnancy outcome. *Journal of the American Dietetic Association, 108,* 553–561.

later in life. In the long term, children born to mothers with diabetes are at increased risk for hypertension and high BMI in childhood.

Diabetes mellitus requires nutrition management regardless of whether it was present before conception or developed during gestation as a result of the metabolic changes of pregnancy. Women with preexisting diabetes should achieve glycemic control prior to conception. All women should be screened for gestational diabetes between 24 and 28 weeks of pregnancy. Nutrition recommendations for managing diabetes during pregnancy appear in Box 11.3.

Gestational Hypertension

Gestational Hypertension: systolic blood pressure of 140 mmHg or greater or diastolic blood pressure of 90 mmHg or greater that develops in the second half of pregnancy and ends with childbirth.

Preeclampsia: a toxemia of pregnancy characterized by hypertension accompanied by proteinuria or edema, or both.

Eclampsia: a toxemia of pregnancy that develops with the occurrence of one or more convulsions resulting from preeclampsia.

Gestational hypertension develops in approximately 6% to 17% of nulliparous women and 2% to 4% of multiparous women (Sibai, 2003). It is defined as a systolic blood pressure of greater than or equal to 140 mmHg or a diastolic reading of greater than or equal to 90 mmHg with onset after 20 weeks of gestation and without proteinuria. Often gestational hypertension does not occur until 30 weeks or later.

Approximately 50% of women with gestational hypertension diagnosed before 30 weeks of gestation develop **preeclampsia**, a potentially serious syndrome involving gestational hypertension plus proteinuria (Borzychowski, Sargent, and Redman, 2006). The causes of preeclampsia are unknown but believed to be related to an inadequate placental blood supply, possibly from maternal hypertension and involving an inflammatory response (ADA, 2009a). It is twice as prevalent in overweight women and approximately three times as high in obese women (Catalano, 2007).

Although most cases are mild and asymptomatic, edema of the hands and face, weight gain greater than or equal to 5 pounds a week, visual disturbances, severe headaches, dizziness, and pain in the upper right abdominal quadrant may occur. Preeclampsia increases maternal and infant morbidity and mortality (ADA, 2008). In rare cases, preeclampsia progresses to **eclampsia**, characterized by grand mal seizures and sometimes coma.

Risk factors for eclampsia include a history of chronic hypertension or preeclampsia in a prior pregnancy, primiparity, multiple pregnancy, maternal age of less than 20 years or greater than 35 years, African American race, and maternal obesity (ADA, 2008).

Nutrition interventions aimed at reducing the risk of gestational hypertension or preeclampsia have primarily involved nutrient supplements. Data show that calcium supplements reduce the risk of preeclampsia by approximately 50% in women with low calcium intakes without adverse effects (ADA, 2009a). No benefit was observed in women with adequate calcium intakes. Randomized controlled studies using vitamin C and vitamin E failed to demonstrate benefit (Poston, Briley, Seed, Kelly, and Shennan, 2006). Although omega-3 fatty acids lower blood pressure in nonpregnant people, a recent study found that docosahexaenoic acid (DHA) supplements in the second half of pregnancy did not reduce the risk of preeclampsia or gestational diabetes (Zhou et al., 2012). A salt-restricted diet has not been shown to be beneficial (Duley, Henderson-Smart, and Meher, 2005). Thus, except for calcium supplements for calcium-deficient women, no nutrition interventions are efficacious. In most cases, delivery "cures" preeclampsia.

Maternal Phenylketonuria

Phenylketonuria (PKU): an inborn error of phenylalanine (an essential amino acid) metabolism that results in retardation and physical handicaps in newborns if they are not treated with a low-phenylalanine diet beginning shortly after birth.

Microcephaly: abnormally small head.

Women who have **phenylketonuria (PKU)** and who consume a normal diet before and during pregnancy have very high blood levels of phenylalanine, which are devastating to the developing fetus. As a teratogen, excess serum phenylalanine can cause **microcephaly**, mental retardation, growth retardation, and/or congenital heart abnormalities in any offspring born to a woman with PKU (Lenke and Levy, 1980). The primary determinants of infant outcome are the degree of elevated phenylalanine and the gestational age when phenylalanine control is achieved (van Calcar and Ney, 2012). Most of these infants do not inherit PKU and cannot benefit from a low-phenylalanine diet after birth.

Nutrition plays a key role in the outcome of maternal PKU pregnancies. To prevent mental retardation and other problems associated with maternal PKU, a low-phenylalanine diet is necessary at least 3 months before conception and throughout the duration of the pregnancy to strictly control blood phenylalanine levels and eliminate risks to the developing fetus. However, because phenylalanine is an essential amino acid, it must be provided in the diet in limited amounts to support growth and protein synthesis. Low-phenylalanine diets are very low in total protein, so to prevent protein deficiency, a protein source of synthetic amino acids must be consumed via **medical foods**. An excessive intake of phenylalanine is common without an adequate intake of calories provided by most medical foods (van Calcar and Ney, 2012). Deficiencies of vitamin B_6, vitamin B_{12}, calcium, folate, iron, and omega-3 fatty acids may develop from the restriction of protein foods. The whey protein glycomacropeptide (GMP) may offer a new source of low-phenylalanine dietary protein with greater acceptability and more satiety than traditional amino acid–based medical foods (van Calcar and Ney, 2012). General diet guidelines are listed in Box 11.4.

Medical Foods: a food formulated to be consumed or administered enterally under the supervision of a physician for the specific dietary management of a disease or condition.

Box 11.4   DIET GUIDELINES FOR PREGNANT WOMEN WITH PHENYLKETONURIA (PKU)

Pregnant women with PKU should be advised that

- Complete understanding and strict adherence to the diet are vital.
- Protein foods such as meat, fish, poultry, eggs, dairy products, and nuts are high in phenylalanine and must be eliminated.
- Diet drinks and foods sweetened with aspartame (NutraSweet) are strictly forbidden.
- PKU-appropriate medical foods (e.g., special PKU formula) may be expensive and offensive to adult palates but must be consumed in adequate amounts to support fetal growth and prevent maternal tissue breakdown that would have results similar to those caused by cheating on the diet.
- An adequate calorie intake is necessary for normal protein metabolism.
- Close monitoring of blood phenylalanine levels is essential.

NUTRITION FOR LACTATION

With rare exceptions, breastfeeding is the optimal method of feeding and nurturing infants (ADA, 2009b). The World Health Organization (WHO) recommends that infants be exclusively breastfed for the first 6 months of life with the introduction of complementary foods thereafter as breastfeeding continues up to the age of 2 years or beyond (WHO, 2011). In the United States, both the American Academy of Pediatrics (AAP) and the ADA recommend that infants be exclusively breastfed for the first 6 months of life and that breastfeeding continue with complementary foods until 1 year of age (AAP, 2012; ADA, 2009b). Breastfeeding is an important public health strategy for improving infant and child morbidity and mortality and improving maternal morbidity (ADA, 2009b). The benefits of breastfeeding for both mother and infant are well recognized (Box 11.5).

Box 11.5   BENEFITS OF BREASTFEEDING

For the Mother
- Promotes optimal maternal–infant bonding
- Simulates uterine contractions to help control postpartum bleeding and regain prepregnant uterus size
- Is readily available and requires no mixing or dilution
- Is less expensive than purchasing bottles, nipples, sterilizing equipment, and formula
- Decreases risk of breast and ovarian cancer and type 2 diabetes
- Reduces postpartum bleeding and delays resumption of menstruation, although not reliable for birth control
- Conserves iron stores by prolonging amenorrhea
- Improves bone density and reduces risk for hip fracture
- Reduces risk of postpartum depression
- Enhances self-esteem as a competent mother

For the Infant
- Increases bonding with mother
- Optimal "natural" nutrition that contains no artificial colorings, flavorings, preservatives, or additives
- Safe and fresh
- Reduces risk of acute otitis media, nonspecific gastroenteritis, severe lower respiratory tract infections, and asthma
- Enhances immune system
- Protects against allergies and intolerance
- Promotes better tooth and jaw development than bottle feeding because the infant has to suck harder
- Associated with higher IQ and school performance through adolescence
- Reduces the risk of chronic diseases, such as obesity, type 1 and 2 diabetes, heart disease, hypertension, hypercholesterolemia, and childhood leukemia
- Reduces risk for infant morbidity and mortality

Source: American Dietetic Association. (2009). Position of the American Dietetic Association: Promoting and supporting breastfeeding. *Journal of the American Dietetic Association, 109,* 1926–1942.

Promoting Breastfeeding

The United States has seen a steady increase in breastfeeding rates since the late 1970s when the USDHHS set goals for breastfeeding initiation and duration rates (ADA, 2009b). The most current data show a breastfeeding initiation rate of 76.9%, with 47.2% of 6-month-old infants and 25.5% of 12-month-old infants receiving breast milk (CDC, 2012a).

Despite the abundance of reasons to breastfeed, many women choose not to initiate breastfeeding, only partially breastfeed, or breastfeed for only a short duration (ADA, 2009b). Factors influencing a mother's decision not to breastfeed or to breastfeed for a short duration include unsupportive hospital practices, lack of knowledge, personal beliefs, and family attitudes (Brodribb, Fallon, Hegney, and O'Brien, 2007; McCann, Baydar, and Williams, 2007) (Box 11.6). Although breastfeeding for at least 12 weeks is highly beneficial to both the infant and mother (Krummel, 2007), even a short period of breastfeeding is better than not breastfeeding at all. Women should be encouraged to breastfeed for as long as they are able and not be made to feel guilty if they fall short of the recommendations.

Social support and support from health-care professional influence success with breastfeeding. As a learned behavior, not a physiologic response, the ability to successfully breastfeed and the duration of lactation can be positively impacted by counseling. Preparation for breastfeeding should begin prenatally with counseling, guidance, and support for both the woman and her partner and continue throughout the gestational period. Hospital practices that promote breastfeeding appear in Box 11.7. Contraindications to breastfeeding are listed in Box 11.8.

Maternal Diet

Nutritional needs during lactation are based on the nutritional content of breast milk and the energy "cost" of producing milk. Compared with pregnancy, the need for some nutrients increases, whereas the need for other nutrients falls (see Table 11.2). The healthy diet consumed during pregnancy should continue during lactation. Key recommendations during breastfeeding are listed in Box 11.1.

Box 11.6   FACTORS THAT IMPAIR LACTATION

Impaired Letdown, Related to
Embarrassment or stress
Fatigue
Negative attitude, lack of desire, lack of family support
Excessive intake of caffeine or alcohol
Smoking
Drugs

Failure to Establish Lactation, Related to
Delayed or infrequent feedings
Weak infant sucking because of anesthesia during labor and delivery
Nipple discomfort or engorgement
Lack of support especially from baby's father

Decreased Demand, Related to
Supplemental bottles of formula or water
Introduction of solid food
Infant's lack of interest

Box 11.7 HOSPITAL PRACTICES THAT PROMOTE BREASTFEEDING

- Offer the infant the breast within 1 hour of birth. Hospital procedures should allow for immediate maternal–infant contact after delivery.
- Infant rooming-in.
- Inform all pregnant women about the benefits and management of breastfeeding.
- Show mothers how to breastfeed and maintain lactation even if they are separated from their infants.
- Feed only breast milk in the hospital.
- Give no artificial teats or pacifiers (e.g., dummies, soothers) to breastfeeding infants.
- Provide a phone number for breastfeeding help after discharge.

Source: American Dietetic Association. (2009). Position of the American Dietetic Association: Promoting and supporting breastfeeding. *Journal of the American Dietetic Association, 109,* 1926–1942.

Calories

Women use approximately 500 calories above their normal total daily calorie needs to produce breast milk. Approximately 100 to 150 of these calories come from fat stored during pregnancy, and the remaining calories come from extra calories consumed. An extra 330 cal/day are recommended for the first 6 months of lactation and an extra 400 calories for the second 6 months for women who exclusively breastfeed; partial breastfeeding uses fewer calories. In theory, mobilizing fat calories for the production of breast milk can contribute to a calorie deficit and weight loss over time. In reality, breastfeeding is not always associated with return to preconception weight, and some women actually gain weight during lactation (Lovelady, Stephenson, Kuppler, and Williams, 2006).

For the sample woman used for the MyPlate plan in Figure 11.1, the food plan recommended while she exclusively breastfeeds is 2400 calories, a recommended estimate using food groups, not an exact calorie prescription. This calorie level would allow her to mobilize fat accumulated during pregnancy to provide the additional calories needed to produce enough breast milk.

Adequacy of calorie intake is evaluated by changes in a woman's weight. Women who failed to gain enough weight during pregnancy, who have inadequate fat reserves, or who lose too much weight while breastfeeding may need to increase their calorie intake.

Box 11.8 CONTRAINDICATIONS TO BREASTFEEDING

- Galactosemia in the infant
- Illegal drug use in the mother
- Active tuberculosis
- HIV/AIDS (In some countries, the risk of infant mortality from not breastfeeding may outweigh the risk of acquiring HIV through breast milk.)
- Use of certain drugs, such as radioactive isotopes, antimetabolites, cancer chemotherapy agents, lithium, ergotamine

Source: American Dietetic Association. (2009). Position of the American Dietetic Association: Promoting and supporting breastfeeding. *Journal of the American Dietetic Association, 109,* 1926–1942.

Conversely, women who are not losing weight while lactating can reduce their calorie intake. A study by Lovelady, Garner, Moreno, and Williams (2000) showed that a calorie restriction of 500 cal/day in fully breastfeeding overweight women resulted in a 1 pound loss per week without negative impact on infant growth. Studies suggest that after lactation is established, a 500-calorie deficit diet that emphasizes fruits, vegetables, low-fat dairy, whole grains, legumes, and healthy types of fat is appropriate to promote postpartum weight loss in overweight women (Durham, Lovelady, Brouwer, Krause, and Ostbye, 2011).

Fluid

Another nutritional consideration during lactation is fluid intake. It is suggested that breastfeeding mothers drink a glass of fluid every time the baby nurses and with all meals. Thirst is a good indicator of need except among women who live in a dry climate or who exercise in hot weather. Fluids consumed in excess of thirst quenching do not increase milk volume.

Vitamins and Minerals

For many vitamins and minerals, requirements during lactation are higher than during pregnancy. In general, an inadequate maternal diet decreases the *quantity* of milk produced, not the *quality*. The exceptions are thiamin, riboflavin, vitamin B_6, vitamin B_{12}, vitamin A, and iodine: prolonged inadequate maternal intake of these nutrients reduces their amount in breast milk and may compromise infant nutrition (Allen, 2005). While maternal supplements can correct inadequacies, there are no consistent recommendations concerning the use of supplements during lactation (Zeisel, 2009). Women are encouraged to obtain nutrients from food, not supplements; however, iron supplements may be needed to replace depleted iron stores, not to increase the iron content of breast milk.

Other Considerations

Other considerations concerning maternal diet and breast milk are as follows:

- Highly flavored or spicy foods may impact the flavor of breast milk but need only be avoided if infant feeding is affected.
- Consistent evidence shows that when a lactating mother consumes alcohol, it easily enters breast milk and results in reduced milk production (MacNeil, Lyon, McGrane, and Spahn, 2012). Although alcohol was traditionally recommended to promote let down, there is no scientific evidence to support this practice. An occasional drink of alcohol may be safe, but women should not breastfeed for at least 4 hours afterward.
- Caffeine enters breast milk. Maternal intake should be moderate, such as the equivalent of one to two cups of coffee daily.
- Lactating women should follow the same guidelines for seafood consumption as pregnant women: avoid shark, swordfish, king mackerel, and tilefish; limit albacore tuna to 6 oz/week, eat up to 12 oz/week of fish and shellfish that are lower in mercury; and check with authorities for advisories about fish from local waters.

Attaining Healthy Weight

The highest incidence of obesity in women is during the childbearing years (Krummel, 2007). In a study by Rooney, Schauberger, and Mathiason (2005), excess weight gain during pregnancy, insufficient weight loss at 6 months postpartum, and high prepregnancy BMI were predictive of BMI 15 years later as well as for risk of diabetes, heart disease, and hypertension. Women who had lost most of their pregnancy weight by 6 months postpartum, had breastfed, and/or had participated in regular aerobic exercise tended to gain the least weight over the 15-year follow-up period. Many women do not realize that weight gained during their reproductive years affects their health in midlife (Krummel, 2007).

For many women, the last visit to the obstetrician is at 6 weeks postpartum in the absence of complications. At that time, more than two-thirds of women have not achieved their prepregnancy weight (Krummel, 2007). Some women gain additional weight during the postpartum period. Increased food intake, greater access to food during the day, less exercise, an increase in television viewing, and less social support may all contribute to postpartum weight gain (Johnson, Gerstein, Evans, and Woodward-Lopez, 2006).

Suggestions for managing postpartum weight are as follows (Krummel, 2007):

- Assess readiness to change. Many women say they want to lose weight but are not ready to make behavioral changes, such as avoiding high-fat foods, eating more fiber, and exercising at least three times per week.
- Assess lactation status, dietary intake, and activity levels. Many women may overeat based on the assumption that breastfeeding promotes weight loss and therefore calorie intake is not important (Durham et al., 2011).
- Assess for stress or depressive symptoms, which complicate weight management.

NURSING PROCESS: *Normal Pregnancy*

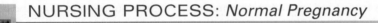

Jana is a 33-year-old professional who is 20 weeks pregnant with her first baby. Her prepregnancy BMI was 19.2. She has gained 7 pounds and complains of constipation. She plans on returning to work 6 weeks after delivery and wants to limit her weight gain so that she can fit into her clothes by the time she returns to work. She has asked you what she should eat that will be good for the baby but not cause her to get fat.

Assessment	
Medical–Psychosocial History	Medical history such as diabetes, hypertension, lactose intolerance, PKU, or other chronic disease
	■ Use of medications and over-the-counter drugs
	■ Adequacy of sunlight exposure
	■ Symptoms of constipation, including frequency, interventions attempted, and results
	■ Other complaints related to pregnancy, such as heartburn
	■ Usual frequency and intensity of physical activity
	■ Attitude about pregnancy and weight gain; knowledge about normal amount and pattern of weight gain during pregnancy
	■ Attitude/plan regarding breastfeeding
	■ Level of family/social support
Anthropometric Assessment	Height, prepregnancy weight, pattern of 7-pound weight gain during pregnancy

NURSING PROCESS: *Normal Pregnancy* (continued)

Biochemical and Physical Assessment	▪ Hemoglobin to screen for iron deficiency anemia. (Many laboratory values change during pregnancy related to normal changes in maternal physiology and so cannot be validly compared with nonpregnancy standards.)
	▪ Glucose, other laboratory values as available
	▪ Blood pressure
Dietary Assessment	▪ How does the client describe her appetite?
	▪ Does the client follow a balanced and varied diet that includes all food groups from MyPlate in reasonable amounts?
	▪ Does the client eat at regular intervals?
	▪ How has the client modified her intake since becoming pregnant?
	▪ Does the client eat nonfoods or have unusual eating habits?
	▪ Does the client take a vitamin and/or mineral supplement?
	▪ Does the client use alcohol, tobacco, caffeine, or herbal supplements?
	▪ Is the client knowledgeable about nutrient needs during pregnancy?
	▪ What cultural, religious, and ethnic influences affect the client's food choices?

Diagnosis

Possible Nursing Diagnoses	▪ Constipation related to pregnancy
	▪ Knowledge deficits of appropriate diet for pregnancy
	▪ Altered nutrition: eating less than the body needs related to voluntary food restriction to limit weight gain

Planning

Client Outcomes	The client will
	▪ Avoid constipation
	▪ Identify measures that prevent constipation
	▪ Explain the importance of nutrition for her health and for fetal growth and development
	▪ Consume an adequate, varied, and balanced diet based on MyPlate
	▪ Explain the amount and pattern of recommended weight gain
	▪ Gain approximately 1 pound of weight per week

Nursing Interventions

Nutrition Therapy	▪ Increase fiber intake gradually to prevent constipation
	▪ Provide an eating plan that includes all food groups and emphasizes ample fruits and vegetables, whole grains, lean protein, fat-free dairy, and healthy fats with total amounts per day based on her calorie needs
	▪ Encourage adequate fluid intake due to increased fiber intake

(continues on page 278)

NURSING PROCESS: *Normal Pregnancy* (continued)

Client Teaching	Instruct the client on ■ The role of nutrition and weight gain in the outcome of pregnancy ■ The role of fiber and fluids in preventing and alleviating constipation Eating plan essentials, including ■ Choosing a variety of foods within each major food group ■ Selecting the appropriate number of servings from each major food group ■ Consuming sources of fiber such as bran and whole-grain breads and cereals, dried peas and beans, fresh fruits, and vegetables Behavioral matters including ■ Abandoning the idea of limiting weight gain to fit into clothes after pregnancy ■ Eating small, frequent meals ■ The importance of maintaining physical activity Where to find more information (see websites at the end of this chapter)

Evaluation

Evaluate and Monitor	■ Monitor for complaints of constipation ■ Monitor amount and pattern of weight gain ■ Suggest changes in the food plan as needed ■ Provide periodic feedback and support

 ## HOW DO YOU RESPOND?

Why don't pregnant women need to increase their calcium intake during pregnancy? The RDA for women age 19 to 50 years—whether pregnant or not—is 1000 mg. The reason why the RDA for calcium does not increase during pregnancy is that the body compensates for the increased need by more than doubling the rate of calcium absorption. If calcium intake was adequate before pregnancy, the amount consumed does not need to increase.

Is it true that pregnant and breastfeeding women should avoid certain foods to prevent allergies from developing in their children? According to a clinical report published by the AAP, there is insufficient evidence of a significant protective effect of maternal dietary restriction during pregnancy or lactation (Greer, Sicherer, Burks, and the Committee on Nutrition and Section on Allergy and Immunology, 2008). There is no convincing evidence that women who avoid eating peanuts or other foods during pregnancy or lactation lower their child's risk of allergies.

CASE STUDY

Sarah is 28 years old and 7 months pregnant with her third child. Her other children are aged 2½ and 1½ years. She had uncomplicated pregnancies and deliveries. Sarah is 5 ft 6 in tall; she weighed 142 pounds at the beginning of this pregnancy, which made her prepregnancy BMI 23. She has gained 24 pounds so far. Prior to her first pregnancy, her BMI was 20 (124 pounds). She is unhappy about her weight gain, but the stress of having two young children and being a stay-at-home mom made losing weight impossible.

She went online for her MyPlate plan, which recommends she consume 2400 cal/ day. She doesn't think she eats that much because she seems to have constant heartburn. She takes a prenatal supplement, so feels pretty confident that even if her intake is not perfect, she is getting all the nutrients she needs through her supplement. A typical day's intake for her is as follows:

Breakfast:	Cornflakes with whole milk (because the children drink whole milk) Orange juice
Snack:	Bran muffin and whole milk
Lunch:	Either a peanut butter and jelly sandwich or tuna fish sandwich with mayonnaise Snack crackers Whole milk Pudding or cookies
Snack:	Ice cream
Dinner:	Macaroni and cheese Green beans Roll and butter Whole milk Cake or ice cream for dessert
Evening:	Chips and salsa

- Does she have any risk factors for a high-risk pregnancy?
- Evaluate her prepregnancy weight and weight gain thus far. How much total weight should she gain?
- Based on the 2400-calorie meal pattern in Figure 11.1, what does Sarah need to eat more of? What is she eating in more than the recommended amounts? How would you suggest she modify her intake to minimize heartburn?
- What would you tell her about weight gain during pregnancy? What strategies would you suggest to her after her baby is born that would help her regain her healthy weight?
- Is her attitude about supplements appropriate? What would you tell her about supplements?

▶ Devise a 1-day menu for her that would provide all the food she needs in the recommended amounts and alleviate her heartburn.

STUDY QUESTIONS

1. A woman trying to become pregnant was told by her physician to take a daily supplement containing 400 μg of folic acid. She asks why a supplement is better than eating folic acid through food. Which statement is the nurses' best response?
   a. "There are few natural sources of folate in food."
   b. "Synthetic folic acid in supplements and fortified foods is better absorbed, more available, and a more reliable source than the folate found naturally in food."
   c. "Folate in food is equally as good as folic acid in supplements. It is just easier to take it in pill form and then you don't have to worry about how much you're getting in food."
   d. "If you are sure that you eat at least five servings of fruits and vegetables every day, you don't really need to take a supplement of folic acid."

2. A woman who was at her healthy weight when she got pregnant is distraught by her 5-pound weight gain between 20 and 24 weeks of gestation. At this point in her pregnancy, her weight gain is right on target. What is the nurse's best response?
   a. "A 5-pound per month weight gain at this point in your pregnancy is normal."
   b. "Although it is considerably less than the recommended amount, it is not a cause for concern. Just be sure to follow your meal plan next month so you get enough calories and nutrients."
   c. "I recommend you write down everything you eat for a few days so we can identify where the problem lies."
   d. "A 5-pound weight gain in 1 month at this point in your pregnancy may be a sign that you are at risk of preeclampsia. You should cut back on the 'extras' in your diet to limit your weight gain for next month."

3. Which of the following conditions are associated with a high-risk pregnancy? Select all that apply.
   a. Prepregnancy BMI of 20
   b. Prepregnancy BMI of greater than 25
   c. Maternal age of 30
   d. Pregnancies spaced less than 18 months apart

4. At her first prenatal visit, an overweight woman asks how much weight she should gain during the course of her pregnancy. What is the nurse's best response?
   a. "You should not gain any weight during your pregnancy. You have adequate calorie reserves to meet all the energy demands of pregnancy without gaining additional weight."
   b. "You should try to gain less than 15 pounds."
   c. "Aim for a 15- to 25-pound weight gain."
   d. "The recommended weight gain for your weight is 25 to 35 pounds."

5. Which of the following statements indicates that the pregnant woman understands the recommendations about caffeine intake during pregnancy?
   a. "I have to give up drinking coffee and cola."
   b. "I will limit my intake of coffee to about 2 cups a day and avoid other sources of caffeine."
   c. "As long as I don't drink coffee, I can eat other sources of caffeine because they don't contain enough to cause any problems."
   d. "Caffeine is harmless during pregnancy, so I am allowed to consume as much as I want."

6. What nutrient is not likely to be consumed in adequate amounts during pregnancy so a supplement is recommended?
   a. Iron
   b. Calcium
   c. Vitamin B_{12}
   d. Vitamin C

7. A woman at 5 weeks of gestation is complaining of nausea throughout the day. What should the nurse recommend?
   a. Small, frequent meals of easily digested carbohydrates
   b. Small, frequent meals that are high in protein
   c. A liquid diet until the nausea subsides
   d. A low fiber intake

8. Which of the following statements is true?
   a. "Women who breastfeed almost always achieve their prepregnancy weight at 6 weeks postpartum."
   b. "Weight loss during lactation is not recommended because it lowers the quantity and quality of breast milk produced."
   c. "Breastfeeding women do not have to increase their intake by the full amount of calories it 'costs' to produce milk because they can mobilize fat stored during pregnancy for some of the extra energy required."
   d. "Women do not need to increase their calorie intake at all for the first 6 months of breastfeeding because they can use calories stored in fat to produce milk."

KEY CONCEPTS

■ Although proper nutrition before and during pregnancy cannot guarantee a successful pregnancy outcome, it does profoundly affect fetal development and birth.

■ A healthy diet based on MyPlate food patterns is recommended before, during, and after pregnancy, with few modifications.

■ All women of childbearing age who are capable of becoming pregnant are urged to consume 400 μg of synthetic folic acid daily—through fortified foods or supplements—to reduce the risk of neural tube defects. The most critical period for the development of neural tube defects is the first month after conception when a woman may not even know she is pregnant.

■ Screening for iron deficiency anemia should occur prior to conception. Women should be encouraged to consume adequate heme iron, calcium, essential fatty acids, and iodine. The potential risks of using dietary supplements should be discussed.

■ Ideally, women should attain a healthy weight prior to conception.

■ Weight gain recommendations during pregnancy are based on a woman's BMI: 25 to 35 pounds for women of normal weight, 28 to 40 pounds for underweight women, 15 to 25 pounds for overweight women, and 11 to 20 pounds for obese women.

■ The recommended pattern of weight gain for normal-weight women is 1.1 to 4.4 pounds in the first trimester and approximately 1 pound/week for the rest of pregnancy. This pattern is adjusted up or down for women who are not within their healthy weight range at the time of conception.

■ Calorie requirements do not increase during the first trimester. In the second trimester, calorie needs increase by 340 cal/day and in the third trimester by 452 cal/day.

■ A woman who eats a varied diet with adequate calories should be able to meet her increased need for vitamins and minerals through food alone except for iron. Iron supplements are recommended. Folic acid requirements increase to 600 μg during pregnancy; supplements and/or fortified foods can provide this amount. Multivitamin and minerals are recommended for specific situations, such as during iron deficiency, for women carrying two or more fetuses, and when intake is poor.

■ Women are urged to avoid alcohol before and during pregnancy because a safe level is not known.

■ The consequences of foodborne illness can be devastating for a developing fetus. Pregnant women are urged to take precautions to avoid foodborne illness.

■ Pregnant women are advised to limit their caffeine intake to 300 mg/day or less—the equivalent of approximately 2 cups of coffee. Caffeine is associated with LBW but not with birth defects.

■ Nonnutritive sweeteners are safe to use during pregnancy with the amounts specified by the FDA.

■ Herbal supplements should not be used during pregnancy because their safety has not been tested during pregnancy or lactation.

■ Women are advised to limit their intake of predatory fish and to heed local advisories for fish consumption to limit their exposure to methylmercury. Mercury poisoning in a fetus can result in developmental delays, cerebral palsy, seizures, and mental retardation.

■ Pregnant woman should engage in moderate physical activity for at least 30 min/day on most days of the week. Safe activities include those that do not have a risk of fall or require lying down in the supine position after the second trimester of pregnancy.

■ Diabetes, gestational hypertension, and maternal PKU are maternal health conditions that can greatly impact fetal development and the course of pregnancy. Women with these conditions must be closely monitored.

■ A screening preformed at the first prenatal visit can identify women at potential nutritional risk during pregnancy and provides baseline data for ongoing monitoring. Adequacy of weight gain is related to adequacy of calorie intake.

■ Nutrition counseling should be initiated early in prenatal care and continue throughout the pregnancy. It should stress the importance of appropriate weight gain, ways to improve overall intake, and the benefits of breastfeeding.

■ Breastfeeding is recommended for the first 12 months of life. In addition to being uniquely suited to infant growth and development, it imparts other significant benefits to both infant and mother.

■ Almost all women are capable of breastfeeding.

■ The healthy diet recommended during pregnancy should be continued during lactation. Although more calories are needed during lactation than pregnancy once lactation is well established, women can eat less than the total calories needed and mobilize calories stored as fat to help regain prepregnancy weight.

■ Thirst is a reliable indicator of fluid need for most women during lactation.

■ Generally, when maternal intake of nutrients is inadequate, the quantity, not the quality, of breast milk is diminished.

■ In the postpartum period, attaining a healthy BMI is important for avoiding obesity and its health risks later in life.

Check Your Knowledge Answer Key

1. **FALSE** The amount of weight a woman gains during pregnancy is an important indicator of fetal growth. However, adequate weight gain during pregnancy cannot by itself ensure the delivery of a normal-birth-weight infant.

2. **FALSE** Obese women should gain 11 to 20 pounds during pregnancy. It is not known how much weight severely obese women should gain during pregnancy.

3. **TRUE** Fortified cereals are a significant source of folic acid. In fact, the recommended amount of folic acid could easily be exceeded with fortified cereal.

4. **TRUE** Both inadequate and excessive maternal weight gain during pregnancy are associated with overweight or obesity in the offspring later in life.

5. **FALSE** The RDA for calcium does not increase during pregnancy because calcium absorption greatly increases. Calcium needs can be met with the equivalent of 3 cups of milk daily.

6. **FALSE** Pregnant and lactating women as well as women who may become pregnant are advised to eliminate only shark, swordfish, king mackerel, and tilefish from their

diets; white albacore tuna should be limited to 6 oz/week, and other fish and shellfish can be consumed in amounts up to 12 oz/week as long as any one particular type of fish is not eaten more than once a week. Local advisories about fish caught in local waters should also be heeded.

7. **TRUE** Calorie requirements do not increase until the second trimester, and even then, the increase is small: an additional 340 calories for the second trimester and an additional 452 calories in the third trimester.

8. **TRUE** Lactation increases calorie recommendations by 500 for the first 6 months of breastfeeding and by 400 for the second 6 months. Women may eat fewer calories than this and still produce enough milk by mobilizing calories stored as fat.

9. **TRUE** An inadequate maternal intake of nutrients decreases the quantity of breast milk produced, not the quality.

10. **TRUE** Thirst is a good indicator of the need for fluids except among women who live in a dry climate or exercise in hot weather.

Student Resources on thePoint

For additional learning materials, activate the code in the front of this book at
http://thePoint.lww.com/activate

Websites

Academy of Nutrition and Dietetics at **www.eatright.org**
American Academy of Pediatrics at **www.aap.org**
American College of Obstetricians and Gynecologists at **www.acog.org**
Government nutrition information center at **www.nutrition.gov**
La Lèche League International at **www.lalecheleague.org**
March of Dimes at **www.marchofdimes.com**
MyPlate for Pregnancy and Breastfeeding at **www.choosemyplate.gov**
Supplemental Nutrition Program for Women, Infants, and Children (WIC) at **www.fns.usda.gov/fns**

References

Allen, L. (2005). Multiple micronutrients in pregnancy and lactation: An overview. *American Journal of Clinical Nutrition, 81*(Suppl.), 1206S–1212S.
American Academy of Pediatrics. (2012). *Breastfeeding and the use of human milk: Policy statement.* Available at www.pediatrics.org/cgi/doi/10.1542/peds.2011-3552. Accessed on 11/8/12.
American College of Obstetricians and Gynecologists. (2009). *ACOG Committee Opinion Number 267. Exercise during pregnancy and the postpartum period.* Available at http://www.acog.org/~/media/Committee%20Opinions/Committee%20on%20Obstetric%20Practice/co267.pdf?dmc=1&ts=20121108T1114276200. Accessed on 11/8/12.
American Dietetic Association. (2008). Position of the American Dietetic Association: Nutrition and lifestyle for a healthy pregnancy outcome. *Journal of the American Dietetic Association, 108,* 553–560.
American Dietetic Association. (2009a). Position of the American Dietetic Association and American Society for Nutrition: Obesity, preproduction, and pregnancy outcomes. *Journal of the American Dietetic Association, 109,* 918–927.
American Dietetic Association. (2009b). Position of the American Dietetic Association: Promoting and supporting breastfeeding. *Journal of the American Dietetic Association, 109,* 1926–1942.
Andres, A., Shankar, K., & Badger, T. (2012). Body fat mass of exclusively breastfed infants born to overweight mothers. *Journal of the Academy of Nutrition and Dietetics, 112,* 991–995.
Barker, D., & Osmond, C. (1986). Infant mortality, childhood nutrition, and ischemic heart disease in England and Wales. *The Lancet, 1,* 1077–1081.
Bloomingdale, A., Guthrie, L., Price, S., Wright, R. O., Platek, D., Haines, J., & Oken, E. (2010). A qualitative study of fish consumption during pregnancy. *American Journal of Clinical Nutrition, 92,* 1234–1240.

Borzychowski, A., Sargent, I., & Redman, C. (2006). Inflammation and pre-eclampsia. *Seminars in Fetal and Neonatal Medicine, 11*, 309–316.

Brodribb, W., Fallon, A., Hegney, D., & O'Brien, M. (2007). Identifying predictors of the reasons women give for choosing to breastfeed. *Journal of Human Lactation, 23*, 338–344.

Catalano, P. (2007). Management of obesity in pregnancy. *Obstetrics and Gynecology, 109*, 419–433.

Centers for Disease Control and Prevention. (2012a). *Breastfeeding report card—United States, 2012.* Available at www.cdc.gov/breastfeeding/data/reportcard.htm. Accessed on 11/9/12.

Centers for Disease Control and Prevention. (2012b). *Clinical Care for women. Health promotion. Family planning and reproductive life plan.* Available at www.cdc.gov/preconception/careforwomen/promotion.html. Accessed on 11/2/12.

Centers for Disease Control and Prevention. (2012c). *Preconception care and health care. Clinical care for women. Nutrition.* Available at www.cdc.gov/preconception/careforwomen/nutrition.html. Accessed on 11/2/12.

Corbett, R., Ryan, C., & Weinrich, S. (2003). Pica in pregnancy: Does it affect pregnancy outcomes? *Maternal Child Nursing, 28*, 183–191.

Crozier, S., Inskip, H., Godfrey, K., Cooper, C., Harvey, N. C., Cole, Z. A., & Robinson, S. M. (2010). Weight gain in pregnancy and childhood body composition: Findings from the Southampton Women's Survey. *American Journal of Clinical Nutrition, 91*, 1745–1751.

Duley, L., Henderson-Smart, D., & Meher, S. (2005). Altered dietary salt for preventing pre-eclampsia, and its complications. *Cochrane Database System Reviews,* (4), CD005548.

Durham, H., Lovelady, C., Brouwer, R., Krause, K. M., & Ostbye, T. (2011). Comparison of dietary intake of overweight postpartum mothers practicing breastfeeding or formula feeding. *Journal of the American Dietetic Association, 111*, 67–74.

Englund-Ogge, L., Brantsaeter, A., Haugen, M., Sengpiel, V., Khatibi, A., Myhre, R., . . . Jacobsson, B. (2012). Association between intake of artificially sweetened and sugar-sweetened beverages and preterm delivery: A large prospective cohort study. *American Journal of Clinical Nutrition, 96*, 552–559.

Godfrey, K., & Barker, D. (2001). Fetal programming and adult health. *Public Health Nutrition, 4*, 611–624.

Greer, F. R., Sicherer, S. H., Burks, A. W., & the Committee on Nutrition and Section on Allergy and Immunology. (2008). Effects of early nutritional interventions on the development of atopic disease in infants and children: The role of maternal dietary restriction, breastfeeding, timing of introduction of complementary foods, and hydrolyzed formulas. *Pediatrics, 121*, 183–191.

Institute of Medicine. (1998). *Dietary reference intakes for thiamin, riboflavin, niacin, vitamin B$_6$, folate, vitamin B$_{12}$, pantothenic acid, biotin, and choline.* Washington, DC: National Academies Press.

Institute of Medicine. (2005). *Dietary reference intakes for energy, carbohydrates, fiber, fat, fatty acids, cholesterol, protein, and amino acids (macronutrients).* Washington, DC: National Academies Press.

Johnson, D. B., Gerstein, D. E., Evans, A. E., & Woodward-Lopez, G. (2006). Preventing obesity: A life cycle perspective. *Journal of the American Dietetic Association, 106*, 97–102.

Josefson, J. (2011). The impact of pregnancy nutrition on offspring obesity. *Journal of the American Dietetic Association, 111*, 50–52.

Kim, H., & Nelson, L. (2012). Are you what you eat? Pica in pregnancy. *Emergency Medicine.* Available at http://www.emedmag.com/PDF/044070004.pdf. Accessed on 11/12/12.

Krummel, D. (2007). Postpartum weight control: A vicious cycle. *Journal of the American Dietetic Association, 107*, 37–40.

Lenke, R., & Levy, H. (1980). Maternal phenylketonuria and hyperphenylalaninemia. An international survey of the outcome of untreated and treated pregnancies. *The New England Journal of Medicine, 303*, 1201–1208.

Lovelady, C. A., Garner, K. E., Moreno, K. L., & Williams, J. P. (2000). The effect of weight loss in overweight, lactating women on the growth of their infants. *The New England Journal of Medicine, 342*, 449–453.

Lovelady, C. A., Stephenson, K. G., Kuppler, K. M., & Williams, J. P. (2006). The effects of dieting on food and nutrient intake of lactating women. *Journal of the American Dietetic Association, 106*, 908–912.

MacNeil, P., Lyon, J., McGrane, M., & Spahn, J. (2012). A systematic review of the health effects of alcohol consumption on lactation performance. *Journal of the Academy of Nutrition and Dietetics, 112*, A93.

Mamun, A., Kinarivala, M., O'Callaghan, M., Williams, G. M., Najman, J. M., & Callaway, L. K. (2010). Associations of excess weight gain during pregnancy with long-term maternal overweight and obesity: Evidence from 21 y postpartum follow-up. *American Journal of Clinical Nutrition, 91,* 1336–1341.

March of Dimes. (2012). *Folic acid for a healthy pregnancy and baby.* Available at http://www .marchofdimes.com/pregnancy/folicacid.html. Accessed on 11/8/12.

Maslova, E., Bhattacharya, S., Lin, S., & Michels, K. (2010). Caffeine consumption during pregnancy and risk of preterm birth: A meta-analysis. *American Journal of Clinical Nutrition, 92,* 1120–1132.

McCann, M., Baydar, N., & Williams, R. (2007). Breastfeeding attitudes and reported problems in a national sample of WIC participants. *Journal of Human Lactation, 23,* 314–324.

National Research Council. (2009). *Weight gain during pregnancy: Reexamining the guidelines.* Washington, DC: The National Academies Press.

Njiru, H., Elchalal, U., & Paltiel, O. (2011). Geophagy during pregnancy in Africa: A literature review. *Obstetrical and Gynecological Survey, 66,* 452–459.

Poston, L., Briley, A., Seed, P., Kelly, F. J., & Shennan, A. H. (2006). Vitamin C and vitamin E in pregnant women at risk for pre-eclampsia (VIP trial): Randomized placebo-controlled trial. *The Lancet, 367,* 1145–1154.

Ricciotti, H. (2008). Nutrition and lifestyle for a healthy pregnancy. *American Journal of Lifestyle Medicine, 2,* 151–158.

Rooney, B., Schauberger, C., & Mathiason, M. (2005). Impact of perinatal weight change on long-term obesity and obesity-related illnesses. *Obstetrics and Gynecology, 106,* 1349–1356.

Sibai, B. (2003). Diagnosis and management of gestational hypertension and preeclampsia. *Obstetrics and Gynecology, 102,* 181–102.

U.S. Department of Agriculture, U.S. Department of Health and Human Services. (2010). *Dietary guidelines for Americans, 2010* (7th ed.). Available at www.health.gov/dietaryguidelines. Accessed on 11/12/12.

U.S. Food and Drug Administration. (2004). *What you need to know about mercury in fish and shellfish. 2004 EPA and FDA advice for women who might become pregnant, nursing mothers, and young children.* Available at. http://www.fda.gov/Food/FoodSafety/Product-SpecificInformation/ Seafood/FoodbornePathogensContaminants/Methylmercury/ucm115662.htm. Accessed on 11/12/12.

van Calcar, S., & Ney, D. (2012). Food products made with glycomacropeptide, a low-phenylalanine whey protein, provide a new alternative to amino acid-based medical foods for nutrition management of phenylketonuria. *Journal of the Academy of Nutrition and Dietetics, 112,* 1201–1210.

World Health Organization. (2011). *Exclusive breastfeeding for six months best for babies everywhere.* Available at http://www.who.int/mediacentre/news/statements/2011/breastfeeding_ 20110115/en/#. Accessed on 11/8/12.

Wrotniak, B., Shults, J., Butts, S., & Stettler, N. (2008). Gestational weight gain and risk of overweight in the offspring at age 7 y in a multicenter, multi-ethnic cohort study. *American Journal of Clinical Nutrition, 87,* 1818–1824.

Yogev, Y., & Catalano, P. (2009). Pregnancy and obesity. *Obstetrics and Gynecology Clinics of North America, 36,* 285–300.

Zeisel, S. (2009). Is maternal diet supplementation beneficial? Optimal development of infant depends on mother's diet. *American Journal of Clinical Nutrition, 89*(Suppl.), 685S–687S.

Zhou, S., Yelland, L., McPhee, A., Quinlivan, J., Gibson, R., & Makrides, M. (2012). Fish-oil supplementation in pregnancy does not reduce the risk of gestational diabetes or preeclampsia. *American Journal of Clinical Nutrition, 95,* 1378–1384.

12 Nutrition for Infants, Children, and Adolescents

CHECK YOUR KNOWLEDGE

TRUE	FALSE		
☐	☐	**1**	Infants have higher requirements per kilogram of body weight for calories and most nutrients than adults do.
☐	☐	**2**	If breastfeeding is discontinued before the infant's first birthday, nutrition should be supplied with iron-fortified infant formula.
☐	☐	**3**	Protein is the nutrient of most concern when solids are introduced into the diet.
☐	☐	**4**	A potential problem with early introduction of solid foods is overfeeding.
☐	☐	**5**	The risk of nutrient deficiencies among American toddlers is low.
☐	☐	**6**	The *Dietary Guidelines for Americans, 2010* do not apply to children, only adolescents and adults.
☐	☐	**7**	Iron deficiency in young children may be related to drinking too much milk.
☐	☐	**8**	Children who regularly skip breakfast have lower intakes of vitamins and minerals than children who normally eat breakfast.
☐	☐	**9**	Overweight youth are at risk for the same complications from overweight that afflict adults—namely, type 2 diabetes, high blood pressure, and metabolic syndrome.
☐	☐	**10**	Among 2- to 18-year-olds, the intake of empty calories far exceeds empty calorie allowance for all age–sex groups.

LEARNING OBJECTIVES

Upon completion of this chapter, you will be able to

1 Compare breastfeeding to formula feeding.
2 Explain how adequacy of intake is assessed for the pediatric population.
3 Give examples of feeding skills seen throughout the first year of life.
4 Describe common eating practices of children that may place them at nutritional risk.
5 Summarize nutritional concerns that arise during childhood and adolescence.
6 Evaluate a youth's diet according to MyPlate food intake recommendations.

The health of American children is improving by some aspects and deteriorating in others. Deficiency diseases and infant mortality have declined over recent decades; however, the prevalence of obesity among children and adolescents has almost tripled since 1980 (Centers for Disease Control and Prevention [CDC], 2012). The statistics are alarming:

- Ten percent to 20% of infants and toddlers in the United States are overweight (≥85th body mass index [BMI] percentile for age) (Ogden, Carroll, Curtin, Lamb, and Flegal, 2010).
- Almost 10% of infants and toddlers from birth to the age of 2 years are obese (≥95th percentile of weight for length) (Ogden et al., 2010).
- Twenty-one percent of children age 2 to 5 years are overweight or obese (Ogden et al., 2010).
- An overweight child between age 2 and 4 years has a fivefold greater risk of being overweight at age 12 years compared to children who are not overweight as preschoolers (De Kroon, Renders, Van Wouwe, Van Buuren, and Hirasing, 2010).
- Approximately 17% of children and adolescents from ages 2 to 19 years old are obese (CDC, 2012).

The goals of nutrition and physical activity for children are to promote optimal physical and cognitive development, a healthy weight, an enjoyment of food, and a decreased risk of chronic disease (American Dietetic Association [ADA], 2008). Actual nutrient requirements vary according to health status, activity pattern, and growth rate. The greater the rate of growth, the more intense are the nutritional needs. Meeting needs is essential; also important is avoiding nutrient and calorie excesses.

INFANCY (BIRTH TO 1 YEAR)

Excluding fetal growth, growth in the first year of life is more rapid than at any other time in the life cycle. Birth weight doubles by 4 to 6 months of age and triples by the first birthday. Length increases by approximately 10 in during the first year. Adequate calories and nutrients are needed to support the unprecedented rate of growth.

Recommendations for the amount of calories, macronutrients, vitamins, and minerals infants should consume are based on the average intakes of healthy full-term newborns who are exclusively breastfed by well-nourished mothers. Although the total amount of calories and nutrients are generally far less than what adults need, the infant's needs are much higher per kilogram of body weight. Proportionately, infants use large amounts of energy and nutrients to fuel their body processes and growth.

Breast Milk

Breast milk is specifically designed to support optimal growth and development in the newborn, and its composition makes it uniquely superior for infant feeding (Box 12.1) (American Academy of Pediatrics [AAP], 2012a). Breastfeeding is credited with numerous potential health benefits for the infant, including lower risks of otitis media, upper respiratory tract infection, lower respiratory tract infection, asthma, atopic dermatitis, gastroenteritis, obesity, celiac disease, type 1 and type 2 diabetes, certain types of leukemia, and sudden infant death syndrome (AAP, 2012a). Although many of these benefits are linked to breastfeeding for 3 months of more, some benefits occur with any duration of breastfeeding, such as the reduced risk of obesity and type 2 diabetes. The AAP contends that because

Box 12.1   COMPOSITION OF BREAST MILK

- The protein content of breast milk is adequate to support growth and development without contributing to an excessive renal solute load.
- The majority of the protein is easy-to-digest whey.
- Breast milk contains small amounts of amino acids that may be harmful in large amounts (e.g., phenylalanine) and high levels of amino acids that infants cannot synthesize well (e.g., taurine).
- The fat in breast milk is easily digested because of fat-digesting enzymes contained in the milk.
- The content of linoleic acid (an essential fatty acid) is high.
- The high level of cholesterol is believed to help infants develop enzyme systems capable of handling cholesterol later in life.
- Breast milk contains amylase (a starch-digesting enzyme), which may promote starch digestion in early infancy when pancreatic amylase is low or absent.
- Breast milk contains enough minerals to support adequate growth and development but not excessive amounts that would burden immature kidneys with a high renal solute load.
- The minerals are mostly protein bound and balanced to enhance bioavailability. For instance, the rate of iron absorption from breast milk is approximately 50% compared with about 4% for iron-fortified formulas. Zinc absorption is better from breast milk than from either cow's milk or formula.
- All vitamins needed for growth and health are supplied in breast milk, but the vitamin content of breast milk varies with the mother's diet.
- The renal solute load of breast milk is approximately one-half that of commercial formulas. The low renal solute load is suited to the immature kidneys' inability to concentrate urine.
- Athough they are more abundant in colostrum, antibodies and anti-infective factors are present in mature breast milk. Bifidus factor promotes the growth of normal gastrointestinal (GI) flora (e.g., *Lactobacillus bifidus*) that protect the infant against harmful GI bacteria.

of the short- and long-term medical and neurodevelopmental benefits of breastfeeding, infant nutrition should be considered a public health issue and not simply a lifestyle choice (AAP, 2012a). The AAP recommends exclusive breastfeeding for the first 6 months of life, which, with few exceptions (Box 12.2), is considered adequate to meet the needs of healthy, full-term infants. Even after solid foods are introduced, breastfeeding should continue for at least the first 12 months of age. What the breastfeeding mother needs to know appears in Box 12.3.

Box 12.2   AMERICAN ACADEMY OF PEDIATRICS RECOMMENDATIONS FOR SUPPLEMENTS FOR BREASTFED, HEALTHY, FULL-TERM INFANTS

- Intramuscular vitamin K after the first feeding and within the first 6 hours of life.
- 400 IU/day of vitamin D beginning at hospital discharge for breastfed and partially breastfed infants. Supplementation should continue daily until daily intake of vitamin D–fortified formula or milk is approximately 1 quart.
- Fluoride should not be given during the first 6 months of life; from age 6 months to 3 years, the decision to provide supplemental fluoride should be based on the fluoride content of the drinking water and other sources, including toothpaste.
- Oral iron drops may be needed before 6 months to support iron stores.

Source: American Academy of Pediatrics. (2012). Policy statement. Breastfeeding and the use of human milk. *Pediatrics, 129,* e827–e841.

Box 12.3   TEACHING POINTS FOR BREASTFEEDING

- The infant should be allowed to nurse for 5 minutes on each breast on the first day to achieve letdown and milk ejection. By the end of the first week, the infant should be nursing up to 15 minutes per breast.
- In the first few weeks of breastfeeding, the infant may nurse 8 to 12 times every 24 hours. Mothers should offer the breast whenever the infant shows early signs of hunger, such as increased alertness, physical activity, mouthing, or rooting. After breastfeeding is well established, eight feedings every 24 hours may be appropriate.
- The first breast offered should be alternated with every feeding so both breasts receive equal stimulation and draining.
- Even though the infant will be able to virtually empty the breast within 5 to 10 minutes once the milk supply is established, the infant needs to nurse beyond that point to satisfy the need to suck and to receive emotional and physical comfort.

- The supply of milk is equal to the demand—the more the infant sucks, the more milk is produced. Infants age 6 weeks or 12 weeks who suck more are probably experiencing a growth spurt and so need more milk.
- Water and juice are unnecessary for breastfed infants in the first 6 months of life, even in hot climates.
- Early substitution of formula or introduction of solid foods may decrease the chance of maintaining lactation.
- Infants weaned before 12 months of age should be given iron-fortified formula, not cow's milk.
- Both feeding the infant more frequently and manually expressing milk will help to increase the milk supply.
- Breast milk can be pumped, placed in a sanitary bottle, and immediately refrigerated or frozen for later use. Milk should be used within 24 hours if refrigerated or within 3 months if stored in the freezer compartment of the refrigerator.

Infant Formula

Infant formulas may be used in place of breastfeeding, as an occasional supplement to breastfeeding, or when exclusively breastfed infants are weaned before 12 months of age. Term formulas contain cow's milk protein and lactose and are made to resemble human milk. The Infant Formula Act regulates the levels of nutrients in formulas, specifying both minimum and maximum amounts of each essential nutrient. Almost all formula used in the United States is iron fortified, a practice that has greatly reduced the risk of iron deficiency in older infants (Krebs and Hambidge, 2007). Because the minimum recommended amount of each nutrient is more than the amount provided in breast milk, nutrient supplements are unnecessary. There are no data to support the use of one term formula over another; they are all nutritionally interchangeable (O'Connor, 2009).

Recently, formulas with long-chain polyunsaturated fatty acids (arachidonic acid and docosahexaenoic acid [DHA], an omega-3 fatty acid) have been marketed to promote eye and brain development (O'Connor, 2009). They are more costly than routine formulas, and most well-conducted randomized trials show no benefit to using them.

A variety of other formulas are available (Table 12.1):

- Preterm formula is intended for infants born before 34 weeks of gestation. Designed to promote "catch-up" growth, these formulas are higher in calories, protein, calcium, magnesium, and phosphorus than routine formulas. Hospital discharge before 34 weeks of gestational age is rare, so these formulas are typically only used in the hospital.
- Enriched formula for infants 34 to 36 weeks of gestation—these formulas contain more calories than term formula but less than preterm formula.

Table 12.1 Infant Formulas

Category	Carbohydrate Source	Protein Source	Indications
Formulas providing 20 cal/oz			
Term formula (e.g., Enfamil with iron, Similac with iron)	Lactose	Cow's milk	Routine
Term formula with added long-chain fatty acids (e.g., Enfamil Lipid, Similac Advance)	Lactose	Cows' milk	Claims to promote eye and brain development
Soy formula (e.g., Enfamil ProSobee, Similac Isomil)	Corn based	Soy	Congenital lactase deficiency, galactosemia
Lactose-free formula (e.g., Enfamil Lactofree, Similac Sensitive)	Corn based	Cow's milk	Congenital and primary lactase deficiency, galactosemia; gastroenteritis in at-risk infants
Hypoallergenic formula (e.g., Enfamil Nutramigen, Similac Alimentum)	Corn or sucrose	Extensively hydrolyzed protein	Milk protein allergy
Antireflux formula (e.g., Similac Sensitive RS)	Lactose thickened with rice starch	Cow's milk	Gastroesophageal reflux
Formulas providing 24 cal/oz			
Preterm formula (e.g., Enfamil 24 Premature, Similac 24 Special Care)	Lactose	Cow's milk	Less than 34 weeks of gestation; weight less than 3 pounds 15 oz
Formulas providing 22 cal/oz			
Enriched formula (e.g., Enfacare, Similac Neosure)	Lactose	Cow's milk	34–36 weeks of gestation; weight of 3 pounds 15 oz or greater

Source: O'Connor, N. (2009). Infant formula. *American Family Physician, 79,* 565–570.

- Soy formula that is intended to be used only for infants with galactosemia or congenital lactase deficiency or from strict vegan families. However, soy formula accounts for almost 25% of formulas sales in the United States (Bhatia and Greer, 2008). Recently, an expert panel was convened to evaluate the safety of soy formula on infant and child development arising from laboratory animal studies that showed the isoflavones found in soy formulas had an adverse effect on development (National Institute of Environmental Health Sciences, National Institutes of Health, U.S. Department of Health and Human Services [USDHHS], 2010). The National Toxicology Program concurred with the opinion of the expert panel that there is minimal concern for adverse effects on development in infants who consume soy formula.
- Lactose-free formula that contains a corn-based carbohydrate for infants with congenital or primary lactase deficiency, galactosemia, or gastroenteritis in at-risk infants
- Hypoallergenic and nonallergenic formulas for infant with an allergy to milk protein
- Antireflux formulas for infants with gastroesophageal reflux
- Specialty formulas for infants with inborn errors of metabolism, such as phenylketonuria (PKU) or maple syrup urine disease. These specialized formulas are intentionally lacking or deficient in one or more nutrients, so they do not supply adequate nutrition for normal infants. They must be supplemented with small amounts of regular formula.

The amount of formula provided per feeding and the frequency of feeding depend on the infant's age and individual needs. General parameters are provided in Table 12.2. Overfeeding is one of the biggest hazards of formula feeding. Caregivers should recognize

Table 12.2 General Parameters for Formula Feeding

Age	Number of Feedings in 24 Hours	Amount per Feeding (oz)
1 month	6–8	2–4
2 months	5–6	5–6
3–5 months	4–5	6–7

that infants cry for reasons other than hunger and should not be fed every time they cry, nor should an infant be forced to finish her or his bottle. To avoid nursing bottle caries, infants and children should not be put to bed with a bottle of formula, milk, juice, or other sweetened liquid (Fig. 12.1). Teaching points for formula feeding are summarized in Box 12.4.

Infant Feeding and Obesity

Many overweight infants remain overweight as children; childhood obesity has long been known as a strong predictor of adult obesity (Whitaker, Wright, Pepe, Seidel, and Dietz, 1997). Research suggests that the critical period for establishing dietary intake patterns, eating habits, and food preferences begins in infancy and, although inconsistent, may be set as early as 2 years of age (Cashdan, 1994). Strategies to reduce rates of overweight in very young children are gaining greater attention, particularly parental feeding practices that may promote obesity, such as inattention to hunger and satiety cues or using controlling, rewarding, or restrictive feeding (Dattilo et al., 2012).

Breastfeeding duration and/or exclusivity has been inversely related to the rate of weight gain during infancy and with weight and risk of overweight and obesity in toddlers and preschoolers (Gillman, 2008; Griffiths, Smeeth, Hawkins, Cole, and Dezateux, 2009; Gunnarsdottir, Schack-Neilsen, Michaelsen, Sørensen, and Thorsdottir, 2010; USDHHS, 2011). Exclusive breastfeeding for at least the first 6 months of age is recommended (Dattilo et al., 2012). Exactly how breastfeeding is protective against obesity in later life is not clear. Potential explanations have been suggested:

- Formula-fed infants generally grow quicker than breastfed infants during infancy (Nommsen-Rivers and Dewey, 2009), and at 1 year of age, formula-fed infants tend to have a higher body weight and weight for length (Kramer et al., 2004). A number of studies show that high postnatal weight gain increases the risk of later obesity (Chomtho et al., 2008; Stettler et al., 2005).

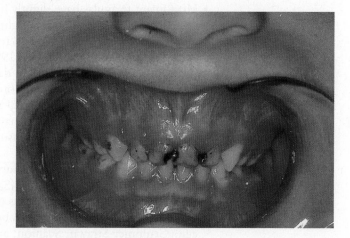

■ FIGURE 12.1 Nursing bottle caries. Notice the extensive decay in the upper teeth. (© K. L. Boyd, DDS/Custom Medical Stock Photo)

Box 12.4 TEACHING POINTS FOR FORMULA FEEDING

One of the greatest hazards of formula feeding is overfeeding. Never force the infant to finish a bottle or to take more than he or she wants. Signs that an infant is finished include biting the nipple, puckering the face, and turning away from the bottle. Discourage the misconception that "a fat baby = a healthy baby = good parents."

Each feeding should last 20 to 30 minutes.

Formula may be given at room temperature, slightly warmed, or directly from the refrigerator; however, always give formula at approximately the same temperature.

Spitting up of a small amount of formula during or after a feeding is normal. Feed the infant more slowly and burp more frequently to help alleviate spitting up.

Hold the infant closely and securely. Position the infant so that the head is higher than the rest of the body.

Avoid jiggling the bottle and making extra movements that could distract the infant from feeding.

Check the flow of formula by holding the bottle upside down. A steady drip from the nipple should be observed. If the flow is too rapid because of a too large nipple opening, the infant may overfeed and develop indigestion. If the flow rate is too slow because of a too small nipple opening, the infant may tire and fall asleep without taking enough formula. Discard any nipples with holes that are too large, and enlarge holes that are too small with a sterilized needle.

Reassure caregivers that there is no danger of "spoiling" an infant by feeding him or her when the infant cries for a feeding.

Burp the infant halfway through the feeding, at the end of the feeding, and more often if necessary to help get rid of air swallowed during feeding. Burping can be accomplished by gently rubbing or patting the infant's back as he or she is held on the shoulder, lies on his or her stomach over the caregiver's lap, or sits in an upright position.

After the teeth erupt, the baby should be given only plain water for a bedtime bottle-feeding. Never prop the bottle or put the infant to bed with a bottle.

- Formula-fed infants have different feeding patterns than breastfed infants, which may impact later obesity risk (Koletzko et al., 2009). Formula-fed infants have a lower frequency of meals and a longer interval between feedings than typically found in breastfed infants.
- The nutrient content and taste of human milk vary. It is postulated that early exposure to differences in taste may program infants to different food selection and dietary habits later in life compared to formula-fed infants (Mennella, Jagnow, and Beauchamp, 2001).
- Most infant formulas have slightly higher calorie density than breast milk, and calories consumed per kilogram of body weight in formula-fed infants ages 3 to 12 months have been reported to be approximately 10% to 18% higher than breastfed infants (Heinig, Nommsen, Peerson, Lonnerdal, and Dewey, 1993).
- Even more striking than calorie density is the difference in protein intake: formula-fed infants consume 55% to 80% more protein per kilogram than breastfed infants (Alexy, Kersting, Sichert-Hellert, Manz, and Schöch, 1999). Some proposed mechanisms by which a higher protein intake may predispose infants to obesity later in life include its effect on energy expenditure, insulin secretion, and human growth hormone secretion (Koletzko et al., 2009).
- Studies suggest breastfeeding during early infancy is associated with greater appetite regulation later in childhood (DiSantis, Collins, Fisher, and Davey, 2011). Breastfed infants are not subjected to parents urging them to "finish the bottle."
- Breastfed infants are less likely to be given complementary foods at less than 4 months of age (Grummer-Strawn, Scanlon, and Fein, 2008). Late introduction of complementary

feedings may protect against adult overweight (Schack-Nielsen, Sorensen, Mortensen, and Michaelsen, 2010).

Complementary Foods: Introducing Solids

Introducing complementary foods earlier than 4 months of age is associated with early or excessive weight in infants, toddlers, and preschoolers (Hawkins, Cole, and Law, 2009; Huh, Rifas-Shiman, Taveras, Oken, and Gillman, 2011; Sloan, Gildea, Stewart, Sneddon, and Iwaniec, 2008). Parents are urged to delay introducing solid foods until the infant exhibits developmental readiness.

Physiologically, complementary foods become a necessary source of nutrients at around 6 months of age because neonatal nutrient reserves become depleted and the concentrations of some nutrients in breast milk, such as zinc, decline over time (Krebs and Hambidge, 2007). Developmentally, most infants exhibit readiness to spoon-feed around 4 to 6 months of age as reflexes disappear, head control develops, and the infant is able to sit. Over time, control of the head, neck, jaw, and tongue; hand–eye coordination; and the ability to sit, grasp, chew, drink, and self-feed evolve. The eruption of teeth indicates readiness to progress from strained to mashed to chopped fine to regular consistency foods. Guidelines for introducing solids on the basis of developmental readiness appear in Table 12.3.

For both breastfed and formula-fed infants, iron-fortified infant cereal is traditionally the first solid food introduced. To increase the likelihood of acceptance, parents are urged to give a small amount of formula or breast milk to take the edge off hunger before beginning the cereal. Iron-fortified infant cereals are recommended until the infant is 12 to 18 months old because the iron in these cereals is absorbed more readily than that from other cereals.

Traditionally, the order of foods introduced after iron-fortified cereals was vegetables, fruits, meats, and then eggs. The order is no longer considered important, and some experts recommend offering meat as one of the first complementary foods because of its iron and zinc content (AAP, 2012b). Although easily chewed red meats, such as baby food meat and home-pureed cooked meats are recommended, relatively few infants under 9 months are fed baby or nonbaby meats of any kind (Siega-Riz et al., 2010). Commercial baby food dinners are more commonly consumed. Chicken and turkey, which provide less heme iron than red meats, are the most popular meats, followed by hot dogs, sausages, and cold cuts, which are higher in fat and sodium and lower in iron and zinc than plain meats.

New foods should be introduced in plain and simple form one at a time for a period of 5 to 7 days to identify allergic reactions, such as rashes, fussiness, vomiting, diarrhea, or constipation. If there is a positive family history for food allergies, milk, eggs, wheat, and citrus fruits should be introduced cautiously. Peanuts and peanut butter should be avoided because of the potential for severe allergic reaction.

Infants differ in the amount of food they want or need at each feeding. The amount of solid food taken at a feeding may vary from 1 to 2 tsp initially to ¼ to ½ cup as the infant gets older. To avoid overfeeding, infants and children should be allowed to self-regulate the amount of food consumed. Only healthy foods should be introduced; it may take 15 to 20 exposures before a new food is accepted (Johnson, 2000). Parents should be cautioned against introducing empty-calorie foods simply to provide calories. The high nutritional requirements for healthy growth and development leave little room for foods with low nutritional value (May and Dietz, 2010). Tips for creating a positive eating environment are listed in Box 12.5.

Fruit juices were once considered essential complementary foods. The AAP Committee on Nutrition (2001) recommends that 100% fruit juice not be introduced until after 6 months of age, recognizing that it provides no nutritional benefits over whole fruit. Excessive amounts of juice may displace the intake of nutrient-rich food and milk in the diet and contribute to an excessive calorie intake.

Table 12.3 Sequence of Infant Development and Feeding Skills in Normal, Healthy, Full-Term Infants*

Developmental Skills			
Baby's Approximate Age	Mouth Patterns	Hand and Body Skills	Feeding Skills or Abilities
Birth through 5 months	▪ Suck/swallow reflex ▪ Tongue thrust reflex ▪ Rooting reflex ▪ Gag reflex	▪ Poor control of head, neck, trunk ▪ Brings hands to mouth around 3 months	▪ Swallows liquids but pushes most solid objects from the mouth
4 months through 6 months	▪ Draws in upper or lower lip as spoon is removed from mouth ▪ Up-and-down munching movement ▪ Can transfer food from front to back of tongue to swallow ▪ Tongue thrust and rooting reflexes begin to disappear ▪ Gag reflex diminishes ▪ Opens mouth when sees spoon approaching	▪ Sits with support ▪ Good head control ▪ Uses whole hand to grasp objects (palmar grasp)	▪ Takes in a spoonful of pureed or strained food and swallows it without choking ▪ Drinks small amounts from cup when held by another person, with spilling
5 months through 9 months	▪ Begins to control the position of food in the mouth ▪ Up-and-down munching movement ▪ Positions food between jaws for chewing	▪ Begins to sit alone unsupported ▪ Follows food with eyes ▪ Begins to use thumb and index finger to pick up objects (pincer grasp)	▪ Begins to eat mashed foods ▪ Eats from a spoon easily ▪ Drinks from a cup with some spilling ▪ Begins to feed self with hands
8 months through 11 months	▪ Moves food from side-to-side in mouth ▪ Begins to curve lips around rim of cup ▪ Begins to chew in rotary pattern (diagonal movement of the jaw as food is moved to the side or center of the mouth)	▪ Sits alone easily ▪ Transfers objects from hand to mouth	▪ Begins to eat ground or finely chopped food and small pieces of soft food ▪ Begins to experiment with spoon but prefers to feed self with hands ▪ Drinks from a cup with less spilling
10 months through 12 months	▪ Rotary chewing (diagonal movement of the jaw as food is moved to the side or center of the mouth)	▪ Begins to put spoon in mouth ▪ Begins to hold cup ▪ Good eye-hand-mouth coordination	▪ Eats chopped food and small pieces of soft, cooked table food ▪ Begins self-spoon feeding with help

*Developmental stages may vary with individual babies.

Source: U.S. Department of Agriculture Food Nutrition Service. (n.d.). *Feeding infants. A guide for use in child nutrition programs.* Available at www.fns.usda.gov/tn/Resources/feedinginfants-ch2.pdf. Accessed on 11/13/12.

Box 12.5   TIPS TO CREATE A POSITIVE EATING ENVIRONMENT

- Keep in mind that it is not important if a child refuses to eat a particular food (e.g., spinach), so long as the child has a reasonable intake from each major food group.
- Offer a variety of foods, not just the ones you like. Repeated exposures may be needed before a child accepts a new food.
- Fat and cholesterol should not be limited in the diets of very young children, who need fat and cholesterol for their developing brains and nervous systems.
- Never force a child to eat; if a healthy child is hungry, he or she will eat.
- Do not use food to reward, punish, bribe, or convey love.

- Let toddlers explore and enjoy food, even if it means eating with their fingers.
- Space meals further apart and limit snacking so the child will be hungry at mealtimes.
- Keep mealtime relaxed, pleasant, and unhurried, allowing 20 to 30 minutes per meal.
- Eat with the child.
- Children may refuse to eat because they are (1) too excited or distracted, (2) seeking attention, (3) expressing independence, (4) too tired, or (5) simply not hungry. When any of these instances occur, remove the child's plate without comment. If the child wants a snack later, make it nutritious.

NUTRITION FOR TODDLERS AND PRESCHOOLERS

Evidence suggests that dietary habits acquired in early childhood persist through to adulthood (Kelder, Perry, Klepp, and Lytle, 1994). Parents are the primary gatekeepers and role models for their young children's food intake and habits; their feeding practices and style have been shown to affect children's eating behavior and their weight status (de Lauzon-Guillain et al., 2012). Parents should decide what foods the child is offered, when the child eats, and where eating takes place; the child should decide whether he or she wants to eat. Although it is commonly assumed that children who are allowed to self-serve consume fewer calories, results of a recent study showed that this is not necessarily true (Savage, Haisfield, Fisher, Marini, and Birch, 2012). Some children need guidance and rules to learn how to self-select appropriate portion sizes. Tips for getting children on the path to healthy eating appear in Figure 12.2.

Calories and Nutrients

There is very little research on the best ways to achieve optimal nutritional intakes from 1 to 2 years of age, the transition period between infancy and childhood. The dramatic decrease in growth rate is reflected in a disinterest in food, a "physiologic anorexia" due to lower calorie needs per kilogram of body weight. Two-year-olds should eat approximately 1000 calories per day in three meals with one to two snacks.

The *Dietary Guidelines for Americans, 2010* are intended for people who are age 2 years and older; thus, the content of childhood diets should be similar to that of adult diets. The basic messages are to choose whole grains for at least half the total grain intake; eat plenty of colorful fruit and vegetables; choose low-fat or nonfat milk; choose lean proteins; and limit solid fats, added sugars, and sodium (U.S. Department of Agriculture [USDA], USDHHS, 2010). The AAP recommends that fruit juice be limited to 4 to 6 oz/day (AAP, Committee on Nutrition, 2001). A daily food plan guide for

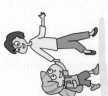

Get your child on the path to healthy eating.

Focus on the meal and each other.
Your child learns by watching you.' Children are likely to copy your table manners, your likes and dislikes, and your willingness to try new foods.

Offer a variety of healthy foods.
Let your child choose how much to eat. Children are more likely to enjoy a food when eating it is their own choice.

Be patient with your child.
Sometimes new foods take time. Give children a taste at first and be patient with them. Offer new foods many times.

Let your children serve themselves.
Teach your children to take small amounts at first. Let them know they can get more if they are still hungry.

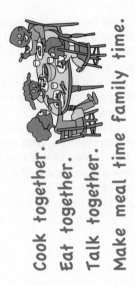

Cook together.
Eat together.
Talk together.
Make meal time family time.

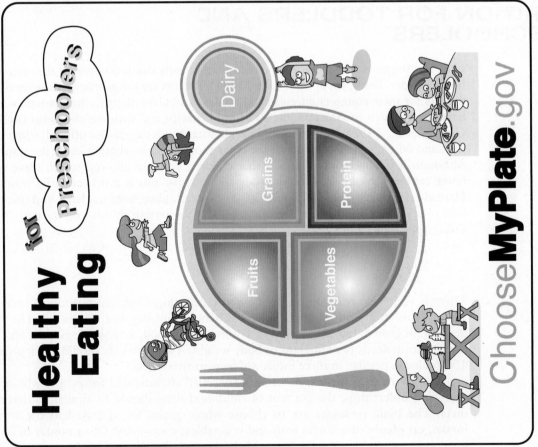

■ **FIGURE 12.2** Healthy eating for preschoolers. Get your child on the path to healthy eating. (Available at www.choosemyplate.gov)

2- to 5-year-olds is featured in Figure 12.3. Figure 12.4 features sample 1000-calorie and 1600-calorie meal patterns.

Although the food children need is the same as adults, the portion sizes are not. A rule-of-thumb guideline to determine age-appropriate serving sizes is to provide 1 tbsp of food per year of age (e.g., the serving size for a 3-year-old is 3 tbsp). By ages 4 to 6 years, recommended serving sizes are similar to those for adults. A study by Looney and Raynor (2011) found that the portion sizes of snacks offered to preschoolers, more so than the caloric density of the snacks, impact energy intake. This finding suggests that limiting snack sizes may be an effective strategy for reducing excessive calorie intake in children.

Eating Practices

Milk Anemia: an iron deficiency anemia related to excessive milk intake, which displaces the intake of iron-rich foods from the diet.

At age 1 year, the child should be drinking from a cup and eating many of the same foods as the rest of the family. Whole milk becomes a major source of nutrients, including fat; children between the ages of 1 and 2 years have a relatively higher need for fat to support rapid growth and development (Daniels and Greer, 2008). However, milk intake should not exceed 2 to 3 cups per day because, in greater amounts, it may displace the intake of iron-rich foods from the diet and promote **milk anemia**. The AAP recommends that the introduction of reduced-fat milk be delayed until after the age of 2 years. However, in children between 1 and 2 years old who are overweight or obese or who have a family history of obesity, dyslipidemia, or cardiovascular disease, the use of reduced-fat milk is considered appropriate (Daniels and Greer, 2008).

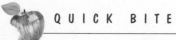

QUICK BITE

Foods that may cause choking in small children

Hot dogs	Tough meat
Candy	Watermelon with seeds
Nuts	Celery
Grapes	Popcorn
Raw carrots	Peanut butter

Beginning around 15 months of age, a child may develop food jags as a normal expression of autonomy as the child develops a sense of independence. By the end of the second year, children can completely self-feed and can seek food independently.

Until the age of 4 years, young children are at risk of choking. To decrease the risk of choking, foods that are difficult to chew and swallow should be avoided; meals and snacks should be supervised; foods should be prepared in forms that are easy to chew and swallow (e.g., cut grapes into small pieces and spread peanut butter thinly); and infants should not be allowed to eat or drink from a cup while lying down, playing, or strapped in a car seat.

Nutrients of Concern

Data from the Feeding Infants and Toddlers Study (FITS) 2008 show that American infants and toddlers meet or exceed their calorie and protein requirements with minimal risk of vitamin and mineral deficiencies, with the exception of iron and zinc in a small subset of older infants (Butte et al., 2010). However, the FITS also showed the following (Dwyer, Butte, Beming, Siega-Riz, and Reidy, 2010):

- Intakes of folic acid, preformed vitamin A, zinc, and sodium exceeded the Tolerable Upper Intake Levels (ULs) in a significant proportion of toddlers and preschoolers.
- Many toddlers consume diets below the Estimated Average Requirement (EAR) for vitamin E, and mean potassium and fiber intakes are under the Adequate Intake (AI).
- Many toddlers between the ages of 1 and 3 years are consuming diets with a lower percentage of total fat than recommended.

Healthy Eating for preschoolers

Daily Food Plan

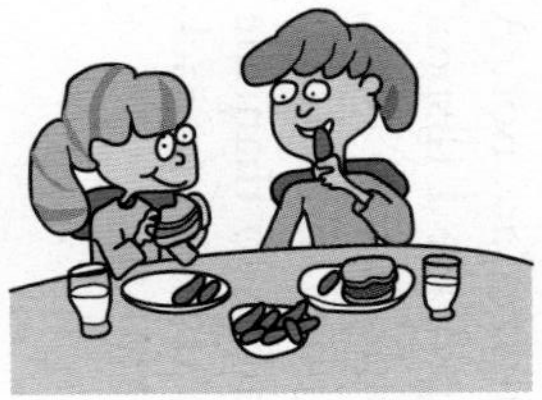

Use this Plan as a general guide.

- These food plans are based on average needs. Do not be concerned if your child does not eat the exact amounts suggested. Your child may need more or less than average. For example, food needs increase during growth spurts.

- Children's appetites vary from day to day. Some days they may eat less than these amounts; other days they may want more. Offer these amounts and let your child decide how much to eat.

Food group	2 year olds	3 year olds	4 and 5 year olds	What counts as:
Fruits	1 cup	1 – 1 1/2 cups	1 – 1 1/2 cups	**1/2 cup of fruit?** 1/2 cup mashed, sliced, or chopped fruit; 1/2 cup 100% fruit juice; 1/2 medium banana; 4-5 large strawberries
Vegetables	1 cup	1 1/2 cups	1 1/2 – 2 cups	**1/2 cup of veggies?** 1/2 cup mashed, sliced, or chopped vegetables; 1 cup raw leafy greens; 1/2 cup vegetable juice; 1 small ear of corn
Grains Make half your grains whole	3 ounces	4 – 5 ounces	4 – 5 ounces	**1 ounce of grains?** 1 slice bread; 1 cup ready-to-eat cereal flakes; 1/2 cup cooked rice or pasta; 1 tortilla (6" across)
Protein Foods	2 ounces	3 – 4 ounces	3 – 5 ounces	**1 ounce of protein foods?** 1 ounce cooked meat, poultry, or seafood; 1 egg; 1 Tablespoon peanut butter; 1/4 cup cooked beans or peas (kidney, pinto, lentis)
Dairy Choose low-fat or fat free	2 cups	2 1/2 cups	2 1/2 cups	**1/2 cup of dairy?** 1/2 cup milk; 4 ounces yogurt; 3/4 ounce cheese; 1 string cheese

There are many ways to divide the Daily Food Plan into meals and snacks. View the "Meal and Snack Patterns and Ideas" to see how these amounts might look on your preschooler's plate at www.choosemyplate.gov/preschoolers.html.

Some foods are easy for your child to choke on while eating. Skip hard, small, whole foods, such as popcorn, nuts, seeds, and hard candy. Cut up foods such as hot dogs, grapes, and raw carrots into pieces smaller than the size of your child's throat — about the size of a nickel.

FIGURE 12.3 Healthy eating for preschoolers daily food plan. (Available at www.choosemyplate.gov)

Meal and Snack Pattern

These patterns show one way a 1000 and 1600 calorie Daily Food Plan can be divided into meals and snacks for a preschooler. Sample food choices are shown for each meal or snack.

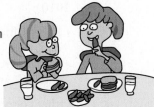

1000 Calorie Plan

Breakfast	
1 ounce grains 1/2 cup fruit 1/2 cup dairy*	Cereal and banana *1 cup crispy rice cereal* *1/2 cup sliced banana* *1/2 cup milk**

Morning Snack	
1/2 ounce grains 1/2 cup fruit	1/2 slice cinnamon bread 1/2 large orange

Lunch	
1 ounce grains 1/4 cup vegetables 1/2 cup dairy* 1 ounce protein foods	Open-faced chicken sandwich and salad *1 slice whole wheat bread* *1 slice American cheese** *1 ounce sliced chicken* *1/4 cup baby spinach (raw)* *2 Tbsp. grated carrots*

Afternoon Snack	
1/4 cup vegetables 1/2 cup dairy*	1/4 cup sugar snap peas 1/2 cup yogurt*

Dinner	
1/2 ounce grains 1/2 cup vegetables 1/2 cup dairy* 1 ounce protein foods	Chicken & potatoes *1 ounce chicken breast* *1/4 cup mashed potato* 1/4 cup green peas 1/2 small whole wheat roll 1/2 cup milk*

1600 Calorie Plan

Breakfast	
1 ounce grains 1/2 cup fruit 1/2 cup dairy*	Cereal and banana *1 cup crispy rice cereal* *1/2 cup sliced banana* *1/2 cup milk**

Morning Snack	
1 ounce grains 1/2 cup fruit 1 ounce protein foods	Egg sandwich *1 slice bread* *1 hard cooked egg* 1/2 large orange

Lunch	
1 ounce grains 1/2 cup vegetables 1/2 cup fruit 1/2 cup dairy* 1 ounce protein foods	Open-faced chicken sandwich and salad *1 slice whole wheat bread* *1 slice American cheese** *1 ounce sliced chicken* *1/2 cup baby spinach (raw)* *1/4 cup grated carrots* *1 small frozen banana*

Afternoon Snack	
1/2 cup vegetables 1/2 cup dairy*	1/2 cup sugar snap peas 1/2 cup yogurt*

Dinner	
2 ounce grains 1 cup vegetables 1 cup dairy* 3 ounces protein foods	Chicken & potatoes *3 ounces chicken breast* *1/2 cup mashed potato* 1/2 cup green peas 2 small whole wheat rolls 1 cup milk*

*Offer your child fat-free or low-fat milk, yogurt, and cheese.
Source: choosemyplate.gov

■ FIGURE 12.4   Meal and snack pattern. (Available at www.choosemyplate.gov)

The FITS 2008 study also revealed troubling food consumption patterns (Dwyer et al., 2010):

- French fries remain the most popular vegetable among toddlers older than 12 months of age.
- Thirty percent of toddlers did not eat any vegetables on the day of the food intake survey, and 25% ate no fruit.

Other concerns are the use of cow's milk before age 1 year and the use of reduced-fat milk during the second year of life (Siega-Riz et al., 2010).

NUTRITION FOR CHILDREN

Childhood represents a more latent period of growth compared to infancy and adolescence. Before puberty, children annually grow 2 to 3 in in height and gain about 5 pounds on average. Although there are individual differences, usually a larger child eats more than a smaller one; an active child eats more than a quiet one; and a happy, content child eats more than an anxious one. School-age children maintain a relatively constant intake in relation to their age group; children who are considered big eaters in second grade are also big eaters in sixth grade.

Calories and Nutrients

Total calorie needs steadily increase during childhood, although calorie needs per kilogram of body weight progressively fall. The challenge in childhood is to meet nutrient requirements without exceeding calorie needs. MyPlate food and calorie level guidelines for ages 6 to 18 years are shown in Table 12.4.

Table 12.4 MyPlate Food and Calorie Intake Levels Recommended for 6- to 18-Year-Olds

Daily Amount of Calories and Food Recommended by Age and Gender for Moderately Active Individuals*							
Age							
Males	6–8	9–10	11	12–13	14	15	16–18
Females	7–9	10–11	12–18				
Calorie Level	**1600**	**1800**	**2000**	**2200**	**2400**	**2600**	**2800**
Daily amount of food							
Fruits (cups)	1.5	1.5	2	2	2	2	2.5
Vegetables (cups)	2	2.5	2.5	3	3	3.5	3.5
Grains (oz-eq)	5	6	6	7	8	9	10
Protein Foods (oz-eq)	5	5	5.5	6	6.5	6.5	7
Dairy (cups)	3	3	3	3	3	3	3
Oils (tsp)	5	5	6	6	7	8	8
Empty calorie allowance	120	160	260	270	330	360	400

*Calorie needs generally increase by 200/day at each age for active individuals and decrease by 200/day for people who are sedentary.

Source: www.choosemyplate.gov

The Dietary Reference Intakes (DRIs) for children are divided into two age groups: 1- to 3-year-olds and 4- to 8-year-olds. Thereafter, age groups are further divided by gender: for males and females, the age groups through adolescence are 9- to 13-year-olds and 14- to 18-year-olds. Generally, nutrient needs increase with each age grouping, and most nutrient requirements reach their adult levels at the 14- to 18-year age group.

Eating Practices

As children get older, they consume more foods from nonhome sources and have more outside influences on their food choices. School, friends' houses, childcare centers, and social events present opportunities for children to make their own choices beyond parental supervision. Children who are home alone after school prepare their own snacks and, possibly, meals. The "ideal" of children eating breakfast, dinner, and a snack at home, with a nutritious brown-bag or healthy cafeteria lunch at school, is not representative of what most children are eating.

Children who eat dinner with their families at home tend to have higher intakes of fruits, vegetables, vitamins, and minerals and lower intakes of saturated and trans fatty acids, soft drinks, and fried foods (ADA, 2008). Family meals promote social interaction and allow children to learn food-related behaviors. Parents should provide and consume healthy meals and snacks and avoid or limit empty-calorie foods (Fig. 12.5). Snacks, especially sweetened beverages, should be limited during sedentary activities. Healthy snack ideas are listed in Box 12.6. Forbidding the intake of certain foods and pressuring children to eat are counterproductive in that they may lead to overeating, dislikes, and an interest in eating forbidden foods (Fisher and Birch, 1999). The food groups most likely to be consumed in inadequate amounts are fruits, vegetables, and whole grains.

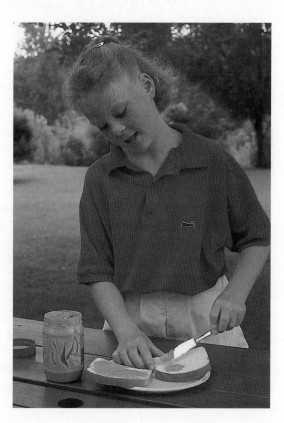

■ FIGURE 12.5   Good nutritional habits, such as eating healthy snacks, develop early in life. (© Bob Kramer)

Box 12.6   HEALTHY SNACKS

Unsweetened cereal with or without milk
Meat or cheese on whole-grain bread or crackers
Graham crackers, fig bars
Whole-grain cookies or muffins made with oatmeal, dried fruit, or iron-fortified cereal
Quick breads such as banana, date, pumpkin bread
Raw vegetables, vegetable juices
Fresh, dried, or canned fruits without sugar
Pure fruit juice as a drink or frozen on a stick
Low-fat yogurt with or without fresh fruit added
Air-popped popcorn (not before age 4 years)
Peanut butter on bread, crackers, celery, apple slices
Pretzels
Milk shakes made with fruit and low-fat ice cream or frozen yogurt
Low-fat ice cream, frozen yogurt, sherbet, sorbet, fruit ice
Animal crackers, ginger snaps
Skim or 1% milk (after age 2 years)
Low-fat cheese, low-fat cottage cheese
Rice cakes or popcorn cakes

Nutrients of Concern

Important concerns during childhood include excessive intakes of calories, sodium, and fat, especially saturated fat. Nutrients most likely to be consumed in inadequate amounts are calcium, fiber, vitamin E, magnesium, and potassium (ADA, 2008). The percentage of children with usual nutrient intakes below the EAR tends to increase with age and is greater among females than males. The AAP recommends that children who consume less than 1 L/day of vitamin D–fortified milk take a supplement of 400 IU/day (Wagner, Greer, and the Section on Breastfeeding and Committee on Nutrition, 2008).

NURSING PROCESS: *Well Child*

Amanda is a 24-month-old girl who is seen regularly in the Well Baby Clinic for her checkups and immunizations. At this visit, you discover that her height and weight are in the 25th percentile for her age. Records indicate that previously she had consistently ranked in the 75th percentile for weight and 50th percentile for height. The change has occurred over the last 6 months. Her mother complains that Amanda is "fussy" and has lost interest in eating.

Assessment

Medical–Psychosocial History

- Medical history including prenatal, perinatal, and birth history; specifically assess for gastrointestinal (GI) problems such as slow gastric emptying, constipation, diarrhea, and allergies
- Use of medications that can cause side effects such as delayed gastric emptying, diarrhea, constipation, or decreased appetite
- Level of development for age
- Elimination and reflux patterns, if applicable

NURSING PROCESS: *Well Child* (continued)

	▪ Caregiver's ability to understand; attitude toward health and nutrition and readiness to learn
	▪ Psychosocial and economic issues such as the living situation, who does the shopping and cooking, adequacy of food budget, need for food assistance, and level of family and social support
	▪ Use of vitamins, minerals, and nutritional supplements: what, how much, and why they are given
Anthropometric Assessment	▪ Obtain height and weight to calculate BMI; determine BMI-for-age percentile
	▪ Head circumference for age
	▪ Pattern of weight gain and growth
Biochemical and Physical Assessment	▪ Laboratory values, including hemoglobin and hematocrit, and the significance of any other values that are abnormal
Dietary Assessment	▪ Food records, if available
	▪ Interview the primary caregiver to assess the following:
	▪ What does Amanda usually eat in a 24-hour period, including types and amounts of food, frequency and pattern of eating, and texture of foods eaten?
	▪ How does her intake compare to a 1000-calorie (the calorie level appropriate for 2-year-olds) MyPlate intake pattern?
	▪ What food groups is she consuming less than recommended amounts of?
	▪ Are self-feeding skills appropriate for Amanda's age?
	▪ Is the mealtime environment positive?
	▪ What is the caregiver's attitude about Amanda's current weight, recent weight loss, and eating behaviors?
	▪ Are the caregiver's expectations about how much Amanda should eat reasonable and appropriate? What is the problem according to the caregiver?
	▪ Are there cultural, religious, and ethnic influences on the family's eating habits?

Diagnosis

Possible Nursing Diagnoses	Altered nutrition: eating less than the body needs as evidenced by change of two percentile channels in growth charts

Planning

Client Outcomes	The client will
	▪ Experience appropriate growth in height and weight
	▪ Consume, on average, an intake consistent with MyPlate recommendations for a 1000-calorie diet by eating a variety of foods within each food group
	▪ Achieve or progress toward age-appropriate feeding skills

(continues on page 304)

NURSING PROCESS: *Well Child* (continued)

Nursing Interventions

Nutrition Therapy

Client Teaching

Promote MyPlate food plan of 1000 calories, which is appropriate for her age

Instruct the caregiver

- On the role of nutrition in maintaining health and promoting adequate growth and development, including the importance of adequate calories and protein
- On eating-plan essentials, including the importance of
  - Choosing a varied diet to help ensure an adequate intake
  - Providing foods of appropriate texture for age
  - Providing three meals plus three or more planned snacks to maximize intake
  - Providing liquids after meals, instead of with meals, to avoid displacing food intake
  - Limiting low-nutrient-dense foods (e.g., fruit drinks, carbonated beverages, sweetened cereals) because they displace the intake of more nutritious foods
  - The need to modify the diet, as appropriate, to improve elimination patterns

Address behavioral matters, such as

- Providing a positive mealtime environment (e.g., limiting distractions, having the child well rested before mealtime)
- Not using food to punish, reward, or bribe the child
- Promoting eating behaviors and skills appropriate for the age
- Keeping accurate food records
- Modifying foods to increase their nutrient density, such as by fortifying milk with skim milk powder; using milk in place of water in recipes; melting cheese on potatoes, rice, or noodles; and so on

Evaluation

Evaluate and Monitor

- Monitor growth in height and weight
- Evaluate food records to assess adequacy of intake according to a 1000-calorie MyPlate plan
- Progress toward age-appropriate feeding skills

NUTRITION FOR ADOLESCENTS (12–18 YEARS)

The slow growth of childhood abruptly and dramatically increases with pubescence until the rate is as rapid as that of early infancy. Adolescence is a period of physical, emotional, social, and sexual maturation. Approximately 15% to 20% of adult height and 50% of adult weight are gained during adolescence. Fat distribution shifts and sexual maturation occurs.

Subsequently, calorie and nutrient needs increase, as does appetite, but exactly when those increases occur depends on the timing and duration of the growth spurt. Because there are wide variations in the timing of the growth spurt among individuals, chronological age is a poor indicator of physiologic maturity and nutritional needs.

Gender differences are obvious. For instance, girls generally experience increases in growth between 10 and 11 years of age and peak at 12 years. Because peak weight occurs before peak height, many girls and parents become concerned about what appears to be excess weight. In contrast, boys usually begin the growth spurt at about 12 years of age and peak at 14 years. Stature growth ceases at a median age of approximately 21 years. Nutritional needs increase later for boys than for girls.

Calories and Nutrients

QUICK BITE

Sources of calcium
Milk
Yogurt
Hard cheeses, such as cheddar
Calcium-fortified orange juice
Calcium-fortified breakfast cereals
Canned fish with bones, such as salmon
"Greens," such as bok choy, collard greens, turnip greens, kale
Broccoli
Chinese/Napa cabbage
Okra
Tofu, soymilk
Tortillas made from lime-processed corn

Table 12.4 lists MyPlate recommended calorie intakes for adolescents, which are based on DRI estimated energy expenditure calculations that account for age, gender, weight, height, physical activity level, and energy deposition. Generally, nutrient requirements are higher during adolescence than at any other time in the life cycle, with the exception of pregnancy and lactation. Notice that the calories suggested for moderately active females aged 12 to 18 years is 2000, whereas for males, the need ranges from 2200 to 2800 calories. Females require fewer calories than males because they have proportionally more fat tissue and less muscle mass from the effects of estrogen. Girls also experience less bone growth than boys.

Eating Practices

In early adolescence, peer pressure overtakes parental influence on food choices. As the adolescent becomes increasingly independent, more self-selected meals and snacks are purchased and eaten outside the home. A natural increase in appetite combined with fast-food marketing practices geared toward adolescents and a decrease in physical activity increase the risk of overeating. Few adolescents consume recommended amounts of fruits, vegetables, dairy foods, and whole grains (Bruening et al., 2012). A study by Bowman (2002) found that from the mid-1970s to the mid-1990s, milk intake in adolescents decreased by 36% and the intake of sodas and fruit drinks almost doubled.

Nutrients of Concern

Adolescents are at risk of consuming inadequate amounts of several nutrients, such as calcium, potassium, magnesium, vitamin A, and fiber, because they are underconsuming several food groups. Because adolescents consume much less vitamin D–fortified milk than recommended, the AAP recommends a multivitamin or vitamin D–only supplement of 400 IU for adolescents who do not consume adequate vitamin D per day through vitamin D–fortified milk (100 IU/8 oz) and/or vitamin D–fortified foods (e.g., fortified cereals and orange juice) (Wagner et al., 2008).

Calcium intake is also a concern because milk intake is low (Bowman, 2002) and need is high. For males and females from age 9 to 18 years, the Recommended Dietary Allowance (RDA) for calcium is 1300 mg—higher than at any other time in the life cycle. Approximately half of adult bone mass is accrued during adolescence; optimizing calcium intake during adolescence increases bone mineralization and may decrease the risk of fracture and osteoporosis later in life. In reality, mean calcium intake is less than the RDA for both males and females from age 9 years onward.

Iron is a concern because adolescents have increased needs for iron related to an expanding blood volume, the rise in hemoglobin concentration, and the growth of muscle mass. In boys, peak iron requirement occurs between 14 and 18 years of age as muscle mass expands. The requirement for iron in adolescent girls increases from 8 to 15 mg/day at the age of 14 years to account for menstrual losses. For girls who are not menstruating at 14 years old, the requirement for iron is 10.5 mg/day, not 15 mg/day. Girls tend to develop an iron deficiency slowly after puberty, particularly if menstrual losses are compounded by poor eating habits or chronic fad dieting. Heme iron, found in meats, is better absorbed than nonheme iron. Nonheme iron absorption increases when a source of vitamin C, such as orange juice or tomatoes, is consumed at the same time.

Adolescents consume an excess of calories, solid fat, and added sugars. The mean sodium intake among 12- to 19-year-olds is more than 3000 mg, which far exceeds the AI of 1500 mg (USDA, Agricultural Research Service, 2010). The five major sources of calories among 14- to 18-year-olds, in descending order, are soda, pizza, grain desserts, yeast breads, and chicken (Reedy and Krebs-Smith, 2010).

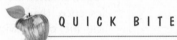

QUICK BITE

Sources of nonheme iron
Iron-fortified, ready-to-eat cereals
Whole wheat, enriched, or fortified bread
Noodles, rice, or barley
Canned plums
Cooked dried apricots
Raisins
Bean dip
Peanut butter

NUTRITION CONCERNS DURING CHILDHOOD AND ADOLESCENCE

Indicators of nutrition risk for children and adolescents appear in Box 12.7. Nutrition concerns discussed next include overweight and obesity, breakfast skipping, and adolescent pregnancy. Eating disorders are discussed in Chapter 14.

Overweight and Obesity

More than 23 million children and adolescents are overweight or obese in the United States (Ogden et al., 2010). Weight gain occurs when calorie intake exceeds calorie expenditure over time. Factors that contribute to an excessive calorie intake include large portion sizes, snacking, away-from-home meals, and sugar-sweetened beverage consumption (Brownell, Schwartz, Puhl, Henderson, and Harris, 2009). A study to identify the top food sources of

Box 12.7   INDICATORS OF NUTRITION RISK IN CHILDREN AND ADOLESCENTS

- Meal skipping three or more times per week
- Frequent breakfast skipping
- Eating fast food more than three times per week
- Eating from only one food group
- Poor appetite
- Frequently eating without family supervision

Source: Melanson, K. (2008). Lifestyle approaches to promoting healthy eating for children. *American Journal of Lifestyle Medicine, 2,* 26–36.

calories and empty calories (solid fats and added sugars) among children and adolescents revealed the following (Reedy and Krebs-Smith, 2010):

- The top sources of calories for 2- to 18-year-olds are grain desserts (139 cal/day), pizza (136 cal/day), and soda (118 cal/day).
- Empty calories provide almost 40% of total calories consumed daily.
- Empty calorie intake far exceeds empty calorie allowance in all age–sex groups.
- Half of empty calories come from six foods: soda, fruit drinks, dairy desserts, grain desserts, pizza, and whole milk.

Overweight and obese children and adolescents are developing complications of excess weight seen in adults, such as prediabetes, diabetes, hypertension, and hyperlipidemia (May, Kuklina, and Yoon, 2012). Overweight and obesity in childhood or adolescence increase the risk of several diseases in adulthood, such as insulin resistance, stroke, cardiovascular disease, and renal failure (LaFontaine, 2008). Among obese girls, the risk of premature death as an adult increases threefold (van Dam, Willet, Manson, and Hu, 2006). Eighty percent of overweight and obese adolescents become obese adults (Dietz, 2004).

Overweight and obesity can have negative social and psychological consequences. A study that followed almost 11,000 American adolescents found that obese girls were half as likely to attend college, were more likely to consider committing suicide and use alcohol and marijuana, and had a more negative self-image than normal-weight girls (Crosnoe, 2007). Teasing and psychological abuse by peers and adults can lead to social isolation, depression, and low self-esteem. Overweight children may actually consume fewer calories than their thin counterparts. Because they are social outcasts though, a perpetuating cycle of weight gain, inactivity, and further weight gain makes weight control difficult.

Although multifactorial in origin, the fundamental cause of overweight and obesity is an imbalance between calorie intake and calorie expenditure. Over the last 25 years, the average calorie intake of American children has increased, and portion sizes have grown. On the other side of the energy equation, physical inactivity is seen as a major contributor to weight gain in children.

Healthy Lifestyles and Obesity Prevention

Prevention of obesity is critical because data on long-term successful treatment is limited (AAP, 2003). Parental support for a more healthful lifestyle is vital to initiating and sustaining changes in eating and exercise behaviors. Parents often recognize that they need to set an example for their children but lack the time to do so. Still other parents who are overweight may feel they cannot set a good example because they do not practice what they preach. Other barriers to parents taking action are (1) a belief that children will outgrow their excess weight, (2) a lack of knowledge about how to help children control their weight, and (3) a fear they will cause eating disorders in their children. Even among adolescents, parents still have a major impact on food intake.

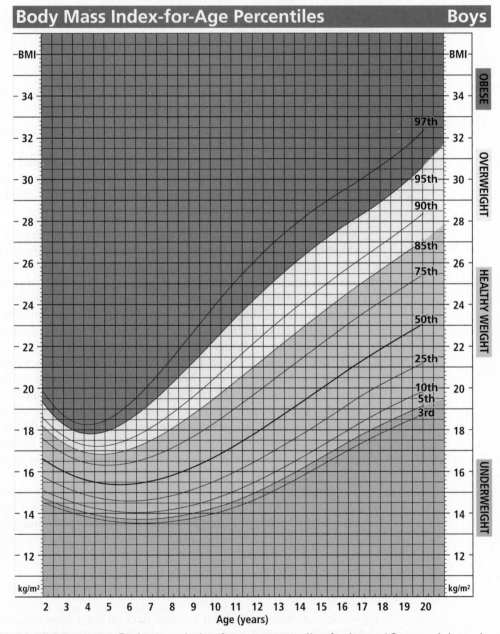

■ **FIGURE 12.6**   Body mass index-for-age percentiles for boys. (**Source:** Adapted from the Centers for Disease Control and Prevention [CDC] Growth Chart, New York State Department of Health.)

The AAP recommends all children be targeted for obesity prevention beginning at birth (Barlow and the Expert Committee, 2009). At minimum, BMI should be calculated and plotted at each well visit. Gender-specific, BMI-for-age percentiles are used to screen for overweight childhood because BMI varies by age and gender (Figs. 12.6 and 12.7). All children and adolescents who are not in the healthy weight range should undergo further assessment of medical risks, behavior risks, and attitudes (Barlow and the Expert

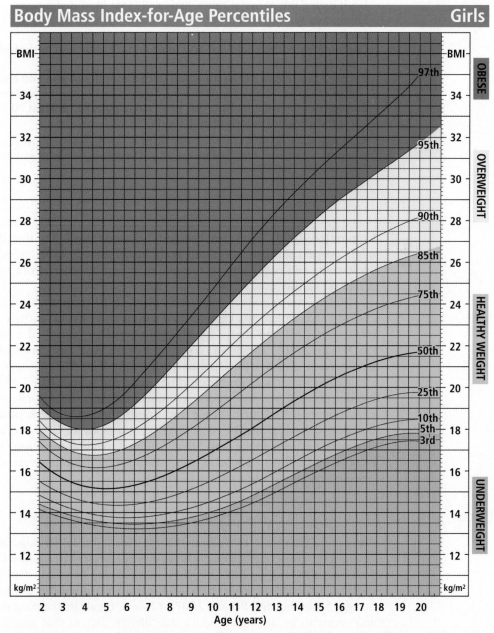

Body Mass Index-for-Age Percentiles   **Girls**

■ FIGURE 12.7   Body mass index-for-age percentiles for girls. (**Source:** Adapted from the Centers for Disease Control and Prevention [CDC] Growth Chart, New York State Department of Health.)

Box 12.8	HEALTHY BEHAVIORS THAT MAY HELP PREVENT EXCESSIVE WEIGHT GAIN

Limit intake of sugar-sweetened beverages.

Encourage the intake of more fruits and vegetables to the levels recommended in MyPlate.

Limit TV viewing and screen time to a maximum of 2 hours/day after the age of 2 years. TV viewing is not appropriate for children younger than 2 years.

Eat breakfast daily.

Limit eating out at restaurants, especially fast-food restaurants.

Encourage family meals.

Limit portion size.

Consume adequate calcium and fiber and a balance of carbohydrates, protein, and fat.

Encourage exclusive breastfeeding until 6 months of age and continue breastfeeding after complementary foods are introduced to 12 months and beyond.

Engage in moderate to vigorous physical activity for at least 60 minutes daily.

Limit the intake of calorie-dense foods.

Source: Barlow, S., & the Expert Committee. (2007). Expert Committee recommendations regarding the prevention, assessment, and treatment of child and adolescent overweight and obesity: Summary report. *Pediatrics, 120,* S164–S192.

Committee, 2009). However, the AAP notes the possibility that BMI screening programs might worsen stigmatization and body image already experienced by obese children and adolescents and may increase the risk of eating disorders from inappropriate weight loss practices (Nihiser et al., 2009).

The *Dietary Guidelines for Americans, 2010* recommends that overweight or obese children and adolescents change their eating and physical activity behaviors to prevent an increase in BMI and that a health professional be consulted to manage weight (USDA, USDHHS, 2010). The expert committee of the AAP has identified healthy habits that may help prevent excessive weight gain (Box 12.8). The ADA takes the position that pediatric overweight requires a combination of family and school-based programs that include promoting physical activity, parent training/modeling, behavioral counseling, and nutrition education (ADA, 2006). While the importance of implementing obesity interventions for adolescents is clear, the most effective strategies for doing so are unknown (Shepherd, Neumark-Sztainer, Beyer, and Story, 2006). Providing nutrition- and calorie-related information, especially to adolescent girls, has the potential to inadvertently lead to weight preoccupation and unhealthful calorie counting.

Breakfast Skipping

Among children age 6 to 13 years, an estimated 8% to 15% skip breakfast (Affenito, 2007). Adolescent females are more likely to skip breakfast than males of similar age, and African American adolescents (24%) are more likely to skip breakfast than White adolescents (13%) (Nicklas, O'Neil, and Myers, 2004). Breakfast is missed more than any other meal (Utter, Scragg, Mhurchu, and Schaaf, 2007). Overall, breakfast skipping tends to increase with age and seems to be associated with other lifestyle factors that may be detrimental to health, such as dieting and infrequent exercise (Rampersaud, Pereira, Girard, Adams, and Metzl, 2005). Children who regularly skip breakfast have lower intakes of vitamins and minerals than those who routinely eat breakfast, and those nutrients are not made up for at other meals.

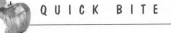

QUICK BITE

Nontraditional breakfast ideas
Pizza
Peanut butter sandwich
Soup with crackers
Yogurt parfait
Smoothies
Baked potato with cottage cheese
Dinner leftovers

In the Bogalusa Heart Study, 10-year-old breakfast skippers failed to meet two-thirds of the reference standards for vitamin A, vitamin B_6, vitamin D, riboflavin, folate, calcium, iron, magnesium, phosphorus, riboflavin, and zinc (Nicklas, O'Neil, and Berenson, 1998). Eating breakfast is linked to better academic performance (Kleinman et al., 2002) and cognition among children (Pollitt and Mathews, 1998). Children who skip breakfast are significantly less likely to meet recommendations for fruit and vegetable intake and more likely to frequently eat unhealthy snacks (Utter et al., 2007). Breakfast skipping has been reported to be associated with a higher BMI in children (Berkey, Rockett, Gillman, Field, and Colditz, 2003) and also with larger waist circumference and higher levels of fasting insulin, total cholesterol, and low-density lipoprotein cholesterol compared to children who eat breakfast (Smith et al., 2010). Although a high-fiber, nutrient-fortified, ready-to-eat cereal with skim milk and fruit may be an optimal choice for breakfast, nontraditional breakfasts may be more appealing to people who "don't like breakfast."

Adolescent Pregnancy

Adolescent pregnancy is associated with physiologic, socioeconomic, and behavioral factors that increase health risks to both infant and mother. Infants born to adolescent mothers are at higher risk of low birth weight (LBW) and preterm birth and are more likely to die within the first year of life than infants whose mothers are in their 20s or 30s (March of Dimes, 2007). Pregnant adolescents are at higher risk for anemia, high blood pressure, and excessive postpartum weight retention (Nielsen, Gittelsohn, Anliker, and O'Brien, 2006).

Compared with adult women, pregnant adolescents

- Are more likely to be physically, emotionally, financially, and socially immature. Low socioeconomic status may be a major reason for the high incidence of LBW infants and other complications of adolescent pregnancy.
- May not have adequate nutrient stores because they need large amounts of nutrients for their own growth and development. Although female adolescent growth is usually complete by the age of 15 years, physical maturity is not reached until 4 years after menarche, which usually occurs by age 17 years.
- May give low priority to healthy eating. Dieting, erratic eating patterns, reliance on fast foods, and meal skipping (especially breakfast) are common adolescent practices.
- May have poor intake and status of certain micronutrients, such as folate, iron, and vitamin D, which increases the risk of small-for-gestational-age births in pregnant adolescents (Baker et al., 2009).
- Often need to gain more weight for their BMI than older women to improve birth outcomes (Institute of Medicine [IOM], 2009).
- Are more concerned with body image and confused about weight gain recommendations. Many do not understand why they should gain more than 7 pounds, the weight of the average baby at birth.
- Are more likely to smoke during pregnancy. Smoking doubles a woman's risk of delivering an LBW baby and increases the risk of complications, premature delivery, and stillbirth (USDHHS, 2004).
- Seek prenatal care later and have fewer total visits during pregnancy.

Appropriate weight gain and adequate nutrition are among the most important controllable factors that contribute to a healthful outcome of pregnancy for both mother and infant (Nielsen et al., 2006). Good nutrition has the potential to decrease the incidence of LBW infants and to improve the health of infants born to adolescents. Teenagers within the healthy BMI range should gain 25 to 35 pounds or more if they are very young (IOM, 2009). The MyPlate recommendations in Table 12.4 can also be used by pregnant teens. MyPlate is useful both in assessing dietary strengths and weaknesses and in providing a framework for implementing dietary changes in a way the teenager can understand. Because teens living with one or more adults may have little control over what food is available to them, parents and significant others should also be encouraged to attend counseling sessions.

How Do You Respond?

Does early introduction of solid foods help infants sleep through the night?
A frequently given reason for introducing solids before 4 months of age is the unsupported belief that it will help infants to sleep through the night. A major objection to the early introduction of solids is that it may interfere with establishing sound eating habits and may contribute to overfeeding because infants less than 4 months old are unable to communicate satiety by turning away and leaning back.

What foods are most likely to cause allergies? Ninety percent of food allergy reactions are caused by these eight foods: milk, eggs, soy, peanuts, nuts (cashews, almonds), wheat, fish, and shellfish. Most people who have a food allergy are allergic to only one food.

Does chocolate cause or aggravate acne? Scientific evidence does not demonstrate that diet causes acne, but it may aggravate it. The implicated dietary factors are a high glycemic load diet and dairy products. Further research is needed to clarify the link between diet and acne and determine if nutrition therapy can play a role in acne treatment.

Can diet be blamed for attention-deficit and hyperactivity disorder (ADHD)?
In the 1970s, the late Dr. Ben Feingold proposed that food additives and salicylates may be responsible for about 25% of cases of hyperactivity with learning disability among school-age children. Most controlled studies do not support the hypothesis that avoiding artificial colors and flavors; the preservatives beta-hydroxytheophylline [BHT] and butylated hydroxyanisole [BHA]; and salicylate-containing fruits, vegetables, and spices (the Feingold diet) helps to control hyperactivity (Marcason, 2005). Likewise, there is a lack of evidence that removing sugar from the diet of a child with ADHD results in fewer symptoms (Ballard, Hall, and Kaufmann, 2010). However, it is possible that a very small subset of children with ADHD have food sensitivities.

Case Study

Andrew is 16 years old and sedentary. He is 5 ft 8 in tall, weighs 218 pounds, and has a BMI of 33. He has been overweight for most of his life, as is most of his extended paternal family. His mother has tried "everything" over the years to get him to lose weight, from putting him on her own weight loss diet to hiding foods he shouldn't have, such as soft drinks and chips, to limit his access. He has a part-time job in a fast-food restaurant and is able to leave the school property at lunchtime to have lunch where he works.

He is not good at sports but loves to play video games and watch movies. He hates that he's so big but feels hopeless about changing. His normal day's intake is as follows:

Breakfast:	Two doughnuts and a large glass of apple juice
Lunch:	A double cheeseburger, large fries, and a large shake
Snacks:	Frozen mini pizzas, a large soft drink, and a handful of cookies
Dinner:	The same as lunch on nights he works. If he's home, he eats whatever is available, often pizza or sandwiches and chips, ice cream, and a soft drink
Snacks:	Chips and salsa, and a soft drink

- Using the BMI-for-age percentile for boys, what is Andrew's weight status? Is it an appropriate approach to limit Andrew's calories to outgrow his current weight status?
- How many calories should Andrew consume daily? Based on the MyPlate intake levels, which food groups is he consuming the appropriate amounts of? Which groups is he overeating? Which groups is he not eating enough of? What are the sources of empty calories in his diet?
- What specific goals would you encourage Andrew to set regarding his intake, activity, and weight?
- What would you suggest his mother do to support better eating habits and a healthier weight?

STUDY QUESTIONS

1. Which statement indicates the mother understands the nurse's instructions about breastfeeding?
   a. "Breastfeeding should only last 5 minutes on each breast."
   b. "Sometimes babies cry just because they are thirsty, so a bottle of water should be offered before breastfeeding begins to see if the infant is just thirsty."
   c. "The longer the baby sucks, the less milk I will have for the next feeding."
   d. "The first breast offered should be alternated with each feeding."

2. A mother asks why toddlers shouldn't drink all the milk they want. Which of the following is the nurse's best response?
   a. "Consuming more than the recommended amount of milk can displace the intake of iron-rich foods from the diet and increase the toddler's risk of iron deficiency anemia."
   b. "Consuming more than the recommended amount of milk increases the risk of milk allergy."
   c. "Too much milk can lead to overhydration."
   d. "Consuming more than the recommended amount of milk will provide too much protein."

3. The nurse knows her instructions about introducing solids into the infant's diet have been effective when the mother states
   a. "Babies should be introduced to solid foods at 1 to 3 months of age."
   b. "New foods should be given for 5 to 7 days so that allergic responses can be easily identified."
   c. "Infants are more likely to accept infant cereal for the first time if it is mixed with breast milk or formula and given from a bottle."
   d. "The appropriate initial serving size for solids is 1 to 2 tbsp."

4. Which of the following would be the best snack for a 2-year-old?
   a. Popcorn
   b. Banana slices
   c. Fresh cherries
   d. Raw celery

5. Which groups are adolescents most likely to eat in inadequate amounts? Select all that apply.
   a. Whole grains
   b. Vegetables
   c. Fruits
   d. Meat

6. The client asks if her 10-year-old daughter needs a weight loss diet. Which of the following would be the nurse's best response?
   a. "Rather than a diet at this age, you should just forbid her to eat sweets and empty calories."
   b. "Because prevention of overweight is more effective than treatment, you should start to limit her calorie intake by only serving low-fat and artificially sweetened foods."
   c. "Ten-year-old girls are about to enter the growth spurt of puberty, and it is natural for her to gain weight before she grows taller. Diets are not recommended for children, although healthy eating and moderation are always appropriate."
   d. "She needs extra calories for the upcoming growth spurt, so you should be encouraging her to eat more than she normally does."

7. Calorie and nutrient requirements during adolescence
   a. Are higher than during adulthood because of growth and developmental changes.
   b. Peak early and then fall until adulthood is reached.
   c. Are lower than during childhood.
   d. Cannot be generalized because individual variations exist.

8. Nutrients most likely to be deficient in an adolescent's diet are
   a. Vitamin A and folate
   b. Protein and vitamin C
   c. Zinc and phosphorus
   d. Iron and calcium

KEY CONCEPTS

■ An optimal diet supports normal growth and development within calorie and nutrient guidelines.

■ Because of varying rates of growth and activity, nutritional requirements are less precise for children and adolescents than they are for adults.

■ Exclusive breastfeeding is recommended for the first 6 months of life. Breastfeeding should continue up to the age of 1 year.

■ Iron-fortified infant formula is an acceptable alternative or supplement to breastfeeding. The biggest hazard of formula feeding is overfeeding.

■ Adequacy of growth (height and weight) is the best indicator of whether or not an infant's intake is nutritionally adequate.

■ Complementary foods should not be introduced before the infant is developmentally ready, usually around 6 months of age. Iron-fortified infant cereal is traditionally the first food introduced. New foods should be introduced one at a time for a period of 5 to 7 days so that any allergic reaction can be easily identified.

■ Nutritional guidelines on how to achieve optimal nutritional intakes for toddlers do not exist. Infants and toddlers are at low risk of nutrient deficiencies, yet their diets may already be beginning to be high in added sugars and fats and low in fruits and vegetables.

■ Parents are the primary gatekeepers of their children's nutritional intake. They should make healthy foods available and not introduce foods into their children's diet that have no value other than calories.

■ The food groups most likely to be consumed in inadequate amounts by children and adolescents are fruits, vegetables, whole grains, and dairy products, increasing their risk of inadequate intakes of calcium, potassium, fiber, and other nutrients.

■ The *Dietary Guidelines for Americans, 2010* are intended for all Americans age 2 years and older.

■ Compared to breakfast eaters, youth who skip breakfast eat less vitamins and minerals, have lower academic performance, frequently eat unhealthy snacks, and are more likely to be overweight.

■ Overweight and obesity among youth are a major public health concern. Children suffer greater social and psychological effects of obesity than adults. Disorders common in adults who are overweight, such as glucose intolerance, type 2 diabetes, hypertension, hyperlipidemia, and metabolic syndrome, may also develop in children who are overweight. Childhood overweight may increase the risk of insulin resistance, stroke, cardiovascular disease, and renal failure in adulthood. All children are targets for obesity prevention beginning at birth.

■ Adolescents may have unhealthy eating habits that increase their risk of poor pregnancy outcome, such as a high intake of sugar and inadequate intakes of iron and folate.

Check Your Knowledge Answer Key

1. **TRUE** The amount of calories and protein needed per unit of body weight is greater for infants than for adults because growth in the first year of life is more rapid than at any other time in the life cycle (excluding the fetal period).

2. **TRUE** If breastfeeding is discontinued before the infant's first birthday, it should be replaced with iron-fortified infant formula. Cow's milk is not recommended before the age of 1 year.

3. **FALSE** Iron is the nutrient of most concern when solids are introduced into the diet.

4. **TRUE** Overfeeding is a potential problem with early introduction of solid foods because young infants are unable to communicate satiety, the feeling of fullness.

5. **TRUE** The risk of nutrient deficiencies among American toddlers is negligible. However, the risks of overfeeding and eating empty calories are real.

6. **FALSE** The *Dietary Guidelines for Americans, 2010* are intended for all Americans over the age of 2 years.

7. **TRUE** Milk can displace the intake of iron-rich foods, increasing the risk of iron deficiency.

8. **TRUE** Children who regularly skip breakfast have lower intakes of vitamins and minerals than children who normally eat breakfast.

9. **TRUE** An overweight child is more likely to develop complications of adult overweight, such as diabetes, hypertension, and metabolic syndrome.

10. **TRUE** Among 2- to 18-year-olds, the intake of empty calories far exceeds empty calorie allowance for all age–sex groups.

Student Resources on thePoint

For additional learning materials, activate the code in the front of this book at
http://thePoint.lww.com/activate

Websites

American Academy of Pediatrics at **www.aap.org**
A parent website backed by the American Academy of Pediatrics at **www.healthychildren.org**
Children's Nutrition Research Center at Baylor College of Medicine at **www.bcm.edu/cnrc/**
Food and Nutrition Information Center for information on child care nutrition, WIC, and healthy school meals at **www.nal.usda.gov/fnic**
Kids Food CyberClub at **www.kidsfood.org**
KidsHealth at **www.kidshealth.org**
Nutrition Explorations at **www.nutritionexplorations.org**

References

Affenito, S. (2007). Breakfast: A missed opportunity. *Journal of the American Dietetic Association, 107*, 565–569.

Alexy, U., Kersting, M., Sichert-Hellert, W., Manz, F., & Schöch, G. (1999). Macronutrient intake of 3- to 36-month old German infants and children: Results of the DONALD Study. Dortmund Nutrition and Anthropometric Longitudinally Designed Study. *Annals of Nutrition and Metabolism, 43*, 14–22.

American Academy of Pediatrics. (2003). Policy statement. Prevention of pediatric overweight and obesity. *Pediatrics, 112*, 424–430.

American Academy of Pediatrics. (2012a). Policy statement. Breastfeeding and the use of human milk. *Pediatrics, 129*, e827–e841.

American Academy of Pediatrics. (2012b). *Switching to solid foods.* Available at http://www .healthychildren.org/English/ages-stages/baby/feeding-nutrition/Pages/Switching-To-Solid-Foods.aspx. Accessed on 11/13/12.

American Academy of Pediatrics, Committee on Nutrition. (2001). The use and misuse of fruit juice in pediatrics. *Pediatrics, 107*, 1210–1213.

American Dietetic Association. (2006). Position of the American Dietetic Association: Individual-, family-, school-, and community-based interventions for pediatric overweight. *Journal of the American Dietetic Association, 106*, 925–945.

American Dietetic Association. (2008). Position of the American Dietetic Association: Nutrition guidance for healthy children ages 2 to 11 years. *Journal of the American Dietetic Association, 108*, 1038–1047.

Baker, P., Wheeler, S., Sanders, T., Thomas, J. E., Hutchinson, C. J., Clarke, K., . . . Poston, L. (2009). A prospective study of micronutrient status in adolescent pregnancy. *American Journal of Clinical Nutrition, 89*, 1114–1124.

Ballard, W., Hall, M., & Kaufmann, L. (2010). Clinical inquiries. Do dietary interventions improve ADHD symptoms in children? *Journal of Family Practice, 59*, 234–235.

Barlow, S., & the Expert Committee. (2007). Expert Committee recommendations regarding the prevention, assessment, and treatment of child and adolescent overweight and obesity: Summary report. *Pediatrics, 120*(Suppl. 4), S164–S192.

Berkey, C., Rockett, H., Gillman, M., Field, A. E., & Colditz, G. A. (2003). Longitudinal study of skipping breakfast and weight change in adolescents. *International Journal of Obesity and Related Metabolic Disorders, 27*, 1258–1266.

Bhatia, J., & Greer, F. (2008). Use of soy protein-based formulas in infant feeding. *Pediatrics, 121*, 1062–1068.

Bowman, S. (2002). Beverage choices of young females: Changes and impact on nutrient intakes. *Journal of the American Dietetic Association, 102*, 1234–1239.

Brownell, K., Schwartz, M., Puhl, R., Henderson, K. E., & Harris, J. L. (2009). The need for bold action to prevent adolescent obesity. *Journal of Adolescent Health, 45*, S8–S17.

Bruening, M., Eisenberg, M., MacLehose, R., Nanney, M. S., Story, M., & Neumark-Sztainer, D. (2012). Relationship between adolescents' and their friends' eating behaviors: Breakfast, fruit, vegetables, whole-grain, and dairy intake. *Journal of the Academy of Nutrition and Dietetics, 112*, 1608–1613.

Butte, N., Fox, M., Briefel, R., Siega-Riz, A. M., Dwyer, J. T., Deming, D. M., & Reidy, K. C. (2010). Nutrient intakes of US infants, toddlers, and preschoolers meet or exceed Dietary Reference Intakes. *Journal of the American Dietetic Association, 110*(Suppl. 3), S27–S37.

Cashdan, E. (1994). A sensitive period for learning about food. *Human Nature, 5*, 279–291.

Centers for Disease Control and Prevention. (2012). *Obesity rates among all children in the United States.* Available at www.cdc.gov/obesity/data/childhood.html. Accessed on 11/13/12.

Chomtho, S., Wells, J., Williams, J., Davies, P. S., Lucas, A., & Fewtrell, M. S. (2008). Infant growth and later body composition: Evidence from the 4-component model. *American Journal of Clinical Nutrition, 87*, 1776–1784.

Crosnoe, R. (2007). Gender, obesity, and education. *Sociology of Education, 80*, 241–260.

Daniels, S., & Greer, F. (2008). Lipid screening and cardiovascular health in childhood. *Pediatrics, 122*, 198–208.

Dattilo, A., Birch, L., Krebs, N., Lake, A., Taveras, E. M., & Saavedra, J. M. (2012). Need for early interventions in the prevention of pediatric overweight: A review and upcoming directions. *Journal of Obesity, 2012*, 123023.

De Kroon, M., Renders, C., Van Wouwe, J., Van Buuren, S., & Hirasing, R. A. (2010). The Terneuzen Birth Cohort: BMI changes between 2 and 6 years correlated strongest with adult overweight. *PLoS One, 5*, e9155.

de Lauzon-Guillain, B., Oliveria, A., Charles, M., Grammatikaki, E., Jones, L., Rigal, N., . . . Monnery-Patris, S. (2012). A review of methods to assess parental feeding practices and preschool children's eating behavior: The need for further development of tools. *Journal of the Academy of Nutrition and Dietetics, 112*, 1578–1602.

Dietz, W. (2004). Overweight in childhood and adolescence. *The New England Journal of Medicine, 350*, 855–857.

DiSantis, K., Collins, B., Fisher, J., & Davey, A. (2011). Do infants fed directly from the breast have improved appetite regulation and slower growth during early childhood compared with infants fed from a bottle? *International Journal of Behavioral Nutrition and Physical Activity, 8*, 89.

Dwyer, J., Butte, N., Beming, D., Siega-Riz, A. M., & Reidy, K. C. (2010). Feeding Infants and Toddlers Study 2008: Progress, continuing concerns, and implications. *Journal of the American Dietetic Association, 110*(Suppl. 3), S60–S67.

Fisher, J., & Birch, L. (1999). Restricting access to palatable foods affects children's behavioral response, food selection, and intake. *American Journal of Clinical Nutrition, 69*, 1264–1272.

Gillman, M. (2008). The first months of life: A critical period for development of obesity. *American Journal of Clinical Nutrition, 87*, 1587–1589.

Griffiths, L., Smeeth, L., Hawkins, S. S., Cole, T. J., & Dezateux, C. (2009). Effects of infant feeding practice on weight gain from birth to 3 years. *Archives of Disease in Childhood, 94*, 577–582.

Grummer-Strawn, L., Scanlon, K., & Fein, S. (2008). Infant feeding and feeding transitions during the first year of life. *Pediatrics, 122*, S36–S42.

Gunnarsdottir, I., Schack-Neilsen, L., Michaelsen, K., Sørensen, T. I., & Thorsdottir, I. (2010). Infant weight gain, duration of exclusive breast-feeding and childhood BMI—Two similar follow-up cohorts. *Public Health Nutrition, 13*, 201–207.

Hawkins, S., Cole, T., & Law, C. (2009). An ecological systems approach to examining risk factors for early childhood overweight: Findings from the UK Millennium Cohort Study. *Journal of Epidemiology and Community Health, 63*, 147–155.

Heinig, M., Nommsen, L., Peerson, J., Lonnerdal, B., & Dewey, K. G. (1993). Energy and protein intakes of breastfed and formula-fed infants during the first year of life and their association with growth velocity: The DARLING study. *American Journal of Clinical Nutrition, 58*, 152–161.

Huh, S., Rifas-Shiman, L., Taveras, E., Oken, E., & Gillman, M. W. (2011). Timing of solid food introduction and risk of obesity in preschool-aged children. *Pediatrics, 127*, e544–e551.

Institute of Medicine. (2009). *National Research Council. Weight gain during pregnancy: Reexamining the guidelines.* Washington, DC: The National Academies Press.

Johnson, R. (2000). Changing eating and physical activity patterns of US children. *The Proceedings of the Nutrition Society, 59*, 295–301.

Kelder, S., Perry, C., Klepp, K., & Lytle, L. (1994). Longitudinal tracking of adolescent smoking, physical activity, and food choice behaviors. *American Journal of Public Health, 84*, 1121–1126.

Kleinman, R. E., Hall, S., Green, H., Korzec-Ramirez, D., Patton, K., Pagano, M. E., & Murphy, J. M. (2002). Diet, breakfast, and academic performance in children. *Annals of Nutrition and Metabolism, 46*(Suppl. 1), 24–30.

Koletzko, B., von Kries, R., Closa, R., Escribano, J., Scaglioni, S., Giovannini, M., . . . Grote, V. (2009). Can infant feeding choices modulate later obesity risk? *American Journal of Clinical Nutrition, 89*(Suppl.), 1502S–1508S.

Kramer, M., Guo, T., Platt, R., Vanilovich, I., Sevkovskaya, Z., Dzikovich, I., . . . Dewey, K. (2004). Feeding effects on growth during infancy. *Journal of Pediatrics, 145,* 600–605.

Krebs, N., & Hambidge, M. (2007). Complementary feeding: Clinically relevant factors affecting timing and composition. *American Journal of Clinical Nutrition, 85*(Suppl.), 639S–645S.

LaFontaine, T. (2008). The epidemic of obesity and overweight among youth: Trends, consequences, and interventions. *American Journal of Lifestyle Medicine, 2,* 30–36.

Looney, S., & Raynor, H. (2011). Impact of portion size and energy density on snack intake in preschool-aged children. *Journal of the American Dietetic Association, 111,* 414–418.

Marcason, W. (2005). Can dietary intervention play a part in the treatment of attention deficit and hyperactivity disorder? *Journal of the American Dietetic Association, 105,* 1161–1162.

March of Dimes. (2007). *Professionals and researchers. Quick reference: Fact sheets: Teenage pregnancy.* Available at www.marchofdimes.com/printableArticles/14332_1159.asp. Accessed on 4/21/08.

May, A., & Dietz, W. (2010). The Feeding Infants and Toddlers Study 2008: Opportunities to assess parental, cultural, and environmental influences on dietary behaviors and obesity prevention among young children. *Journal of the American Dietetic Association, 110,* S11–S15.

May, A., Kuklina, E., & Yoon, P. (2012). Prevalence of cardiovascular disease risk factors among US adolescents, 1999–2008. *Pediatrics, 129,* 1035–1041.

Mennella, J., Jagnow, C., & Beauchamp, G. (2001). Prenatal and postnatal flavor learning by human infants. *Pediatrics, 107,* E88.

National Institute of Environmental Health Sciences, National Institutes of Health, U.S. Department of Health and Human Service. (2010). *National Toxicology Program brief on soy infant formula.* Available at http://ntp.niehs.nih.gov/ntp/ohat/genistein-soy/SoyFormulaUpdt/FinalNTPBriefSoyFormula_9_20_2010.pdf#search=soy. Accessed on 11/14/12.

Nicklas, T., O'Neil, C., & Berenson, G. (1998). Nutrient contribution of breakfast, secular trends, and the role of ready-to-eat cereals: A review of data from the Bogalusa Heart Study. *American Journal of Clinical Nutrition, 67*(Suppl.), 757–763S.

Nicklas, T., O'Neil, C., & Myers, L. (2004). The importance of breakfast consumption to nutrition of children, adolescents, and young adults. *Nutrition Today, 1,* 30–39.

Nielsen, J. N., Gittelsohn, J., Anliker, J., & O'Brien, K. (2006). Interventions to improve diet and weight gain among pregnant adolescents and recommendations for future research. *Journal of the American Dietetic Association, 106,* 1825–1840.

Nihiser, A., Lee, S., Wechesler, H., McKenna, M., Odom, E., Reinold, C., . . . Grummer-Strawn, L. (2009). BMI measurement in schools. *Pediatrics, 124*(Suppl. 1), S89–S97.

Nommsen-Rivers, L., & Dewey, K. (2009). Growth of breastfed infants. *Breastfeeding Medicine, 4*(Suppl. 1), S45–S49.

O'Connor, N. (2009). Infant formula. *American Family Physician, 79,* 565–570.

Ogden, C., Carroll, M., Curtin, L., Lamb, M. M., & Flegal, K. M. (2010). Prevalence of high body mass index in US children and adolescents, 2007–2008. *Journal of American Medical Association, 303,* 242–249.

Pollitt, E., & Mathews, R. (1998). Breakfast and cognition: An integrative summary. *American Journal of Clinical Nutrition, 67*(Suppl.), 804S–813S.

Rampersaud, G. C., Pereira, M. A., Girard, B. L., Adams, J., & Metzl, J. D. (2005). Breakfast habits, nutritional status, body weight, and academic performance in children and adolescents. *Journal of the American Dietetic Association, 105,* 743–760.

Reedy, J., & Krebs-Smith, S. (2010). Dietary sources of energy, solid fats, and added sugars among children and adolescents in the US. *Journal of the American Dietetic Association, 110,* 1477–1484.

Savage, J., Haisfield, L., Fisher, J., Marini, M., & Birch, L. L. (2012). Do children eat less at meals when allowed to serve themselves? *American Journal of Clinical Nutrition, 96,* 36–43.

Schack-Nielsen, L., Sorensen, T., Mortensen, E., & Michaelsen, K. (2010). Late introduction of complementary feeding, rather than duration of breastfeeding, may protect against adult overweight. *American Journal of Clinical Nutrition, 91,* 610–627.

Shepherd, L. M., Neumark-Sztainer, D., Beyer, K. M., & Story, M. (2006). Should we discuss weight and calories in adolescent obesity prevention and weight-management programs? Perspectives of adolescent girls. *Journal of the American Dietetic Association, 106,* 1454–1458.

Siega-Riz, A., Deming, D., Reidy, K., Fox, M. K., Condon, E., & Briefel, R. R. (2010). Food consumption patterns of infants and toddlers: Where are we now? *Journal of the American Dietetic Association, 110*(Suppl. 3), S38–S51.

Sloan, S., Gildea, A., Stewart, M., Sneddon, H., & Iwaniec, D. (2008). Early weaning is related to weight and rate of weight gain in infancy. *Child: Care, Health and Development, 34,* 59–64.

Smith, K., Gall, S., McNaughton, S., Blizzard, L., Dwyer, T., & Venn, A. J. (2010). Skipping breakfast: Longitudinal associations with cardiometabolic risk factors in the Childhood Determinants of Adult Health Study. *American Journal of Clinical Nutrition, 92,* 1316–1325.

Stettler, N., Stallings, V., Troxel, A., Zhao, J., Schinnar, R., Nelson, S. E., . . . Strom, B. L. (2005). Weight gain in the first week of life and overweight in adulthood: A cohort study of European American subjects fed infant formula. *Circulation, 111,* 1897–1903.

U.S. Department of Agriculture, Agricultural Research Service. (2010). *Nutrient intakes from food: Mean amounts consumed per individual, by gender and age. What We Eat in American, NHANES 2007–2008.* Available at www.ars.usda.gov/ba/bhnrc/fsrg. Accessed on 6/9/12.

U.S. Department of Agriculture, U.S. Department of Health and Human Services. (2010). *Dietary guidelines for Americans, 2010* (7th ed.). Available at www.health.gov/dietaryguidelines. Accessed on 6/9/12.

U.S. Department of Health and Human Services. (2004). *The health consequences of smoking: A report of the Surgeon General.* Atlanta, GA: CDC, Office on Smoking and Health. Available at www.cdc.gov/tobacco/data_statistics/sgr/sgr_2004/highlights/3.htm. Accessed on 7/21/08.

U.S. Department of Health and Human Services. (2011). *The Surgeon General's call to action to support breastfeeding.* Washington, DC: U.S. Department of Health and Human Services, Office of the Surgeon General.

Utter, J., Scragg, R., Mhurchu, C. N., & Schaaf, D. (2007). At-home breakfast consumption among New Zealand children: Associations with body mass index and related nutrition behaviors. *Journal of the American Dietetic Association, 107,* 570–576.

van Dam, R. M., Willet, W. C., Manson, J. E., & Hu, F. B. (2006). The relationship between overweight in adolescents and premature death in women. *Annals of Internal Medicine, 145,* 91–97.

Wagner, C., Greer, F., & the Section on Breastfeeding and Committee on Nutrition. (2008). Prevention of rickets and vitamin D deficiency in infants, children, and adolescents. *Pediatrics, 122,* 1142–1152.

Whitaker, R., Wright, J., Pepe, M., Seidel, K. D., & Dietz, W. H. (1997). Predicting obesity in young adulthood from childhood and parental obesity. *New England Journal of Medicine, 337,* 869–873.

13 Nutrition for Older Adults

CHECK YOUR KNOWLEDGE

TRUE	FALSE		
☐	☐	**1**	The majority of people 65 years and older rate their health as good or better.
☐	☐	**2**	In general, calorie needs in older adults decrease while the need for other nutrients stays the same or increases.
☐	☐	**3**	Older adults have higher fluid requirements than younger adults.
☐	☐	**4**	Older adults should get vitamin B_{12} from supplements or fortified foods.
☐	☐	**5**	Older adults generally do not consume enough iron.
☐	☐	**6**	Sarcopenia is inevitable and irreversible.
☐	☐	**7**	Weight loss in older adults is associated with mortality.
☐	☐	**8**	The RDA for calcium is highest in early adulthood when peak bone mass is being attained.
☐	☐	**9**	The prevalence of malnutrition in long-term care facilities is 10%.
☐	☐	**10**	A major cause of undernutrition in long-term care is loss of appetite.

LEARNING OBJECTIVES

Upon completion of this chapter, you will be able to

1 Give examples of physiologic changes that occur with aging and that have an impact on nutrition.
2 Compare calorie and nutrient needs of older adults to those of younger adults.
3 Compare modified MyPlate for Older Adults with intake guidelines for younger adults.
4 Explain why older adults may need supplements of calcium, vitamin D, and vitamin B_{12}.
5 Screen an older person for risk of nutrition problems.
6 Debate the benefits of using a liberal diet in long-term care facilities.
7 Propose strategies for enhancing food intake in long-term care residents.

With the exception of Chapters 11 and 12, which cover infants, children, and adolescents, this book implicitly addresses nutrition as it pertains to adults—nutrient and calorie basics in Unit 1; food intake guidelines and consumer and cultural nutrition issues in Unit 2; and the role of nutrition in the prevention and treatment of illness and disease in Unit 3. Yet adulthood represents a wide age range, from young adults at 18 years to the "oldest old."

Adults over 50 years, and especially those over 70 years, have different nutritional needs than do younger adults. This chapter focuses on how aging impacts nutrition for older adults.

AGING AND OLDER ADULTS

Aging is a gradual, inevitable, complex process of progressive physiologic, cellular, cultural, and psychosocial changes that begin at conception and end at death. As cells age, they undergo degenerative changes in structure and function that eventually lead to impairment of organs, tissues, and body functioning. Box 13.1 outlines the changes in physiology, income, health, and psychosocial well-being associated with aging that have nutritional implications.

Box 13.1   CHANGES THAT MAY OCCUR WITH AGING

Composition and Energy Expenditure Changes
- Decrease in lean body mass
- Increase in fat tissue
- Decrease in basal metabolic rate
- Decrease in physical activity

Oral and Gastrointestinal (GI) Changes
- Difficulty in chewing related to loss of teeth and periodontal disease
- Constipation is more common and may be related to decreased peristalsis from loss of abdominal muscle tone, inadequate fluid and fiber intake, secondary reaction to drug therapy, or a decrease in physical activity.
- Digestive disorders may occur from a decreased secretion of HCl in the stomach and digestive enzymes, decreased GI motility, and decreased organ function.
- Prevalence of atrophic gastritis increases.
- Nutrient absorption may decrease because of decreased mucosal mass and decreased blood flow to and from the mucosal villi.

Metabolic Changes
- Altered glucose tolerance; the underlying reason may be a decrease in insulin secretion or a decrease in tissue sensitivity to insulin.
- Synthesis of vitamin D in the skin decreases with age.

Central Nervous System Changes
- Tremors, slowed reaction time, short-term memory deficits, personality changes, and depression may occur secondary to a decrease in the number of brain cells or the decrease in blood flow to the brain.

Renal Changes
- Ability to concentrate urine decreases

Sensory Losses
- Hearing loss, loss of visual acuity, decreased sense of smell, decreased number of taste buds, and decreased sensation of thirst

Other Changes
- Change in income related to retirement
- Reliance on medications
- Social isolation related to death of spouse, living alone, impaired mobility
- Poor self-esteem related to change in body image, lack of productivity, feelings of aimlessness

Exactly how and why aging occurs is unknown, although most theories are based on genetic or environmental causes.

Aging Demographics

Older adults, especially those older than 85 years of age, represent the fastest growing segment of the American population (Federal Interagency Forum on Aging-Related Statistics, 2012). In 2010, an estimated 40.3 million people, or 13% of the population, were age 65 years and over. By the year 2030, it is estimated that 72.1 million Americans, nearly 20% of the population, will be over age 65 years. The number of Americans age 85 years and older is expected to increase from 5.5 million in 2010 to 8.7 million in 2030.

Life expectancies at both 65 and 85 years have increased. People who live to age 65 years can expect to live an average of 19.2 more years; among people who live to age 85 years, women will survive another 7 years on average and men will survive another 5.9 years (Federal Interagency Forum on Aging-Related Statistics, 2012). Adopting a healthy lifestyle early in life and maintaining it throughout life along with a healthy body weight and physically active lifestyle may help the elderly avoid physical and mental deteriorations associated with aging (Bernstein and Munoz, 2012).

Despite the misconceptions and stereotypes that people have of older adults, they are a heterogeneous group that varies in age, marital status, social background, financial status, living arrangements, and health status. Most adults older than age 65 years have one chronic health problem, such as hypertension, arthritis, heart disease, or diabetes (Fig. 13.1) (Federal Interagency Forum on Aging-Related Statistics, 2012). Yet during 2008–2010, 76% of people 65 years and older considered their health to be good or better (Federal Interagency Forum on Aging-Related Statistics, 2012), possibly because people define

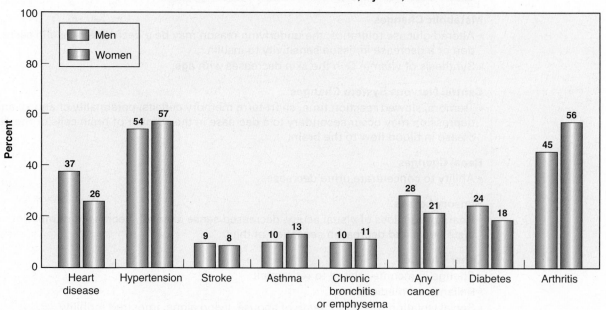

■ FIGURE 13.1 Chronic health conditions. (**Source:** Interagency Forum on Aging-Related Statistics. [2012]. *Older Americans 2008: Key indicators of well-being.* Washington, DC: U.S. Government Printing Office.)

wellness and illness differently as they age and may accept changes in health as a normal aspect of aging. Certainly differences exist between the "well" and the "frail" elderly, the latter group consisting of those with defined needs for support for activities of daily living. In 2009, only 4.1% of people 65 years and older lived in an institutional setting (Federal Interagency Forum on Aging-Related Statistics, 2012).

Healthy Aging

Genetic and environmental "life advantages"—such as genetic potential for longevity, intelligence, motivation, curiosity, good socialization, religious affiliation, marriage and family, avoidance of substance abuse, availability of health care, adequate sleep, and sufficient rest and relaxation—have positive effects on both length and quality of life. Other major determinants of successful aging are physical activity and healthy eating. Older adults are urged to follow the adult guidelines for physical activity or as their abilities allow (Box 13.2). Strong evidence shows that for adults and older adults, physical activity lowers the risk of heart disease, stroke, type 2 diabetes, hypertension, dyslipidemia, metabolic syndrome, and weight gain in addition to improving cardiovascular and muscular fitness, preventing falls, reducing depression, and improving cognitive function (U.S. Department of Health and Human Services [USDHHS], 2008). Healthy eating can enhance wellness, improve nutritional status, help avoid illness, and prevent or delay diseases and disability. Although the earlier in life a healthy diet and lifestyle are adopted the better, evidence shows that even initiating healthy changes in one's 60s and 70s provides definite benefits in many categories of chronic disease (Rivlin, 2007).

Box 13.2   2008 PHYSICAL ACTIVITY GUIDELINES FOR AMERICANS

Adults (Age 18–64 Years)
- Adults should do 2 hours and 30 minutes a week of moderate-intensity or 1 hour and 15 minutes (75 minutes) a week of vigorous-intensity aerobic physical activity, or an equivalent combination of moderate- and vigorous-intensity aerobic physical activity. Aerobic activity should be performed in episodes of at least 10 minutes, preferably spread throughout the week.
- Additional health benefits are provided by increasing to 5 hours (300 minutes) a week of moderate-intensity aerobic physical activity, or 2 hours and 30 minutes a week of vigorous-intensity physical activity, or an equivalent combination of both.
- Adults should also do muscle-strengthening activities that involve all major muscle groups performed on 2 or more days per week.

Older Adults (Age 65 Years and Older)
- Older adults should follow the adult guidelines. If this is not possible due to limiting chronic conditions, older adults should be as physically active as their abilities allow. They should avoid inactivity. Older adults should do exercises that maintain or improve balance if they are at risk of falling.

For all individuals, some activity is better than none. Physical activity is safe for almost everyone, and the health benefits of physical activity far outweigh the risks. People without diagnosed chronic conditions (e.g., diabetes, heart disease, or osteoarthritis) and who do not have symptoms (e.g., chest pain or pressure, dizziness, or joint pain) do not need to consult with a health care provider about physical activity.

Source: U.S. Department of Health and Human Services. (2008). *Physical activity guidelines for Americans. At-a-glance: A fact sheet for professionals.* Available at www.health.gov/paguidelines/factsheetprof.aspx. Accessed on 11/20/12.

Nutritional Needs of Older Adults

Knowledge of the nutritional needs of older adults is growing. However, health status, physiologic functioning, physical activity, and nutritional status vary more among older adults (especially people older than 70 years) than among individuals in any other age group, so nutrient recommendations may not be appropriate for all elderly individuals at all times. In general, calorie needs decrease, yet vitamin and mineral requirements stay the same or increase. Two Dietary Reference Intake (DRI) groupings exist for mature adults, one for people age 51 to 70 years and another for adults over the age of 70 years. Calories and selected nutrients are discussed in the following sections.

Calories

Calorie needs decrease with age, attributed in large part to progressive decreases in physical activity (Table 13.1) (Bernstein and Munoz, 2012). A decrease in physical activity directly lowers calorie expenditure. Indirectly, a decrease in physical activity leads to a loss of lean body mass. It is changes in body composition—namely, a decrease in muscle and bone mass and an increase in percentage of body fat—that account for the decrease in metabolic rate of approximately 2% per decade beginning around the age of 30 years (Elmadfa and Meyer, 2008). Taken together, the decrease in physical activity and lower metabolic rate lead to an estimated 5% decrease in total calorie needs each decade. However, neither the changes in body composition nor the decrease in physical activity is inevitable (Rivlin, 2007). Studies show that with appropriate weight training exercises, muscle loss can be prevented and reversed, even among 90-year-old frail institutionalized men and women (Fiatarone et al., 1990; Kerksick et al., 2007; Kryger and Andersen, 2007; Pratley et al., 1994).

Protein

The Recommended Dietary Allowance (RDA) for protein remains constant at 0.8 g/kg for both men and women from the age of 19 years on (National Research Council, 2005a). This

Table 13.1 MyPlate Calorie Levels Based on Sex, Age, and Activity Level

MyPlate assigns individuals to a calorie level based on their sex, age, and activity level.

	Males				Females		
Activity Level	Sedentary*	Moderately Active*	Active*	Activity Level	Sedentary*	Moderately Active*	Active*
Age (Years)				Age (Years)			
51–55	2200	2400	2800	51–55	1600	1800	2200
56–60	2200	2400	2600	56–60	1600	1800	2200
61–65	2000	2400	2600	61–65	1600	1800	2000
66–70	2000	2200	2600	66–70	1600	1800	2000
71–75	2000	2200	2600	71–75	1600	1800	2000
76 and up	2000	2200	2400	76 and up	1600	1800	2000

*Calorie levels are based on the Estimated Energy Requirements (EER) and activity levels from the Institute of Medicine Dietary Reference Intakes Macronutrients Report, 2002.

Sedentary = less than 30 minutes a day of moderate physical activity in addition to daily activities.

Moderately Active = at least 30 minutes but up to 60 minutes a day of moderate physical activity in addition to daily activities.

Active = 60 or more minutes a day of moderate physical activity in addition to daily activities.

Lean Body Mass: skeletal muscle and bone mass.

National Health and Nutrition Examination Survey (NHANES): a survey conducted by the National Center for Health Statistics designed to assess the health and nutritional status of adults and children in the United States via personal interviews and physical examinations.

level represents the minimum protein intake necessary to avoid progressive loss of **lean body mass** as determined by nitrogen balance studies (Wolfe, Miller, and Miller, 2008). However, the data were gathered almost entirely in college-aged men who can maintain nitrogen balance on less protein than can older adults (Wolfe et al., 2008). Physiologic changes and less lean body mass in older adults leads to decreases in total body protein and contributes to increased frailty, impaired wound healing, and decreased immune function (Bernstein and Munoz, 2012). Evidence suggests that older adults need more protein than younger adults and that a protein intake between 1.0 and 1.6 g/kg/day is safe and adequate to meet the needs of healthy older adults (Houston et al., 2008). (See section on Sarcopenia.)

According to data from the **National Health and Nutrition Examination Survey (NHANES)** 2007–2008, mean protein intake exceeds the RDA for both men and women among all age groups, although a steady decline in intake occurs with aging (U.S. Department of Agriculture [USDA], Agricultural Research Service [ARS], 2010). An estimated 7.2% to 8.6% of older adult women consume protein below their estimated average requirement (Fulgoni, 2008). Factors that may contribute to a decrease in protein intake include the cost of high-protein foods, the decreased ability to chew meats, lower overall intake of food, and changes in digestion and gastric emptying (Paddon-Jones, Short, Campbell, Volpi, and Wolfe, 2008).

Water

The Adequate Intake (AI) for water, which includes total water from drinking water, other beverages, and water in solid foods, is constant from 19 years of age through more than 70 years old, with 3.7 L/day of total water recommended for men and 2.7 L/day for women (Institute of Medicine, 2005). Both of these figures represent a level of intake necessary to replace normal daily losses and prevent the effects of dehydration (National Research Council, 2005b). Like younger adults, the elderly are able to maintain fluid balance over a wide range of intakes.

Most older adults do not meet the recommended intake for water (Bernstein and Munoz, 2012). A number of physiologic changes and other factors increase the risk of dehydration in the elderly, including an impaired sensation of thirst, alterations in mental status and cognition, adverse effects of medications, impaired mobility, and an age-related decrease in the ability to concentrate urine. Fear of incontinence and pain from arthritis may cause voluntary restriction in fluid intake. Dehydration can contribute to constipation, cognitive impairment, functional decline, and death (Bernstein and Munoz, 2012).

Fiber

For all age groups, the AI for fiber is based on median intake levels observed to protect against coronary heart disease (CHD) (National Research Council, 2005a). From the age of 1 year on and for both genders, the AI for fiber is set at 14 g/1000 cal of intake. Based on median calorie intakes, the AI for fiber is 38 g/day for men through age 50 years and 30 g/day thereafter. A similar decrease occurs in women, whose AI is 25 g/day from 19 to 50 years and 21 g/day thereafter.

Intake surveys consistently show that older adults consume approximately half the recommended amount of fiber (USDA, ARS, 2010). Increasing fiber intake may help prevent constipation, improve glycemic control, and reduce serum cholesterol levels (Bernstein and Munoz, 2012).

Vitamins and Minerals

Most recommended levels of intake for vitamins and minerals do not change with aging. Significant exceptions to this generalization are calcium and vitamin D and, for women, the

Table 13.2 Important Nutrients Whose RDAs Change with Aging*

Nutrient	Age 31–50 Years	Age 51–70 Years	Age 71+ Years	Rationale for Change
Calcium (mg/day)	1000	1200 (female) 1000 (male)	1200	The efficiency of calcium absorption decreases with age.
Vitamin D (IU/day)	600	600	800	The ability to synthesize vitamin D on the skin from sunlight decreases with age.
Iron (mg/day) Females only	18	8	8	Cessation of menstruation

*Values are for both males and females unless otherwise indicated.

Source: Institute of Medicine. (2010). *Dietary Reference Intakes for calcium and vitamin D.* Available at http://www.iom.edu/Reports/2010/Dietary-Reference-Intakes-for-Calcium-and-Vitamin-D.aspx. Accessed 2/1/13.

recommendation for iron (Table 13.2). The DRI for sodium decreases with aging because the AI is extrapolated from younger adults based on median calorie intakes from food surveys. Although the total amount of vitamin B_{12} recommended does not change with aging, people over 50 years are advised to consume most of their requirement from fortified food or supplements because 10% to 30% of older adults may not be able to absorb natural vitamin B_{12} from food (National Research Council, 1998).

According to NHANES data from 2007–2008, the mean intake of several micronutrients is deficient in the diets of older adults—namely, vitamins A, D, and E; calcium; magnesium; and potassium (Table 13.3) (USDA, ARS, 2010). Conversely, their intake of sodium is too high.

Table 13.3 Sources of Food Components That May Be Lacking in the Diets of Older Adults

Food Component	Sources
Vitamin A	Green and orange vegetables, especially **green leafy vegetables**; orange fruits, liver, **milk**
Vitamin D	**Milk**, fortified soy milk, fatty fish, some fortified ready-to-eat cereals
Vitamin E	Vegetable oils, margarine, salad dressing made with vegetable oil, nuts, seeds, **whole grains**, **green leafy vegetables**, fortified cereals
Calcium	**Milk**, yogurt, cheese, fortified orange juice, **green leafy vegetables**, **legumes**
Magnesium	**Green leafy vegetables**, nuts, **legumes**, **whole grains**, seafood, chocolate, **milk**
Potassium	Fruit and **vegetables**, **legumes**, **whole grains**, **milk**, meats
Fiber	**Whole grains**; **legumes**; fruit and **vegetables**, especially the skin and seeds

Note: **Bold** type used to illustrate the commonality of sources among these nutrients.

Healthy Eating Guidelines

MyPlate for Older Adults, produced by Tufts University, is designed to help healthy, older adults who are living independently choose a diet that is consistent with the *Dietary Guidelines for Americans, 2010* (Fig. 13.2). The graphic features a variety of colorful fruits and vegetables, whole and fortified grains, low-fat and nonfat dairy milk and dairy products, lean proteins, and liquid vegetable oils. Noteworthy features are as follows:

- Nutrient-dense food choices are used to illustrate each food group. As calorie needs decrease, there is less room for empty-calorie foods that are high in solid fats or added sugar.
- The examples of foods featured on the plate are convenient, affordable, and readily available. For instance, peaches canned in natural juice are shown because they are easy to prepare, are more affordable, and have a longer shelf life than fresh peaches.
- Low-sodium canned vegetables appear as an option to help lower sodium intake.
- Eight beverage servings are featured next to the plate to highlight the importance of adequate fluid intake.
- Older adults engaged in common activities appear in an icon across the top of the placemat as a reminder that there are a variety of options for engaging in physical activity.

Food Intake of Older Adults

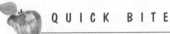

QUICK BITE

Fruits and vegetables that are easily consumed by people who have difficulty chewing

Ripe bananas	Canned fruit
Baked winter squash	Soft melon
Mashed potatoes	Citrus sections
Stewed tomatoes	Cooked carrots
Baked apples	

Like younger adults, older Americans consume less fruit and vegetables than recommended, and starchy vegetables account for about 80% of total vegetable intake on any given day (USDA, Center for Nutrition Policy and Promotion, 2007). Major improvements in the nutritional health of older adults could be realized if older adults increased their intakes of whole grains, dark green and orange vegetables and legumes, and fat-free or low-fat milk products (Federal Interagency Forum on Aging-Related Statistics, 2012). Notice in Table 13.3 that for the nutrients most likely to be consumed in inadequate amounts by older adults, whole grains, vegetables (especially green leafy vegetables), legumes, and milk are listed as sources for three or more of these nutrients. Other changes to improve the quality of older adults' intake are to incorporate foods and beverages that are lower in sodium and to consume fewer calories from solid fats, alcoholic beverages, and added sugars. Frequently, food choices of older adults are based on considerations other than food preferences, such as income; the client's physical ability to shop, prepare, chew, and swallow food; and the occurrence of food intolerances related to chronic disease or side effects of medication. Box 13.3 features tips for eating well as you get older.

While snacking may contribute to an excess calorie intake and obesity in other age groups, snacking in older adults may help ensure an adequate intake. A study by Zizza, Tayie, and Lino (2007) found that as older adults' frequency of snacking increased, their daily intakes of vitamins A, C, and E; beta-carotene; magnesium; copper; and potassium improved. For older adults at risk of inadequate intake, encouraging snacking between meals may be more effective than urging them to eat more at each meal.

My Plate for Older Adults

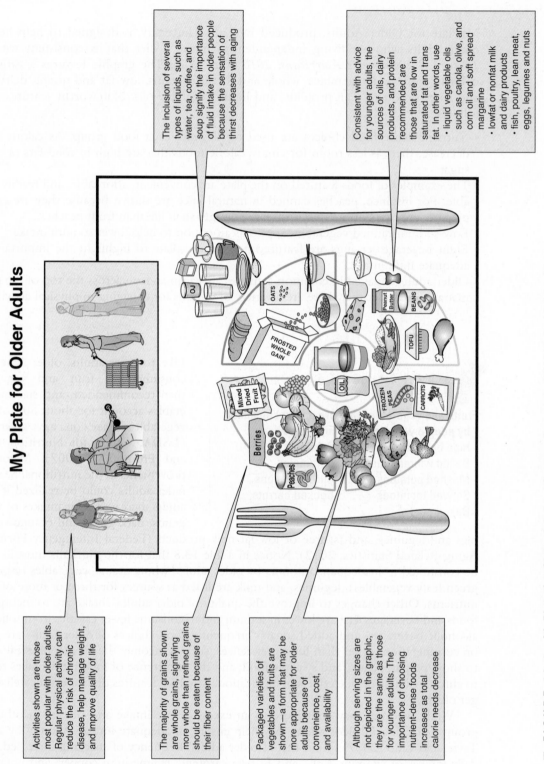

The inclusion of several types of liquids, such as water, tea, coffee, and soup signify the importance of fluid intake in older people because the sensation of thirst decreases with aging

Consistent with advice for younger adults, the sources of oils, dairy products, and protein recommended are those that are low in saturated fat and trans fat. In other words, use
- liquid vegetable oils such as canola, olive, and corn oil and soft spread margarine
- lowfat or nonfat milk and dairy products
- fish, poultry, lean meat, eggs, legumes and nuts

Activities shown are those most popular with older adults. Regular physical activity can reduce the risk of chronic disease, help manage weight, and improve quality of life

The majority of grains shown are whole grains, signifying more whole than refined grains should be eaten because of their fiber content

Packaged varieties of vegetables and fruits are shown—a form that may be more appropriate for older adults because of convenience, cost, and availability

Although serving sizes are not depicted in the graphic, they are the same as those for younger adults. The importance of choosing nutrient-dense foods increases as total calorie needs decrease

■ **FIGURE 13.2** MyPlate for Older Adults. (**Source:** Copyright 2011 Tufts University. For details about the MyPlate for Older Adults, please see http://nutrition.tufts.edu/research/myplate-older-adults)

Box 13.3   TIPS FOR EATING WELL AS YOU GET OLDER

Enjoy Your Meals

Eating is one of life's pleasures, but some people lose interest in eating and cooking as they get older. They may find that food no longer tastes good. They may find it harder to shop for food or cook, or they don't enjoy meals because they often eat alone. Others may have problems chewing or digesting the food they eat.

Why Not Eating Can Be Harmful

If you don't feel like eating because of problems with chewing, digestion, or gas, talk with your doctor or a registered dietitian. Avoiding some foods could mean you miss out on needed vitamins, minerals, fiber, or protein. Not eating enough could mean that you don't consume enough nutrients and calories.

Problems with Taste or Smell?

One reason people lose interest in eating is that their senses of taste and smell change with age. Foods you once enjoyed might seem to have less flavor when you get older. Some medicines can change your sense of taste or make you feel less hungry. Talk with your health care provider if you have no appetite, or if you find that food tastes bad or has no flavor.

If you don't feel like eating because food no longer tastes good, you can enhance the flavor of food by cooking meals in new ways or adding different herbs and spices.

Problems Chewing?

If you have trouble chewing, you might have a problem with your teeth or gums. If you wear dentures, not being able to chew well could also mean that your dentures need to be adjusted. Talk to your health care provider or dentist if you're finding it hard to chew food.

Chewing problems can sometimes be resolved by eating softer foods. For instance, you could replace raw vegetables and fresh fruits with cooked vegetables or juices. Also choose foods like applesauce and canned peaches or other fruits.

Meat can also be hard to chew. Instead, try eating ground or shredded meat, eggs, or dairy products like fat-free or low-fat milk, cheese, and yogurt. You could also replace meat with soft foods like cooked beans and peas, eggs, tofu, tuna fish, etc.

Problems with Digestion?

If you experience a lot of digestive problems, such as gas or bloating, try to avoid foods that cause gas or other digestive problems. If you have stomach problems that don't go away, talk with your health care provider. If you do not have an appetite or seem to be losing weight without trying, talk to your health care provider or ask to see a registered dietitian.

Try New Dishes

Making small changes in the way you prepare your food can often help overcome challenges to eating well. These changes can help you to enjoy meals more. They can also help make sure that you get the nutrients and energy you need for healthy, active living.

■ Look for ways to combine foods from the different food groups in creative ways. You can do this while continuing to eat familiar foods that reflect your cultural, ethnic, or family traditions.

(continues on page 330)

Box 13.3   Tips for Eating Well as You Get Older (continued)

- Experiment with ethnic foods, regional dishes, or vegetarian recipes.
- Try out different kinds of fruits, vegetables, and grains that add color to your meals.
- Try new recipes from friends, newspapers, magazines, television cooking shows, or cooking websites.
- Take a cooking class to learn new ways to prepare meals and snacks that are good for you. Grocery stores, culinary schools, community centers, and adult education programs offer these classes.

Eat with Others

Eating with others is another way to enjoy meals more. For instance, you could share meals with neighbors at home or dine out with friends or family members. You could also join or start a breakfast, lunch, or dinner club.

Many senior centers and places of worship host group meals. You might also arrange to have meals brought to your home.

When Eating Out

When you eat out, you can still eat well if you choose carefully, know how your food is prepared, and watch portion sizes. Here are some tips.

- Eat reasonable amounts of food and stay within your calorie needs for the day.
- Select main dishes that include vegetables, such as salads, vegetable stir fries, or kebobs.
- Order your food baked, broiled, or grilled instead of fried.
- Make sure it is thoroughly cooked, especially dishes with meat, poultry, seafood, or eggs.
- Choose dishes without gravies or creamy sauces.
- Ask for salad dressing on the side so you can control the amount you eat.
- Ordering half portions or splitting a dish with a friend can help keep calorie intake down.

Ask for Substitutions

Also, don't be afraid to ask for substitutions. Many restaurants and eating establishments not only offer healthful choices but let you substitute healthier foods. For example, you might substitute fat-free yogurt for sour cream on your baked potato. Instead of a side order of onion rings or French fries, you could have the mixed vegetables. Ask for brown rice instead of white rice. Try having fruit for dessert.

Meals are an important part of our lives. They give us nourishment and a chance to spend time with friends, family members, and others. If physical problems keep you from eating well or enjoying meals, talk with a health care professional. If you need help shopping or preparing meals or want to find ways to share meals with others, look for services in your community. Your area Agency on Aging can tell you about these services. To contact your area Agency on Aging, call the Eldercare Locator toll-free at 1-800-677-1116.

Source: National Institute on Aging, National Institutes of Health, U.S. Department of Health and Human Services. (n.d.). Available at http://nihseniorhealth.gov/eatingwellasyougetolder/enjoyyourmeals/01.html

Vitamin and Mineral Supplements

In theory, older adults should be able to obtain adequate amounts of all essential nutrients through well-chosen foods. In practice, a large percentage of older adults do not obtain recommended amounts of many nutrients from food alone (Sebastian, Cleveland, Goldman, and Moshfegh, 2007). According to 2003–2006 survey data, 70% of adults older than 70 years reported taking at least one supplement in the previous month, with 33% taking a multivitamin/multimineral supplement (Albright et al., 2012). A study by Fabian, Bogner, Kickinger, Wagner, and Elmadfa (2012) showed that the use of supplements significantly improved the status of several vitamins in elderly people, particularly for vitamins B_1, B_2, and B_{12}, folate, and vitamin D. While food is the preferred vehicle for providing nutrients, low-dose multivitamin and mineral supplements can be valuable in helping older adults achieve nutritional adequacy (Sebastian et al., 2007). Interestingly, supplement users generally tend to eat more nutrient-dense diets than nonsupplement users.

Undernutrition and Malnutrition

Older adults represent the largest demographic group at disproportionate risk for inadequate intake and protein–calorie malnutrition (PCM) (Skates and Anthony, 2012). Cross-sectional and longitudinal studies indicate that the quantity of food and calorie intake decreases substantially with age (Bernstein and Munoz, 2012). As calorie intake decreases, so does micronutrient intake. Numerous physiologic, psychosocial, cultural, and medical factors may contribute to a decrease in intake and appetite in older adults (Wernette, White, and Zizza, 2011). Weight loss, functional dependence, cognitive impairment, loneliness, living without a partner, history of lung or heart disease, and the presence of acute vomiting are among the risk factors for malnutrition in older adults (Jurschik et al., 2010).

The exact prevalence of undernutrition and malnutrition is unknown because there is currently no gold standard for diagnosis. Recent data show an overall prevalence of malnutrition at 23% of older adults, and an additional 43% of older adults are at risk for malnutrition (Kaiser et al., 2010). These figures translate to nearly two-thirds of older adults with malnutrition or risk for malnutrition. Malnutrition is reported to affect 91% of older adults in rehabilitation facilities, 86% in hospitals, 67% in nursing homes, and 38% living in the community (Kaiser et al., 2010).

Malnutrition impairs quality of life and increases morbidity and mortality. It is linked to diminished cognitive function, physical weakness, and muscle wasting, which increase the risk of falls, fractures, and infections (Skates and Anthony, 2012). Among hospitalized older adults, malnutrition is associated with longer hospitalizations (Pichard et al., 2004) and higher rates of complications and death (Thomas et al., 2002). In nursing homes, malnutrition increases the risk of pressure ulcers, cognitive deficits, and infections (Barrett-Connor, Edelstein, Corey-Bloom, and Wiederhold, 1996; Horn et al., 2004; Hudgens, Langkam-Henken, Stechmiller, Herrlinger-Garcia, and Nieves, 2004). Selected factors that may contribute to malnutrition are discussed in the following sections.

Anorexia of Aging

"Anorexia of aging" is a term used to describe the natural decrease in food intake that occurs even in healthy older adults in response to a decrease in physical activity and metabolic rate. Older adults exhibit less hunger and earlier satiety than younger adults (Bernstein and Munoz, 2012). Diminished appetite contributes to undernutrition in both community and institutional settings and can lead to unintentional weight loss, which is often associated with poor health outcomes and is a marker for deteriorating well-being in older adults

(Bernstein and Munoz, 2012). Loss of appetite is a key predictor of malnutrition in older adults (Bernstein and Munoz, 2012).

Functional Limitations

Instrumental Activities of Daily Living (IADL) Limitations: difficulty performing (or unable to perform for a health reason) one or more of the following tasks: using the telephone, light housework, heavy housework, meal preparation, shopping, or managing money.

Activities of Daily Living (ADL) Limitations: difficulty performing (or unable to perform for a health reason) one or more of the following tasks: bathing, dressing, eating, getting in/out of chairs, walking, or using the toilet.

Aging causes a progressive decline in physical function that is related to a decrease in muscle mass and strength (Villareal, Apovian, Kushner, and Klein, 2005). In community-dwelling elderly, sarcopenic obesity is independently associated with functional instrumental activities of daily living disability (Baumgartner et al., 2004). In 2009, the percentage of Medicare enrollees age 65 years and older with a functional limitation (previously called disability) was 42% (Federal Interagency Forum on Aging-Related Statistics, 2012). Twelve percent of this population had one or more **instrumental activities of daily living (IADL) limitations** without any **activities of daily living (ADL) limitations**, and almost 18% had difficulty with one to two ADL. Diseases that increase the risk of functional limitations include cerebrovascular accident, diabetes, ischemic heart disease, and arthritis (Bernstein and Munoz, 2012).

Social Isolation

Eating alone is a risk factor for poor nutritional status among older adults; therefore, efforts should be made to eat with friends and relatives whenever possible. Other potential options are the federally funded nutrition programs—congregate meals and Meals on Wheels. These programs are designed to provide low-cost, nutritious, hot meals; education about food and nutrition; opportunities for socialization and recreation; and information on other health and social assistance programs. The congregate meal program provides a hot, balanced, midday meal and the opportunity to socialize in senior citizen centers and other public or private facilities. Those who choose to pay may do so; otherwise, the meal is free. Meals on Wheels is a home-delivered meal program for elderly persons who are unable to get to congregate meal centers because they live in an isolated area or have a chronic illness or physical limitations. Usually, a hot meal is served at midday and a bagged lunch is included to be used as the evening meal. Modified diets, such as carbohydrate-controlled diets and low-sodium diets, are provided as needed.

Polypharmacy

Both prescription and over-the-counter drugs have the potential to affect and be affected by nutritional status. Sometimes, drug–nutrient interactions are the intended actions of the drug, such as the effect of warfarin on vitamin K status. At other times, alterations in nutrient intake, metabolism, or excretion may be an unwanted side effect of drug therapy. Although well-nourished individuals on short-term drug therapy may easily withstand the negative effects of drug–nutrient interactions, people who are malnourished or those on long-term drug regimens may experience significant nutrient deficiencies and decreased tolerance to drug therapy.

The elderly are at risk for developing drug-induced nutrient deficiencies because they have more chronic illnesses, are often on long-term drug therapy, and polypharmacy increases with age. In a study by Heuberger and Caudell (2011), the prevalence of polypharmacy in participants (average age 75.5 years) was 43%, with 51.5% of those participants using five or more medications. Polypharmacy was associated with poorer nutritional status. Overall, as the number of medications used increased, the intake of

- Fiber decreased
- Cholesterol, carbohydrates, and sodium increased
- Fat-soluble vitamins, B vitamins, and minerals decreased

Nutrition Screening for Older Adults

Nutrition screening to identify presence or risk of malnutrition is appropriate in any setting where older adults receive services or care, such as in hospitals, long-term care facilities, community-based care, home health, and physician offices (Kamp, Wellman, and Russell, 2010). Screening is often the responsibility of the nurse.

A widely used quick and easy tool for screening older adults is the Mini Nutritional Assessment–Short Form (MNA-SF) (Fig. 13.3). It is the newest version of a nutrition screening tool designed and validated as a stand-alone tool to identify PCM in people 65 years and older (Skates and Anthony, 2012). It consists of six questions with a maximum possible score of 14. A score from 12 to 14 indicates normal nutritional status, 8 to 11 indicates at risk for malnutrition, and 7 or less indicates malnutrition. Scores less than 12 warrant further assessment by a dietitian.

NUTRITION-RELATED CONCERNS IN OLDER ADULTS

Overall goals of nutrition therapy for older adults are to maintain or restore maximal independent functioning and health and to maintain the client's sense of dignity and quality of life by imposing as few dietary restrictions as possible. Nutrition therapy for older adults should consider the individual's physiologic, pathologic, and psychosocial conditions.

Arthritis

An estimated 50 million American adults have some form of doctor-diagnosed arthritis (Cheng, Hootman, Murphy, and Helmick, 2010). Osteoarthritis (OA), the most common form of arthritis, can lead to joint degeneration, chronic pain, muscle atrophy, impaired mobility, and poor balance. Arthritis is the leading cause of disability (Centers for Disease Control and Prevention [CDC], 2007).

OA is associated with aging and normal "wear and tear" on joints; the knee is the most commonly affected joint. Excess body weight, which creates chronic mechanical stress on the weight-bearing joints, is a well-established risk factor; 66% of adults with doctor-diagnosed arthritis are overweight or obese (CDC, 2011). Other risk factors for OA include genetics, age, gender, occupation, exercise, trauma, and muscle weakness (Arthritis Foundation, 2012). Symptoms of OA usually appear after the age of 45 years.

The objective of treatment is to control pain, improve function, and reduce physical limitations. Currently, there is no diet or specific food or food component known to effectively prevent or treat arthritis (Bernstein and Munoz, 2012). However, weight loss and appropriate exercise seem to have a positive effect on preventing and treating OA (Greenstone, 2007). Data from the Arthritis, Diet, and Activity Promotion Trial (ADAPT) study of overweight and obese older adults with OA of the knee showed that the combination of a weight loss diet and exercise improved both subjective and objective measures of physical function and quality of life, and the benefits were greater than when either diet or exercise was used alone (Messier et al., 2004). Losing weight reduces strain on the weight-bearing joints; exercise improves strength, mobility, and joint stability and may also reduce pain and improve function (Roddy et al., 2005).

Osteoporosis

Throughout life, bone tissue is constantly being destroyed and rebuilt, a process known as remodeling. In the first few decades of life, net gain exceeds net loss as bone mass and

Mini Nutritional Assessment
MNA®

Nestlé NutritionInstitute

Last name:		First name:	

Sex:	Age:	Weight, kg:	Height, cm:	Date:

Complete the screen by filling in the boxes with the appropriate numbers. Total the numbers for the final screening score.

Screening

A Has food intake declined over the past 3 months due to loss of appetite, digestive problems, chewing or swallowing difficulties?
0 = severe decrease in food intake
1 = moderate decrease in food intake
2 = no decrease in food intake ☐

B Weight loss during the last 3 months
0 = weight loss greater than 3 kg (6.6 lbs)
1 = does not know
2 = weight loss between 1 and 3 kg (2.2 and 6.6 lbs)
3 = no weight loss ☐

C Mobility
0 = bed or chair bound
1 = able to get out of bed / chair but does not go out
2 = goes out ☐

D Has suffered psychological stress or acute disease in the past 3 months?
0 = yes   2 = no ☐

E Neuropsychological problems
0 = severe dementia or depression
1 = mild dementia
2 = no psychological problems ☐

F1 Body Mass Index (BMI) (weight in kg) / (height in m^2) ☐
0 = BMI less than 19
1 = BMI 19 to less than 21
2 = BMI 21 to less than 23
3 = BMI 23 or greater ☐

IF BMI IS NOT AVAILABLE, REPLACE QUESTION F1 WITH QUESTION F2.
DO NOT ANSWER QUESTION F2 IF QUESTION F1 IS ALREADY COMPLETED.

F2 Calf circumference (CC) in cm
0 = CC less than 31
3 = CC 31 or greater ☐

Screening score
(max. 14 points) ☐☐

12-14 points: ☐ Normal nutritional status
8-11 points: ☐ At risk of malnutrition
0-7 points: ☐ Malnourished

Save
Print
Reset

Ref.   Vellas B, Villars H, Abellan G, et al. *Overview of the MNA® - Its History and Challenges*. J Nutr Health Aging 2006;10:456-465.
        Rubenstein LZ, Harker JO, Salva A, Guigoz Y, Vellas B. *Screening for Undernutrition in Geriatric Practice: Developing the Short-Form Mini Nutritional Assessment (MNA-SF)*. J. Geront 2001;56A: M366-377.
        Guigoz Y. *The Mini-Nutritional Assessment (MNA®) Review of the Literature - What does it tell us?* J Nutr Health Aging 2006; 10:466-487.
        Kaiser MJ, Bauer JM, Ramsch C, et al. *Validation of the Mini Nutritional Assessment Short-Form (MNA®-SF): A practical tool for identification of nutritional status.* J Nutr Health Aging 2009; 13:782-788.
        ® Société des Produits Nestlé, S.A., Vevey, Switzerland, Trademark Owners

For more information: www.mna-elderly.com

■ **FIGURE 13.3** Mini Nutrition Assessment screening tool.

Peak Bone Mass:
the most bone mass a
person will ever have.

density are accrued. Around the age of 30 years, **peak bone mass** is attained (USDHHS, 2012). Thereafter, more bone is lost than is gained. During the first 5 years or so after onset of menopause, women experience rapid bone loss related to estrogen deficiency. After that, bone loss continues at a slower rate.

Osteoporosis is a disease characterized by a decrease in total bone mass and deterioration of bone tissue, which leads to increased bone fragility and risk of fracture. An estimated 10 million Americans have osteoporosis, and another 34 million have low bone mass, which puts them at risk for osteoporosis (National Osteoporosis Foundation [NOF], 2012). It is predicted that one in two women and up to one in four men over the age of 50 years will break a bone due to osteoporosis (NOF, 2012). Older adults, white women, postmenopausal women, people with low body weight, and those with a low calcium intake are most at risk for osteoporosis. Cigarette smoking, heavy alcohol intake, physical inactivity, and certain medications also reduce bone mass.

Osteoporosis prevention begins early in life with an adequate intake of calcium and vitamin D combined with daily weight-bearing physical activity to promote peak bone mass: the greater the peak bone mass attained, the less damaging the inevitable loss of bone mass. Adequate calcium and vitamin D and daily weight-bearing physical activity are vitally important throughout life for strengthening and protecting bones (USDHHS, 2012).

Once bone mass has deteriorated to the point where osteoporosis is diagnosed, medications are necessary to stop bone loss and increase bone density. Nutrition plays a supportive role, with adequate calcium and vitamin D being the most prominent concerns. People who cannot or will not consume the equivalent of 3 cups of milk daily should obtain the remaining calcium they need from calcium supplements. Calcium from supplements is absorbed best in doses of 500 mg or less, so if multiple doses are required, they should be spread out over the day. Other nutrients that are important for bone health include vitamin A, vitamin K, magnesium, and vitamin C—nutrients that can be obtained through a healthy diet that contains at least five servings of fruits and vegetables daily (Nieves, 2005). High-protein diets are often cited as a risk for osteoporosis because they may increase calcium excretion. However, cross-sectional studies indicate that high-protein diets do not adversely affect calcium retention (Roughead, Johnston, Lykken, and Hunt, 2003) and that protein undernutrition is associated with low bone mineral density and greater risk of fracture (Heaney, 2002). Excess sodium should be avoided; high sodium intakes have been shown to increase urinary calcium losses. Limited evidence suggests that a low-sodium diet may positively impact bone density (Carbone et al., 2005).

Sarcopenia

Sarcopenia: the loss
of muscle mass with
aging.

Age-related loss of lean body mass is a normal part of aging; **sarcopenia** occurs when age-related loss of skeletal muscle mass is accompanied by loss of muscle strength and function. Advanced sarcopenia is characterized by physical frailty, increased likelihood of falls, impaired ability to perform ADL, and diminished quality of life (Paddon-Jones et al., 2008). Sarcopenia is estimated to affect 8% to 40% of adults over the age of 60 years and approximately 50% of those over the age of 75 years (Berger and Doherty, 2010). Sarcopenia should be considered in all older adults with observed declines in physical function, strength, or overall health and especially in older adults who are bedridden, who cannot rise independently from a chair, or who have a slow gait (Evans, 2010).

At around 50 years of age, loss of muscle mass averages 1% to 2% per year, but because of the large reserve of muscle, function is not impaired. In the early 60s, a person's loss of muscle becomes evident as muscle strength declines an average of 3% per year. An estimated 20% to 40% of muscle strength may be lost by the time a person reaches the 70s. Loss of muscle strength, rather than mass, is associated with mortality risk (Newman et al., 2006).

Although sarcopenia is a complex and multifactorial process associated with numerous age-related changes, it is facilitated in large part by a sedentary lifestyle and less than optimal diet (Paddon-Jones et al., 2008). As of now, the only option to improve body composition is a balanced diet with adequate protein and strength-training exercises using progressive resistance (Fig. 13.4) (Benton, Whyte, and Dyal, 2011).

There is no consensus on how much protein is necessary to manage or prevent sarcopenia. A protein intake greater than the RDA has been shown to improve muscle mass, strength, and function in older adults and may also improve immune status, wound healing, blood pressure, and bone health (Wolfe et al., 2008). In the Healthy ABC Study cohort, community-dwelling adults age 70 to 79 years who consumed the highest quintile of protein intake lost approximately 40% less lean body mass over a 3-year period than participants in the lowest quintile of protein intake (Houston et al., 2008). A protein intake of 1.5 g/kg/day or approximately double the current RDA of 0.8 g/kg may be a reasonable goal for optimal health and function in older adults (Wolfe et al., 2008). Some experts recommend older adults consume 25 to 30 g of high-quality protein at each of three meals, the equivalent of 3 to 4 oz of protein foods (Symons, Sheffield-Moore, Wolfe, and Paddon-Jones, 2009). Also recommended is a liberal intake of proteins that are rich in leucine, an essential amino acid that stimulates the majority of protein synthesis (Schardt, 2011).

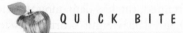

QUICK BITE

Proteins richest in essential amino acids and leucine

Eggs	Meat	Fish
Dairy	Poultry	Soy

Obesity

Dietary excesses and physical inactivity have led to an increase in overweight and obesity among older adults in the past two decades. In 2009–2010, 38% of people age 65 years and

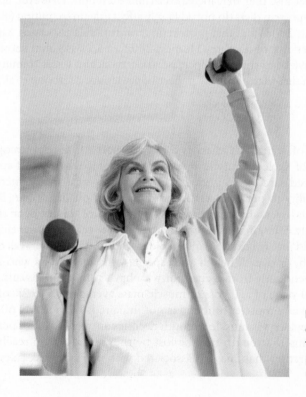

■ **FIGURE 13.4** An older woman exercising with dumbbells. Resistance training, such as weight lifting, is important for maintaining and building muscle mass.

over were obese; in the 75 years and older category, 30% of women and 27% of men were obese (Federal Interagency Forum on Aging-Related Statistics, 2012).

Obesity is a major cause of preventable disease and premature death. It increases the risk of hypertension, diabetes, cardiovascular disease, certain cancers, and osteoarthritis—disorders that become more prevalent with aging. Obesity impairs quality of life by exacerbating age-related declines in health and physical function, which lead to increased dependence, disability, and morbidity (Bernstein and Munoz, 2012).

Sarcopenic obesity is obesity characterized by loss of muscle mass and strength combined with an increase in body fat mass. Sarcopenic obesity results in worse physical functional declines than just sarcopenia or obesity alone (Houston, Nicklas, and Zizza, 2009).

Weight loss in overweight and obese older adults has been shown to improve quality of life, lower risk of chronic disease, reduce disability and frailty, and improve physical functioning and mobility (Houston et al., 2009; Villareal, Banks, Sinacore, Siener, and Klein, 2006; Vincent, Vincent, and Lamb, 2010). However, there are significant health risks of weight loss in older adult (Bernstein and Munoz, 2012). Loss of weight is not synonymous with, nor does it have the same benefit as, loss of fat. Intentional weight loss causes loss of muscle—even when the goal is fat loss—which has a negative impact on functional capacity. Several observational studies have linked weight loss with an increased risk of mortality (Knudtson, Klein, Klein, and Shankar, 2005). Benefits of weight loss must be weighed against the potential risks.

Promoting weight loss in obese older adults presents unique challenges. Many older people may not feel a need to make changes at this point in life. Active participation in physical activity may be difficult because of medical problems, financial limitations, or impaired hearing or vision. Diminished sense of taste, living alone, depression, and limited food budget may impede changes in intake. Other factors that impact the appropriateness of weight management include the presence of comorbidities, cognitive function, lifestyle, and quality of life (Bernstein and Munoz, 2012).

The goal of weight loss therapy for older adults should be to improve physical function and quality of life. A lifestyle approach that combines modest calorie restriction with exercise appears to be the optimal method of decreasing fat mass and preserving muscle mass (Han, Tajar, and Lean, 2011). Careful attention must be given to ensure an adequate intake of protein, fluid, fiber, vitamin D, and vitamin B_{12} (Houston et al., 2009). Randomized controlled trials are needed to determine the benefits and risks of long-term weight management in obese older adults (Han et al., 2011).

Alzheimer Disease

Alzheimer disease (AD) is the most common form of dementia among older adults, affecting an estimated 5.1 million Americans (National Institute on Aging [NIA], National Institutes of Health, 2012). Although not a normal consequence of aging, the risk of AD increases with age, and symptoms usually appear after the age of 60 years (NIA, 2012).

The cause of AD is unknown, and there is no cure. AD appears to result from a complex series of events in the brain that occur over time. Disruptions in nerve cell communication, metabolism, and repair eventually cause many nerve cells to stop functioning, lose connections with other nerve cells, and die. Genetic and nongenetic factors (e.g., inflammation of the brain, stroke) have been identified in the etiology of AD. Like CHD, AD is at least partially a vascular problem, but plaques that form with AD are filled with beta-amyloid, an indissoluble protein, not fat and cholesterol.

Cerebrovascular and cardiovascular disease and their risk factors, such as hypercholesterolemia, hypertension, diabetes, and overweight, increase the likelihood of developing AD as well as other dementias (DeKosky et al., 2006). Interventions that lower serum cholesterol levels or other risk factors and improve cardiovascular health, such as diet, physical activity, and medications, may possibly have beneficial effects related to the risk of AD (Dwyer and Donoghue, 2010). For instance, the Zutphen Elderly Study showed that people who eat fish had less cognitive decline than people who do not eat fish (vanGelder, Tijhuis, and Kalmijn, 2007). It may be that omega-3 fatty acids provide protection against AD through their **antithrombosis** and anti-inflammatory activity, because inflammation is part of the AD syndrome. In addition, complying with "healthy" diet recommendations at midlife, such as consuming a diet high in fruits and vegetables, whole grains, and seafood while limiting the intake of salt, added fats, added sugars, and alcohol, is associated in older adults with better verbal memory, a cognitive domain particularly vulnerable to AD (Kesse-Guyot et al., 2011).

Antithrombosis: against the formation of a thrombosis or blood clot.

There is little evidence that dietary supplements can prevent or treat AD (Dwyer and Donoghue, 2010). A study by Kroger et al. (2009) found no association between omega-3 fatty acids and AD. Multivitamins do not reduce the risk of dementia (Huang et al., 2006). Combinations of vitamin B_{12} and folic acid in large doses failed to slow cognitive decline in older adults with moderate AD (Aisen et al., 2008). In people with mild cognitive impairment, large doses of vitamin E failed to slow progression of AD (Isaac, Quinn, and Tabet, 2008). Evidence of efficacy in humans is lacking for riboflavin, vitamin B_6, vitamin C, blueberry extract, and alpha-lipoic acid (Dwyer and Donoghue, 2010).

AD can have a devastating impact on an individual's nutritional status. Compared with healthy older adults, older adults diagnosed with cognitive impairment or AD may have lower intakes of all nutrients (Bernstein and Munoz, 2012). Early in the disease, impairments in memory and judgment may make shopping, storing, and cooking food difficult. The client may forget to eat or may forget that he or she has already eaten and consequently may eat again. Changes in the sense of smell may develop, a preference for sweet and salty foods may occur, and unusual food choices are not uncommon. Agitation increases energy expenditure, and weight loss is common. Choking may occur if the client forgets to chew food sufficiently before swallowing or hoards food in the mouth. Eating of nonfood items may occur, and eventually self-feeding ability is lost. Clients in the latter stage of AD no longer know what to do when food is placed in the mouth. When this occurs, a decision regarding the use of other means of nutritional support (e.g., nasogastric or percutaneous endoscopic gastrostomy tube feedings) must be made.

LONG-TERM CARE

Long-term care residents tend to be frail elderly with multiple diseases and conditions, including psychosocial, functional, and medical problems. The prevalence of malnutrition or risk for malnutrition is estimated at 67% of nursing home residents and 91% for older adults in rehabilitation facilities (Kaiser et al., 2010). Malnutrition has a negative impact on both the quality and length of life and is an indicator of risk for increased mortality (American Dietetic Association [ADA], 2005). As previously stated, Figure 13.3 is an appropriate screening tool for all older adults in all settings. In addition to the screening criteria, additional risks among long-term care residents include the following:

- Pressure ulcers may be a symptom of inadequate food and fluid intake. They produce a fourfold increase in the risk of death (ADA, 2005).
- Dysphagia can lead to inadequate food intake, dehydration, weight loss, and malnutrition. Quality of life is impaired, and the risk of aspiration pneumonia increases.
- The loss of independence, depression, altered food choices, and cognitive impairments can negatively impact food intake.

The Downhill Spiral

Loss of appetite is a key indicator for malnutrition (Bernstein and Munoz, 2012). An inadequate intake of food means the supply of calories, protein, vitamins, and minerals is reduced, which can lead to weight loss and depletion of essential nutrients. Undernutrition increases the risk of illness and infection. If an infection develops, metabolic rate increases, which increases the need for calories and protein. Undernutrition is exacerbated, and a downward spiral ensues.

To prevent malnutrition, ongoing monitoring of residents' intakes is vital so that prompt action can be taken. The **Minimum Data Set (MDS)** requires food intake be assessed so that residents at risk from inadequate intake (e.g., eating ≤75% of food at most meals) can be identified. Usually, nursing assistants assess food items on a meal tray as a whole and assign a value to the amount eaten, such as 0%, 25%, 50%, or 100%. In practice, this system is fraught with many shortcomings, including the following:

> **Minimum Data Set (MDS):** a component of a federally mandated process of comprehensive assessment of the functional capabilities of all residents living in Medicare- and Medicaid-certified long-term care facilities for the purpose of identifying health problems.

- Food intake records may be neglected because of time constraints or personnel shortages.
- Lack of skill in accurately judging percentage of food consumed. Without adequate training, the reliability of a judgment cannot be guaranteed.
- A practical approach to convert individual item estimates into meaningful estimates of overall meal intake has yet to be determined. For instance, 50% may mean the resident ate half of everything served *or* ate all of half the items served (e.g., all the fruit punch, diced peaches, and green beans) and none of the other half (e.g., chicken rice casserole, milk, and whole-grain muffin). In terms of estimating calories and nutrients consumed, there are significant differences between these two scenarios.

Although the system is far from perfect, it has the potential to yield accurate estimations of individual food and fluid intake when staff is adequately trained and the importance of monitoring intake is understood by the whole health-care team.

Promoting an Adequate Intake

Preventing malnutrition is a quality of life issue. Efforts should be made to optimize food and fluid intake at each meal and snack. Mealtime should be made as enjoyable experience as possible. Encourage independence in eating, and supervise dining areas so that proper feeding techniques are used when residents are assisted or fed by certified nursing assistants. Food preferences should be honored whenever possible. Family involvement increases residents' intake. Additional strategies to promote food intake appear in Box 13.4.

Residents at risk of malnutrition or with poor intakes may be given oral supplements to boost overall calorie and protein intake. Although they may be useful, these supplements may not be well accepted or tolerated on a long-term basis. Taste fatigue and lack of hunger for the meal that follows may occur. Use of supplements as a substitute for food deprives residents of the enjoyment of eating foods of their choice. The potential benefits must be weighed against the potential negative consequences. Another option is to increase the nutrient density of foods served with commercial modules or added ingredients: the nutritional value increases while the volume of food served remains the same.

Restrictive Diets

The use of restrictive diets as part of medical care in long-term care facilities is controversial. Although carbohydrate- or calorie-controlled diets may be theoretically beneficial for older adults with diabetes or obesity, the goals of preventing malnutrition and maintaining

Box 13.4 STRATEGIES TO PROMOTE INTAKE IN LONG-TERM CARE RESIDENTS

Provide a neat and comfortable dining environment.
Use simple verbal prompts to eat.
Provide small, frequent meals rather than three large meals.
Provide specialized utensils such as a scoop plate, nosey cup, etc.
Place food on placemat directly in front of resident.
Avoid staff interruptions during feeding of residents.
Minimize noise and distractions in the dining room.
Use tactile prompt such as hand-over-hand.
Offer finger foods.
Encourage family involvement.
Honor individual preferences.

quality of life are of greater priority for most long-term care residents. Restrictive diets have the potential to negatively affect quality of life by eliminating personal choice in meals, dulling appetite, and promoting unintentional weight loss, thereby compromising functional status. Restrictive diets should be used only when a significant improvement in health can be expected, such as in cases of ascites or constipation.

A Liberal Diet Approach

To meet the needs of individual residents, a holistic approach is advocated that includes the individual's personal goals, overall prognosis, risk/benefit ratio, and quality of life. A liberalized approach has been shown to promote a better intake, lower the incidence of unintentional weight loss, and improve quality of life in long-term care residents (ADA, 2005). A liberal diet is basically a healthy diet of nutrient-dense foods that contains neither excessive nor restrictive amounts of fat, cholesterol, sugar, and sodium (Box 13.5). The risks of a restrictive diet (e.g., decreased intake and weight loss) must be weighed against

Box 13.5 SAMPLE LIBERAL DIET FOR OLDER ADULTS

Breakfast
Orange juice
Oatmeal
One soft cooked egg
One slice buttered whole wheat toast
Low-fat milk
Coffee/tea

Lunch
Turkey sandwich made with two slices whole wheat bread, tomato, romaine lettuce, and low-fat salad dressing
Vegetable soup
Sliced strawberries over angel food cake
One cup low-fat milk
Coffee/tea

Dinner
Roast pork
Oven roasted potatoes
Baked acorn squash
Fresh fruit salad
Ice cream
Coffee/tea

Snack
One cup low-fat yogurt

the potential benefits, especially when potential benefits may be lacking in older adults. Consider the following:

- Low-sodium diets used in treating hypertension are often poorly tolerated by older adults and may lead to loss of appetite, hyponatremia, or confusion (ADA, 2005).
- According to the American Diabetes Association, imposing dietary restrictions on long-term care residents with diabetes is unwarranted (Bantle et al., 2008). It recommends that residents receive a regular diet that is consistent in the amount and timing of carbohydrates. The use of "no concentrated sweets" or "no sugar added" diets is not supported by evidence. Caution is urged in the use of weight loss diets because undernutrition is common.
- The relationship between high cholesterol and all-cause mortality in older people is still under debate (Darmon, Kaiser, Bauer, Sieber, and Pichard, 2010). Several studies have failed to find a positive association between total cholesterol and cardiovascular mortality after age 70 years (Krumholz et al., 1994). Thus, the validity of a low-cholesterol diet in treating long-term care residents is questionable. Malnutrition is a greater threat to the majority of older adults than is hypercholesterolemia. Prudent measures for long-term residents with cardiac disease include using 1% or lower fat milk, substituting trans fat–free margarines for regular margarine and butter, and providing lean cuts of meat in place of fatty meats.

QUICK BITE

Examples of foods made more nutrient/calorie dense
Mashed potatoes made with a glucose module
Milk fortified with nonfat dry milk powder
Oatmeal made with added butter, nonfat dry milk, and sugar
Coffee with a commercial supplement similar to cream that adds calories and protein
Scrambled eggs with added cheese
Fruit juice with a glucose module added

A liberal diet can be modified to meet the requirements of residents with increased needs, such as those who have pressure ulcers. A liberal diet with extra meat and/or milk will provide increased amounts of calories, protein, and fluid. Foods may be made more nutrient dense with the addition of skim milk powder, cream in place of milk, or through modular products. Supplemental vitamin C and zinc may be ordered to promote healing. As with any nutritional intervention, frequent and accurate monitoring of the resident's intake, weight, and hydration status is vital to prevent or treat nutrition-related problems.

NURSING PROCESS: *Older Adult*

Harold Hausman is a regular participant of the monthly congregational nursing program sponsored at his church. He is a sedentary 82-year-old widower who lives alone. You have noticed that he has lost weight over the last several months. He has asked you to answer a few questions he has about the low-sodium, low-cholesterol diet his doctor recommended.

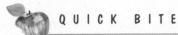

Assessment

Medical–Psychosocial History
- Medical history including hyperlipidemia, hypertension, cardiovascular disease, or gastrointestinal complaints
- Ability to understand, attitude toward health and nutrition, and readiness to learn
- Attitude about his present weight and recent weight loss

(continues on page 342)

NURSING PROCESS: *Older Adult* (continued)

- Usual activity patterns
- Use of prescribed and over-the-counter drugs
- Functional limitations such as impaired ability to shop, cook, and eat
- Psychosocial and economic issues such as who does the shopping and cooking, adequacy of food budget, need for food assistance, and level of family and social support

Anthropometric Assessment

- Height, current and usual weight
- Percent weight change
- Determine BMI

Biochemical and Physical Assessment

- Cholesterol level, if available
- Blood pressure
- Dentition and ability to swallow

Dietary Assessment

- Why did your doctor give you this low-sodium, low-cholesterol diet?
- How many daily meals and snacks do you usually eat?
- What is a normal day's intake for you?
- What changes have you made in implementing this diet? For instance, did you stop using the saltshaker at the table or are you reading labels for sodium content? Did you change the type of butter/margarine you use? The type of salad dressing?
- Do you prepare food with added fat, or do you bake, broil, steam, or boil your food?
- How does your intake compare to a 2000-cal/day meal plan recommended by MyPlate for people your age?
- Do any cultural, religious, or ethnic considerations influence your eating habits?
- Do you use vitamins, minerals, or nutritional supplements? If so, which ones, how much, and why are they taken?
- Do you use alcohol, tobacco, and caffeine?
- How is your appetite?

Diagnosis

Possible Nursing Diagnoses   Altered nutrition: eating less than the body needs

Planning

Client Outcomes

The client will

- Attain/maintain a "healthy" weight
- Consume, on average, a varied and balanced diet that meets the recommended number of servings from the 2000-calorie MyPlate meal plan
- Implement healthy low-sodium, low-cholesterol changes to his usual intake without compromising nutritional or caloric adequacy

NURSING PROCESS: *Older Adult* (continued)

Nursing Interventions	
Nutrition Therapy	Encourage a varied and balanced diet that meets the recommended number of servings from each of the major MyPlate food groups for a 2000-calorie diet
Client Teaching	Instruct the client on

- The role of nutrition in maintaining health and quality of life, including the following:
    - A balanced diet based on the major food groups helps maximize the quality of life
    - Avoiding excess salt is prudent for all people; recommendations on sodium intake should be made on an individual basis according to the client's cardiac and renal status, appetite, and use of medications
    - Although it is wise to avoid high-fat, nutrient-poor foods such as most cakes, cookies, pastries, pies, chips, full-fat dairy products, and fried foods, observing too severe a fat restriction compromises calorie intake and may result in undesirable weight loss
- Eating plan essentials, including the importance of
    - Choosing a varied diet to help ensure an average adequate intake; limiting food choices or skipping a food group increases the risk of both nutrient deficiencies and excesses
    - Eating enough food to avoid unfavorable weight loss
    - Eating enough high-fiber foods such as whole-grain breads and cereals, dried peas and beans, and fresh fruits and vegetables
    - Drinking adequate fluid
- Behavioral matters, including
    - The importance of discussing the rationale for the low-sodium, low-cholesterol diet with his physician, particularly because he has had an unfavorable weight loss
    - How to read labels to identify low-sodium foods
- Physical activity goals that may help improve appetite and intake

Evaluation	
Evaluate and Monitor	<ul><li>Monitor weight and blood pressure</li><li>Provide periodic feedback and reinforcement on food intake and questions about diet</li></ul>

How Do You Respond?

Do glucosamine and chondroitin work for arthritis pain? These two products have been used for more than 40 years to prevent or treat OA based on the premise that the disease is caused by a deficiency of these components of cartilage (Fouladbakhsh, 2012). However, recent results from a comprehensive meta-analysis concluded that glucosamine

(continues on page 344)

and chondroitin, used alone or together, did not decrease joint pain or influence joint-space narrowing over time (Wandel et al., 2010). At best, evidence is inconclusive that these supplements are effective.

What makes weight change "significant"? Significant weight change is defined as 5% or more in 30 days or 10% or more in 180 days. Most often, significant unintentional *weight gain* reflects fluid accumulation, not weight per se, and although it may indicate a serious health threat, eating too many calories is not to blame. Conversely, significant unintentional *weight loss* is much more common, and even if nutrition is not the cause, it is part of the solution. Because weight loss is one of the most important and sensitive indicators of malnutrition, it is vital to accurately weigh residents at least on a monthly basis.

CASE STUDY

Annie is an 80-year-old widow who lives alone. She has a long history of hypertension and diabetes and suffers from the complications of CHD and neuropathy. She has diabetic retinopathy, which has left her legally blind. She has never been compliant with a diabetic diet but takes insulin as directed. She is 5 ft 5 in tall and weighs 170 pounds, down from her usual weight of 184 pounds 5 months ago.

Annie reluctantly agreed to receive Meals on Wheels so she does not have to prepare lunch and dinner except on weekends. Her daughter buys groceries for Annie every week, and her grocery list generally consists of milk, oatmeal, two cans of soup, two bananas, a bag of chocolate candy, a layer cake, two doughnuts, and mixed nuts. Her weekend meals consist of whatever she has available to eat.

- What is Annie's BMI? How would you assess her weight status?
- Is her recent weight loss significant? Is it better for her to lose weight, maintain her present weight, or try to regain what she has lost?
- What would you recommend Annie eat for breakfast? For snacks? For weekend meals? Would you discourage her from eating sweets?
- What arguments would you make for her to eat better?

STUDY QUESTIONS

1. A 68-year-old man who has steadily gained excess weight over the years complains that it is too late for him to make any changes in diet or exercise that would effectively improve his health, particularly the arthritis he has in his knees. Which of the following would be the nurse's best response?
   a. "You're right. You should have made changes long ago. You cannot benefit from a change in diet and exercise now."
   b. "It is too hard for older people to change their habits. You should just continue what you've been doing and know that it's a quality of life issue to enjoy your food."
   c. "It may not help to change your diet and exercise, but it certainly wouldn't hurt. Why don't you give it a try and see what happens?"
   d. "It is not too late to make changes, and losing weight through diet and exercising are more effective at relieving arthritis pain than either strategy is alone. And older people often are better at making lifestyle changes than are younger adults."

2. The nurse knows her instructions about vitamin B_{12} are effective when the client verbalizes he will
   a. Consume more meat.
   b. Consume more fruits and vegetables.
   c. Eat vitamin B_{12}–fortified cereal.
   d. Drink more milk.

3. A client complains that she is not eating any more than she did when she was 30 years old and yet she keeps gaining weight. Which of the following would be the nurse's best response?
   a. "As people get older, they lose muscle mass, which lowers their calorie requirements, and physical activity often decreases too. You can increase the number of calories you burn by building muscle with resistance exercises and increasing your activity."
   b. "You may not think you are eating more calories but you probably are because the only way to gain weight is to eat more calories than you burn."
   c. "Weight gain is an inevitable consequence of getting older related to changes in your body composition. Do not worry about it because older people are healthier when they are heavier."
   d. "You need fewer calories now than when you were 30. The only way to lose weight is to eat less than you are currently eating."

4. A mineral likely to be consumed in inadequate amounts by older adults is
   a. Iron
   b. Potassium
   c. Zinc
   d. Sodium

5. The best dietary advice for the possible prevention of Alzheimer disease is to
   a. Consume a high-fiber diet.
   b. Eat a heart healthy diet of fruits, vegetables, whole grains, and seafood.
   c. Take a multivitamin every day.
   d. Avoid foods with a high glycemic index.

6. Risk factors for malnutrition in older adults include (select all that apply)
   a. A decrease in food intake in the last 3 months due to loss of appetite
   b. Weight loss
   c. Acute disease
   d. Neuropsychological problems
   e. Impaired mobility
   f. BMI of 23

7. Older adults doing resistance exercises to rebuild lost muscle may also need to increase their intake of what nutrient to achieve their objective?
   a. Calories
   b. Carbohydrate
   c. Protein
   d. Iron

8. Which of the following may help promote the intake of a resident in long-term care? Select all that apply.
   a. Use simple verbal prompts to eat.
   b. Provide three meals a day; avoid snacks.
   c. Minimize noise and distractions in the dining room.
   d. Offer finger foods.
   e. Honor individual preferences; solicit input from resident and family.

KEY CONCEPTS

■ Aging begins at birth and ends in death. Exactly how and why aging occurs is not known.

■ Good eating habits developed early in life promote health in old age.

■ As a group, older adults are at risk for nutritional problems because of changes in physiology (including changes in body composition, gastrointestinal tract, metabolism, central nervous system, renal system, and the senses), changes in income, changes in health, and psychosocial changes.

■ Older adults represent a heterogeneous population that varies in health, activity, and nutritional status. Generalizations about nutritional requirements are less accurate for this age group than for others.

■ Generally, calorie needs decrease, but the need for nutrients stays the same or increases with aging. Requirements increase for calcium and vitamin D. Older adults need to obtain their RDA for vitamin B_{12} from the synthetic form found in supplements or fortified foods. The DRI for sodium decreases due to the decrease in calorie requirement. The RDA for iron in women decreases when menses stops.

■ MyPlate for Older Adults is designed to help community-dwelling older adults consume a healthy diet based on the *Dietary Guidelines for Americans, 2010* (see Fig. 13.2). Nutrient-dense fruits and vegetables, whole and fortified grains, low-fat and nonfat dairy milk and dairy products, lean proteins, and liquid vegetable oils are depicted on a dinner plate to show variety and proportion. Physical activity is featured at the top of the placemat to illustrate that normal daily activities count; a variety of fluids occupy a place next to the dinner plate.

■ Generally, older adults do not consume enough vitamin E, magnesium, fiber, calcium, potassium, and probably vitamin D. They should be encouraged to eat more whole grains, dark green and orange fruits and vegetables, legumes, and milk and milk products.

■ Screening for nutritional problems is appropriate for all older adults and in all settings. Screening is essential so that timely nutrition intervention can be instituted.

■ Weight loss is the most effective dietary strategy against osteoarthritis. The benefits of weight loss and exercise combined are greater than when either method is used alone. Benefits include improvements in physical function and quality of life.

■ Even interventions begun late in life can slow or halt bone loss characteristic of osteoporosis. The equivalent of three glasses of milk is needed to meet calcium requirement in older adults. Calcium supplements may be necessary to achieve the recommended amount. Other nutrients important for bone health include vitamin D, vitamin A, vitamin K, magnesium, vitamin C, and phytoestrogens.

■ Sarcopenia is the loss of muscle mass and strength that occurs with aging. It is not inevitable and can be reversed with resistance training and adequate protein intake. To build muscle in older adults, more protein than the RDA may be required.

■ The treatment of obesity in older adults is not without risk. Weight loss can be counterproductive if it comes from a loss of muscle and bone, not fat. For many older adults, malnutrition presents more of a risk than overweight.

■ Many known risk factors for Alzheimer disease (AD) are similar to those for CHD. Although the role of diet has not clearly been established, a heart healthy diet may help reduce the risk of AD.

■ Long-term care residents are at risk for malnutrition. Preventive efforts should focus on maintaining an adequate calorie and protein intake. Honor special requests, encourage food from home, and provide assistance with eating as needed.

■ Goals of diet intervention for older adults are to maintain or restore maximal independent functioning and to maintain quality of life. Restrictive diets may not be appropriate for older adults and may actually promote malnutrition; they should be used only when a significant improvement in health can be expected.

■ A liberal diet approach may help prevent malnutrition and improve quality of life.

■ Pressure ulcers increase the need for calories, protein, and other nutrients. Increasing nutrient density without increasing the volume of food served may be the most effective method of delivering additional nutrients. Between-meal supplements may also be needed to maximize intake.

Check Your Knowledge Answer Key

1. **TRUE** Seventy-four percent of adults age 65 years and older rated their health as good or better during the period 2004–2006. Self-assessment of health status is important because poor ratings correlate with higher risks of mortality (Federal Interagency Forum on Aging-Related Statistics, 2012).

2. **TRUE** In general, calorie needs in older adults decrease due to a decrease in lean body mass and physical activity while the need for other nutrients stays the same or increases.

3. **FALSE** The AI for water does not change for men or women from the age of 19 years onward. Older adults have a blunted sense of thirst, yet if they are healthy, normal drinking and eating habits are considered adequate to guide fluid intake.

4. **TRUE** Older adults do not need more vitamin B_{12} than younger adults, but their ability to absorb the natural form of B_{12} from food may be impaired. Adults over the age of 50 years are urged to consume the RDA for vitamin B_{12} from fortified foods or supplements to ensure adequacy.

5. **FALSE** Most older adults consume adequate amounts of iron. In fact, they are cautioned against consuming supplements that contain iron so as not to exceed the upper limit for iron.

6. **FALSE** Although loss of lean body mass is a normal consequence of aging, muscle mass can be replaced with resistance exercises and a diet adequate in protein.

7. **TRUE** Weight loss in older adults is associated with functional limitations, nursing home admissions, and mortality.

8. **FALSE** While it is true that peak calcium retention—the period when calcium intake has the greatest impact on bone density—occurs between the ages of 4 and 20 years, the efficiency of absorption decreases with age, so the AI for calcium for older adults is higher than that of younger adults.

9. **FALSE** The prevalence of malnutrition or dehydration among residents of long-term care facilities is from 23% to 85%.

10. **TRUE** A major cause of undernutrition among long-term care residents is loss of appetite. Monitoring of intake is essential to identify problems early, before a downhill spiral develops.

Student Resources on thePoint

For additional learning materials, activate the code in the front of this book at
http://thePoint.lww.com/activate

Websites

Alzheimer's Association at **www.alz.org**
American Association of Retired Persons at **www.aarp.org**
American Geriatrics Society at **www.americangeriatrics.org**
Arthritis Foundation at **www.arthritis.org**
National Institute of Aging Information Office at **www.nih.gov/nia**

References

Aisen, P., Schneider, L., Sano, M., Diaz-Arrastia, R., van Dyck, C., Weiner, . . . Thal, L. J. (2008). Alzheimer Disease Cooperative Study. High-dose B vitamin supplementation and cognitive decline in Alzheimer disease: A randomized controlled trial. *Journal of the American Medical Association, 300,* 1774–1783.

Albright, C., Schembre, S., Steffen, A., Wilkens, L. R., Monroe, K. R., Yonemori, K. M., & Murphy, S. P. (2012). Differences by race/ethnicity in older adults' beliefs about the relative importance of dietary supplements vs prescription medications: Results from the SURE study. *Journal of the Academy of Nutrition and Dietetics, 112,* 1223–1229.

American Dietetic Association. (2005). Position of the American Dietetic Association: Liberalization of the diet prescription improves quality of life for older adults in long-term care. *Journal of the American Dietetic Association, 105,* 1955–1965.

Arthritis Foundation. (2012). *Osteoarthritis.* Available at www.arthritis.org/who-gets-osteoarthritis.php. Accessed on 11/27/12.

Bantle, J., Wylie-Rosett, J., Albright, A. L., Apovian, C. M., Clark, N. G., Franz, M. J., . . . Wheeler, M. L. (2008). Nutrition recommendations and interventions for diabetes. A position statement of the American Diabetes Association, *Diabetes Care, 31,* S61–S78.

Barrett-Connor, E., Edelstein, S., Corey-Bloom, J., & Wiederhold, W. (1996). Weight loss precedes dementia in community-swelling older adults. *Journal of the American Geriatrics Society, 44,* 1147–1152.

Baumgartner, R., Wayne, S., Walters, D., Janssen, I., Gallagher, D., & Morley, J. E. (2004). Sarcopenic obesity predicts instrumental activities of daily living disability in the elderly. *Obesity Research, 12,* 1995–2004.

Benton, M., Whyte, M., & Dyal, B. (2011). Sarcopenic obesity: Strategies for management. *American Journal of Nursing, 111,* 38–44.

Berger, M., & Doherty, T. (2010). Sarcopenia: Prevalence, mechanisms and functional consequences. *Interdisciplinary Topics in Gerontology, 37,* 94–114.

Bernstein, M., & Munoz, N. (2012). Position of the Academy of Nutrition and Dietetics: Food and nutrition for older adults: Promoting health and wellness. *Journal of the Academy of Nutrition and Dietetics, 112,* 1255–1277.

Carbone, L., Barrow, K., Bush, A., Boatright, M., Michelson, J., Pitts, K., . . . Watsky, M. (2005). Effects of a low sodium diet on bone metabolism. *Journal of Bone and Mineral Metabolism, 23,* 506–513.

Centers for Disease Control and Prevention. (2007). National and state medical expenditures and lost earnings attributable to arthritis and other rheumatic conditions—United States, 2003. *Morbidity and Mortality Weekly Report, 56,* 4–7.

Centers for Disease Control and Prevention. (2011). *Arthritis-related statistics.* Available at www.cdc.gov/arthritis/data_statistics/arthritis_related_stats. htm#2. Accessed on 11/27/12.

Cheng, Y., Hootman, J., Murphy, L., & Helmick, C. G. (2010). Prevalence of doctor-diagnosed arthritis and arthritis-attributable activity limitation—United States, 2007-2008. *Morbidity and Mortality Weekly Report, 59,* 1261–1265.

Darmon, P., Kaiser, M., Bauer, J., Sieber, C. C., & Pichard, C. (2010). Restrictive diets in the elderly: Never say never again? *Clinical Nutrition, 29,* 170–174.

DeKosky, S., Fitzpatrick, A., Ives, D., Saxton, J., Williamson, J., Lopez, O. L., . . . Furberg, C. (2006). The Ginkgo Evaluation of Memory (GEM) study: Design and baseline data of a randomized trial of ginkgo biloba extract in the prevention of dementia. *Contemporary Clinical Trials, 27,* 238–253.

Dwyer, J., & Donoghue, M. (2010). Is risk of Alzheimer disease a reason to use dietary supplements? *American Journal of Clinical Nutrition, 91,* 1155–1156.

Elmadfa, I., & Meyer, A. (2008). Body composition, changing physiological functions and nutrient requirements of the elderly. *Annals of Nutrition and Metabolism, 52*(Suppl. 1), 2–5.

Evans, W. (2010). Skeletal muscle loss: Cachexia, sarcopenia, and inactivity. *American Journal of Clinical Nutrition, 91*(Suppl.), 1123S–1127S.

Fabian, E., Bogner, M., Kickinger, K., Wagner, K. H., & Elmadfa, I. (2012). Vitamin status in elderly people in relation to the use of nutritional supplements. *Journal of Nutrition, Health, and Aging, 16,* 206–212.

Federal Interagency Forum on Aging-Related Statistics. (2012). *Older Americans 2012. Key indicators of well-being.* Washington, DC: U.S. Government Printing Office.

Fiatarone, M., Marks, E., Ryan, N., Meredith, C. N., Lipsitz, L. A., & Evans, W. J. (1990). High-intensity strength training in nonagenarians. Effects on skeletal muscle. *Journal of the American Medical Association, 26,* 3029–3034.

Fouladbakhsh, J. (2012). Complementary and alternative modalities to relieve osteoarthritis symptoms. *American Journal of Nursing, 112,* S44–S41.

Fulgoni, V. (2008). Current protein intake in America: Analysis of the National Health and Nutrition Examination Survey, 2003–2004. *American Journal of Clinical Nutrition, 87,* S1554–S1557.

Greenstone, C. (2007). Osteoarthritis: A lifestyle medicine assessment of risks, prevention, and treatment. *American Journal of Lifestyle Medicine, 1,* 256–259.

Han, R., Tajar, B., & Lean, M. (2011). Obesity and weight management in the elderly. *British Medical Bulletin, 97,* 169–196.

Heany, R. (2002). Protein and calcium: Antagonists or synergists? *American Journal of Clinical Nutrition, 75,* 609–610.

Heuberger, R., & Caudell, K. (2011). Polypharmacy and nutritional status in older adults: A cross-sectional study. *Drugs and Aging, 28,* 315–323.

Horn, S., Bender, S., Ferguson, M., Smout, R. J., Bergstrom, N., Taler, G., . . . Voss, A. C. (2004). The National Pressure Ulcer Long-Term Care Study: Pressure ulcer development in long-term care residents. *Journal of the American Geriatrics Society, 52,* 359–367.

Houston, D. K., Nicklas, B., Ding, J., Harris, T. B., Tylavsky, F. A., Newman, A. B., . . . Kritchevsky, S. B. (2008). Dietary protein intake is associated with lean mass change in older, community-dwelling adults: The Health, Aging, and Body Composition (Health ABC) Study. *American Journal of Clinical Nutrition, 87,* 150–155.

Houston, D., Nicklas, B., & Zizza, C. (2009). Weighty concerns: The growing prevalence of obesity among older adults. *Journal of the American Dietetic Association, 109,* 1886–1895.

Huang, H., Caballero, B., Chang, S., Alberg, A. J., Semba, R. D., Schneyer, C., . . . Bass, E. B. (2006). Multivitamin mineral supplements and prevention of chronic disease: Executive summary. *American Journal of Clinical Nutrition, 85*(Suppl.), 265S–269S.

Hudgens, J., Langkam-Henken, B., Stechmiller, J., Herrlinger-Garcia, K. A., & Nieves, C., Jr. (2004). Immune function is impaired with a Mini Nutritional Assessment score indicative of malnutrition in nursing home elders with pressure ulcers. *Journal of Parenteral and Enteral Nutrition, 28,* 416–422.

Institute of Medicine. (2005). *Dietary reference intakes for energy, carbohydrates, fiber, fat, fatty acids, cholesterol, protein, and amino acids (macronutrients).* Washington, DC: The National Academies Press.

Isaac, M., Quinn, R., & Tabet, N. (2008). Vitamin E for Alzheimer disease and mild cognitive impairment. *Cochrane Database System Reviews, (3),* CD002854.

Jurschik, P., Torres, J., Sola, R., Nuin, C., Botigué, T., & Lavedán, A. (2010). High rates of malnutrition in older adults receiving different levels of health care in Lleida, Catalonia: An assessment of contributory factors. *Journal of Nutrition for the Elderly, 29,* 410–422.

Kaiser, M., Bauer, J., Ramsch, C., Uter, W., Guigoz, Y., Cederholm, T., . . . Sieber, C. C. (2010). Frequency of malnutrition in older adults: A multinational perspective using the Mini Nutrition Assessment. *Journal of the American Geriatrics Society, 58,* 1734–1738.

Kamp, B., Wellman, N., & Russell, C. (2010). Position of the American Dietetic Association, American Society for Nutrition, and Society for Nutrition Education: Food and nutrition programs for community-residing older adults. *Journal of the American Dietetic Association, 11,* 463–472.

Kerksick, C., Thomas, A., Campbell, B., Taylor, L., Wilborn, C., Marcello, B., . . . Kreider, R. B. (2009). Effects of a popular exercise and weight loss program on weight loss, body composition, energy expenditure and health in obese women. *Nutrition and Metabolism, 6,* 23.

Kesse-Guyot, E., Amieva, H., Castebon, K., Henegar, A., Ferry, M., Jeandel C., . . . Galan, P. (2011). Adherence to nutritional recommendations and subsequent cognitive performance: Findings from the prospective Supplementation with Antioxidant Vitamins and Minerals 2 (SU. VI.MAX 2) study. *American Journal of Clinical Nutrition, 93,* 200–210.

Knudtson, M., Klein, B., Klein, R., & Shankar, S. (2005). Associations with eight loss and subsequent mortality risk. *Annals of Epidemiology, 15,* 483–491.

Kroger, E., Verreault, R., Carmichael, P., Lindsay, J., Julien, P., Dewailly, E., . . . Laurin, D. (2009). Omega-3 fatty acids and risk of dementia: The Canadian Study of Health and Aging. *American Journal of Clinical Nutrition, 90,* 184–192.

Krumholz, H., Seeman, T., Merrill, S., Mendes de Leon, C. F., Vaccarino, V., Silverman, D. I., . . . Berkman, L. F. (1994). Lack of association between cholesterol and coronary heart disease mortality and morbidity and all-cause mortality in persons older than 70 years. *Journal of the American Medical Association, 47,* 961–969.

Kryger, A., & Andersen, J. (2007). Resistance training in the older old: Consequences for muscle strength, fiber types, fiber size, and MHC isoforms. *Scandinavian Journal of Medicine and Science in Sports, 17,* 422–430.

Messier, S. P., Loeser, R. F., Miller, G. D., Morgan, T. M., Rejeski, W. J., Sevick, M., . . . Williamson, J. D. (2004). Exercise and dietary weight loss in overweight and obese older adults with knee osteoarthritis: The Arthritis, Diet, and Activity Promotion Trial. *Arthritis and Rheumatism, 50,* 1501–1510.

National Institute on Aging, National Institutes of Health. (2012). *Alzheimer's disease fact sheet.* Available at /www.nia.nih.gov/alzheimers/publication/alzheimers-disease-fact-sheet. Accessed on 11/29/12.

National Osteoporosis Foundation. (2012). *Learn about osteoporosis.* Available at http://www.nof.org/learn. Accessed on 11/28/12.

National Research Council. (1998). *Dietary reference intakes for thiamin, riboflavin, niacin, vitamin B$_6$, folate, vitamin B$_{12}$, pantothenic acid, biotin, and choline.* Washington, DC: The National Academies Press.

National Research Council. (2005a). *Dietary reference intakes for energy, carbohydrate, fiber, fat, fatty acids, cholesterol, protein, and amino acids (macronutrients).* Washington, DC: The National Academies Press.

National Research Council. (2005b). *Dietary reference intakes for water, potassium, sodium, chloride, and sulfate.* Washington, DC: The National Academies Press.

Newman, A., Kupelian, V., Visser, M., Simonsick, E., Goodpaster, B., Kritchevsky, S., . . . Harris, T. (2006). Strength, but not muscle mass, is associated with mortality in the health, aging, and body composition study cohort. *Journals of Gerontology. Series A, Biological Sciences and Medical Sciences, 61,* 72–77.

Nieves, J. (2005). Osteoporosis: The role of micronutrients. *American Journal of Clinical Nutrition, 81*(Suppl.), 1232S–1239S.

Paddon-Jones, D., Short, K., Campbell, W., Volpi, E., & Wolfe, R. R. (2008). Role of dietary protein in the sarcopenia of aging. *American Journal of Clinical Nutrition, 87*(Suppl.), 1562S–1566S.

Pichard, C., Kyle, U., Morabia, A., Perrier, A., Vermeulen, B., & Unger, P. (2004). Nutritional assessment: Lean body mass depletion at hospital admission is associated with an increased length of stay. *American Journal of Clinical Nutrition, 79,* 613–618.

Pratley, R., Nicklas, B., Rubin, M., Miller, J., Smith, A., Smith, M., . . . Goldberg, A. (1994). Strength training increases resting metabolic rate and norepinephrine levels in healthy 50- to 65-yr-old men. *Journal of Applied Physiology, 76,* 133–137.

Rivlin, R. (2007). Keeping the young-elderly healthy: Is it too late to improve our health through nutrition? *American Journal of Clinical Nutrition, 86*(Suppl.), 1572S–1576S.

Roddy, E., Zhang, W., Doherty, M., Arden, N. K., Barlow, J., Birrell, F., . . . Richards, S. (2005). Evidence-based recommendations for the role of exercise in the management of osteoarthritis of the hip or knee—The MOVE consensus. *Rheumatology, 44,* 67–73.

Roughead, Z., Johnston, L., Lykken, G., & Hunt, J. (2003). Controlled high meat diets do not affect calcium retention or indices of bone status in healthy postmenopausal women. *Journal of Nutrition, 133,* 1020–1026.

Schardt, D. (2011). Staying strong. How exercise and diet can help preserve your muscles. *Nutrition Action Health Letter, 38*(1), 3–6.

Sebastian, R. S., Cleveland, L. E., Goldman, J. D., & Moshfegh, A. J. (2007). Older adults who use vitamin/mineral supplements differ from nonusers in nutrient intake adequacy and dietary attitudes. *Journal of the American Dietetic Association, 107,* 1322–1332.

Skates, J., & Anthony, P. (2012). Identifying geriatric malnutrition in nursing practice: The Mini Nutritional Assessment (MNA®)—An evidence-based screening tool. *Journal of Gerontological Nursing, 38,* 18–27.

Symons, T., Sheffield-Moore, M., Wolfe, R., & Paddon-Jones, D. (2009). A moderate serving of high-quality protein maximally stimulates skeletal muscle protein synthesis in young and elderly subjects. *Journal of the American Dietetic Association, 109,* 1582–1586.

Thomas, D., Zdrowski, C., Wilson, M., Conright, K. C., Lewis, C., Tariq, S., & Morley, J. E. (2002). Malnutrition in sub-acute care. *American Journal of Clinical Nutrition, 75,* 308–313.

U.S. Department of Agriculture, Agricultural Research Service. (2010). *Nutrient intakes from food: Mean amounts consumed per individual, by gender and age. What We Eat in American, NHANES 2007-2008.* Available at www.ars.usda.gov/ba/bhnrc/fsrg. Accessed on 6/9/12.

U.S. Department of Agriculture, Center for Nutrition Policy and Promotion. (2007). *Fruit and vegetable consumption by older Americans. Nutrition Insight 34.* Available at http://www.cnpp.usda.gov. Accessed on 5/1/08.

U.S. Department of Health and Human Services. (2008). *Physical activity guidelines for Americans. At-a-glance: A fact sheet for professionals.* Available at www.health.gov/paguidelines/factsheetprof .aspx. Accessed on 11/20/12.

U.S. Department of Health and Human Services. (2012). *The Surgeon General's report on bone health and osteoporosis: What it means to you.* Washington, DC: U.S. Department of Health and Human Services, Office of the Surgeon General.

vanGelder, B., Tijhuis, M., & Kalmijn, S. (2007). Fish consumption, n-3 fatty acids, and subsequent 5-y cognitive decline in elderly men: The Zutphen Elderly Study. *American Journal of Clinical Nutrition, 85,* 1142–1147.

Villareal, D. T., Apovian, C. M., Kushner, R. F., & Klein, S. (2005). Obesity in older adults: Technical review and position statement of the American Society for Nutrition and NAASO, the Obesity Society. *American Journal of Clinical Nutrition, 82,* 923–934.

Villareal, D., Banks, M., Sinacore, D., Siener, C., & Klein, S. (2006). Effect of weight loss and exercise on frailty in obese older adults. *Archives of Internal Medicine, 166,* 860–866.

Vincent, H., Vincent, K., & Lamb, K. (2010). Obesity and mobility disability in the older adult. *Obesity Reviews, 11,* 568–579.

Wandel, S., Juni, P., Tendel, B., Nüesch, E., Villiger, P. M., Welton, N. J., . . . Trelle, S. (2010). Effects of glucosamine, chondroitin, or placebo in patients with osteoarthritis of hip or knee: Network meta-analysis. *British Medical Journal, 341,* c4675.

Wernette, C., White, B., & Zizza, C. (2011). Signaling proteins that influence energy intake may affect unintentional weight loss in elderly persons. *Journal of the American Dietetic Association, 111,* 864–873.

Wolfe, R., Miller, S., & Miller, K. (2008). Optimal protein intake in the elderly. *Clinical Nutrition, 27,* 675–684.

Zizza, C., Tayie, F., & Lino, M. (2007). Benefits of snacking in older Americans. *Journal of the American Dietetic Association, 107,* 800–806.

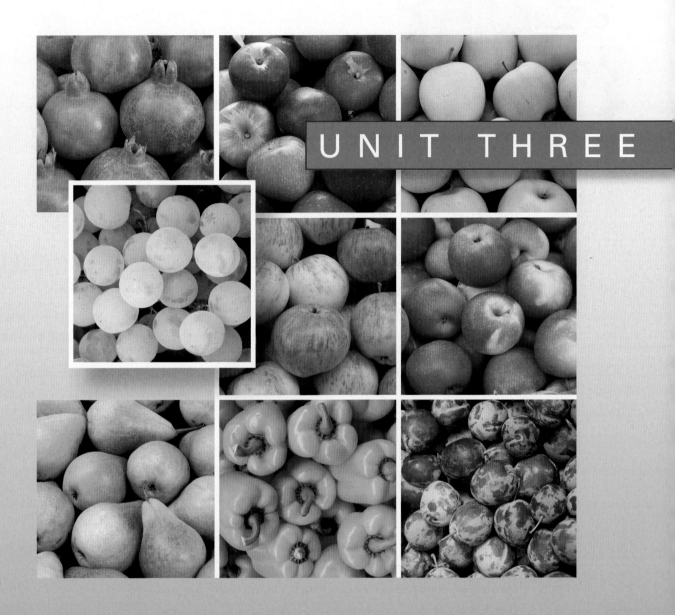

UNIT THREE

Nutrition in
Clinical Practice

14 Obesity and Eating Disorders

TRUE **FALSE**

☐	☐	**1** Eating in the evening causes weight gain.
☐	☐	**2** Skipping meals is an effective strategy for cutting calories.
☐	☐	**3** It is easier to lose weight than to maintain a lower weight after weight loss.
☐	☐	**4** Keeping a food diary can help improve eating habits.
☐	☐	**5** Obesity-related health problems improve only after the body mass index (BMI) is lowered to normal.
☐	☐	**6** If a person will try only one strategy, lowering calories is more effective at promoting short-term weight loss than increasing activity.
☐	☐	**7** Even if weight loss does not occur, increasing activity helps to lower blood pressure and improves glucose tolerance.
☐	☐	**8** People who eat fewer than 1200 calories may need a multivitamin and mineral supplement.
☐	☐	**9** For weight loss, it is better to cut carbohydrates than to cut fat grams.
☐	☐	**10** Bulimia poses fewer nutritional problems than anorexia does.

LEARNING OBJECTIVES

Upon completion of this chapter, you will be able to

1 Discuss the impact an obesogenic environment has on the prevalence of obesity.
2 Propose obesity treatment recommendations based on an individual's BMI and the presence of comorbidities.
3 Suggest an appropriate calorie intake to promote weight loss based on gender.
4 Discuss optimal macronutrient distribution for weight loss.
5 Create a sample weight loss meal plan based on MyPlate intake patterns.
6 Compare strategies to promote weight loss with those that are effective in maintaining weight loss.
7 Contrast nutrition therapy for anorexia nervosa with that of bulimia nervosa.

Obesity has reached epidemic proportions: since 1976–1980, the prevalence of obesity (BMI ≥30) in American adults age 20 to 74 years has more than doubled from 14.5% to 35.7% in 2009–2010 (Fig. 14.1) (Fryar, Carroll, and Ogden, 2012). The prevalence of obesity has climbed in both men and women; in all age groups; and in all racial, ethnic, and socioeconomic groups. Extreme obesity (BMI ≥40) is increasing at a faster rate than any other class of obesity in the United States (Sturm, 2007).

A far less common weight issue is disordered eating manifested as anorexia nervosa or bulimia. Historically, the study of obesity and eating disorders has been separate: The former has been rooted in medicine, and the latter has been the focus of psychiatry and psychology. Yet there are commonalities between them, such as questions of appetite regulation, concerns with body image, and similar etiologic risk factors.

This chapter focuses on obesity—its causes, complications, and treatment approaches, including nutrition therapy, behavior modification, physical activity, pharmacology, and surgery. Eating disorders and their nutrition therapy are described.

OBESITY

Overweight: a BMI of 25 or greater.

Obesity: a BMI of 30 or greater.

Overweight is defined as having a BMI ≥25. It is related to an excessive body weight, not necessarily excessive body fat. Muscle, bone, fat, and water all contribute to body weight. **Obesity,** on the other hand, is defined as having a BMI ≥30, a condition characterized by excess accumulation of body fat.

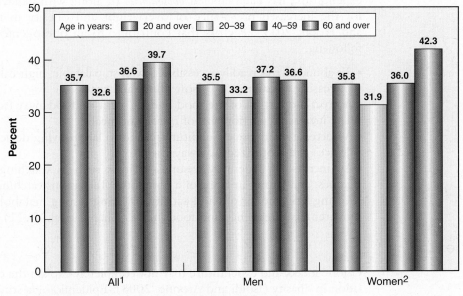

[1]Significant increasing linear trend by age ($p < 0.01$).
[2]Significant increasing linear trend by age ($p < 0.001$).
NOTE: Estimates were age adjusted by the direct method to the 2000 U.S. Census population using the age groups 20–39, 40–59, and 60 and over.
Source: CNC/NCHS, NHANES, 2009-2010

■ **FIGURE 14.1** Prevalence of obesity in the United States, 2009–2010.

Causes of Obesity

Obesity occurs when calorie intake exceeds calorie expenditure (i.e., people eat more calories than they expend over time). Although we know *how* obesity occurs, *why* it occurs is not fully understood despite intensive study. Increasingly, obesity is viewed as a metabolic disease with a cause far more complicated than a simple lack of willpower to control eating (Allison et al., 2008). Clearly, certain individuals are more susceptible to weight gain than others (Blackburn, Wollner, and Heymsfield, 2010). Several studies show that body weight is maintained at a stable "set-point" range despite variations in calorie intake and expenditure. Unfortunately, it appears that the body is more efficient in protecting against weight loss when calories are restricted than it is at preventing weight gain when calorie intake is excessive (Farias, Cuevas, and Rodrigues, 2011). It is likely that obesity results from a dynamic interaction between an increasingly **obesogenic environment**, behavior, and genetics (Laddu, Dow, Hingle, Thomson, and Going, 2011).

> **Obesogenic Environment**: an environment that produces and supports overweight and obesity.

Obesogenic Environment

The dramatic rise in obesity in the U.S. population over the last four decades has occurred without changes in the gene pool, suggesting that the root cause is lifestyle and environment, not biology (Chaput, Klingenberg, Astrup, and Sjodin, 2011). Swinburn et al. (2009) estimate that Americans today, compared with Americans in the 1970s, have a positive energy balance of 400 cal/day, although other researchers have estimated the "**energy gap**" at about 100 cal/day (Hill, Wyatt, Reed, and Peters, 2003). Swinburn et al. (2009) contend that this imbalance is due in large part to an increased intake in food. A decrease in physical activity has also contributed to the calorie imbalance.

> **Energy Gap**: the difference between calories consumed and calories expended.

The current environment, which encourages energy intake and discourages energy expenditure, has been labeled *obesogenic*. It, along with behavior, is believed to account for the increased prevalence of overweight and obesity in the world today (Corsica and Hood, 2011). Factors that contribute to an obesogenic environment include the following:

- An abundance of readily accessible, low-cost, palatable, high-calorie foods in large portions
- Increasing consumption of soft drinks and snacks
- A great proportion of the food budget spent on food away from home
- The increasing portion size of restaurant meals
- A decrease in energy expenditure related to labor-saving devices, such as remote control devices and motorized walkways
- An increase in sedentary leisure activities, such as watching television, playing video games, and sitting in front of a computer. Television watching may promote obesity by leaving less time for physical activity, lowering resting metabolic rate, and/or promoting greater meal frequency and food intake (Chaput et al., 2011).

Genetics

Calorie intake and expenditure may not completely explain the complexity of weight regulation in obesity (Isoldi and Aronne, 2008). Epidemiologic studies point to a genetic susceptibility (Herrera and Lindgren, 2010). Genetics does not cause obesity but is involved in how likely a person is to gain or lose weight in response to changes in calorie intake by influencing basal metabolic rate, where body fat is distributed, and response to overeating (O'Neil and Nicklas, 2007). Genetics may also account for the individual differences in weight loss that occur in response to calorie restriction (Loos and Rankinen, 2005) and may even account for nutrient-specific food preferences (Bauer et al., 2009). Supporting the case for a genetic basis to weight status is the tendency of adopted children to have similar weights to their biological parents, not their adoptive parents (Moll, Burns, and Lauer, 1991; Stunkard et al., 1986). Estimates on the heritability of BMI range from 40% to 70% (Herrera and Lindgren, 2010).

Gene–Environment Interaction

Clearly there is a gene–environment interaction. Even when a genetic susceptibility exists, exposure to an obesogenic environment is necessary for obesity to develop (Herrera and Lindgren, 2010). Likewise, in people with a genetic predisposition to obesity, the severity of the disease is largely determined by lifestyle and environmental conditions (Loos and Rankinen, 2005).

Complications of Obesity

Abdominal Obesity: waist circumference exceeding 35 inches in women or 40 inches in men.

Metabolic Syndrome: a cluster of interrelated symptoms, including obesity, insulin resistance, hypertension, and dyslipidemia, which together increase the risk of cardiovascular disease and diabetes.

Obesity significantly increases mortality and morbidity. It is associated with a wide variety of comorbidities, including diabetes, hyperlipidemia, fatty liver disease, obstructive sleep apnea, gastroesophageal reflux disease, vertebral disk disease, osteoarthritis, and increased risk of certain cancers (Guh et al., 2009). **Abdominal obesity**, part of the **metabolic syndrome**, increases the risk of coronary heart disease and type 2 diabetes (see Chapter 20). Obesity increases the risk of complications during and after surgery and the risk of complications during pregnancy, labor, and delivery. Higher body weights are associated with higher mortality from all causes. Overweight-obesity and physical inactivity are estimated to be responsible for nearly 1 in 10 deaths in the United States (Danaei et al., 2009).

Obesity presents psychological and social disadvantages. In a society that emphasizes thinness, obesity leads to feelings of low self-esteem, negative self-image, depression, and hopelessness (Valtonen, Laaksonen, and Tolmunen, 2008). Negative social consequences include stereotyping; prejudice; stigmatization; social isolation; and discrimination in social, educational, and employment settings.

Goals of Treatment

Ideally, treatment would "cure" overweight and obesity; that is, weight would fall into the healthy BMI category and would be maintained there permanently. This would be gradually accomplished with a 1- to 2-pound loss every week for the first 6 months of weight loss therapy, for a total of 10% weight loss. After 6 months, when the rate of weight loss usually decreases, then plateaus, the focus would shift to maintaining that weight loss. After 6 months of weight maintenance, weight loss efforts would be repeated. The cycle would continue until healthy weight is achieved.

In reality, this ideal is seldom achieved. On an individual level, treating obesity with lifestyle modification—namely, nutrition therapy and physical activity—has proven to be extremely difficult (Tsai and Wadden, 2005). People who have successfully lost weight have done so by making drastic changes in their eating and exercise habits (Wyatt, Wing, and Jill, 2002). Over time, most people who lose weight through lifestyle modification regain most of the weight lost (Tsai and Wadden, 2005).

The goal of losing large amounts of weight may be unrealistic and overwhelming and, from a health perspective, not necessary to achieve medically significant health benefits (Blackburn, 1995). A modest weight loss of 5% to 10% of usual body weight is associated with significant improvements in blood pressure, cholesterol and plasma lipid levels, and blood glucose levels and may prevent or delay the onset of type 2 diabetes and hypertension in high-risk people, even if "healthy" weight is not achieved (Seagle and Strain, 2009). Compared with dramatic weight loss, modest weight loss is more attainable, easier to maintain over the long term, and sets the stage for subsequent weight loss.

Setting a modest weight loss goal and keeping that weight off are far more realistic than striving for thinness. Yet for some people, even modest weight loss may be unattainable. A more appropriate weight management goal for clients unable to lose weight is to prevent additional weight gain. Although this may sound like a passive approach, it requires active intervention, not simply maintenance of the status quo.

Evaluating Motivation to Lose Weight

Objectively identifying who may benefit from weight loss is not the only criterion to be considered before beginning treatment; assessing the client's level of motivation is crucial because weight loss is not likely to occur in people who are not motivated or not ready to change (Fig. 14.2). Even worse, imposing treatment on an unmotivated or unwilling client may preclude subsequent attempts at weight loss when the client may be more likely to succeed. It is essential to assess the client's level of motivation before beginning weight loss therapy. Factors to consider appear in Box 14.1.

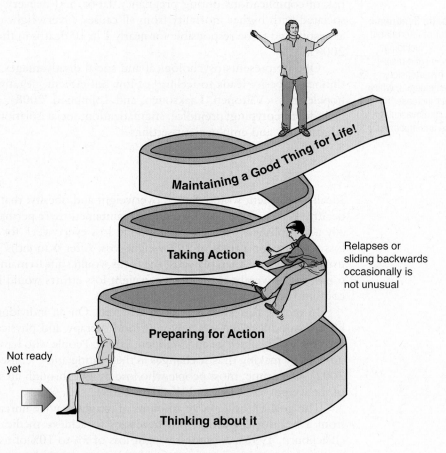

Relapses or sliding backwards occasionally is not unusual

Not ready yet

■ FIGURE 14.2 Stages of change graphic.

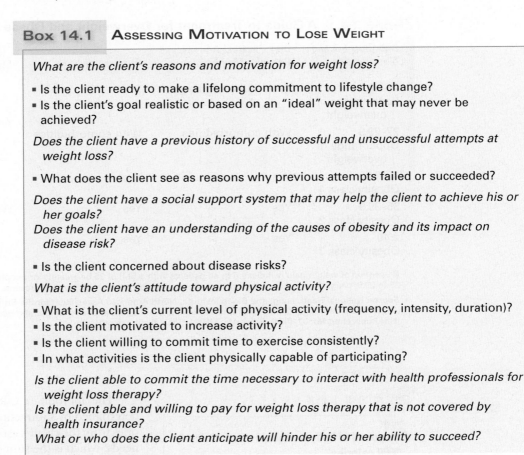

Box 14.1   ASSESSING MOTIVATION TO LOSE WEIGHT

What are the client's reasons and motivation for weight loss?

- Is the client ready to make a lifelong commitment to lifestyle change?
- Is the client's goal realistic or based on an "ideal" weight that may never be achieved?

Does the client have a previous history of successful and unsuccessful attempts at weight loss?

- What does the client see as reasons why previous attempts failed or succeeded?

Does the client have a social support system that may help the client to achieve his or her goals?

Does the client have an understanding of the causes of obesity and its impact on disease risk?

- Is the client concerned about disease risks?

What is the client's attitude toward physical activity?

- What is the client's current level of physical activity (frequency, intensity, duration)?
- Is the client motivated to increase activity?
- Is the client willing to commit time to exercise consistently?
- In what activities is the client physically capable of participating?

Is the client able to commit the time necessary to interact with health professionals for weight loss therapy?

Is the client able and willing to pay for weight loss therapy that is not covered by health insurance?

What or who does the client anticipate will hinder his or her ability to succeed?

WEIGHT MANAGEMENT

A lifestyle approach that includes nutrition therapy, physical activity, and behavior modification is the basis of comprehensive weight management. Pharmacotherapy and surgery may be used in conjunction with lifestyle interventions, based on the individual's BMI and the presence of comorbidities (Table 14.1).

Nutrition Therapy

The first priority in obesity treatment is to decrease calorie intake, usually by 500 to 1000 cal/day to achieve a weekly weight loss of 1 to 2 pounds (Seagle and Strain, 2009). This recommendation is based on the assumption that 1 pound of fat mass is approximately equivalent to 3500 calories and that this rate of weight loss remains constant over a period of time. However, metabolic adaptations occur during weight loss (e.g., fewer calories expended during daily activities because body weight is lower) that require a further decrease in calorie intake to achieve a negative calorie balance and continued weight loss (Finkler, Heymsfield, and St-Onge, 2012). This is one factor that contributes to the decreasing rate of weight loss that occurs as the duration of a diet increases (Finkler et al., 2012).

Table 14.1 A Guide to Treatment for Overweight and Obese People

BMI Category and Classification	Diet, Physical Activity, and Behavior Modification	Pharmacotherapy	Surgery
25–26.9 Lower range of overweight	With comorbidities		
27–29.9 Upper range of overweight	With comorbidities	With comorbidities	
30–34.5 Obesity class 1	Yes	Yes	
35–39.9 Obesity class 2	Yes	Yes	With comorbidities
≥40 Obesity class 3	Yes	Yes	

Prevention of weight gain is indicated in all patients with a BMI of 25 or greater; for people with a BMI of 25 to 29.9, weight loss is not necessarily recommended unless comorbidities are present.

Source: National Heart, Lung, and Blood Institute, North American Association for the Study of Obesity. (2002). *The practical guide: Identification, evaluation, and treatment of overweight and obesity in adults* (NIH Publication No. 02-4084). Bethesda, MD: National Institutes of Health.

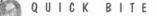

QUICK BITE

One pound of body fat equals approximately 3500 calories

To lose 1 pound per week, 3500 fewer calories per week should be consumed 3500 calories ÷ 7 days/week = 500 calorie deficit per day

To lose 2 pounds per week, 7000 fewer calories per week should be consumed 7000 calories ÷ 7 days/week = 1000 calorie deficit per day

The appropriate calorie intake may be determined by subtracting 500 to 1000 calories from the client's estimated total energy needs, which is the sum of calories used for basal metabolic rate and physical activity (see Chapter 7). A more general approach is to choose a specific calorie level based on gender. The National Institutes of Health (NIH) recommends low-calorie diets of 1000 to 1200 cal/day for overweight women and 1200 to 1600 cal/day for overweight men and heavier (>165 pounds) or more active women (National Heart, Lung, and Blood Institute, 1998). This level of calorie restriction can promote up to an 8% loss of body weight when followed for 3 to 12 months (Cannon and Kumar, 2009). Table 14.2 lists the amount of food in each of these calorie levels based on MyPlate intake recommendations. A multivitamin and mineral supplement is recommended whenever calorie intake falls to 1200 calories or less.

If 1200 calories can promote a 1 to 2 pound loss per week, will a more drastic calorie reduction speed the weight loss process? Clients often think that the greater the calorie deficit, the quicker the weight loss. In reality, cutting calories too much, particularly when protein intake is low, may result in higher proportions of lean tissue loss, leading to a compensatory decrease in basal energy expenditure and a reduction in exercise tolerance (Blackburn et al., 2010). This makes weight loss and eventual weight maintenance more difficult.

Very-low-calorie diets (VLCDs) provide approximately 800 cal/day in a liquid formulation enriched with high biologic value protein and 100% of the Daily Value for

Table 14.2 MyPlate Intake Patterns for Low-Calorie Diets

Group	1000 Calories	1200 Calories	1400 Calories	1600 Calories
Grains (oz equivalents)	3	4	5	6
Vegetables (cups)	1	1.5	1.5	2
Fruits (cups)	1	1	1.5	1.5
Dairy (cups)	2	2	2	3
Protein foods (oz equivalents)	2	3	4	5
Oils (tsp)	2	3	4	5

Source: www.choosemyplate.gov

micronutrients. Weight loss is quick and significant in the short term; long-term weight loss is similar between VLCD and routine low-calorie diets (Tsai and Wadden, 2006). VLCDs are not appropriate when BMI is less than 30, are not recommended for long-term use, and should be used only under the supervision of a physician (Cannon and Kumar, 2009; Turk et al., 2009). VLCDs are often used prior to bariatric surgery to reduce overall surgical risk in clients with severe obesity (Seagle and Strain, 2009). Using VLCDs for at least 2 weeks reduces liver size, and longer use (e.g., 6 weeks) results in clinically significant decreases in abdominal obesity (Colles, Dixon, Marks, Strauss, and O'Brien, 2006).

Macronutrient Composition

The optimal macronutrient composition for weight loss has been extensively studied (Hession et al., 2009). Weight loss diets are typically classified as low carbohydrate, low fat, or balanced. Sample menus for each type of diet appear in Table 14.3.

Low-Carbohydrate Diets (Atkins Type). A low carbohydrate intake causes liver glycogen depletion and subsequent diuresis, which produces a quick and dramatic weight loss. When carbohydrate intake is very low (e.g., <20 g/day), ketones are produced from fat metabolism. Ketones help dampen hunger (Johnstone, Horgan, Murison, Bremner, and Lobley, 2008). Randomized controlled trials show that weight loss at 6 months is greater in people on a low-carbohydrate weight loss diet than in people who follow a low-fat weight loss diet, but the difference is not significant after 12 months (Gardner et al., 2007; Nordmann et al., 2006).

Low-carbohydrate diets that severely limit fruit, vegetables, and whole grains may be deficient in fiber and micronutrients, particularly thiamin, folic acid, vitamin C, and magnesium (Gardner et al., 2010). A study by Brinkworth, Noakes, Buckley, Keogh, and Clifton (2009) showed that weight loss and improvements in blood pressure, glucose, insulin, and insulin resistance were the same after 12 months on a low-carbohydrate diet compared to an isocaloric low-fat diet. However, participants on the low-carbohydrate diet achieved greater decreases in serum triglyceride levels and increases in serum high-density lipoprotein (HDL) cholesterol levels (favorable) but also greater increases in their low-density lipoprotein (LDL) cholesterol levels (unfavorable). The long-term safety of very-low-carbohydrate diets (e.g., <35% of total calories) has not been determined (Seagle and Strain, 2009). They should be used with caution, even over a short term, in people with osteoporosis, kidney disease, or high levels of LDL cholesterol (Seagle and Strain, 2009).

Low-Fat Diets (Ornish Diet). A low-fat weight loss diet is the best studied and most frequently recommended diet by leading health authorities (Lichtenstein et al., 2006; Seagle and Strain, 2009). Fat has more than twice the calories as an equivalent amount of

Table 14.3 A Comparison of Weight Loss Diet Plans and Sample Menus

	Low Fat	Balanced (Moderate-Fat/High-Carbohydrate Diet)	Low Carbohydrate
	Composition of sample plans and menus		
Total calories	1475	1490	1479
Carbohydrate	74%	50%	22%
Protein	17%	20%	20%
Fat	9%	30%	58%
	Intake patterns		
Total servings from each group per day			
Grains	8	7	2
Vegetables	5	2	2
Fruits	7	3	2
Milk or yogurt	2 fat-free	2 fat-free	1
Protein foods	2 oz fat-free meat	5 oz lean meat	8 oz medium fat
Oils	3	5	11
	Sample menu		
Breakfast	½ cup orange juice 1 small banana ¼ cup scrambled egg beaters 2 slices whole wheat toast 2 tsp butter	½ cup orange juice 1 oz shredded wheat 2 slices whole wheat toast 1 cup skim milk 2 tsp butter	½ cup orange juice 2 scrambled eggs cooked in 2 tsp butter 1 oz pork sausage
Snack	⅔ cup plain yogurt with ¾ cup blueberries 3 graham crackers		⅔ cup artificially sweetened yogurt
Lunch	1 cup lentil soup (counts as 1 oz meat and 1 grain) Grilled vegetable sandwich on 2 slices whole wheat bread 1 cup tossed salad Fat-free dressing 1 slice watermelon	2 slices whole wheat bread 2 oz deli turkey 1 tsp mayonnaise 1 cup salad made with greens, carrots, onions, and mushrooms 1 tbsp Italian dressing	2 oz canned tuna mixed with 2 tsp mayonnaise 4 pieces melba toast ½ cup sliced tomatoes 1 tbsp Italian dressing
Snack	½ cup fat-free pudding	1 small apple	20 peanuts (counts as 2 fats)
Dinner	½ cup black beans with ⅓ cup rice and tomatoes (counts as 2 grains and 1 vegetable) 1 cup salad 1 tbsp Italian dressing ½ cup steamed broccoli ¾ cup canned mandarin oranges 1 cup skim milk	3 oz grilled skinless chicken breast ⅓ cup brown rice ½ cup steamed broccoli 1 tsp butter 1¼ cup strawberries	3 oz steak ⅓ cup rice 1 cup salad topped with 8 large olives 1 tbsp Italian dressing 1¼ cup strawberries with 2 tbsp whipped cream
Snack	1 frozen 100% juice bar	1 oz whole wheat crackers	6 almonds

protein or carbohydrate, so it is an effective target for lowering calorie intake. A low-fat diet generally means saturated fat and trans fat intakes are lower; the *Dietary Guidelines for Americans, 2010* and nutrition recommendations from the American Diabetes Association and American Heart Association urge Americans to reduce their intake of saturated and trans fats (Bantle et al., 2008; Lichtenstein et al., 2006; U.S. Department of Agriculture, U.S. Department of Health and Human Services [USDHHS], 2010). Clinical trials have demonstrated that low-fat weight loss diets, when used in combination with lifestyle counseling and physical activity, promote a 5% to 10% weight loss and prevent or reduce diabetes and/or hypertension (Pi-Sunyer et al., 2007). When fat intake is very low and the diet is primarily vegetarian, the intakes of vitamins E (found in oils) and B_{12} and zinc (found in animal sources) may be inadequate (Gardner et al., 2010).

Balanced Diets (LEARN Diet). A balanced weight loss diet is patterned after MyPlate guidelines with a calorie distribution of approximately 50% carbohydrate, 30% fat, and 20% protein—intakes within the ranges recommended by the Dietary Reference Intakes. A similar diet, the Zone diet, is approximately 40% carbohydrate, 30% fat, and 30% protein. A study by Gardner et al. (2010) showed no risk of vitamin or mineral inadequacies in participants consuming a low-calorie diet similar to the Zone diet. In fact, the study noted that participants had higher intakes of vitamins A, C, and E while on the Zone diet compared to their baseline intakes. Tips for making healthy food choices while following a balanced low-calorie plan are featured in Box 14.2.

The Bottom Line. Low-calorie diets produce weight loss regardless of which macronutrients they emphasize (Sacks et al., 2009). When total calories are the same, the macronutrient distributions of the diet do not affect the amount of weight lost over time. However,

- Low-carbohydrate diets produce a greater weight and fat loss than low-fat or balanced weight loss diets during the first 6 months and may be preferred by some people who want to see quick results.
- There is a risk of not consuming adequate amounts of all micronutrients with either a very-low-carbohydrate diet or a very-low-fat diet.
- Although weight loss and fat loss do not appear related to the percentage of protein consumed, lean muscle mass is better preserved among dieters who consume a higher protein intake (e.g., 27% of total calories from protein vs. 16%) (Farnsworth et al., 2003). Weight loss diets with 25% to 30% of protein may also provide greater **satiety** (Schoeller and Buchholz, 2005).
- The "best" type of diet is individualized to the client's preference and health status.

Satiety: the feeling of fullness.

Portion Control

Marketplace food and beverage portions are at least two times bigger than standard serving sizes (Young and Nestle, 2003), leading people to have an altered perception of appropriate portion size. The Academy of Nutrition and Dietetics recognizes portion control as an important strategy to prevent weight gain as well as an integral component of weight loss programs (Seagle and Strain, 2009). Providing clients with common household equivalents to estimate portion sizes is a useful tool. While clients may not have any idea what 3 oz of meat looks like, they can visual the size of a deck of cards to estimate reasonable meat portions. Proportioned 100-calorie packages and smaller dinner plates, serving utensils, and glassware may also help "right size" portions.

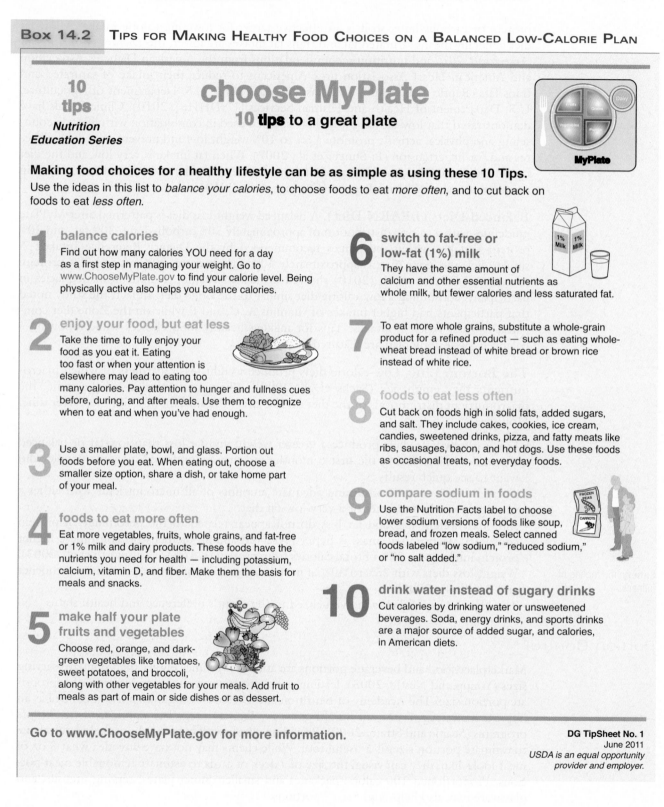

10 tips

Nutrition Education Series

choose MyPlate

10 **tips** to a great plate

MyPlate

Making food choices for a healthy lifestyle can be as simple as using these 10 Tips.

Use the ideas in this list to *balance your calories*, to choose foods to eat *more often*, and to cut back on foods to eat *less often*.

1 balance calories

Find out how many calories YOU need for a day as a first step in managing your weight. Go to www.ChooseMyPlate.gov to find your calorie level. Being physically active also helps you balance calories.

2 enjoy your food, but eat less

Take the time to fully enjoy your food as you eat it. Eating too fast or when your attention is elsewhere may lead to eating too many calories. Pay attention to hunger and fullness cues before, during, and after meals. Use them to recognize when to eat and when you've had enough.

3 Use a smaller plate, bowl, and glass. Portion out foods before you eat. When eating out, choose a smaller size option, share a dish, or take home part of your meal.

4 foods to eat more often

Eat more vegetables, fruits, whole grains, and fat-free or 1% milk and dairy products. These foods have the nutrients you need for health — including potassium, calcium, vitamin D, and fiber. Make them the basis for meals and snacks.

5 make half your plate fruits and vegetables

Choose red, orange, and dark-green vegetables like tomatoes, sweet potatoes, and broccoli, along with other vegetables for your meals. Add fruit to meals as part of main or side dishes or as dessert.

6 switch to fat-free or low-fat (1%) milk

They have the same amount of calcium and other essential nutrients as whole milk, but fewer calories and less saturated fat.

7 To eat more whole grains, substitute a whole-grain product for a refined product — such as eating whole-wheat bread instead of white bread or brown rice instead of white rice.

8 foods to eat less often

Cut back on foods high in solid fats, added sugars, and salt. They include cakes, cookies, ice cream, candies, sweetened drinks, pizza, and fatty meats like ribs, sausages, bacon, and hot dogs. Use these foods as occasional treats, not everyday foods.

9 compare sodium in foods

Use the Nutrition Facts label to choose lower sodium versions of foods like soup, bread, and frozen meals. Select canned foods labeled "low sodium," "reduced sodium," or "no salt added."

10 drink water instead of sugary drinks

Cut calories by drinking water or unsweetened beverages. Soda, energy drinks, and sports drinks are a major source of added sugar, and calories, in American diets.

Go to www.ChooseMyPlate.gov for more information.

DG TipSheet No. 1
June 2011
USDA is an equal opportunity provider and employer.

Eating Frequency

The Academy of Nutrition and Dietetics Evidence Library considers the strength of the evidence "fair" in recommending calories be distributed throughout the day in four to five meals and snacks, including breakfast (Seagle and Strain, 2009). Regular, frequent meals and snacks may help clients avoid periods of hunger, thereby increasing the likelihood of dietary adherence. Breakfast may play a role in weight management by affecting appetite control, diet quality, and metabolism. An individualized pattern that prevents periods of hunger is recommended.

Meal Replacements

If self-selection or portion control is difficult, meal replacements can be an effective weight loss and weight loss maintenance strategy (Seagle and Strain, 2009). Commercial diet programs, such as Jenny Craig and Nutrisystem, feature one to two meals per day of vitamin- and mineral-fortified, low-calorie "meals," which may be in the form of a shake, frozen entrée, or meal bar. Because choices are restricted and meals are portion controlled, the risk of poor food choices is reduced. A study by Levitsky and Pacanowski (2011) found that using one meal substitute per day is sufficient to cause a 250-calorie daily decrease in calorie intake and weight loss.

Behavior Modification

Behavior modification focuses on changing the client's eating and exercise behaviors thought to contribute to obesity and closely monitoring those behaviors. Box 14.3 lists behavior modification ideas that may help change eating behaviors. Key behavior modification strategies are discussed in the following text.

Self-monitoring involves keeping a detailed record of the time, amount, description, preparation, and calorie content of all foods and beverages consumed. Recording additional information, such as the client's emotional state, intensity of hunger, and activities at the time of eating, may help identify "problem" behaviors. The primary purpose of using food records is to increase awareness of how often and under what circumstances the client engages in behaviors that support or sabotage weight loss efforts. The act of recording food eaten causes people to alter their intake. Self-monitoring of activity establishes a record of the type and amount (in minutes) of daily programmed activity. Lifestyle activity can be monitored with the use of a pedometer. Self-monitoring is often considered one of the most essential components of behavior modification.

Goal setting may involve specific calorie, fat gram, and physical activity goals designed to achieve a 1- to 2-pound weight loss per week, or it may involve specific eating behaviors in need of improvement. Goals should be realistic, specific, and measurable so that success can be achieved, thereby engendering a sense of accomplishment and bolstering motivation. Instead of a goal to "eat better," a goal may be to "eat oatmeal and fruit for breakfast 5 days per week."

Stimulus control involves restructuring the environment to avoid or change cues that trigger undesirable behaviors (e.g., keeping "problem" foods out of sight or out of the house) or instituting new cues to elicit positive behaviors (e.g., putting walking shoes by the front door as a reminder to go walking).

Problem solving involves identifying eating problems or high-risk situations, planning alternative behaviors, implementing the alternative behaviors, and evaluating the plan to determine whether or not it reduces problem eating behaviors.

Box 14.3   BEHAVIOR MODIFICATION IDEAS

Think Thin
- Make a list of reasons why you want to lose weight.
- Set long-term goals; avoid crash dieting based on getting into a particular dress or weighing a certain weight for an upcoming event or occasion.
- Give yourself a nonfood reward (e.g., new clothes, a night of entertainment) for losing weight.
- Enlist the support of family and friends.
- Learn to distinguish hunger from cravings.

Plan Ahead
- Keep food only in the kitchen, not scattered around the house.
- Stay out of the kitchen except when preparing meals and cleaning up.
- Avoid tasting food while cooking; don't take extra portions to get rid of a food.
- Place the low-calorie foods in the front of the refrigerator; keep the high-calorie foods hidden.
- Remove temptation to better resist it: "Out of sight, out of mind."
- Plan meals, snacks, and grocery shopping to help eliminate hasty decisions and impulses that may sabotage dieting.

Eat Wisely
- Wait 10 minutes before eating when you feel the urge; hunger pangs may go away if you delay eating.
- Never skip meals.
- Eat before you're starving and stop when satisfied, not stuffed.
- Eat only in one designated place, and devote all your attention to eating. Activities such as reading and watching television can be so distracting that you may not even realize you ate.
- Serve food directly from the stove to the plate instead of family style, which can lead to large portions and second helpings.
- Eat the low-calorie foods first.
- Drink water with meals.
- Use a small plate to give the appearance of eating a full plate of food.
- Chew food thoroughly and eat slowly.
- Put utensils down between mouthfuls.
- Leave some food on your plate to help you feel in control of food rather than feeling that food controls you.
- Eat before attending a social function that features food; while there, select low-calorie foods to nibble on.
- Eat satisfying foods and do not restrict particular foods.

Shop Smart
- Never shop while hungry.
- Shop only from a list; resist impulse buying.
- Buy food only in the quantity you need.
- Don't buy foods you find tempting.
- Stock upon fruits and vegetables for low-calorie snacking.

Box 14.3   BEHAVIOR MODIFICATION IDEAS (continued)

Change Your Lifestyle
- Keep busy with hobbies or projects that are incompatible with eating to take your mind off eating.
- Brush your teeth immediately after eating.
- Trim recipes of extra fat and sugar.
- Keep food and activity records.
- Keep hunger records.
- Give yourself permission to enjoy an occasional planned indulgence and do so without guilt; don't let disappointment lure you into a real eating binge.
- Exercise.
- Get more sleep if fatigue triggers eating.
- Weigh yourself regularly.

Cognitive restructuring involves reducing negative self-talk, increasing positive self-talk, setting reasonable goals, and changing inaccurate beliefs.

Relapse prevention focuses on teaching clients how to prevent lapses from becoming relapses.

Promoting Dietary Adherence

Motivation to stick to a restrictive diet typically decreases over time (Ebbeling et al., 2012). According to National Health and Nutrition Examination Survey (NHANES) data from 1999–2006, only one in six overweight and obese adults report ever having maintained weight loss of at least 10% of their body weight for 1 year (Kraschnewski et al., 2010). Even highly motivated and nutritionally informed people struggle to avoid highly palatable, calorie-dense foods (Appelhans, Whited, Schneider, and Pagoto, 2011). Biologic adaptations to weight loss, such as a decrease in energy expenditure and an increase in hunger, make weight loss increasingly difficult (Sumithran et al., 2011).

Neurobiology, and not simply willpower, may also impact dietary adherence. For instance, the human tendency to pursue instant gratification (e.g., palatable, calorie-dense food) over delayed rewards (e.g., health benefits of weight loss) has a neural basis (Appelhans et al., 2011). In practical terms, a greater emphasis on behavior modification strategies may be needed to overcome the neurobiologic influences that make it so difficult to maintain a low-calorie intake (Appelhans et al., 2011). Adding structure to a low-calorie diet may improve adherence by limiting food choices, which reduces temptation and the potential for overeating (Fabricatore, 2007). Structure can be added by providing meal plans and actual grocery lists, menus, and recipes or reliable websites where they may be found.

Physical Activity

In most studies, physical activity and improved fitness reduce the health risks of obesity regardless of the degree of obesity or baseline health status (Lee, Sui, and Blair, 2009). Increasing activity during weight loss helps preserve or increase lean body mass, which favorably impacts metabolic rate. With or without weight loss, increasing activity lowers blood pressure and triglycerides, increases HDL cholesterol, and improves glucose tolerance and cardiorespiratory fitness. Subjectively, increased activity improves the sense of well-being, reduces tension, increases agility, and improves alertness. Current physical activity guidelines recommend the following (Donnelly et al., 2009):

- Approximately 30 minutes of moderate to vigorous physical activity (MVPA) 5 to 7 days per week to prevent weight gain
- 150 to 420 minutes/week of MVPA for weight loss
- 200 to 400 minutes/week of MVPA to maintain weight loss

Physical activity and calorie restriction work synergistically when paired together (Blackburn et al., 2010). Weight loss via diet alone involves loss of lean mass, which lowers metabolic rate and therefore calorie needs. To achieve weight loss via exercise alone is more difficult than by diet alone; a weekly exercise expenditure of 2000 calories may be necessary (Saris et al., 2003). The amount of weight loss at this level of activity is modest and likely to be frustrating; however, the health benefits are significant (Laddu et al., 2011). Compared to weight loss from dieting, weight loss from exercise produces a greater percentage of fat loss as well as a greater decrease in abdominal and visceral fat (Ross et al., 2000). After weight loss, regular exercise is the primary predictor of weight maintenance (USDHHS, 2008).

Moderate-intensity aerobic activity (e.g., walking, cycling, swimming) is most commonly recommended for weight loss and maintenance. Clients with severe obesity may struggle to achieve levels of aerobic exercise that are sufficient to reap health benefits (Blackburn et al., 2010). A better option may be progressive strength training, a safe and effective form of exercise that improves insulin sensitivity and increases muscle strength. There is evidence that resistance training combined with higher protein intake promotes weight loss and fat loss while maintaining muscle mass, which is especially important in obese people losing large amounts of weight (Donnelly et al., 2009).

Promoting Exercise Adherence

Unlike dietary adherence, exercise adherence seems to improve with less structure, possibly by eliminating the barriers of lack of time or financial expense (Fabricatore, 2007). Strategies that may promote exercise adherence include encouraging clients to

- Exercise at home rather than at on-site or supervised exercise sessions.
- Exercise in multiple short bouts (10 minutes each), instead of one long session.
- Adopt a more active lifestyle, such as taking the stairs instead of the elevator or pacing while on the phone instead of sitting down.

Pharmacotherapy

In conjunction with lifestyle changes of diet, behavior modification, and physical activity, pharmacotherapy is recommended for people with a BMI of 30 or greater or for people with a BMI of 27 or greater with comorbid conditions, such as hypertension, type 2 diabetes, or dyslipidemia (see Table 14.1). According to the National Institutes of Health, average weight loss with medication is 10 pounds more than with nondrug treatments (National Institute of Diabetes and Digestive and Kidney Diseases and Weight-Control Information Network, 2010). Maximum weight loss occurs within 6 months and then levels off or increases. Medications are more effective when combined with a low-calorie diet, physical activity, and behavior modification. The drugs approved by the U.S. Food and Drug Administration (FDA) for weight loss are appetite suppressants or lipase inhibitors (Table 14.4). Appetite suppressants work by slowing gastric emptying, which provides a

Table 14.4 Drugs Approved for Weight Loss

Generic Name	Food and Drug Administration Approval for Weight Loss	Drug Type	Common Side Effects
Phentermine	Yes; short term (up to 12 weeks) for adults	Appetite suppressant	Increased blood pressure and heart rate, sleeplessness, nervousness
Diethylpropion	Yes; short term (up to 12 weeks) for adults	Appetite suppressant	Dizziness, headache, sleeplessness, nervousness
Phendimetrazine	Yes; short term (up to 12 weeks) for adults	Appetite suppressant	Sleeplessness, nervousness
Orlistat	Yes; long term (up to 1 year) for adults and children age 12 and older	Lipase inhibitor	Gastrointestinal issues (cramping, diarrhea, oily spotting), rare cases of severe liver injury reported
Lorcaserin	Yes; long-term use if tolerated and effective	Appetite suppressant	Headache, dizziness, fatigue, nausea, dry mouth, and constipation
Qsymia (trade name for the combination drug of phentermine and topiramate)	Yes; long-term use	Appetite suppressant; seizure treatment	As listed for phentermine plus numbness of skin, change in taste, birth defects, suicidal thoughts

Source: National Institute of Diabetes and Digestive and Kidney Disease and Weight-Control Information Network. (2010). *Prescription medications for the treatment of obesity*. Bethesda, MD: National Institute of Diabetes and Digestive and Kidney Diseases, National Institutes of Health. Available at http://win.niddk.nih.gov/publications/prescription.htm#meds. Accessed 12/11/12; and Food and Drug Administration Consumer. (2012). *Medications target long-term weight control*. Available at http://www.fda.gov/downloads/ForConsumers/ConsumerUpdates/UCM312391.pdf. Accessed 12/11/12.

feeling of fullness (Laddu et al., 2011). Tolerance may develop after only a few weeks, and there is risk of abuse. Common side effects are generally increased heart rate and blood pressure, dry mouth, agitation, insomnia, nausea, diarrhea, and constipation. Box 14.4 contains selected supplements that may be used for weight loss.

Lipase inhibitors work by reducing dietary fat absorption. Orlistat is approved for long-term use in severely obese adults, although its safety and efficacy have been established only up to 2 years. Over-the-counter Alli is a lower dose of the prescription version of Orlistat.

The FDA recently approved two new drugs that are considered lifelong therapies in people who respond to and tolerate them. Lorcaserin works by suppressing appetite. It should be discontinued if a patient fails to lose 5% of their weight after 12 weeks. Qsymia is a combination of phentermine and topiramate. The FDA recommends Qsymia be discontinued gradually if it fails to produce a 3% weight loss after 12 weeks on the recommended dose or after another 12 weeks on the highest dose (FDA, 2012).

Bariatric Surgery

Bariatric surgery is the most effective treatment for severe obesity, producing a 30% to 70% loss of excess weight that is largely maintained over time (Mechanick et al., 2009). Additional benefits include high remission rates of many obesity-related comorbidities, including diabetes, dyslipidemia, and hypertension as well as improved quality of life and a reduction in mortality (Mechanick et al., 2009). Because of its effectiveness, some researchers suggest the current criteria for performing the surgery (BMI of ≥40 or BMI of 35–39.9 for clients who have major comorbidities) be lowered to possibly a BMI of 30 (O'Brien et al., 2006). Surgical procedures for obesity work by (1) restricting the stomach's capacity, (2) creating

---

Box 14.4 SELECTED WEIGHT LOSS SUPPLEMENTS

Ephedra (ma huang): shown to promote a modest but significant increase in weight loss when used for 6 months or less; long-term efficacy untested. Associated with serious adverse events, such as seizures, stroke, and death. Sale banned in the United States since 2004.

Bitter orange: claims state bitter orange is a substitute for ephedra. Little evidence of efficacy; more research is needed. Safety concerns have been raised.

Chromium picolinate: little evidence that it increases lean body mass or decreases body fat; few or no adverse events.

Conjugated linoleic acid: little evidence of benefit; few data available on safety.

Chitosan: little evidence of benefit; there are no long-term safety trials in humans

Yohimbine: insufficient evidence on efficacy and safety to support its use in weight loss.

L-Carnitine: studies are limited and do no support its use for weight loss.

Calcium: diets rich in dairy products may lower the risk for obesity or promote weight loss in people who are overweight; to date, there is less evidence that calcium supplements have a similar effect on weight loss.

Green tea extract: a few, small studies suggest that regular consumption of green tea/extract may promote weight control. More studies are needed.

Source: Dwyer, J., Allison, D., & Coates, P. (2005). Dietary supplements in weight reduction. *Journal of the American Dietetic Association, 105*, S80–S86.

---

malabsorption of nutrients and calories, or (3) combining both. Intensive nutritional counseling is needed to help clients minimize gastrointestinal (GI) distress after eating and optimize effectiveness of the surgery. The two most common procedures worldwide are adjustable gastric banding (AGB) and Roux-en-Y gastric bypass (RYGB). Sleeve gastrectomy is relatively new as a stand-alone procedure. All procedures are performed laparoscopically.

Adjustable Gastric Banding

AGB works purely by restricting the capacity of the stomach. An inflatable band encircles the uppermost stomach to create a 15- to 30-mL capacity gastric pouch with a limited outlet between the pouch and the main section of the stomach (Fig. 14.3). The outlet diameter can be adjusted by inflating or deflating a small bladder inside the "belt" through a small subcutaneous reservoir. The size of the outlet can be repeatedly changed as needed. Clients must understand the importance of eating small meals, eating slowly, chewing food thoroughly, and progressing the diet gradually from liquids, to puréed foods, to soft foods.

Laparoscopic AGB is generally considered to be more flexible, less invasive, and safer than RYGB, but its results are less reliable and less effective (Nagle, 2010). Risks include band slippage or erosion into the stomach and reflux esophagitis (Laddu et al., 2011). Weight loss is usually less than with bypass surgeries, and the long-term outcomes beyond 5 to 7 years are unclear (Nagle, 2010).

Roux-en-Y Gastric Bypass

Dumping Syndrome: symptoms (e.g., nausea, abdominal cramping, diarrhea, hypoglycemia) that occur from rapid emptying of an osmotic load from the stomach into the small intestine.

Gastric bypass reduces storage capacity of the stomach to approximately 5% of normal with ingested food bypassing approximately 95% of the stomach, the entire duodenum, and a small portion of the proximal jejunum (Fig. 14.4) (Laddu et al., 2011). Weight loss is typically thought to occur from malabsorption and **dumping syndrome**. However, malabsorption, as measured by prealbumin and fecal fat, is not observed after the standard RYGB

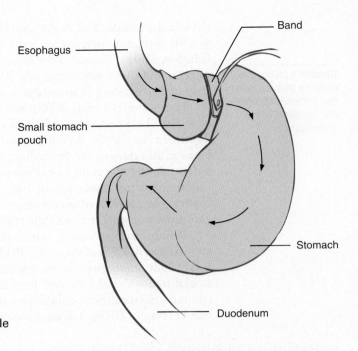

FIGURE 14.3 Adjustable gastric banding.

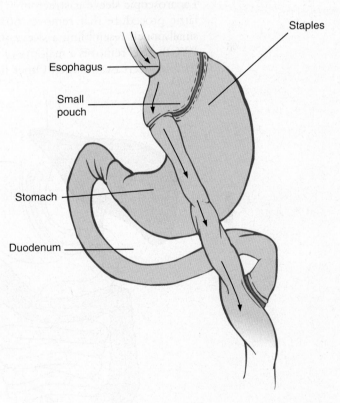

FIGURE 14.4 Roux-en-Y gastric bypass.

(MacLean, Rhode, and Nohr, 2001). Likewise, although dumping sometimes occurs, its severity does not correlate with the efficacy of RYGB (Cummings, Overduin, and Foster-Schuber, 2004). Because of a greater loss of appetite secondary to altered regulation of **ghrelin** and other gut hormones, RYGB may be more effective at producing weight loss than gastric banding (Cummings et al., 2004).

In randomized trials, RYGB has caused 50% to 80% loss of excess body weight (Laddu et al., 2011). Long-term (15 years or more) maintenance of weight loss is good (Jones, 2000). In the 1990s, RYGB in morbidly obese clients was found to improve type 2 diabetes within days of the procedure, suggesting that improved insulin sensitivity occurred independently of weight loss (Pories et al., 1995). Cohen, Pinheiro, Correa, and Schiavon (2006) reported resolution of type 2 diabetes and dyslipidemia in 100% of clients and hypertension in 97% of clients after RYGB. These findings extend the field of bariatric surgery from just weight loss to the realm of metabolic surgery (Nagle, 2010).

Perioperative mortality, which occurs mostly from pulmonary embolism or sepsis, is approximately 1% (Laddu et al., 2011). Postoperative complications occur in 10% of cases and include anastomotic leaks, internal hernias, GI bleeding, ulcers in the bypass segments, stomal stenosis, and gallstone formation with rapid weight loss (Jones, 2000). The most common micronutrient deficiencies after RYGB include iron, folate, vitamin B_{12}, and vitamin D (Nagle, 2010). Lifelong use of micronutrient supplements is required.

> **Ghrelin:** a protein produced by stomach cells that enhances appetite and decreases energy expenditure.

Laparoscopic Sleeve Gastrectomy

Laparoscopic sleeve gastrectomy (LSG) has recently been promoted as a stand-alone bariatric procedure that removes 60% to 85% of the stomach longitudinally, resulting in a small pouch resembling a sleeve (hence the name) or long thin banana (Fig. 14.5). Like RYGB, LSG removes a majority of the stomach, which reduces ghrelin hormone levels and thereby decreases hunger. Other hormones involved in food intake and insulin sensitivity

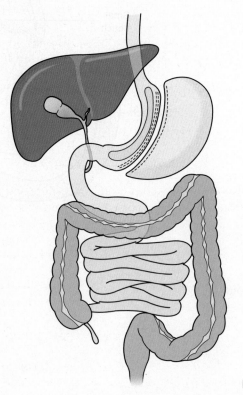

■ FIGURE 14.5 Sleeve gastrectomy.

are also altered. Malabsorption and dumping syndrome do not occur because the pylorus is preserved. Excess body weight loss resulting from LSG is generally described as superior to weight loss from AGB and comparable to weight loss after RYGB: at 2 years after surgery, weight loss averages 61% for LSG, 53% for AGB, and 67% for RYGB (Nocca et al., 2008). There are no long-term data on the use of LSG as a stand-alone procedure (Snyder-Marlow, Taylor, and Lenhard, 2010).

Nutrition Therapy

Bariatric surgery is not a magical cure for weight loss but rather a tool that works best when combined with diet and lifestyle changes. Bariatric surgery requires dramatic and dynamic changes in intake. Nutrition therapy is important presurgically, postsurgically, and long-term for weight management and overall health.

Presurgical Phase. A weight loss of 10% of excess body weight in the few weeks prior to surgery reduces liver size, which can shorten surgery time and may prevent surgical complications (Van Nieuwenhove et al., 2011) Presurgical weight loss may also improve long-term weight loss results (Alvarado et al., 2005). Most presurgical diets last for 2 weeks and consist of low-carbohydrate protein shakes and low-calorie beverages. Controlled portions of lean proteins, low-carbohydrate vegetables, and fruit may be permitted. Often the presurgical weight loss diet is a VLCD with or without pharmacology, depending on the client's clinical status and history of dieting (Kulick, Hark, and Deen, 2010).

Even if a VLCD is not used, bariatric clients can benefit from making healthful eating changes prior to surgery. Simple changes may be recommended, such as eating more fruits and vegetables, eliminating sweetened beverages, or avoiding fried foods. Clients should be screened for problematic eating behaviors that are barriers to postsurgical success, such as binge eating, emotional eating, and boredom eating (Tempest, 2012).

Counseling should give clients a realistic expectation of the postoperative phase, dispelling any notions that the surgery guarantees success. Topics to address include the need to drastically reduce portion sizes, the unpredictability of food intolerances, and the necessity of regular physical activity (Tempest, 2012). Clients should be given a copy of the postsurgical diet so they can have the appropriate food items available at home after discharge.

Postsurgical Phase. Nutrition goals after surgery are to create a substantial calorie deficit while meeting macronutrient and micronutrient requirements. Guidelines (Mechanick et al., 2009) recommend

- A clear liquid meal within 24 hours after any bariatric procedure, as ordered by the physician. Low-sugar or sugar-free, noncarbonated, caffeine-free beverages are provided, such as decaffeinated tea and Crystal Light.
- A progression of the meal pattern, based on the procedure and as defined by facility protocol (Table 14.5). Protein shakes may be added within 48 hours after surgery. The diet progresses to pureed and soft consistencies (Box 14.5). Dietary modifications are needed for the rest of the client's life.
- Ongoing nutrition and meal planning, counseling during hospitalization, and outpatient follow-up.
- Small, frequent meals. Clients are advised to chew food thoroughly and to avoid fluids for at least 30 minutes before or after eating. Clients are advised to eat slowly and to stop eating when they feel full.
- A balanced plan that includes more than five servings of fruits and vegetables to ensure an adequate intake of fiber and phytochemicals.
- Between 60 and 120 g of protein daily. Clients are advised to begin each "meal" with protein. Low-carbohydrate, liquid-protein supplements may be used in place of a meal.

Table 14.5 Bariatric Surgery Diet Guidelines

Time After Surgery	Diet Recommendations
1–2 days	Drink clear liquids that are sugar free, noncarbonated, and caffeine free. Sip liquids; avoid using a straw to avoid swallowing air.
3–7 days	Ingest a minimum of 48–64 oz/day of total fluids with 24–32 oz of clear liquids plus 24–32 oz of full liquids. Clear liquids should be sugar free or artificially sweetened and include salty fluids. Use full liquids ■ With ≤15 g sugar per serving ■ That are protein rich but limit to 20 g protein/serving when using added protein/whey powders Examples include ■ Lactaid milk or soy milk with added soy or whey powder ■ Plain or blended yogurt ■ Greek yogurt ■ Blended soup
2–3 Weeks	Increase clear liquids; total fluid intake/day should be 48–64+ oz. Replace full liquids with soft, moist, diced, ground, or pureed protein foods as tolerated, such as scrambled eggs; ground meats, poultry, or fish with gravy, broth, or light mayonnaise (to moisten); bean soups; cottage cheese; low-fat cheese; yogurt; sugar-free liquid protein supplements (e.g., sugar-free instant breakfast) or milk fortified with sugar-free whey (protein powder may be used in place of a meal). Consume protein at the beginning of each of 4–6 meals/snacks per day with limited portion sizes. Chew food thoroughly. Avoid fluids with meals and until at least 30 minutes after eating. Use small plates and utensils to help control portion sizes.
4 weeks	Continue with guidelines above and advance diet by adding well-cooked, soft vegetables and soft and/or peeled or canned fruit, such as ■ Whipped winter squash ■ Soft cooked carrots ■ Banana ■ Water-packed canned peaches ■ Unsweetened applesauce Adequate hydration is vital during rapid weight loss phase.
5 weeks	Continue to eat protein with some fruit or vegetable at each meal. Consider consuming salads at 1 month postoperatively if tolerated. Avoid rice, bread, and pasta until the 60 g of protein plus fruits and vegetables can be consumed comfortably daily.
As hunger increases and tolerance improves	Remember that a healthy solid food diet consists of adequate protein, fruits, vegetables, and whole grains. Keep in mind that calorie needs are individualized according to height, weight, and age. Avoid raw fruits and vegetables that are highly fibrous, such as celery, corn, tomatoes, and oranges; they may be eaten if well cooked or pureed. Consume 3 meals and 2 snacks per day of limited portion size. Continue with 48–64 oz of clear liquids that are noncarbonated, calorie free, and caffeine free Chew foods thoroughly. Avoid liquids for at least 30 minutes before and after eating.

Sources: Mechanick, J., Kushner, R., Sugerman, H., Gonzalez-Campoy, J. M., Collazo-Clavell, M. L., Spitz, A. F., . . . Guven, S. (2009). American Association of Clinical Endocrinologists, The Obesity Society, and American Society for Metabolic and Bariatric Surgery medical guidelines for clinical practice for the perioperative nutritional, metabolic, and nonsurgical support of the bariatric surgery patient. *Obesity, 17*(Suppl. 1), S1–S70; and Kulick, D., Hark, L., & Deen, D. (2010). The bariatric surgery patient: A growing role for registered dietitians. *Journal of the American Dietetic Association, 110,* 593–599.

Box 14.5   Sample Menu for Pureed/Soft Diet*

After Gastric Bypass Surgery

8 am:	¼ cup sugar-free instant breakfast made with fat-free milk
	¼ cup sugar-free gelatin
9 am:	1 cup skim milk
10 am:	1 cup sugar-free decaffeinated tea
12 noon:	1 cup liquid protein supplement
1 pm:	¼ cup smooth, sugar-free, low-fat vanilla yogurt
	¼ cup broth
2 pm:	Sugar-free popsicle
3 pm:	1 cup liquid protein supplement
5 pm:	½ cup strained cream soup made with fat-free milk
	½ cup low-sodium tomato juice
7 pm:	3 tbsp cottage cheese
8 pm:	1 cup skim milk
9 pm:	1 cup high-protein cream of chicken soup

*All beverages should be sipped slowly at a rate of 2 oz every 15 minutes.

- Avoiding concentrated sweets, which are a source of empty calories for any bariatric client and may aggravate dumping syndrome after malabsorption procedures.
- At least one to two multivitamins daily with additional supplements of iron, calcium with vitamin D, and vitamin B_{12}. Additional supplements may be needed based on the individual's laboratory values and symptoms.
- At least 1.5 L of fluid daily to maintain hydration. Fluids should be consumed slowly.
- Parenteral nutrition should be considered in critically ill clients who are unable to tolerate sufficient enteral nutrition for more than 5 to 7 days or noncritically ill clients who are unable to tolerate sufficient enteral nutrition for more than 7 to 10 days.

Foods that may not be tolerated during the first few months after surgery include red meat, chicken, and turkey (unless finely minced); products made with white flour; foods high in sugar or fat; and raw fruits and vegetables (Kulick et al., 2010). To promote continued weight loss, portion sizes should remain small. At 2 months after surgery, total food intake is approximately 1 cup per meal. At least 60 g of protein per day is needed to avoid protein malnutrition. Clients should eat at scheduled times instead of grazing, and meals should take at least 30 minutes. Food should be thoroughly chewed. Clients should participate in physical activity on most days of the week. To aggressively prevent nutrient deficiencies, lifelong vitamin supplementation and monitoring are required. Weight regain is another long-term challenge; significant regain occurs in up to 20% of clients following RYGB (Nagle, 2010). This may be due to anatomic and physiologic adaptations that allow the client to gradually resume bad old habits (Nagle, 2010).

Weight Maintenance After Loss

While losing weight may be difficult, keeping it off is even harder. Most evidence suggests that the majority of people who lose weight eventually regain the weight over subsequent months or years (Hill and Wyatt, 2005). Diets that lead to weight loss are not necessarily effective for maintaining weight loss. A negative calorie balance cannot be maintained indefinitely; learning how to achieve energy balance after weight loss is vital. Most people fail to maintain their new lower weight because they try to do so through calorie restriction alone (Hill and Wyatt, 2005). Data suggest that weight loss maintenance is most likely to succeed when physical activity increases significantly.

The National Weight Control Registry (NWCR) was founded in 1994 to identify and investigate behavioral and psychological characteristics of people who are successful in maintaining significant weight loss (NWCR, 2012). To be eligible, participants must have lost a minimum of 30 pounds and kept it off for more than 1 year. The NWCR is currently tracking more than 10,000 people in the registry; the average participant has lost an average of 66 pounds and kept it off for 5½ years. Moreover, 98% of participants modified their intake to lose weight, and 94% increased physical activity. Participants are surveyed annually to identify the strategies they use to maintain their weight loss. According to Rena Wing, cofounder of the NWCR, the single best predictor of who will be successful at maintaining weight loss is how long the individual has kept his or her weight off (Schardt, 2008). After maintaining weight loss for 2 years, the risk of regain is less than half. Weight regain is most likely to occur in people who ease up on physical activity, increase their fat intake, or start watching more television (Schardt, 2008). Once people start to regain weight, few are able to fully reverse it. The characteristics of successful weight maintainers appear in Box 14.6.

Obesity Prevention

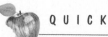

QUICK BITE

What 100 calories look like
12 oz light beer
5 oz white wine
8 oz soft drink
3 Buffalo wings
½ cup sweetened applesauce
1 fun-size Almond Joy
½ small McDonald's French fries
12 cashew nuts

It is suggested that small changes in diet and exercise that total a mere 100 cal/day may be enough to prevent obesity in most of the population (Hill and Wyatt, 2005). Consider that for most people, obesity develops insidiously without a conscious change in food intake or activity. For instance, even a seemingly insignificant 1 oz of cheddar cheese that supplies 100 calories will produce a 10-pound weight gain in a year if consumed daily and not offset by an increase in activity:

$$100 \text{ cal} \times 365 \text{ days/year} = 36,500 \text{ excess cal/year}$$

$$36,500 \text{ cal/year divided by } 3500 \text{ cal/lb} = \text{slightly over 10 lb/year weight gain}$$

Research suggests that it may take more behavior change to prevent weight regain after loss than to prevent weight gain in those who have never been obese, making prevention efforts imperative (Hill and Wyatt, 2005).

Box 14.6   SUCCESSFUL WEIGHT MAINTENANCE

Based on participants in the National Weight Control Registry (NWCR), people who are successful at maintaining weight loss

- Eat a low-calorie diet. Most people eat a low-fat diet to maintain their loss.
- Eat 4 to 5 times per day.
- Eat a consistent diet from day to day. Eating a limited number of foods may make the diet boring, which helps limit eating.
- 78% eat breakfast every day, which may help control hunger later in the day.
- Are extremely physically active. Ninety percent of registrants exercise, on average, approximately 1 hour per day. Walking is the exercise of choice for most people.
- 75% weigh themselves at least once a week.
- 62% watch fewer than 10 hours of TV a week.

Source: NWCR Facts. Available at www.nwcr.ws/default.htm. Accessed on 12/9/12; and Schardt, D. (2008). Secrets of successful losers. *Nutrition Action Health Letter, 35,* 8.

NURSING PROCESS: *Obesity*

Rosa is 37 years old, 5 ft 4 in tall, and the mother of two children. Before her first child was born 10 years ago, her normal weight was 140 pounds. She gained 35 pounds during pregnancy and didn't regain her normal weight before her second pregnancy a year later. She is now at her heaviest weight of 168 pounds. She complains of fatigue and thinks her weight contributes to her asthma. She has tried several diets and has been unable to take weight off and keep it off. Her doctor told her she has prehypertension and encouraged her to lose weight to lower both her blood pressure and serum glucose levels. The fear of needing medication for hypertension or diabetes has motivated her to lose weight.

Assessment

Medical–Psychosocial History	▪ Medical history and comorbidities such as hypertension, dyslipidemia, cardiovascular disease, diabetes, sleep apnea, osteoarthritis, and esophageal reflux
	▪ Medications that may promote weight gain or interfere with weight loss, such as insulin and other antidiabetes agents, steroid hormones, psychotropic drugs, mood stabilizers, antidepressants, and antiepileptic drugs
	▪ Motivation to lose weight including previous history of successful and unsuccessful attempts to lose weight, social support, and perceived barriers to success
Anthropometric Assessment	▪ Height, current weight, BMI
	▪ Weight history; heaviest adult weight, usual body weight
	▪ Waist circumference
Biochemical and Physical Assessment	▪ Lab values related to comorbidities, such as total cholesterol, LDL cholesterol, HDL cholesterol, triglycerides, glucose, hemoglobin A1c
	▪ Triiodothyronine (T_3) and thyroxine (T_4) for thyroid function
	▪ Blood pressure
Dietary Assessment	▪ How many daily meals and snacks do you usually eat?
	▪ What is a typical day's intake?
	▪ How do you think your usual intake needs to change to be healthier or to help you lose weight?
	▪ How often do you eat breakfast?
	▪ How many servings of fruits and vegetables do you eat daily?
	▪ How much sweetened soda do you drink daily?
	▪ Do you watch your fat intake? If so, what do you do to limit fat?
	▪ Do you watch your carbohydrate intake? If so, what do you do to limit carbohydrates?
	▪ How many meals per week do you eat out?
	▪ In regard to diet, what is your "weakness"?
	▪ Do you know if you eat for reasons other than hunger, for example, when you are bored, sad, lonely, or anxious?
	▪ Do you take vitamins, minerals, or supplements to help with weight loss? If so, what?
	▪ What is your goal weight?

(continues on page 378)

NURSING PROCESS: *Obesity* (continued)

- How much moderate-intensity exercise do you do on a daily basis? How active is your lifestyle? How easy would it be for you to become more active?
- How much alcohol do you consume?
- Do you have any cultural, religious, or ethnic food preferences?
- Do you have any food allergies or intolerances?

Diagnosis

Possible Nursing Diagnosis

Altered nutrition: intake exceeds the body's needs as evidenced by excess body weight

Planning

Client Outcomes

The client will
- Gradually increase physical activity to a total of 60 minutes of moderate-intensity activity on most days of the week
- Explain the relationship between calorie intake, physical activity, and weight control
- Consume a nutritionally adequate, hypocaloric diet consisting of healthy carbohydrates, healthy fats, and lean protein
- Eat at least three meals per day
- Practice behavior modification techniques to change undesirable eating habits
- Lose 1 to 2 pounds/week on average until 10% of initial weight is lost
- Improve health status as evidenced by a decrease in total cholesterol, LDL cholesterol, and glucose; an increase in HDL cholesterol; and improved blood pressure, as appropriate

Nursing Interventions

Nutrition Therapy

- Decrease calorie intake to 1200/day in three meals plus two to three snacks throughout the day to prevent intense hunger and subsequent overeating
- Provide a 1200-calorie eating plan that specifies portion sizes and number of servings from each food group recommended for each meal and snack

The daily plan will include

4 grains, preferably all of them whole grains

1½ cups of vegetables

1 cup of fruit

3 oz of protein foods

2 cups of fat-free milk

4 tsp of oil

- Encourage ample fluid intake, preferably water and other noncalorie drinks, to promote excretion of metabolic wastes

NURSING PROCESS: *Obesity* (continued)

Client Teaching	Instruct the client on

Instruct the client on

The interrelationship between a hypocaloric diet, increased physical activity, and behavior change in managing weight

The eating plan essentials, including

- Meal and snack timing and frequency
- The emphasis on high-satiety foods, such as whole grains, fruit and vegetables, and lean protein
- Tips for eating out (Chapter 10), food preparation techniques, and the basics of food purchasing and label reading

Behavioral matters, including

- Eating only in one place while sitting down
- Putting utensils down between mouthfuls
- Monitoring hunger on a scale of 1 to 10 with 1 corresponding to "famished" and 10 corresponding to "stuffed." Encourage clients to eat when the hunger scale is at about 3 and to stop when satisfied (not full) at about 6 or 7.
- Weighing oneself at least once a week
- Periodically keeping a record of food intake and activity
- "Planning" splurges instead of eating on impulse. Planned splurges involve making a conscious decision to eat something, enjoying every mouthful of the food, and then moving on from the experience without feelings of guilt or failure.

Changing eating attitudes by

- Replacing negative self-talk with positive talk
- Replacing the attitude of "always being on a diet" with an acceptance of eating healthier and less as a way of life
- Consulting a physician or dietitian if questions concerning the eating plan or weight loss arise

Evaluation

Evaluate and Monitor

- Monitor weight
- Evaluate food and activity records to assess adherence; suggest changes in the meal plan as needed
- Provide periodic feedback and reinforcement
- Monitor biochemical data for improvements attributable to weight loss

EATING DISORDERS: ANOREXIA NERVOSA, BULIMIA NERVOSA, AND EATING DISORDERS NOT OTHERWISE SPECIFIED

Body Dysmorphic Disorder: excessive preoccupation with a real or imagined defect in physical appearance.

Eating disorders are serious biologically based mental illnesses that can have a profound impact on medical, psychological, and social functioning (Rome and Ammerman, 2003; Swanson, Crow, LeGrange, Swendsen, and Merikangas, 2011). They are generally characterized by abnormal eating patterns, **body dysmorphic disorder** or distorted perceptions of body image, and use of compensatory behaviors, such as excessive physical activity, vomiting, or laxative use (Miller and Golden, 2010) (Fig. 14.6). Eating disorders differ in manifestation, risk factors, nutritional complications, and medical complications (Table 14.6). Treatment approaches also differ.

Etiology

Eating disorders result from interaction between genetics, biology, temperament, and environment (Tholking et al., 2011). Although numerous psychological, physical, social, and cultural risk factors have been identified, it is not known how or why these factors interact to cause eating disorders. Risk factors that precede the diagnosis of an eating disorder include dieting, early childhood eating and GI problems, increased concern about weight and size, negative self-evaluation, sexual abuse, and other traumas (Ozier and Henry, 2011). Major stressors, such as the onset of puberty, parents' divorce, death of a family member, and ridicule of being or becoming fat are frequent precipitating factors. Athletes (e.g., dancers, gymnasts) may develop eating disorders to improve their performance. People with eating disorders often have coexisting mood, anxiety, impulse control, or substance use disorders (Hudson, Hiripi, Pope, and Kessler, 2007). Each person's recovery process is unique; therefore, treatment plans are highly individualized.

Anorexia Nervosa (AN): a condition of self-imposed fasting or severe self-imposed dieting.

A multidisciplinary approach that includes nutrition counseling, behavior modification, psychotherapy, family counseling, and group therapy is most effective. Antidepressant drugs effectively reduce the frequency of problematic eating behaviors but do not eliminate them. Most eating disorders are treated on an outpatient basis; however, severe cases of **anorexia nervosa (AN)** may necessitate hospitalization. Treatment is often time consuming and frustrating.

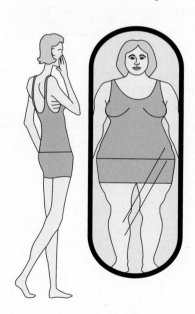

■ FIGURE 14.6 A woman suffering from anorexia sees herself as overweight.

Table 14.6   A Comparison of Anorexia Nervosa and Bulimia Nervosa

	Anorexia Nervosa	Bulimia Nervosa
Major characteristics	Compulsive pursuit of thinness Intense fear of becoming fat; intense preoccupation with food Self-worth based on size and shape	Lack of sense of control regarding eating Fear of being overweight
Onset and population	Usually develops during adolescence or young adulthood; 90%–95% are female	Usually develops during adolescence or young adulthood; is more likely to occur in men than anorexia
Typical eating and exercise behaviors	Semistarvation with compulsive exercise; onset of disorder is usually preceded by dieting behavior	Gorging (e.g., 1200–11,500 calories in a short amount of time) followed by purging, such as self-induced vomiting, excessive exercise, abuse of laxatives, emetics, diuretics, or fasting; "dieting" is a way of life but bingeing may occur several times per day and may be planned
Weight	Less than 85% of expected weight, which is a BMI of 17.5 or less for adults	Fluctuations are normal; weight may be normal or slightly above normal.
Emotional symptoms	Vicarious enjoyment of food; denial of the condition can be extreme; body image disturbance; pronounced emotional changes; low self-esteem	Displays mood swings; full recognition of the behavior as abnormal; ongoing feelings of isolation, self-deprecating thoughts, depression, and low self-esteem
Physical symptoms	Lanugo hair on the face and trunk; brittle listless hair; dry skin, brittle nails, intolerance of cold	May appear normal Swollen salivary glands in cheeks Sores, scars, or calluses on knuckles or hands
Cardiovascular effects	Bradycardia, hypotension, orthostatic hypotension	Arrhythmias; palpitations; weakness
GI effects	Delayed gastric emptying, decreased motility, severe constipation	Bloating, constipation, flatulence; gastric dilation with rupture is a risk
Endocrine/metabolic imbalances	Cold sensitivity; fatigue; hypercholesterolemia, hypoglycemia; amenorrhea or menstrual irregularities	Menstrual irregularities, dehydration, and electrolyte imbalances may occur secondary to vomiting and laxative abuse; rebound fluid retention with edema
Musculoskeletal	Osteopenia, osteoporosis, muscle wasting and weakness	Dental erosion; muscular weakness
Growth status	Arrested growth and maturation	Usually not affected
Nutrient deficiencies	Protein–calorie malnutrition; various micronutrient deficiencies	Varies

Source: Nutrition Care Manual. (2012). *Eating disorders.* Available at www.nutritioncaremanual.org. Accessed on 12/9/12; and *Laureate Eating Disorders Program.* (n.d.). Available at www.eatingdisorders.laureate.com. Accessed on 12/10/12.

Bulimia Nervosa (BN): an eating disorder characterized by recurrent episodes of bingeing and purging.

AN is more difficult to treat than **bulimia nervosa (BN)** because bulimics know their behavior is abnormal and many are willing to cooperate with treatment. People with AN have a greater incidence of relapse and a higher mortality rate compared to people diagnosed with other eating disorders (Tholking et al., 2011). Although "full" and "partial" recovery are not clearly defined, it is estimated that 50% of people diagnosed with AN have a full recovery with treatment, 30% achieve partial recovery, and 20% have lifelong problems and maintain dieting and food fears (Nutrition Care Manual, 2012). The overall mortality rate is reported to range from 5% to 16% (Miller and Golden, 2010).

Nutrition Therapy for Anorexia

Nutritional therapy goals are to reestablish and maintain normal eating behaviors; correct signs, symptoms, and complications of the eating disorder; and promote long-term maintenance of reasonable weight. The initial weight goal may simply be to prevent further weight loss, or a lower-than-normal weight goal may be selected, such as enough weight to regain normal physiologic function and menstruation. When this has been achieved, the goal is reevaluated. Although weight gain is not the only criterion for judging success, a reasonable weight gain goal is 1 to 2 pounds/week (Nutrition Care Manual, 2012). Nutrition therapy guidelines are listed in Box 14.7.

Refeeding Syndrome: a condition characterized by severe shifts in fluid and electrolytes, especially phosphorus, from the extracellular to intracellular fluid when refeeding begins in a person who is severely malnourished and depleted in total body phosphorus.

Even though calorie needs are high to restore body weight, the initial eating plan offered is low in calories (e.g., 1200–1400 cal/day) to avoid overwhelming the client. Also, large amounts of food may not be well tolerated after prolonged semistarvation, and **refeeding syndrome** is a risk in severely malnourished clients. Strategies, such as increasing calories gradually, for example, in increments of 100 to 200 calories, and close monitoring of electrolyte levels are recommended.

Strategies to promote compliance and feelings of trust include involving the client in formulating individualized goals and meal plans; offering rewards linked to the quantity of calories consumed, not to weight gain; and having the client record food intake and exercise activity. A study by Schebendach et al. (2008) showed that among clients who

---

Box 14.7   NUTRITION THERAPY GUIDELINES FOR ANOREXIA NERVOSA

- Help maximize intake and tolerance with small, frequent meals.
- Advance the diet only when the client is able to complete a full meal. Calories may eventually be increased to 3000 or more per day.
- Because gastrointestinal intolerance may exist, limit gassy foods in the early stages of treatment, such as cruciferous vegetables (broccoli, cauliflower, cabbage), dried peas and beans, dried prunes and raisins, carbonated beverages, garlic, onions, melon, and products containing sorbitol. It may also be prudent to limit fatty and fried foods.
- Serve small, attractive meals based on individual food preferences. Foods that are nutritionally dense help to minimize the volume of food needed. Finger foods served cold or at room temperature help to minimize satiety sensations.
- Never force the client to eat, and minimize the emphasis on food. Initially, clients may respond to nutrition therapy better if they are allowed to exclude high-risk binge foods from their diet. However, the binge foods should be reintroduced later so that the "feared food" (trigger food) idea is not promoted.
- Help control symptoms of constipation and fluid retention with a high-fiber or low-sodium diet, respectively.
- Consider prescription of a multivitamin and mineral supplement.
- Avoid caffeine because it is both a stimulant and a mild diuretic.
- Use enteral or parenteral nutrition only if necessary to stabilize the client medically. Overly aggressive nutritional repletion carries medical risks of fluid retention and refeeding syndrome; psychological risks may include a perceived loss of control, loss of identity, increased body distortion, and mistrust of the treatment team. Enteral support should never be used as punishment for difficult clients.

Calorie Density: the amount of calories in a given weight of food.

achieved restoration of weight through treatment for AN, those who consumed diets low in **calorie density** and limited in variety had increased risk of relapse.

Nutrition Therapy for Bulimia Nervosa

BN is characterized by binge eating episodes followed by purging for weight control. Purging is accomplished by self-induced vomiting; laxative, diuretic, or diet pill abuse; excess exercising; or fasting. Contrary to popular opinion, binges do not always consist of large amounts of food; people who are restrictive eaters may consider an eating episode a "binge" even with small amounts of food (Nutrition Care Manual, 2012). The salient characteristic of bingeing is that the food is eaten in secrecy. Clients are left feeling shameful and guilty. Binge foods tend to be soft, easy to swallow, easy to regurgitate, and composed of high-fat or high-sugar foods that the client normally restricts from the diet.

People with BN tend to have similar attitudes about food, weight, and body shapes as people with AN; however, they tend to have fewer serious medical complications because their undernutrition is less severe. Treatment approaches are similar for BN and AN, except that weight restoration is not a goal. Nutritional counseling focuses on identifying and correcting food misinformation and fears and includes discussing normal weight fluctuations, planning meals, establishing a normal pattern of eating, and identifying the dangers of dieting. Bulimics must understand that gorging is only one aspect of a complex pattern of altered behavior; in fact, excessive dietary restriction is a major contributor to the disorder. Although most clients with BN want to lose weight, dieting and recovery from an eating disorder are incompatible. Normalization of eating behaviors is a primary goal.

Initially, nutrition therapy for bulimia is structured and relatively inflexible to promote the client's sense of control. Meal patterns, similar to those used for people with diabetes, may be used to specify portion sizes, to identify food groups to include with each meal and snack, and to denote the frequency of eating. The initial meal plan may be low in calories and may be nutritionally inadequate to avoid overwhelming the client. However, enough calories should be provided to prevent hunger, which can precipitate a binge. A 1500-calorie diet distributed among three balanced meals plus snacks may be used. Adequate fat is provided to help delay gastric emptying and contribute to satiety. Calories are gradually increased as needed. Having the client record intake *before* eating adds to a sense of control. Nutrition therapy guidelines for BN appear in Box 14.8.

Eating Disorders Not Otherwise Specified

Eating disorders not otherwise specified (EDNOS) are at least as common as AN and BN, but prevalence rates are unknown because there is no simple definition of EDNOS. This group represents subacute cases of AN or BN—clients who may meet all the criteria for AN except that they have not missed three consecutive menstrual periods, or clients of normal weight who purge without bingeing. Binge eating disorder, in which bingeing occurs without purging, is also classified as an EDNOS.

Binge eating disorder differs from BN in that binge eating is not accompanied by purging behaviors to control weight. People with binge eating disorder are often obese and, unlike people with BN, do not restrict their eating between binge episodes and overeat without feeling a loss of control (Nutrition Care Manual, 2012). Binge eating episodes are associated with three or more of the following: eating more quickly than normal; eating until uncomfortably full; eating large amounts of food when not physically hungry; eating alone due to embarrassment over how much is eaten; and feeling disgusted, depressed, or guilty about overeating (Nutrition Care Manual, 2012). Bingeing must occur at least twice

---

BOX 14.8   NUTRITION THERAPY GUIDELINES FOR BULIMIA NERVOSA

- To increase awareness of eating and satiety, meals and snacks should be eaten while sitting down; finger foods and foods that are cold or at room temperature should be avoided; and the meal duration should be of appropriate length.
- Dieting should be discouraged.
- Eating strategies that may help to regulate intake include balanced meals at regular intervals.
- A high-protein and/or high-fiber snack slightly before the times of the day when the binge is most likely to occur may help promote satiety and keep blood glucose levels within normal range.
- Clients may be encouraged to gradually introduce forbidden binge foods into their diets. This is a key step in changing the all-or-none behavior of bingeing/purging.
- Clients who are laxative dependent are at risk for bowel obstruction if the protocol for laxative withdrawal is not implemented. A high-fiber diet with plenty of fluids helps to normalize bowel movements while the use of laxatives is gradually decreased. Stool softeners may be ordered.
- A daily multivitamin may be appropriate if intake or variety is low.
- When relapse occurs, the structured meal plan should be resumed immediately.

---

a week over at least 6 months. Risk factors for binge eating include childhood obesity, parental obesity, a high degree of body dissatisfaction, dysfunctional attitudes about weight and shape, poor self-esteem, and impaired social functioning (Nutrition Care Manual, 2012).

Binge eating may be treated with a nondieting approach, which is also referred to as Health at Any Size. Compared to traditional weight loss diets that rely on restrictive eating and increasing physical activity to promote weight loss, the nondiet approach is an internally regulated approach with the primary goal to normalize eating behaviors. Weight loss may or may not be a secondary goal. A nondieting approach emphasizes

- Eating nourishing food and enjoying it
- Self-acceptance and size acceptance
- Awareness of internal cues for hunger and satiety
- Physical activity for enjoyment, not weight management

Clients may feel like the nondiet approach is not an approach at all but rather permission to overeat. Those who insist on following a restrictive diet may still benefit from some of the principles of the nondieting approach.

How Do You Respond?

Is it a good idea to substitute special low-carbohydrate products for regular foods? Choosing reduced-carbohydrate versions of "empty-calorie" foods ignores the big picture: to lose weight, calories have to be decreased. Substituting reduced-carbohydrate muffins or beer for their regular-carbohydrate counterparts is likely to have little or no impact on calorie intake. In addition, specially prepared low-carbohydrate foods do not taste like the original food and may cost two to four times more. A better alternative to choosing low-carbohydrate items is to avoid foods made with white flour and sugar and switch to carbohydrates that provide satiety—namely, whole-grain breads and cereals, fruit, vegetables, and dried peas and beans.

CASE STUDY

CC: "I hate being fat."

Client history: CC is a 43-year-old mother of three who has experienced gradual weight gain after the birth of each of her children. She is 5 ft 7 in tall, weighs 189 pounds, works full time, and does not engage in regular exercise. She is considered pre-diabetic and has prehypertension and appears eager to make lifestyle changes to improve her health and be a better nutritional role model for her children. She has successfully lost weight in the past through Weight Watchers but eventually got bored and regained all of the weight she lost. She does not want to count calories. She wants to know how many servings from each food group she should eat to lose weight and what the best foods from each group are.

Her usual intake is as follows: no breakfast; snacks at a vending machine twice a day; fast food for lunch; and dinner with the family. Her dinner usually consists of about 6 oz of meat, potatoes, sometimes a vegetable, bread with butter, and dessert. CC admits to a weakness for "sweets."

- What is CC's weight status based on her BMI?
- What additional information about her eating behaviors would be helpful?
- What MyPlate calorie level would you recommend for her?
- What food groups does she need to consume more of? Less of? What would you tell her about the "best" foods from each group?
- Create a nursing care plan complete with nursing diagnosis, client goal, interventions, and monitoring recommendations.
- Devise a meal pattern with the calorie allowance you recommend; include three meals per day and two snacks. Prepare a sample menu.
- What behavioral strategies would you recommend for her?

STUDY QUESTIONS

1. The client asks if it is okay for her to follow a low-carbohydrate, Atkins-type diet in the short term to get her started on her weight loss efforts. Which of the following would be the nurse's best response?
   a. "No, low-carbohydrate diets are not healthy and would only sabotage your weight loss efforts."
   b. "Initially, a low-carbohydrate diet can help you lose weight more quickly than other types of diets, but over time, what is most important is the amount of calories you eat, not the macronutrient distribution. You can try it, but discontinue it if you experience any side effects."
   c. "A low-carbohydrate diet is better than any other type of diet and is a good choice for you to use."
   d. "A low-fat diet is easier. Try that instead."

2. A major reason why it becomes increasing difficult to keep losing weight on a weight loss diet is that
   a. The loss of fat tissue lowers metabolic rate.
   b. A lighter body expends fewer calories than a heavier body when doing activity.
   c. Fluid retention becomes an issue over time.
   d. A decrease in food intake means that fewer calories are used to metabolize food.

3. The client asks if meal replacements, such as Jenny Craig products, are a good idea to help with weight loss. Which of the following would be the nurse's best response?
   a. "They are a great way to control portions and can help you adhere to your diet when used as suggested."
   b. "They are gimmicks that fail to teach you how to control your own intake. They are not recommended."
   c. "Most people gain weight while using them. You should stay away from them."
   d. "They are not nutritionally balanced so you actually have to overeat in order to meet your nutritional requirements if you use them."

4. Which of the following strategies promotes adherence to exercise? Select all that apply.
   a. Promote structure by encouraging the client to exercise at on-site or supervised exercise sessions.
   b. Encourage the client to exercise in multiple short bouts (10 minutes each), instead of one long session.
   c. Encourage a more active lifestyle, such as parking far away from the door when going to the mall or work.
   d. Encourage the client to exercise at home.

5. Which of the following calorie level ranges is considered appropriate for weight loss diets for most women?
   a. 800–900 cal/day
   b. 1000–1200 cal/day
   c. 1400–1600 cal/day
   d. 1800–2000 cal/day

6. Which of the following may help to promote adherence to a hypocaloric diet?
   a. A meal plan and recipes
   b. A list of forbidden foods
   c. A calorie counter
   d. A fat gram counter

7. When instituting nutrition therapy for a client diagnosed with bulimia nervosa, the priority is to
   a. Teach the client about nutrient and calorie requirements.
   b. Halt weight loss.
   c. Normalize eating behaviors.
   d. Provide sufficient calories for weight gain.

8. When instituting nutrition therapy for a client diagnosed with anorexia nervosa, the priority is to
   a. Teach the client about nutrient and calorie requirements.
   b. Halt weight loss.
   c. Normalize eating behaviors.
   d. Provide sufficient calories for weight gain.

KEY CONCEPTS

■ Approximately 36% of American adults are obese. The prevalence of obesity has increased in both genders, in all age groups, and among all races and ethnicities.

■ Obesity is a chronic disease of multifactorial origin. It is likely that an obesogenic environment, behavior, and genetics are involved in its development.

■ Obesity is resistant to treatment when success is measured by achieving healthy BMI alone. Rather than concentrating solely on weight loss to measure success, other health benefits, such as lowered blood pressure and lowered serum glucose levels, should also be considered.

- A modest weight loss of 5% to 10% of initial body weight usually effectively lowers disease risks. For some people, a reasonable goal may be to halt weight gain, not to lose weight.
- A hypocaloric intake, increased physical activity, and behavior therapy are the cornerstones to weight loss therapy. Pharmacotherapy and surgery are additional options for some people.
- In theory, a calorie deficit of 500 to 1000 cal/day results in a loss of 1 to 2 pounds/week. In practice, biologic adaptations occur, making it increasingly difficult to continue losing weight without a further reduction in calories.
- Generally, weight loss diets range from 1000 to 1200 cal/day for most women and 1200 to 1600 cal/day for men.
- As long as calories are reduced and healthy sources of fat and carbohydrates are used, the macronutrient composition of the diet does not impact weight loss. What matters is the relationship between calorie intake and calorie output, not the source of calories consumed.
- Because portion sizes have grown over the last few decades, people's perception of what a normal portion size is may be distorted. Estimating portion sizes using common household items may help people "right size." Other recommendations include using a smaller dinner plate, smaller utensils, and prepackaged 100-calorie products.
- Eating at regular, frequent intervals may help prevent extreme hunger and reduce the risk of binge eating. Meal patterns should be individualized.
- Meal replacements eliminate choices in what to eat and how much to eat and have been shown to effectively promote weight loss and weight maintenance after loss.
- Behavior therapy promotes lifelong changes in eating and activity habits. It is a process that involves identifying behaviors that need improvement, setting specific behavioral goals, modifying "problem" behaviors, and reinforcing the positive changes.
- Dietary adherence may be enhanced by providing a structured meal plan with shopping lists and recipe ideas.
- An increase in activity helps to burn calories and has a favorable impact on body composition and weight distribution. Even without weight loss, exercise lowers blood pressure and improves glucose tolerance and blood lipid levels.
- To achieve weight loss, 150 to 420 minutes/week of moderate to vigorous physical activity may be needed. The same amount of activity may be necessary to maintain weight after weight loss.
- People who are severely obese may not be able to achieve the recommended intensity and duration of aerobic benefits to reap weight loss benefits. Progressive strength training may be a better option for physical activity for this population.
- Resistance training combined with higher protein intake promotes weight and fat loss while maintaining muscle mass, which is especially important when weight loss is large.
- Clients may be more likely to adhere to a physical activity program if they are encouraged to participate in physical activity at home and in short bouts, if that is preferred. Moving more throughout the day by reducing sedentary activities is also recommended.
- Pharmacotherapy is adjunctive therapy in the treatment of obesity. Drugs are not effective in all people, and they are only effective for as long as they are used.
- Surgery to promote weight loss therapy involves limiting the capacity of the stomach. Gastric bypass also circumvents a portion of the small intestine to cause malabsorption of calories. Both types effectively promote weight loss but are tools, not magic strategies.
- Bariatric surgeries require lifelong changes in eating behaviors to ensure continued success. The postsurgical diet progresses from clear liquids to pureed food to a soft diet. Small, frequent meals are necessary to avoid overstretching the pouch. Sugars are avoided to decrease the risk of dumping syndrome. Nutritional deficiencies are a lifelong risk, requiring preventative supplementation.

■ Weight maintenance after loss may be more difficult to achieve than weight loss itself. Common characteristics of people who are able to maintain long-term weight loss include consuming a low-calorie diet, eating consistently from day to day, eating breakfast, becoming very physically active, weighing themselves frequently, watching TV for a limited period of time, and not letting a small weight gain become a big weight gain.

■ Anorexia nervosa and bulimia nervosa are characterized by preoccupation with body weight and food and usually are preceded by prolonged dieting. Although their cause is unknown, they are considered to be multifactorial in origin.

■ Anorexia nervosa is a condition of severe self-imposed starvation, often accompanied by a frantic pursuit of exercise. Although they appear to be severely underweight, anorexics have a distorted self-perception of weight and see themselves as overweight. They may have numerous physical and mental symptoms. Anorexia can be fatal.

■ Bulimia, which occurs more frequently than anorexia, is characterized by binge eating (consuming large amounts of food in a short period) and purging (e.g., self-induced vomiting, laxative abuse). Foods consumed tend to be soft and easily regurgitated. Bulimic individuals usually appear to be of normal or slightly above normal weight, and they experience less severe physical symptoms than anorexic individuals do. Bulimia is rarely fatal.

■ Binge eating disorder is similar to bulimia except that it is not accompanied by purging behaviors. A nondieting approach may be used to help normalize eating behaviors.

■ Eating disorders are best treated by a team approach that includes nutritional intervention and counseling to restore normal eating behaviors and adequate nutritional status.

Check Your Knowledge Answer Key

1. **FALSE** Calories eaten during the evening do not "count" more than calories eaten at any other time of day. It comes down to calories in versus calories out. The problem with eating in the evening is that it is frequently "mindless munching" in front of the TV and the calories seem to pile up unconsciously.

2. **FALSE** People who skip meals tend to feel hungrier later on and then eat more than they normally would.

3. **TRUE** Most people are able to lose weight through diet and exercise, but most people eventually regain most or all of the weight they lost.

4. **TRUE** Keeping a food diary, as well as a physical activity diary, can help people improve their eating habits by revealing problematic patterns or trends.

5. **FALSE** Obesity-related problems improve or are resolved with a modest weight loss of 5% to 10% of initial weight even if healthy weight is not achieved.

6. **TRUE** Most short-term weight loss occurs from a decrease in total calorie intake. Physical activity helps to maintain weight loss.

7. **TRUE** With or without weight loss, an increase in physical activity helps to lower blood pressure and improve glucose tolerance.

8. **TRUE** Eating plans that provide less than 1200 calories may not provide adequate amounts of essential nutrients.

9. **FALSE** Neither cutting carbohydrates nor cutting fat grams ensures weight loss unless total calories are reduced. There is no magic combination of nutrients that causes weight loss independent of reducing calories.

10. **TRUE** People affected by bulimia tend to have fewer medical complications than those affected by anorexia because the undernutrition is less severe.

> ## *Student Resources on* thePoint
> ---
> *For additional learning materials, activate the code in the front of this book at*
> **http://thePoint.lww.com/activate**

Websites

For reliable information on weight, dieting, physical fitness, and obesity

American Obesity Association at **www.obesity.org**
Calorie Control Council at **www.caloriecontrol.org**
Centre for Obesity Research and Education at **http://www.core.monash.org/**
Division of Nutrition, Physical Activity, and Obesity, National Center for Chronic Disease
    Prevention and Health Promotion at **www.cdc.gov/nccdphp/dnpa**
International Obesity Taskforce at **www.iotf.org**
National Heart, Lung, and Blood Institute Obesity Education Initiative at **www.nhlbi.nih.gov/
    about/oei/index.htm**
Shape Up America at **www.shapeup.org**
Weight-Control Information Network at **www.niddk.nih.gov/health/nutrit/win.htm**

For free intake/diet analysis

www.fitday.com
www.dietsite.com
www.foodcount.com (offers both free and fee-based subscriptions)
www.nat.uiuc.edu/mynat

For eating disorders

Anorexia Nervosa and Related Eating Disorders (ANRED) at **www.anred.com**
National Eating Disorders Organization at **www.nationaleatingdisorders.org**
Overeaters Anonymous, Inc. at **www.oa.org**
The Renfrew Center at **www.renfrew.org**

References

Allison, D., Downey, M., Atkinson, R., Billington, C. J., Bray, G. A., Eckel, R. H., . . .
    Tremblay, A. (2008). Obesity as a disease: A white paper on evidence and arguments commissioned by the Council of The Obesity Society. *Obesity (Silver Spring), 16,* 1161–1177.
Alvarado, R., Alami, R., Hsu, G., Safadi, B., Sanchez, B., Morton, J., & Curet, M. (2005). The
    impact of preoperative weight loss in patients undergoing laparoscopic Roux-en-Y gastric
    bypass. *Obesity Surgery, 15,* 1282–1286.
Appelhans, B., Whited, M., Schneider, K., & Pagoto, S. (2011). Time to abandon the notion of
    personal choice in dietary counseling for obesity? *Journal of the American Dietetic Association,
    111,* 1130–1136.
Bantle, J., Wylie-Rosett, J., Albright, A. L., Apovian, C. M., Clark, N. G., Franz, M. J., . . .
    Wheeler, M. (2008). Nutrition recommendations and interventions for diabetes. A position
    statement of the American Diabetes Association. *Diabetes Care, 31*(Suppl. 1), S61–S78.
Bauer, F., Elbers, C., Adan, R., Loos, R. J., Onland-Moret, N. C., Grobbee, D. E., . . . van der
    Schouw, Y. T. (2009). Obesity genes identified in genome-wide association studies are associated with adiposity measures and potentially with nutrient-specific food preference. *American
    Journal of Clinical Nutrition, 90,* 951–959.
Blackburn, G. (1995). Effect of degree of weight loss on health benefits. *Obesity Research,
    3*(Suppl. 2), 211S–216S.
Blackburn, G., Wollner, S., & Heymsfield, S. (2010). Lifestyle interventions for the treatment
    of class III obesity: A primary target for nutrition medicine in the obesity epidemic. *American
    Journal of Clinical Nutrition, 91*(Suppl.), 289S–292S.
Brinkworth, G., Noakes, M., Buckley, J., Keogh, J. B., & Clifton, P. M. (2009). Long-term effect of
    a very-low-carbohydrate weight loss diet compared with an isocaloric low-fat diet after 12 months.
    American Journal of Clinical Nutrition, 90, 23–32.
Cannon, C., & Kumar, A. (2009). Treatment of overweight and obesity: Lifestyle, pharmacologic,
    and surgical options. *Clinical Cornerstone, 9,* 55–68.
Chaput, J., Klingenberg, L., Astrup, A., & Sjodin, M. (2011). Modern sedentary activities promote
    overconsumption of food in our current obesogenic environment. *Obesity Review, 12,* e12–e20.

Cohen, R., Pinheiro, J., Correa, J., & Schiavon, C. (2006). Laparoscopic Roux-en-Y gastric bypass for BMI <35 kg/m^2: A tailored approach. *Surgery for Obesity and Related Disease, 2*, 401–404.

Colles, S., Dixon, J., Marks, P., Strauss, B., & O'Brien, P. (2006). Preoperative weight loss with a very-low-energy diet: Quantification of changes in liver and abdominal fat by serial imaging. *American Journal of Clinical Nutrition, 84*, 304–311.

Corsica, J., & Hood, M. (2011). Eating disorders in an obesogenic environment. *Journal of the American Dietetic Association, 111*, 996–1000.

Cummings, D., Overduin, J., & Foster-Schuber, K. (2004). Gastric bypass for obesity: Mechanisms of weight loss and diabetes resolution. *Journal of Clinical Endocrinology and Metabolism, 89*, 2608–2615.

Danaei, G., Ding, E., Mozaffarian, D., Taylor, B., Rehm, J., Murray, C. J., & Ezzati, M. (2009). The preventable cause of death in the United States: Comparative risk assessment of dietary, lifestyle, and metabolic risk factors. *PLoS Medicine, 6*, e1000058.

Donnelly, J., Blair, S., Jakicic, J., Manore, M. M., Rankin, J. W., & Smith, B. K. (2009). American College of Sports Medicine position stand: Appropriate physical activity intervention strategies for weight loss and prevention of weight regain for adults. *Medicine and Science in Sports and Exercise, 41*, 459–471.

Ebbeling, C., Swain, J., Feldman, H., Wong, W., Hachey, D., Garcia-Lago, E., & Ludwig, D. (2012). Effects of dietary composition on energy expenditure during weight-loss maintenance. *Journal of the American Medical Association, 307*, 2627–2634.

Fabricatore, A. (2007). Behavior therapy and cognitive-behavioral therapy of obesity: Is there a difference? *American Journal of Clinical Nutrition, 107*, 92–99.

Farias, M., Cuevas, A., & Rodrigues, F. (2011). Set-point theory and obesity. *Metabolic Syndrome and Related Disorders, 9*, 85–89.

Farnsworth, E., Luscombe, N., Noakes, M., Wittert, G., Argyiou, E., & Clifton, P. (2003). Effect of a high-protein, energy-restricted diet on body composition, glycemic control, and lipid concentrations in overweight and obese hyperinsulinemic men and women. *American Journal of Clinical Nutrition, 78*, 31–39.

Finkler, E., Heymsfield, S., & St-Onge, M. (2012). Rate of weight loss can be predicted by patient characteristics and intervention strategies. *Journal of the Academy of Nutrition and Dietetics, 112*, 75–80.

Fryar, C., Carroll, M., & Ogden, C. (2012). *Prevalence of overweight, obesity, and extreme obesity among adults: United States, trends 1960–1962 through 2009–2010. HCHS Health E-Stat.* Available at http://www.cdc.gov/nchs/data/hestat/obesity_adult_09_10/obesity_adult_09_10.htm. Accessed on 1/15/13.

Gardner, C., Kiazand, A., Alhassan, S., Kim, S., Stafford, R. S., Balise, R. R., . . . King, A. C. (2007). Comparison of the Atkins, Zone, Ornish, and LEARN diet for change in weight and related risk factors among overweight premenopausal women. *Journal of the American Medical Association, 297*, 969–977.

Gardner, C., Kim, S., Bersamin, A., Dopler-Nelson, M., Otten, J., Oelrich, B., & Cherin, R. (2010). Micronutrient quality of weight loss diets that focus on macronutrients: Results from the A TO Z study. *American Journal of Clinical Nutrition, 92*, 304–312.

Guh, D., Zhang, W., Bansback, N., Amarsi, Z., Birmingham, C. L., & Anis, A. H. (2009). The incidence of co-morbidities related to obesity and overweight: A systematic review and meta-analysis. *BMC Public Health, 9*, 88.

Herrera, B., & Lindgren, C. (2010). The genetics of obesity. *Current Diabetes Reports, 10*, 498–505.

Hession, M., Rolland, C., Kulkarni, U., Wise, A., & Broom, J. (2009). Systematic review of randomized controlled trials of low-carbohydrate vs. low-fat/low-calorie diets in the management of obesity and its comorbidities. *Obesity Reviews, 10*, 36–50.

Hill, J., & Wyatt, J. (2005). Role of physical activity in preventing and treating obesity. *Journal of Applied Physiology, 99*, 765–770.

Hill, J., Wyatt, J., Reed, G., & Peters, J. C. (2003). Obesity and the environment: Where do we go from here? *Science, 299*, 835–855.

Hudson, J., Hiripi, E., Pope, H., & Kessler, R. (2007). The prevalence and correlates of eating disorders in the National Comorbidity Survey Replication. *Biological Psychiatry, 61*, 348–358.

Isoldi, K. K., & Aronne, L. J. (2008). The challenge of treating obesity: The endocannabinoid system as a potential. *Journal of the American Dietetic Association, 108*, 823–831.

Johnstone, A., Horgan, G., Murison, S., Bremner, D., & Lobley, G. (2008). Effects of a high-protein ketogenic diet on hunger, appetite, and weight loss in obese men feeding ad libitum. *American Journal of Clinical Nutrition, 87*, 44–55.

Jones, K. (2000). Experience with the Roux-en-Y gastric bypass, and commentary on current trends. *Obesity Surgery, 10*, 183–185.

Kraschnewski, J., Boan, J., Esposito, J., Sherwood, N. E., Lehman, E. B., Kephart, D. K., & Sciamanna, C. N. (2010). Long-term weight loss maintenance in the United States. *International Journal of Obesity (London), 34,* 1644–1654.

Kulick, D., Hark, L., & Deen, C. (2010). The bariatric surgery patients: A growing role for registered dietitians. *Journal of the American Dietetic Association, 110,* 593–599.

Laddu, D., Dow, C., Hingle, M., Thomson, C., & Going, S. (2011). A review of evidence-based strategies to treat obesity in adults. *Nutrition in Clinical Practice, 26,* 512–525.

Lee, D., Sui, X., & Blair, S. (2009). Does physical activity ameliorate the health hazards of obesity? *British Journal of Sports Medicine, 43,* 49–51.

Levitsky, D., & Pacanowski, C. (2011). Losing weight without diet. Use of commercial foods as meal replacements for lunch produces an extended energy deficit. *Appetite, 57,* 311–317.

Lichtenstein, A., Appel, L., Brands, M., Carnethon, M., Daniels, S., Franch, H. A., . . . Wylie-Rosett, J. (2006). Diet and lifestyle recommendations. Revision 2006. A scientific statement from the American Heart Association Nutrition Committee. *Circulation, 114,* 82–96.

Loos, R., & Rankinen, T. (2005). Gene-diet interactions on body weight changes. *Journal of the American Dietetic Association, 105*(Suppl.), S29–S34.

MacLean, D., Rhode, B., & Nohr, C. (2001). Long-or short-limb gastric bypass? *Journal of Gastrointestinal Surgery, 5,* 525–530.

Mechanick, J., Kushner, R., Sugerman, H., Gonzalez-Campoy, J. M., Collazo-Clavell, M. L., Spitz, A. F., . . . Guven, S. (2009). American Association of Clinical Endocrinologists, The Obesity Society, and American Society for Metabolic and Bariatric Surgery medical guidelines for clinical practice for the perioperative nutritional, metabolic, and nonsurgical support of the bariatric surgery patient. *Obesity, 17*(Suppl. 1), S1–S70.

Miller, C., & Golden, N. (2010). An introduction to eating disorders: Clinical presentation, epidemiology and prognosis. *Nutrition in Clinical Practice, 25,* 110–115.

Moll, P., Burns, T., & Lauer, R. (1991). The genetic and environmental sources of body mass index variability: The Muscatine Ponderosity Family Study. *American Journal of Human Genetics, 49,* 1243–1255.

Nagle, A. (2010). Bariatric surgery—A surgeon's perspective. *Journal of the American Dietetic Association, 110,* 520–523.

National Heart, Lung, and Blood Institute (NHLBI) Expert Panel on the Identification, Evaluation, and Treatment of Overweight and Obesity in Adults. (1998). *Executive summary of the clinical guidelines on the identification, evaluation, and treatment of overweight and obesity in adults.* Rockville, MD: NHLBI.

National Institute of Diabetes and Digestive and Kidney Diseases and Weight-Control Information Network. (2010). *Prescription medications for the treatment of obesity.* Bethesda, MD: National Institute of Diabetes and Digestive and Kidney Diseases, National Institutes of Health. Available at http://win.niddk.nih.gov/publications/prescription.hem#meds. Accessed on 12/12/12.

National Weight Control Registry. (2012). Available at http://www.nwcr.ws/. Accessed on 12/12/12.

Nocca, D., Krawczykowsky, D., Bomans, B., Noël, P., Picot, M. C., Blanc, P. M., . . . Fabre, J. M. (2008). A prospective multicenter study of 163 sleeve gastrectomies: Results at 1 and 2 years. *Obesity Surgery, 18,* 560–565.

Nordmann, A. J., Nordmann, A., Briel, M., Keller, U., Yancy, W. S., Jr., Brehm, B. J., & Bucher, H. C. (2006). Effects of low-carbohydrate vs low-fat diets on weight loss and cardiovascular risk factors: A meta-analysis of randomized controlled trials. *Archives of Internal Medicine, 166,* 285–293.

Nutrition Care Manual. (2012). *Eating disorders.* Available at www.nutritioncaremanual.org. Accessed on 12/10/12.

O'Brien, P., Dixon, J., Laurie, C., Skinner, S., Proietto, J., McNeil, J., . . . Anderson, M. (2006). Treatment of mild to moderate obesity with laparoscopic adjustable gastric banding or an intensive medical program: A randomized trial. *Annals of Internal Medicine, 144,* 625–633.

O'Neil, C., & Nicklas, T. (2007). Relationship between diet/physical activity and health. *American Journal of Lifestyle Medicine, 1,* 457–481.

Ozier, A., & Henry, B. (2011). Position of the American Dietetic Association: Nutrition intervention in the treatment of eating disorders. *Journal of the American Dietetic Association, 1111,* 1236–1241.

Pi-Sunyer, X., Blackburn, G., Brancati, F., Bray, G. A., Bright, R., Clark, J. M., . . . Yanovski, S. Z. (2007). Reduction in weight and cardiovascular disease risk factors in individuals with type 2 diabetes: One-year results of the look AHEAD trial. *Diabetes Care, 30,* 1374–1383.

Pories, W., Swanson, M., MacDonald, K., Long, S., Morris, P., Brown, B., . . . Dolezal, J. (1995). Who would have thought it? An operation proves to be the most effective therapy for adult-onset diabetes mellitus. *Annals of Surgery, 222,* 339–352.

Rome, E., & Ammerman, S. (2003). Medical complications of eating disorders: An update. *Journal of Adolescent Health, 33,* 418–426.

Ross, R., Dragnone, D., Jones, P., Smith, H., Paddags, A., Hudson, R., & Janssen, I. (2000). Reduction in obesity and related comorbid conditions after diet-induced weight loss or exercise-induced weight loss in men: A randomized, controlled trial. *Annals of Internal Medicine, 133,* 92–103.

Sacks, F., Bray, G., Carey, V., Smith, S. R., Ryan, D. H., Anton, S. D., . . . Williamson, D. A. (2009). Comparison of weight loss diets with different compositions of fat, protein, and carbohydrates. *New England Journal of Medicine, 360,* 859–873.

Saris, W., Blair, S., Van Baak, M., Eaton, S. B., Davies, P. S., Di Pietro, L., . . . Wyatt, H. (2003). How much physical activity is enough to prevent unhealthy weight gain. Outcome of the IASO 1st Stock Conference and consensus statement. *Obesity Reviews, 4,* 101–114.

Schardt, D. (2008). Secrets of successful losers. *Nutrition Action Health Letter, 35,* 8.

Schebendach, J., Mayer, L., Devlin, M., Attia, E., Contento, I., Wolf, R., & Walsh, B. (2008). Dietary energy density and diet variety as predictors of outcome in anorexia nervosa. *American Journal of Clinical Nutrition, 87,* 810–816.

Schoeller, D., & Buchholz, A. (2005). Energetics of obesity and weight control: Does diet composition matter. *Journal of the American Dietetic Association, 105,* S24–S28.

Seagle, H., & Strain, G. (2009). Position of the American Dietetic Association: Weight management. *Journal of the American Dietetic Association, 109,* 330–346.

Snyder-Marlow, G., Taylor, D., & Lenhard, J. (2010). Nutrition care for patients undergoing laparoscopic sleeve gastrectomy for weight loss. *Journal of the American Dietetic Association, 110,* 600–607.

Stunkard, A., Sorensen, T., Hanis, C., Teasdale, T. W., Chakraborty, R., Schull, W. J., & Schulsinger, F. (1986). An adoption study of human obesity. *New England Journal of Medicine, 314,* 193–198.

Sturm, R. (2007). Increases in morbid obesity in the USA: 2000–2005. *Public Health, 121,* 492–496.

Sumithran, P., Prendergast, L., Delbridge, E., Purcell, K., Shulkes, A., Kriketos, A., & Proietto, J. (2011). Long-term persistence of hormonal adaptations to weight loss. *New England Journal of Medicine, 365,* 1597–1604.

Swanson, S., Crow, S., LeGrange, D., Swendsen, J., & Merikangas, K. (2011). Prevalence and correlates of eating disorders in adolescents: Results from the National Comorbidity Survey Replication Adolescent Supplement. *Archives of General Psychiatry, 68,* 714–723.

Swinburn, B., Sacks, G., Lo, S., Westerterp, K., Rush, C., Rosenbaum, M., . . . Ravussin, E. (2009). Estimating the changes in energy flux that characterize the rise in obesity prevalence. *The American Journal of Clinical Nutrition, 89,* 1723–1728.

Tempest, M. (2012). Counseling the outpatient bariatric client. *Today's Dietitian, 14,* 38–41.

Tholking, M., Mellowspring, A., Eberle, Z., Lamb, R., Myers, E., Scribner, C., . . . Wetherall, K. (2011). American Dietetic Association: Standards of practice and standards of professional performance for registered dietitians (competent, proficient, and expert) in disordered eating and eating disorders. *Journal of the American Dietetic Association, 111,* 1242–1249.

Tsai, A., & Wadden, T. (2005). Systematic review: An evaluation of major commercial weight loss programs in the United States. *Annals of Internal Medicine, 142,* 56–66.

Tsai, A., & Wadden, T. (2006). The evaluation of very-low-calorie diets: An update and meta-analysis. *Obesity Research, 14,* 1283–1293.

Turk, M., Yang, K., Hravnak, M., Sereika, S. M., Ewing, L. J., & Burke, L. E. (2009). Randomized clinical trials of weight loss maintenance: A review. *Journal of Cardiovascular Nursing, 24,* 58–80.

U.S. Department of Agriculture, U.S. Department of Health and Human Services. (2010). *Dietary guidelines for Americans, 2010* (7th ed.). Available at www.health.gov/dietaryguidelines. Accessed 12/12/12.

U.S. Department of Health and Human Services. (2008). *Physical activity guidelines for Americans.* Washington, DC. Available at www.health.gov/paguidelines. Accessed 10/8/12.

U.S. Food and Drug Administration. (2012). Medications target long-term weight control. Available at www.fda.gov/ForConsumers/ConsumerUpdates/ucm312380.htm. Accessed on 12/7/12.

Valtonen, M., Laaksonen, D., & Tolmunen, T. (2008). Hopelessness—A novel facet of the metabolic syndrome in men. *Scandinavian Journal of Public Health, 36,* 795–802.

Van Nieuwenhove, Y., Dambrauskas, Z., Campillo-Soto, A., van Dielen, F., Wiezer, R., Janssen, I., . . . Thorell, A. (2011). Preoperative very low-calorie diet and operative outcome after laparoscopic gastric bypass. *Archives of Surgery, 146,* 1300–1305.

Wyatt, H., Wing, R., & Jill, J. (2002). The National Weight Control Registry. In: D. Bessesen & R. Kushner (Eds.), *Evaluation and management of obesity* (pp. 119–124). Philadelphia, PA: Hanley & Belfus.

Young, L., & Nestle, M. (2003). Expanding portion sizes in the US marketplace: Implications for nutrition counseling. *Journal of the American Dietetic Association, 103,* 231–234.

15 Feeding Patients: Oral Diets and Enteral and Parenteral Nutrition

CHECK YOUR KNOWLEDGE

TRUE   FALSE

☐   ☐   **1** Hospitalized patients are at risk for malnutrition.

☐   ☐   **2** Patient tolerance is improved when oral intake progresses slowly after surgery from a clear liquid diet to regular food.

☐   ☐   **3** Modular products provide a single nutrient and are used to increase the calorie or protein density of food or tube feedings.

☐   ☐   **4** Osmolality is a primary consideration in selecting an appropriate enteral formula.

☐   ☐   **5** The terms *fiber* and *residue* are synonymous.

☐   ☐   **6** The patient's ability to digest nutrients is a primary consideration when deciding the type of enteral formula to use.

☐   ☐   **7** A continuous drip delivered by a pump is recommended for administering tube feedings to patients who are critically ill.

☐   ☐   **8** Parenteral nutrition can be infused through a peripheral or central vein.

☐   ☐   **9** Hyperglycemia is a normal and harmless consequence of parenteral nutrition.

☐   ☐   **10** Coloring tube-feeding formulas with food dye helps to prevent aspiration.

LEARNING OBJECTIVES

Upon completion of this chapter, you will be able to

1 Modify a menu to an altered consistency diet (e.g., clear liquid diet, pureed diet, mechanically altered diet).
2 Give examples of therapeutic diets and their uses.
3 Compare intact enteral formulas with hydrolyzed formulas.
4 Choose the most appropriate enteral formula for a given patient.
5 Evaluate an enteral feeding schedule for appropriateness and adequacy.
6 Propose interventions to combat various nutrition-related problems that may occur with enteral nutrition.
7 Compare enteral nutrition to parenteral nutrition.
8 Discuss the components of parenteral nutrition and the usual concentration of macronutrients provided.

The prevalence of malnutrition among hospitalized adults is estimated at 15% to 60%, depending on the patient population and how malnutrition is defined (Mueller, Compher, and Druyan, 2011). Malnutrition is a major contributor to increased morbidity and mortality, postoperative complications, increased length of hospital stay, and higher health-care costs (Kruizenga et al., 2005). Patients may be malnourished upon admission due to the effects of acute or chronic illness. Ironically, nutritional status tends to worsen among all patients during hospitalization (McWhirter and Pennington, 1994).

In a study by Dupertuis et al. (2003), 85% of patients in an acute care setting who ate three meals in a 24-hour period failed to meet their calorie or protein requirements. Appetite may be impaired by fear, pain, or anxiety. Hospital food may be refused because it is unfamiliar, tasteless (e.g., cooked without salt), inappropriate in texture (e.g., pureed meat), religiously or culturally unacceptable, or served at times when the patient is unaccustomed to eating (Fig. 15.1). Meals may be withheld or missed because of diagnostic procedures or medical treatments. Inadequate liquid diets may not be advanced to a solid food diet in a timely manner. Patients may underestimate the importance of nutrition in their recovery process. Giving the right food to the patient is one thing; getting the patient to eat (most of it) is another. See Box 15.1 for suggestions on how to promote an adequate intake.

This chapter presents the range of feeding options used to meet patients' nutritional needs, from oral diets and nutritional supplements to enteral nutrition and parenteral nutrition. Figure 15.2 depicts a decision-making model for choosing the appropriate type and method of feeding.

Box 15.1 PROMOTING AN ADEQUATE INTAKE

Attention to details can make a big difference in the patient's acceptance of hospital food.

- Let the patient select his or her own menu whenever possible. This gives the patient a greater sense of control, increases the likelihood that the food will be consumed, and may prompt the patient to ask questions about the particular diet or provide information about his or her personal food and nutrition history.
- Offer patients who do not like menu selections the daily "standby" or choices as alternatives. Be aware that "hospital food" is frequently used as a vehicle for patients to vent anger and frustration over their loss of control.
- Be aggressive about diet progressions. Keep in mind that advancing the diet as quickly as possible allows the patient to meet nutritional requirements sooner and increases patient satisfaction.
- Set the stage for a pleasant meal. Be sure trays are delivered promptly to ensure foods are at the proper temperatures. Adjust the lighting and make sure the patient is in an appropriate sitting position. Screen the patient from offensive sights and remove unpleasant odors from the room. Encourage family to visit at mealtime, if appropriate. Offer mouth care to improve appetite, if appropriate.

- Be positive. Refrain from negative comments about the food. Also be aware of what your body language is saying to the patient. A frown or raised eyebrows can speak volumes.
- Provide assistance when necessary. Encourage the patient to self-feed to the greatest extent possible. Some patients may benefit from minor help such as opening milk cartons or buttering bread; others may need to be completely fed. Monitor the patient's ability to self-feed and adjust the intensity of help accordingly.
- Gently motivate the patient to eat. Sometimes, encouragement is all that is needed to get the patient to eat. For other patients, motivation comes from being made aware of the importance of food in the recovery process. Thinking of food as part of treatment instead of a social function may improve intake even when appetite is compromised.
- Identify eating problems. Patients who feel full quickly should be encouraged to eat the most nutritious items first (meat, milk) and save the less dense items for last (juice, soup, coffee). Patients who have difficulty chewing benefit from a mechanical soft diet. Determine if the patient would accept between-meal supplements and a bedtime snack to help maximize intake.

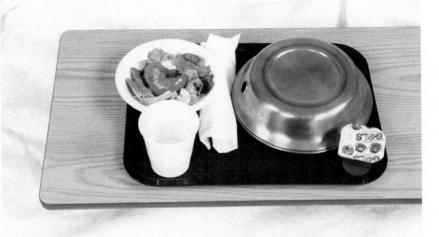

■ **FIGURE 15.1**   Hospital meal.

ORAL DIETS

Oral diets are the easiest and most preferred method of providing nutrition. In most facilities, patients choose what they want to eat from a menu representing the diet ordered by the physician. Oral diets may be categorized as "regular," modified consistency, or therapeutic. Often combination diets are ordered, such as a ground low-sodium diet or a high-protein, soft diet. The actual foods allowed on a diet vary among institutions and the diet manual used.

Private and government regulatory agencies stipulate meal timing, frequency, and nutritional content and require that hospital menus be supervised by a qualified dietitian. Many hospital food service departments offer a room service, cook-to-order menu. Compared to more traditional food service menus, a restaurant-style service allows patients greater control over what and when they eat, provides more menu choices, improves food quality and service temperatures, reduces food waste, and improves patient satisfaction (Fitzpatrick, 2010).

Normal, Regular, and House Diets

Regular diets are used to achieve or maintain optimal nutritional status in patients who do not have altered nutritional needs. No foods are excluded, and portion sizes are not limited on a normal diet. The nutritional value of the diet varies significantly with the actual foods chosen by the patient.

Regular diets are adjusted to meet age-specific needs throughout the life cycle. For instance, a regular diet for a child differs from one for a pregnant woman or an elderly patient. Regular diets are also altered to meet specifications for vegetarian or kosher eating.

Sometimes, physicians order a *diet as tolerated (DAT)* on admission or after surgery. This order is interpreted according to the patient's appetite and ability to eat and tolerate food. The nurse has the authority to advance the diet as tolerated.

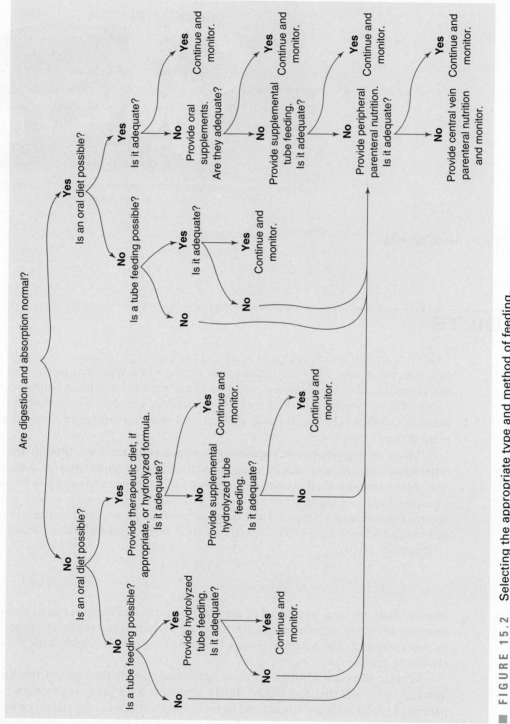
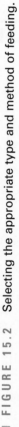

■ **FIGURE 15.2** Selecting the appropriate type and method of feeding.

Are digestion and absorption normal?

No
Is an oral diet possible?

Yes
Provide therapeutic diet, if appropriate, or hydrolyzed formula.
Is it adequate?

Yes
Continue and monitor.

No
Provide supplemental hydrolyzed tube feeding.
Is it adequate?

Yes
Continue and monitor.

No
Is a tube feeding possible?

Yes
Provide hydrolyzed tube feeding.
Is it adequate?

Yes
Continue and monitor.

No

Yes
Is an oral diet possible?

Yes
Is it adequate?

Yes
Continue and monitor.

No
Provide oral supplements.
Are they adequate?

Yes
Continue and monitor.

No
Provide supplemental tube feeding.
Is it adequate?

Yes
Continue and monitor.

No
Provide peripheral parenteral nutrition.
Is it adequate?

Yes
Continue and monitor.

No
Provide central vein parenteral nutrition and monitor.

No
Is a tube feeding possible?

Yes
Is it adequate?

Yes
Continue and monitor.

No

Modified Consistency Diets

Modified consistency diets include clear liquid and mechanically altered diets (Table 15.1). Clear liquid diets may be used to maintain hydration during gastrointestinal illness, such as nausea, vomiting, and diarrhea; in preparation for bowel surgery or procedures; or when oral intake resumes after a prolonged period. A clear liquid diet is the most frequently ordered postoperative meal, based on the rationale that a gradual progression from a clear liquid diet to a regular diet is important for maximizing tolerance when eating resumes. There is little scientific evidence to support this practice. A regular diet as the first meal has been shown to be well tolerated and provides more nutrition and greater patient satisfaction than a clear liquid diet (Warren, Bhalla, and Cresci, 2011).

Mechanically altered diets contain foods that are pureed, chopped/ground, or soft for patients who have difficulty chewing or swallowing. Dysphagia diets are another variation of modified consistency diets that are covered in Chapter 17.

Therapeutic Diets

Therapeutic diets differ from a regular diet in the amount of one or more nutrients or food components for the purpose of preventing or treating disease or illness. The number or timing of meals may also be altered. Table 15.2 outlines the characteristics and indications of selected therapeutic diets.

Nutritional Supplements

Some patients are unable or unwilling to eat enough food to meet their requirements, either because intake is poor or because their nutritional needs are so high that it is difficult to meet requirements in a normal volume of food. For these patients, nutritional supplements with or between meals can significantly boost protein and calorie intakes.

Categories of supplements include clear liquid supplements, milk-based drinks, prepared liquid supplements, and specially prepared foods (Table 15.3). Liquid supplements are easy to consume, are generally well accepted, and tend to leave the stomach quickly, making them a good choice for between-meal snacks.

For nutritional supplements to effectively boost overall nutrient intake, they must be consumed. If possible, allow the patient to taste test several options available and choose the most appealing. Explain the rationale for adding supplements and closely monitor acceptance. A rotation schedule of different types of supplements and various flavors may help forestall or prevent taste fatigue that tends to occur over time. To maximize acceptance, serve liquid supplements cold.

Modular Products

A less frequently used option for maximizing a patient's oral intake is to add a modular product to foods or supplements the patient consumes. Modular products are generally composed of a single nutrient, either carbohydrate (e.g., hydrolyzed cornstarch), protein (e.g., whey protein), or fat (e.g., medium-chain triglycerides [MCT] oil), and increase calorie or nutrient density of the diet without increasing volume. For instance, a patient with chronic renal failure may receive carbohydrate-fortified mashed potatoes to increase calorie intake without increasing protein or altering taste. Disadvantages of using modular products are ineffective quality control (calculation errors), bacterial contamination, and higher costs than standard formulas. Modular products added to tube feedings increase the risk of nutrient imbalances and clogged tubes.

Table 15.1 Characteristics, Indications, and Contraindications of Modified Consistency Diets

Diet Characteristics	Foods Allowed	Indications	Contraindications
Clear liquid			
A short-term, highly restrictive diet composed only of fluids or foods that are transparent and liquid at body temperature (e.g., gelatin). It requires minimal digestion and leaves a minimum of residue. Inadequate in calories and all nutrients except vitamin C if vitamin C–fortified juices are used.	Clear broth or bouillon Coffee, tea, and carbonated beverages, as allowed and as tolerated Fruit juices; clear (apple, cranberry, grape) and strained (orange, lemonade, grapefruit) Fruit ice made from clear fruit juice Gelatin Popsicles Sugar, honey, hard candy Commercially prepared clear liquid supplements	In preparation for bowel surgery or colonoscopy; acute gastrointestinal disorders; transitional feeding after parenteral nutrition Practice of using clear liquids as initial feeding after surgery may not be warranted	Long-term use
Pureed diet			
A diet composed of foods that are blended, whipped, or mashed to pudding-like consistency. All foods should be smooth and free of lumps. Most foods can be liquefied by combining equal parts of solids and liquids; fruits and vegetables need less liquid. Broth, gravy, cream soups, cheese, tomato sauce, milk, and fruit juice are preferable to water for blenderizing due to their higher calorie and nutritional value. Liquids may be thickened to improve ease of swallowing.	All foods are allowed, but consistency is changed to liquid.	Used after oral or facial surgery; for wired jaws; chewing and swallowing problems	None
Mechanically altered diet			
A regular diet modified in texture only. Excludes most raw fruits and vegetables and foods containing seeds, nuts, and dried fruit. Gravies, sauces, milk, and water are used to soften foods that are chopped, ground, mashed, or cooked soft. Sticky foods such as peanut butter are avoided.	Chopped or ground diet: milk; yogurt; pudding; cottage cheese; mashed, soft ripened fruit (peaches, pears, bananas); cooked, mashed soft vegetables (peas, carrots, yams); ground meats; soft casseroles; smooth cooked cereals; soft bite-sized pasta; bread products made into a slurry with the addition of gravy or syrup	Used for patients who have limited chewing ability, such as patients who are edentulous, have illfitting dentures, or have undergone surgery to the head, neck, or mouth	None
Soft diet			
A regular diet that features soft-textured foods that are low in fiber.	Soft cooked vegetables; shredded lettuce; canned fruit; soft, peeled fresh fruit; tender or ground meats; eggs; milk; yogurt; mashed potatoes; white rice; well-cooked pasta; cereals without dried fruits or nuts	Used to limit gastrointestinal irritation and minimize gut activity for healing purposes	Not intended for longterm use because it can cause constipation

Table 15.2   Selected Therapeutic Diets: Characteristics and Indications

Type of Diet	Characteristics	Indications
"Diabetic" or consistent carbohydrate	Total daily carbohydrate content is consistent with emphasis on general nutritional balance. Calories are based on attaining and maintaining healthy weight. A high-fiber intake is encouraged, sodium may be limited, and heart-healthy fats are encouraged over saturated fat.	Type 1 and type 2 diabetes, gestational diabetes; impaired glucose tolerance; impaired fasting glucose
Fat restricted	Fat limited to <50 or <25 g fat/day	Malabsorption syndromes, liver disease, pancreatic disease, chronic cholecystitis, gastroesophageal reflux
High fiber	A general diet with low-fiber foods replaced by foods high in fiber.	To prevent or treat constipation, diabetes, irritable bowel syndrome, hypercholesterolemia, obesity
Low fiber	Fiber limited to <10 g/day	Before surgery to minimize fecal residue; during acute phases of intestinal disorders, such as ulcerative colitis, Crohn disease, and diverticulitis
High calorie, high protein	A diet rich in calorie-dense and/or protein-dense foods	To meet increased nutritional requirements; also used in patients with poor intakes
Calcium rich	Calcium-rich foods are emphasized in a regular diet.	Used for patients with low calcium intake and those at risk for osteoporosis
Iron rich	Iron-rich foods are emphasized in a regular diet.	Used for patients with low iron intake and those with high iron requirements, such as pregnant women and endurance athletes
Potassium modified	Potassium may be increased or restricted by manipulating potassium-rich foods, such as fruits, vegetables, whole grains, milk, and meats.	Low-potassium diets may be used in the treatment of certain renal diseases, in conjunction with certain medications, or in adrenal insufficiency; high-potassium diets may be used in conjunction with certain medications and with certain renal diseases
Sodium restricted	Sodium limit may be set at 500 mg/day, 1000 mg/day, 2000 mg/day, or 3000 mg/day.	Hypertension, congestive heart failure, acute and chronic renal disease, liver disease
Gluten free	Sources of gluten (a protein in wheat, rye, oats, and barley) are eliminated from the diet; gluten-free grains, such as corn, potato, rice, soy, and quinoa are encouraged as sources of complex carbohydrates.	Celiac disease (celiac sprue, nontropical sprue, gluten-sensitive enteropathy) and dermatitis herpetiformis rash
Lactose restricted	Limits foods with lactose ("milk sugar") to the amount tolerated by the individual	Lactose intolerance or lactase insufficiency, which may occur secondary to certain inflammatory gastrointestinal disorders such as ulcerative colitis and Crohn disease

Table 15.3 Examples of Oral Nutritional Supplements

Type	Examples	Characteristics	Comments
Clear liquid	Ensure Enlive! Ensure Clear Resource Breeze	Provide protein and carbohydrates with 0 g fat for patients on clear liquid diets	Although they come in flavors, they are not as well accepted as the other types of supplements.
Milk based	Carnation Instant Breakfast Essentials Ready-to-Drink Carnation Instant Breakfast Essentials Powder Resource Milk Shake Mix	Contain nonfat milk; powdered forms are mixed with milk Provide significant amounts of protein and calories; are relatively inexpensive and palatable	Not suitable for patients with lactose intolerance
Commercially prepared liquid	Ensure products: Regular, High Protein, Plus, and other varieties Boost products: Regular, High Protein, Plus, Glucose Control, and other varieties Carnation Instant Breakfast lactose-free products: Regular, Plus	Regular varieties: 8 g protein, 250 cal/8 oz High protein: 12–15 g protein/8 oz Plus: 14 g protein, 360 cal/8 oz Are lactose free	Generally sweet and flavored Are quick, easy, varied in flavor, often available in grocery stores Most provide complete nutrition, so they can be used as sole source of nutrition
Commercially prepared supplemental foods	Bars Cereal Coffee Coffee creamer Gelatin Pudding	Specially designed to provide a concentrated source of protein and calories	Offer an alternative to sweetened drinks

ENTERAL NUTRITION

Enteral Nutrition (EN): the delivery of nutrients by tube, catheter, or stoma into the gastrointestinal tract beyond the oral cavity; commonly known as tube feeding.

Enteral nutrition (EN) is a way of providing nutrition for patients who are unable to consume an adequate oral intake but have at least a partially functional gastrointestinal (GI) tract that is accessible and safe to use. EN may augment an oral diet or may be the sole source of nutrition. Patients who have problems chewing and swallowing; have a prolonged lack of appetite; have an obstruction, fistula, or altered motility in the upper GI tract; are in a coma; or have very high nutrient requirements are candidates for tube feeding. EN is contraindicated when the GI tract is nonfunctional as in diffuse peritonitis, gastric or intestinal obstruction, paralytic ileus, intractable vomiting, severe diarrhea, and GI ischemia.

According to the Academy of Nutrition and Dietetics Evidence Analysis Library (2012), critically ill adult patients who receive EN experience less septic morbidity and fewer infectious complications than patients who receive parenteral nutrition. EN is also significantly less costly than parenteral nutrition. However, EN has not been proven to impact mortality, and there is little evidence that EN, when compared to parenteral nutrition, reduces length of hospital stay (Academy of Nutrition and Dietetics Evidence

---

Box 15.2 COMPARING NUTRIENT NEEDS TO NUTRIENTS PROVIDED

To calculate calories needed to maintain body weight, a range of 25 to 30 cal/kg actual weight is used. Normal protein RDA is 0.8 g/kg; patients who have increased needs for healing need more, based on the extent of injury or surgery.

Example: Calculate the calorie and protein needs of a patient who weighs his or her healthy body weight of 165 pounds and has normal protein requirements.

1. 165 pounds ÷ 2.2 pounds/kg = 75 kg
2. 75 kg × 25 cal/kg = 1875 calories
   75 × 30 cal/kg = 2250 calories
   Estimated calorie needs: 1875–2250
3. 75 kg × 0.8 g/kg = 60 g protein

If the patient's ability to digest and absorb nutrients is not impaired, a reasonable choice for an enteral formula (for short-term use) would be a standard intact formula such as Nutren 1.0. It would supply adequate calories, protein, and vitamins and minerals when infused over 22 hours/day. Instead of 24 hours/day, 22 hours/day is used to allow "off" time to administer medications. Nutren 1.0 is low in fiber, so if the patient is to receive enteral nutrition for a prolonged period, a fiber-enriched formula may be more suitable.

$$\text{A goal rate of } 90 \text{ mL/hour} \times 22 \text{ hours} = 1980 \text{ mL/day}$$

$$1980 \text{ mL} \times 1.0 \text{ cal/mL} = 1980 \text{ cal/day}$$

$$1.980 \text{ L} \times 40 \text{ g protein/L} = 79.2 \text{ g protein/day}$$

Because the volume of Nutren 1.0 needed to meet RDI for vitamins and minerals is 1500 mL, the patient's estimated nutritional needs would be met with this regimen.

Analysis Library, 2012). More high-quality trials are needed to determine whether EN and parenteral nutrition ultimately reduce morbidity and mortality or simply improve body weight.

Factors that influence how and what is used to feed patients enterally include the patient's calorie and protein requirements (Box 15.2), ability to digest nutrients, feeding route, characteristics of the formula, equipment available, and method of delivery.

Feeding Route

Transnasal Routes: feeding routes that extend from the nose to either the stomach or the small intestine.

Ostomy: a surgically created opening (stoma) made to deliver feedings directly into the stomach or intestines.

The feeding route, or placement of the feeding tube, depends on the patient's medical status and the anticipated length of time tube feeding will be used. **Transnasal routes** include nasogastric (NG), nasoduodenal (ND), and nasojejunal (NJ), of which NG is the most common. They are generally used for tube feedings of relatively short duration (i.e., <3–4 weeks). For permanent or long-term feedings, a surgical incision or needle puncture is used to create an **ostomy** route, either into the stomach (gastrostomy) or jejunum (jejunostomy). The advantages of ostomy routes are that they can be hidden under clothing and eliminate irritation to the mucous membranes. The correct placement of any feeding tube should be verified by radiographs before the first feeding is initiated. Table 15.4 summarizes the advantages and disadvantages of various feeding routes.

Table 15.4 Advantages and Disadvantages of Various Feeding Routes

Route	Indications	Advantages	Disadvantages
Nasogastric (NG)	Inability to safely and adequately consume oral intake Short-term feeding (<6 weeks) with functional gastrointestinal tract	Easy to place and remove tube Uses stomach as reservoir Can use intermittent feedings Dumping syndrome less likely than with NI feedings	Contraindicated for clients at high risk for aspiration Potentially irritating to the nose and esophagus May be removed by uncooperative or confused patients Not appropriate for long-term use Unaesthetic for patient
Nasointestinal (NI)	Short-term feeding for patients at high risk of aspiration, delayed gastric emptying, or gastroesophageal reflux disease (GERD)	Less risk of aspiration, especially important for patients who have impaired gag or cough reflex, decreased consciousness, ventilator dependence, or a history of aspiration pneumonia	Increased risk of dumping syndrome Not appropriate for intermittent or bolus feedings Not appropriate for long-term use Unaesthetic for patient
Gastrostomy	For long-term use in patients with a functional gastrointestinal tract Frequently used for patients with impaired ability to swallow	Same advantages as NG but more comfortable and aesthetic for patient Confirmation of tube placement easier Cannot be misplaced into the trachea	Percutaneous endoscopic gastrostomy insertion contraindicated for clients who cannot have an endoscopy Risk of aspiration pneumonia in clients with GERD Stoma care required Danger of peritonitis Potential for tube dislodgment
Jejunostomy	For long-term use in patients at high risk for aspiration pneumonia and in clients with altered gastrointestinal integrity above the jejunum For short-term use after gastrointestinal surgery	Low risk of aspiration No risk of misplacing tube into the trachea More comfortable and aesthetic for clients than transnasal tubes Because motility resumes more quickly in the intestines than in the stomach after gastrointestinal surgery, feedings can begin sooner than other feedings.	Small-diameter tubes easily become clogged Peritonitis can occur from tube dislodgment. Cannot be used for intermittent or bolus feedings Stoma care required

Formula Characteristics

Most institutions have a formulary of various enteral products available within major categories (Table 15.5). Formulas come in cans or sealed containers to which the tubing is attached for administration. Formulas are designed to provide complete nutrition with nutrient amounts similar to what a normal mixed diet supplies. Virtually all commercially available enteral formulas are gluten and lactose free.

Table 15.5 Selected Standard Tube-Feeding Formulas

Product	Calories per Milliliter	Protein (g/L)	Carbohydrate (g/L)	Fat (g/L)	Volume Needed to Meet 100% RDI* (mL)
Standard (for normal protein and calorie needs)					
Nutren 1.0	1.0	40	127	38	1500
Osmolite 1.0	1.0	44	144	35	1321
High protein					
Isosource HN	1.2	53	160	39	1175
Promote	1.0	63	130	26	1000
High calorie					
Nutren 1.5	1.5	60	169	68	1000
Nutren 2.0	2.0	80	196	104	750
Fiber enriched (each of the formulas below provide 14 g fiber/L)					
Jevity 1.0	1.06	44	155	35	1321
Nutren 1.0 Fiber	1.0	40	127	38	1500
Specialty					
For diabetes:					
Glucerna 1.0	1.0	42	96	54	1420
Nutren Glytrol	1.0	45	100	48	1400
For immune system support:					
Impact	1.0	56	130	28	1500
Impact Glutamine	1.3	78	148	43	1000
For renal failure (after dialysis has been instituted):					
Novasource Renal	2.0	91	183	100	1000
Nepro with Carb Steady	1.8	81	161	96	944
For respiratory insufficiency:					
Pulmocare	1.5	63	106	93	947
Nutren Pulmonary	1.5	68	100	94	1000

*RDI, Reference Daily Intakes, the labeling standard for vitamins, minerals, and protein.

Protein

Standard Formulas: tube-feeding formulas that contain whole molecules of protein; also known as intact or polymeric formulas.

Protein Isolates: semipurified, high biologic value proteins that have been extracted from milk, soybean, or eggs.

Hydrolyzed: broken down.

Enteral formulas are classified by the type of protein they contain. **Standard formulas,** also known as polymeric or intact formulas, are made from whole proteins found in foods (e.g., milk, meat, eggs) or **protein isolates** (see Table 15.5). Because they contain complex molecules of protein, carbohydrate, and fat, standard formulas are intended for patients who have normal digestive and absorptive capacity. Routine standard formulas contain 10% to 25% of total calories from protein or 34 to 43 g protein/L.

Variations of standard formulas include formulas that are high in protein, high in calories, and fiber enriched as well as disease-specific formulas designed for patients with diabetes, immune system dysfunction, renal failure, or respiratory insufficiency (see Table 15.5).

The other category of formulas is **hydrolyzed** or elemental protein formulas (Table 15.6). Completely hydrolyzed formulas contain only free amino acids as their source of protein; partially hydrolyzed formulas contain proteins that are broken down into small peptides and free amino acids. Other nutrients in hydrolyzed formulas are also in simple

Table 15.6 Selected Hydrolyzed Tube-Feeding Formulas

	Calories per Milliliter	Protein (g/L)	Carbohydrate (g/L)	Fat (g/L)	Volume Needed to Meet 100% RDI* (mL)
For impaired gastrointestinal function					
Optimental	1.0	51	139	28	1422
Vivonex RTF	1.0	50	175	12	1500
Specialty formulas					
Liver failure: Nutrihep	1.5	40	290	21	1000
Acutely ill obese: Peptamen Bariatric	1.0	93	78	38	1500
Impaired immune function: Crucial	1.5	94	134	68	1000

*RDI, Reference Daily Intakes, the labeling standard for vitamins, minerals, and protein.

forms that require little or no digestion, such as carbohydrate as hydrolyzed cornstarch or maltodextrin and fat in the form of MCT. Hydrolyzed formulas are intended for patients with impaired digestion or absorption, such as people with inflammatory bowel disease, short-gut syndrome, cystic fibrosis, and pancreatic disorders. Disease-specific formulas are available for a variety of conditions, including liver failure, acute illness in obese patients, and impaired immune system function. Hydrolyzed formulas are more expensive than intact formulas.

Calorie and Nutrient Density

The calorie density of a product determines the volume of formula needed to meet the patient's estimated needs. Routine formulas provide 1.0 to 1.2 cal/mL, whereas high-calorie formulas provide 1.5 to 2.0 cal/mL. A patient who needs 2000 calories can meet her or his calorie needs with 2000 mL of a 1.0 cal/mL formula. If that patient is volume or fluid restricted, a better option is 1000 mL of a 2.0 cal/mL formula.

Nutrient density, as indicated by the amount of formula needed to meet 100% of Reference Daily Intakes (RDIs) for vitamins and minerals, varies among formulas. Generally, the amount of formula needed to meet nutrient RDIs ranges from 1000 to 1500 mL/day. When a tube feeding is the patient's sole source of nutrition, it is important to ensure nutritional adequacy within the volume of formula the patient receives.

Water Content

The water content of tube feedings varies with the caloric concentration. Generally, formulas that provide 1.0 cal/mL provide 850 mL of water per liter. The water content of high-calorie formulas is lower at 690 to 720 mL/L. Adults generally need 30 to 40 mL/kg/day, so most patients who received EN need additional free water to meet fluid requirements. Free water is administered when water is used to flush the tube and as a bolus administration specifically for the purpose of meeting fluid requirements.

Other Nutrients

Corn syrup solids, sucrose, fructose, and sugar alcohol are common carbohydrate sources in standard formulas, providing 30% to 60% of the formula's total calories. Fat, at 10% to 45% of total calories, may come from one or more of the following oils: canola, corn, fish, safflower, or sunflower. The concentrations of fat and carbohydrate are usually not a primary concern, unless they are important because of disease, such as diabetic formulas, high-fat formulas for patients with respiratory disease, and modified-fat formulas for patients with malabsorption.

Fiber and Residue Content

Fiber: the group name for carbohydrates that are not digested in the human GI tract.

Residue: what remains in the GI tract after digestion, namely, fiber, undigested food, intestinal secretions, bacterial cell bodies, and cells shed from the intestinal lining.

Blenderized Formula: a type of standard formula made from blenderized whole foods.

Although they are not synonymous, the terms **fiber** and **residue** are frequently used interchangeably. Fiber stimulates peristalsis, increases stool bulk, and is degraded by GI bacteria to short-chain fatty acids that promote repair and maintenance of the intestinal lining. Fiber combines with undigested food, intestinal secretions, and other cells to make residue. Fiber is one component of residue, but residue encompasses other substances as well.

Hydrolyzed formulas are essentially residue free because they are completely absorbed. Most standard formulas are low in residue because low-residue formulas are not likely to cause gas or abdominal distention and are most suited as an initial feeding in patients who have been on bowel rest, in patients with certain GI disorders, or in patients who have had GI surgery.

The two types of formulas that contain fiber are **blenderized formulas** and formulas supplemented with purified fiber. Blenderized formulas are made from whole foods and thus contain natural sources of fiber. They generally provide approximately 4 g fiber per liter. Fiber-enriched formulas provide 10 to 14 g/L in the form of oat, pea, guar gum, or other fibers. The rationale for adding fiber to enteral formulas was to normalize bowel function; study results do not consistently support the notion that fiber-enriched formulas improve either constipation or diarrhea in tube-fed patients (American Dietetic Association, 2008).

Osmolality

Osmolality: the measure of the number of particles in solution; expressed as milliosmoles per kilogram (mOsm/kg).

Isotonic: a formula that has approximately the same osmolality as blood, about 300 mOsm/kg.

Hypertonic: a formula with an osmolality greater than that of blood (>300 mOsm/kg).

In enteral formulas, **osmolality** is determined by the concentration of sugars, amino acids, and electrolytes. **Isotonic** formulas have approximately the same osmolality as blood and are well tolerated. Generally, the more digested the protein, the greater the osmolality; thus, hydrolyzed formulas are higher in osmolality than standard formulas.

For most people, osmolality does not impact tolerance. However, some patients develop diarrhea when a **hypertonic** formula is infused into the small intestine. Initiating the formula at a slow rate and advancing the rate gradually and slowly improves tolerance.

Equipment

Tubing size and pump availability impact formula selection. Generally, high-fiber formulas have a high viscosity and require a large-bore tube (8 French or greater) to prevent clogging. Adding a modular product to a formula to increase the nutrient or calorie density may also necessitate the use of a larger tube. Hydrolyzed formulas have very low viscosity but should be delivered by pump to ensure controlled administration.

Delivery Methods

Formulas may be given intermittently or continuously over a period of 8 to 24 hours. The rates may be regulated either by a pump or by gravity drip. The type of delivery method to be used depends on the type and location of the feeding tube, the type of formula being administered, and the patient's tolerance.

Intermittent Tube Feedings

Intermittent Feedings: tube feedings administered in equal portions at selected intervals.

Intermittent feedings are administered throughout the day in equal portions of 250 to 400 mL of formula over 30 to 60 minutes every 4 to 6 hours, usually by gravity flow or an electronic pump. The number of feedings given per day depends on the total volume of feeding needed. Feedings may be spaced throughout an entire 24-hour period or may be scheduled only during waking hours to give patients time for uninterrupted sleep. Intermittent feedings are generally used for noncritical patients, home tube feedings, and patients in rehabilitation. They offer the advantage of resembling a more normal pattern of intake, and they allow the client more freedom of movement between feedings. Tolerance of intermittent feedings is optimized by infusing the formula at room temperature. To decrease the risk of aspiration, **gastric residuals** are checked before each feeding until tolerance is clearly established. Although there is no consensus on how much residual is too much, residual volumes of 200 mL or more on two successive assessments suggest poor tolerance (Palmer and Metheny, 2008).

Gastric Residuals: the volume of feeding that remains in the stomach from a previous feeding.

Bolus Feedings

Bolus Feedings: rapid administration of a large volume of formula.

Bolus feedings are a variation of intermittent feedings. The formula is poured into the barrel of a large syringe attached to the feeding tube. A large volume of formula (500 mL maximum; usual volume is 250–400 mL) is delivered relatively quickly, usually in 15 to 30 minutes. These rapid feedings are given four to six times per day. They are used only for feedings into the stomach. Bolus feedings are usually tolerated when infused into the stomach; when infused into the intestine, they may cause *dumping syndrome*: nausea, diarrhea, glycosuria, distention, cramps, and vomiting.

Continuous Drip Method

Continuous drip feedings are given at a constant rate over a 12- to 24-hour period to maximize tolerance and nutrient absorption. Infusion pumps are used to ensure consistent flow rates. This method is recommended for feeding of critically ill clients because it is associated with smaller residual volumes, lower risk for aspiration, and a decrease in the severity of diarrhea when compared to other delivery methods. Continuous feeding is also preferred for feedings delivered into the jejunum; it is frequently used to begin a feeding into the stomach (i.e., NG, gastrostomy, or percutaneous endoscopic gastrostomy [PEG]).

Continuous feedings should be interrupted every 4 hours so that water can be infused into the line to clear the tubing and hydrate the client. Gastric residuals are measured every 4 to 6 hours. If the volume of gastric residual exceeds 500 mL, the feeding should be held and patient tolerance reassessed (Bankhead et al., 2009).

Cyclic Feedings

A variation of continuous drip feedings, cyclic feedings deliver a constant rate of formula over 8 to 12 hours, often during sleeping hours. Extra care must be taken to keep the head of the bed continuously elevated more than 30 degrees to avoid aspiration. Because there is "time off," the rate of infusion tends to be higher than for continuous feedings. Cyclic feedings are usually well tolerated and are often used to maintain a reliable source of nutrition while transitioning from total EN to an oral intake or in noncritical, undernourished patients unable to meet their nutritional needs orally.

Initiating and Advancing the Feeding

Before initiating a feeding, tube placement is verified, ideally by radiography, and the tube is marked with indelible ink or adhesive tape where it exits the nose (Simons and Abdallah, 2012). Other common verification methods, such as auscultation, aspirating gastric contents, and pH testing, are less reliable and not recommended. Elevate the patient's upper body to at least a 30-degree angle, preferably to 45 degrees, for all patients receiving EN, unless it is medically contraindicated (Bankhead et al., 2009) to reduce the risk of aspiration.

Regardless of the access route, tube-feeding formulas are initiated at full strength. The previous practice of diluting hypertonic feedings has not been shown to improve tolerance, prolongs the period of inadequate nutrition support, and may increase the risk of bacterial contamination. Initiating feedings at full strength has not been found to cause tube-feeding intolerance or diarrhea.

To enhance tolerance in critically ill patients and those who have not eaten in a long time, conservative initiation and advancement rates are recommended (Bankhead et al., 2009). Regardless of the type of formula used, the initial rate may begin at 10 to 40 mL/hour and advance by 10 to 20 mL/hour every 8 to 12 hours as tolerated until the desired rate is achieved. The goal rate should be achieved within 24 to 36 hours. Stable patients may tolerate beginning enteral feedings at the goal rate. Other considerations are as follows:

- The commonly recommended maximum flow rate for gastric feedings is 125 mL/hour because higher volumes may increase the risk of aspiration.
- The maximum flow rate for small bowel feedings is determined by individual tolerance. Usually, rates of 140 to 160 mL/hour are well tolerated.
- Using a standard feeding progression schedule helps to ensure timely progression of feedings to the goal rate: the sooner the goal rate is achieved, the sooner the patient's nutritional needs are met.

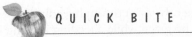

QUICK BITE

Periodic flushing of the tube helps meet water requirements and ensures patency (openness). Although cranberry juice and carbonated beverages may be used, water is the preferred and most commonly used flush (Bankhead et al., 2009). The often-cited standard for maintaining tube patency in adults is to flush with

- at least 15 mL of water before and after administering each medication
- 30 mL of water every 4 hours during continuous feedings or before and after intermittent feedings
- 30 mL of water after residual volume measurements

If a tube becomes clogged, a 60-ml syringe containing 30 to 60 mL of warm water may restore patency. A solution of Viokase (Axcan Pharma, Quebec, Canada) and sodium bicarbonate has also been shown to effectively dissolve clotted formula (Marcuard, Stegall, and Trogdon, 1989) and may help prevent clogging in tubes of home patients when used for 30 minutes per week (Lord, 2003).

Box 15.3 CRITERIA TO MONITOR IN TUBE-FED HOSPITALIZED PATIENTS

- Daily weight to detect fluid shifts
- Daily intake and output
- Gastric residuals every 4 to 6 hours in critically ill patients. Return all aspiration secretions to the stomach because they contain nutrients, electrolytes, and digestive enzymes.
- Character and frequency of bowel movements
- Signs and symptoms of intolerance: vomiting, nausea, distention, constipation
- Daily electrolyte levels, blood urea nitrogen (BUN), and creatinine until goal rate is achieved; thereafter, two to three times per week. Minerals and a weekly blood count may be ordered.
- External length of the tube, to check for displacement
- Tube site for infection

Tube-Feeding Complications

EN is generally considered safe, but GI, metabolic, and mechanical complications are possible. Monitoring ensures that the patient is tolerating the EN regimen and that it is adequately meeting the patient's needs (Box 15.3).

Aspiration is the most serious potential complication with EN (Metheny, 2006). Patients with inhibited cough reflex related to debilitation, unconsciousness, or pulmonary complications are at high risk for aspiration as are those with delayed gastric emptying or gastroesophageal reflux. More common than large-volume aspirations is a series of clinically silent small aspirations. Aspiration increases the risk of aspiration-related pneumonia. Table 15.7 summarizes potential nutrition-related problems in tube-fed patients.

Giving Medications by Tube

Although many medications are frequently given through feeding tubes to patients who are unable to swallow, they should never be given while a feeding is being infused. Some drugs become ineffective if added directly to the enteral formula; also, adding acidic drugs to the formula may cause the protein to coagulate and clog the tube. It is important to stop the feeding before administering drugs and to make sure the tube is flushed with 15 to 30 mL of water before and after the drug is given. If more than one drug is given, flush the tube between doses with 5 mL of water. See Box 15.4 for other drug considerations.

Transition to an Oral Diet

The goal of diet intervention during the transition period between EN and an oral diet is to ensure an adequate nutritional intake while promoting an oral diet. To begin the transition process, the tube feeding should be stopped for 1 hour before each meal. Gradually increase meal frequency until six small oral feedings are accepted. Actual intake should be recorded and evaluated daily. When oral calorie intake consistently reaches 500 to 750 cal/day, tube feedings may be given only during the night. When the patient consistently consumes two-thirds of protein and calorie needs orally for 3 to 5 days, the tube feeding may be totally discontinued.

Table 15.7 Troubleshooting Nutrition-Related Problems in Tube-Fed Patients

Potential Problem	Rationale	Nursing Interventions and Considerations
Aspiration	Feeding infused into the lung	Confirm proper placement of the feeding tube by radiograph prior to initiating a feeding.
	Gastroesophageal reflux	Elevate the bed's headboard 30–45 degrees during feeding and for approximately 1 hour afterward.
	Impaired cough reflex	Consider a nasointestinal or jejunostomy feeding.
	Delayed gastric emptying	Monitor gastric residuals. Switch to a continuous drip delivery method.
Diarrhea	Infusion of a formula that is too cold	Give canned formulas at room temperature. Warm refrigerated formulas to room temperature in a basin of warm water.
	Bacterially contaminated formula	Follow handwashing and sanitation protocol. Refrigerate unused formula promptly. Discard opened cans within 24 hours. Flush the tubing as per protocol. Hang formulas for less than 6 hours. Change extension tubing every 24 hours. Initiate and advance feedings as per protocol.
	Feeding rate too rapid	For existing feedings, decrease the rate to the level tolerated and then advance at half the original increment (e.g., 12 mL/hour instead of 25 mL/hour). Feed smaller volumes more frequently or switch to continuous drip method.
	Volume of formula too great	Consider a high-calorie formula if problem persists.
	Side effect of antibiotics or other medications	Investigate drugs used for possible causes/possible alternatives. Administer antidiarrheals as ordered.
	Malplacement of feeding tube Feeding rate too rapid	Check the position of the tube. Slow the rate of feeding; switch to a continuous drip method of delivery.
Nausea (Discontinue the feeding. Administer antiemetics if ordered by the physician.)	Volume of formula too great → delayed gastric emptying	Check gastric residual and notify the physician if >100 mL. Reduce the volume and then increase gradually. If distention is contributing to nausea, encourage ambulation.
	Feeding too soon after intubation	Allow approximately 1 hour between intubation and the first feeding.
	Anxiety	Explain the procedures to the client and encourage questions. Allow client to verbalize his/her feelings; provide emotional support.
	Intolerance to a specific formula, especially high-fat formulas	Switch to a different formula.
Distention and bloating	High-fat content of formula Decrease in gastrointestinal function, especially among critically ill clients	Switch to lower-fat formula. Check for active bowel sounds; switch to a hydrolyzed formula if bowel sounds are hypoactive.

(continues on page 410)

Table 15.7 Troubleshooting Nutrition-Related Problems in Tube-Fed Patients (continued)

Potential Problem	Rationale	Nursing Interventions and Considerations
Dehydration	Excessive protein intake → compensatory increase in urine output to excrete nitrogenous wastes	Switch to a formula with less protein; increase water intake, if possible.
	Inadequate fluid intake	Provide additional water.
	Glycosuria (glucose in urine)	Test for glucose in the urine; notify physician of glycosuria of 3+ or 4+.
		Administer insulin if ordered by physician.
		Switch to a continuous drip method to avoid giving a high-carbohydrate load with each feeding.
Fluid overload	Excessive use of water to flush tube	Use only 30–50 mL of water to rinse tubing after each feeding.
	Formula too dilute	Check formula preparation for proper dilution.
Constipation	Low residue content of formula	Increase residue content if appropriate (i.e., change to a formula with added fiber or increase fruits and vegetables in a blenderized diet).
	Inactivity	Encourage ambulation as much as possible.
	Dehydration	Monitor intake and output; add free water if intake is not greater than output by 500–1000 mL.
	Obstruction	Stop feeding and notify physician.
Gastric rupture	Dangerous retention of feeding in the stomach related to gastric atony or obstruction	Check for residual before beginning each feeding; observe for signs of impending gastric rupture: distention, epigastric and upper quadrant pain, nausea, a large residual; if observed, discontinue feeding immediately and notify the physician.
Clogged tube	Feeding heated formulas	Do not heat formula.
	Improper cleaning of tube	Replace the feeding tube and bag every 12–24 hours.
		Flush the tube before and after each infusion (regardless of method) with 30–50 mL of water; if flushing fails to remove clog, the tube must be removed and replaced.
		High-viscosity formulas (i.e., blenderized tube feedings or commercial formulas that provide 1.5–2 cal/mL) should be infused by pump and possibly through a large-bore feeding tube to prevent clogging.
		If possible, consider switching to a less calorically dense formula.
		Because it is desirable to use the smallest size tube, viscous formulas may be delivered by a pump to help prevent clogging.
Anxiety	Deprivation of food → lack of sensory, social, and cultural satisfaction from eating	Allow oral intake of food that the client requests, if possible; if oral intake is contraindicated, allow the client to chew his/her favorite food without swallowing.
		If possible, liquefy and add the client's favorite food to the tube feeding.

Table 15.7 **Troubleshooting Nutrition-Related Problems in Tube-Fed Patients** (continued)

Potential Problem	Rationale	Nursing Interventions and Considerations
		Encourage the client to leave the room when others are eating and find other enjoyable activities.
		Encourage client and family to view tube feeding as another way of eating, rather than a form of treatment.
	Altered body image	Encourage client to verbalize his/her feelings.
		Stress positive aspects of tube feeding.
	Loss of control; fear	Encourage client to become involved in preparation and administration of the formula, if possible.
		Inform client of problems that may occur and how to prevent or cope with them.
		Encourage socialization with other well-adapted tube-fed clients.
	Limited mobility	Encourage normal activity.
	Discomfort related to tube or formula intolerance	Control gastrointestinal symptoms, such as diarrhea, nausea, vomiting, and constipation, that interfere with normal activity.
		Observe for intolerances; alleviate with appropriate interventions.
		Be sure to inspect and properly care for the tube exit site to avoid potential complications.
Dry mouth	Irritation of the mucous membranes related to lack of oral intake	Encourage good oral hygiene to alleviate soreness and dryness: mouthwash, warm water rinses, regular brushing.
		Apply petroleum jelly to the lips to prevent cracking.
		Allow ice chips, sugarless gum, and hard candies, if possible, to stimulate salivation.
	Breathing through the mouth	Encourage client to breathe through the nose as much as possible.

Box 15.4 CONSIDERATIONS FOR GIVING MEDICATIONS THROUGH A FEEDING TUBE

- Drugs absorbed from the stomach should never be given through a nasointestinal tube.
- The liquid form of a medication diluted with 30 mL of water should be used for feeding tube administration. If there is no alternative, a drug can be crushed to a fine powder and mixed with water before it is administered. Slow-release drugs should never be crushed.
- Dilute highly viscous and hyperosmolar liquid medications with 10 to 30 mL of water before administering.
- Drugs should be given orally whenever possible.
- Tube feeding may need to be temporarily stopped to permit drug administration on an empty stomach or to avoid drug–nutrient interaction. Some experts recommend stopping a continuous feeding for 15 minutes before and after the delivery of the medication.

NURSING PROCESS: *Enteral Nutrition Support*

Vince is 48 years old, 6 ft tall, and has weighed 170 to 175 pounds throughout his adult life. Two weeks ago, he was admitted to the intensive care unit after an industrial accident caused first- and second-degree burns over 20% of his body. He was initially fed via a nasogastric tube and then started on an oral diet. Vince was only able to achieve 40% of the calorie goal set by the dietitian, so he has reluctantly agreed to be fed by tube for 8 hours during the night to supplement his daytime oral intake.

Assessment

Medical–Psychosocial History	<ul><li>Medical history, such as diabetes or GI disorder</li><li>Medications that may affect nutrition</li><li>Current treatment plan</li><li>Level of tube-feeding acceptance, including fears or apprehension about being tube fed during the night</li><li>If Vince may need a tube feeding after discharge, assess living situation, such as availability of running water, electricity, refrigeration, cooking and storage facilities, employment, social support system, and financial status</li></ul>
Anthropometric Assessment	Height, current weight, body mass index Percentage of usual body weight
Biochemical and Physical Assessment	<ul><li>Check laboratory values—prealbumin (if available), hemoglobin, hematocrit, glucose, electrolytes; other abnormal values for their nutritional significance</li><li>Check tube for proper positioning; check external length of tube every 4 hours to monitor tube placement</li><li>Observe for signs of fluid overload</li><li>Ask if the client has any physical complaints associated with oral food intake or tube feeding, such as nausea or bloating</li><li>Observe abdomen for distention</li><li>Measure residual volumes</li></ul>
Dietary Assessment	<ul><li>How many calories and how much protein are being provided via the tube feeding?</li><li>Do the nocturnal tube feedings affect the amount of food consumed orally during the day?</li><li>Is protocol being followed for administering the tube feeding and documenting administration and tolerance?</li><li>Is Vince able and willing to learn how to use tube feeding at home if necessary?</li></ul>

Diagnosis

Possible Nursing Diagnoses	Altered nutrition: eating less than the body needs r/t inadequate calorie replacement to meet metabolic needs

NURSING PROCESS: *Enteral Nutrition Support* (continued)

Planning	
Client Outcomes	The client will ■ Meet calorie and protein goals via combination of oral and tube feeding ■ Be free of any signs or symptoms of aspiration and other complications ■ Discontinue tube feedings when oral intake is consistently ⅔ of calorie and protein goal

Nursing Interventions	
Nutrition Therapy	■ Administer tube feeding as ordered ■ Encourage oral intake
Client Teaching	Instruct the client ■ On the importance of tube feedings for supplemental nutrition until oral intake meets 75% of goal ■ On the signs and symptoms of intolerance of tube feeding and to alert the nurse if any problems arise ■ Not to adjust the flow rate unless otherwise instructed ■ On formula preparation, administration, and monitoring as well as the rationales and interventions for tube-feeding complications, if home enteral nutrition is indicated

Evaluation	
Evaluate and Monitor	■ Monitor weight ■ Monitor flow rate and administration ■ Monitor for signs and symptoms of intolerance: aspiration, complaints of nausea, bloating, high gastric residuals, and diarrhea

PARENTERAL NUTRITION

Parenteral Nutrition (PN): the delivery of nutrients by vein; parenteral literally means "outside the intestinal tract."

Parenteral nutrition (PN) was developed in the 1960s when researchers from the University of Pennsylvania discovered how to deliver nutrients into the bloodstream via central venous access, thereby bypassing the GI tract (Koretz, 2007). Using a large-diameter central vein allows for the infusion of a nutritionally complete, hypertonic formula because it is quickly diluted; smaller veins are not able to handle such concentrated solutions. PN is a life-saving therapy in patients who have a nonfunctional GI tract, such as in the case of obstruction, intractable vomiting or diarrhea, short bowel syndrome, or paralytic ileus. In practice, PN is used for other clinical conditions, such as critical illness, acute pancreatitis, liver transplantation, and AIDS, and in cancer patients receiving bone marrow transplants.

When PN was first introduced, it was widely and enthusiastically embraced as state-of-the-art therapy. The prevailing school of thought was that "if some is good, more is better" and overfeeding was common practice (Koretz, 2007). At that time, PN was called "hyperalimentation"—literally excessive nourishment. It is now recognized that overfeeding, particularly overfeeding carbohydrates, in nutritionally debilitated patients can lead to a life-threatening complication known as the **refeeding syndrome** (see Chapter 16). The practice of overfeeding has been replaced with a more conservative, lower-in-calories approach.

Because PN is expensive, requires constant monitoring, and has potential infectious, metabolic, and mechanical complications (Box 15.5), it should be used only when an enteral intake is inadequate or contraindicated and when the duration of nutritional support is expected to be 7 days or more (McClave et al., 2009). Current guidelines for the provision and assessment of nutrition support therapy in the adult critically ill patient from the American Society for Parenteral and Enteral Nutrition state that in patients who were previously healthy and well nourished prior to critical illness, the use of PN should be reserved and initiated only after the first 7 days of hospitalization when EN is not feasible (McClave et al., 2009). Two meta-analyses that compared the use of PN and no nutrition support in this population found that no nutrition therapy was associated with lower infectious mortality and a trend toward fewer overall complications than was the use of PN. After the first 14 days of hospitalization, the reverse is true: withholding nutrition therapy is associated with higher mortality and longer length of stay than PN. In patients who have evidence of protein–calorie malnutrition on admission, it is appropriate to initiate PN as soon as

Refeeding Syndrome: a potentially fatal complication that occurs from an abrupt change from a catabolic state to an anabolic state and an increase in insulin caused by a dramatic increase in calories.

Box 15.5   POTENTIAL COMPLICATIONS OF TOTAL PARENTERAL NUTRITION

Infection and Sepsis Related to
Catheter contamination during insertion
Long-term indwelling catheter
Catheter seeding from bloodborne or
   distant infection
Contaminated solution

Mechanical Complications
Dehydration; hypovolemia
Bone demineralization
Hyperglycemia
Rebound hypoglycemia
Hyperosmolar, hyperglycemic, nonketotic
   coma
Azotemia
Electrolyte disturbances
   Hypocalcemia
   Hypophosphatemia, hyperphosphatemia
   Hypokalemia
   Hypomagnesemia
High serum ammonia levels
Deficiencies of
   Essential fatty acids
   Trace elements
   Vitamins and minerals

Altered acid–base balance
Elevated liver enzymes
Fluid overload

**Mechanical Complications Related to
Catheterization**
Catheter misplacement
Hemothorax (blood in the chest)
Pneumothorax (air or gas in the chest)
Hydrothorax (fluid in the chest)
Hemomediastinum (blood in the
   mediastinal spaces)
Subcutaneous emphysema
Hematoma
Arterial puncture
Myocardial perforation
Catheter embolism
Cardiac dysrhythmia
Air embolism
Endocarditis
Nerve damage at the insertion site
Laceration of lymphatic duct
Chylothorax
Lymphatic fistula
Thrombosis

possible after admission and resuscitation when EN is not feasible (McClave et al., 2009). PN is never an emergency procedure, and it should be discontinued as soon as possible.

Catheter Placement

PN may be infused via peripheral or central veins. Peripheral parenteral nutrition (PPN) is not widely used because solutions infused into peripheral veins must be isotonic (i.e., they must have low concentrations of dextrose and amino acids) to prevent phlebitis and increased risk of thrombus formation. Because the caloric and nutritional value of PPN is limited, it is best suited for patients who need short-term nutrition support (7–10 days) and do not require more than 2500 cal/day. PPN is contraindicated in patients who need a fluid restriction, such as in patients with renal failure, liver failure, or congestive heart failure.

Central PN: the infusion of nutrients into the bloodstream by way of a central vein. Central PN solutions are nutritionally complete.

Central PN infuses a hypertonic, nutritionally complete solution through a large-diameter central vein so that it is quickly diluted. A physician threads a central venous catheter through the jugular or subclavian vein until the tip is located just above the heart. Specially trained nurses can place a peripherally inserted central catheter (PICC) at bedside. The line is usually inserted on the inside of the elbow and threaded so the tip of the catheter rests at the superior vena cava.

Composition of PN

PN solutions provide protein, carbohydrate, fat, electrolytes, vitamins, and trace elements in sterile water. They are "compounded" or mixed in the hospital pharmacy, either manually by the pharmacist or through automated compounding equipment, which allows individualization of the solution based on the patient's fluid and nutrient requirements. Automated compounders can mix a 24-hour batch of PN solution into a single container, that is, either a two-in-one formula (dextrose and amino acids) or a three-in-one formula (dextrose, amino acids, and lipids). Most hospitals use a two-in-one system and deliver lipids separately.

Protein

Protein is provided as a solution of crystalline essential and nonessential amino acids with the amounts of specific amino acids varying insignificantly among manufacturers. Amino acid solutions range in concentration from 3.5% to 15%, providing 30 to 150 g protein/L, respectively. Amino acid formulations are available with and without electrolytes. Specially modified amino acid solutions are available for renal failure, liver failure, and high stress, although there is little evidence supporting the use of any of these solutions (Academy of Nutrition and Dietetics Evidence Analysis Library, 2012).

Carbohydrate

Dextrose: another name for glucose.

The carbohydrate used in parenteral solutions in the United States is **dextrose** monohydrate, which provides 3.4 cal/g. It is available in concentrations ranging from 5% to 70%, providing 50 to 700 g/L, respectively. Only concentrations at 10% or less are recommended for PPN so as to avoid damage to the peripheral vein. The minimal amount of dextrose recommended in PN is 100 to 125 g/day for adults; the maximum is 5 mg/kg/min (Academy of Nutrition and Dietetics Evidence Analysis Library, 2012). Although carbohydrate is an important energy source, giving a patient too much can have negative consequences. Hyperglycemia is associated with immune function impairments and increased risk of infectious complications. A high carbohydrate load may also lead to excessive carbon dioxide production, which may complicate weaning from mechanical ventilation. The trend toward less aggressive feeding has decreased the incidence of this complication.

Fat

Lipid emulsions, made from soybean oil or safflower plus soybean oil with egg phospholipid as an emulsifier, are isotonic. They are available in 10%, 20%, and 30% concentrations, supplying 1.1, 2.0, and 2.9 cal/mL, respectively. Lipids are a significant source of calories and so are useful when volume must be restricted or when dextrose must be lowered because of persistent hyperglycemia. Because all lipid emulsions in the United States are composed of mostly proinflammatory omega-6 fatty acids, most experts recommend limiting intravenous lipids to less than 30% of total calories in noncritical patients and that they should be used sparingly in critically ill patients (Academy of Nutrition and Dietetics Evidence Analysis Library, 2012). When PN is used long term, 500 mL of 10% lipids two to three times a week is recommended to prevent fatty acid deficiency (Academy of Nutrition and Dietetics Evidence Analysis Library, 2012). Patients with egg allergies may not tolerate lipid emulsions because they contain egg phospholipids as emulsifiers.

Electrolytes, Vitamins, and Trace Elements

Sodium, potassium, chloride, calcium, magnesium, and phosphorus are the electrolytes added to parenteral solutions. The amounts of these nutrients infused parenterally are lower than Dietary Reference Intake (DRI) recommendations because DRI values take into account the efficiency of intestinal absorption when nutrients are consumed orally. Daily blood tests are used to monitor electrolyte values until the patient is stable.

Standard adult and pediatric preparations exist for vitamins and trace elements. Parenteral multivitamin preparations usually contain all of the vitamins, although a preparation without vitamin K is available for patients on warfarin therapy.

Trace element preparations contain four trace elements (copper, manganese, selenium, and zinc) or seven trace elements (iodine, zinc, manganese, molybdenum, selenium, chromium, and copper). Because iron destabilizes other ingredients in parenteral solutions, a special form of iron must be injected separately as needed.

Medications

Medications are sometimes added to intravenous solutions by the pharmacist or infused into them through a separate port. Patients receiving PN may have insulin ordered if glucose levels are greater than 150 to 200 mg/dL (levels higher than normal are considered acceptable because there is no fasting state with continuous infusions). Heparin may be added to reduce fibrin buildup on the catheter tip. In general, medications should not be added to PN solutions because of the potential incompatibilities of the medication and nutrients in the solution.

Initiation and Administration

PN is initiated and administered according to facility protocol, typically as a 24-hour infusion in critically ill patients. One approach is to initiate PN slowly (i.e., 1 L in the first 24 hours) to give the body time to adapt to the high concentration of glucose and the hyperosmolality of the solution. After the first 24 hours, the rate of delivery is gradually increased by 1 L/day until the optimal volume is achieved. Another approach is to initiate PN at the full volume but with diluted concentrations of macronutrients that are advanced to full concentration as tolerated.

Because rapid changes in the infusion rate can cause severe hyperglycemia or hypo-glycemia and the potential for coma, convulsions, or death, rate changes must be made incrementally. Continuous drip by pump infusion is needed to maintain a slow, constant flow rate. If the rate of delivery falls behind or speeds up, the drip rate is adjusted to the correct hourly rate only; no attempts are made to "catch up" to the ordered volume. Other nursing management considerations appear in Box 15.6.

Cyclic PN: infusing PN at a constant rate for 8 to 12 hours/day.

Overall, studies support the use of **cyclic PN** instead of continuous PN for stable patients who require long-term or home PN (Stout and Cober, 2011). Infusions given over a 10- to 14-hour period offer the patient periodic freedom from the equipment (Stout and Cober, 2011) and allow serum glucose and insulin levels to drop during the periods when PN is not infused, which may reduce the risk of impaired liver function related to excessive glycogen and fat deposition. When it is given during the night, cyclic PN frees the patient to participate in normal activities during the day.

During the switch from continuous to cyclic PN, the infusion time may be gradually decreased by several hours each day, as ordered, and assessment is ongoing for signs of glucose intolerance. To give the pancreas time to adjust to the decreasing glucose load, the infusion rate may be tapered near the end of each cycle to reduce the risk of rebound

---

Box 15.6   NURSING MANAGEMENT CONSIDERATIONS FOR PARENTERAL NUTRITION

- Once parenteral nutrition solutions are prepared, they must be used immediately or refrigerated. It is recommended that solutions be removed from the refrigerator 1 hour before infusion because they must reach approximately room temperature before they are hung. Once hung, the solution is infused or discarded within 24 hours.
- Inspect the solution for "cracking" (appearance of a layer of fat on top or oily globules in the solution), which may occur in three-in-one mixtures if the calcium or phosphorus content is relatively high or if salt-poor albumin has been added. A "cracked" solution cannot be infused; notify the pharmacy and the physician, who may need to adjust the original PN order to eliminate or reduce the offending component.
- Monitor the flow rate to avoid complications and ensure adequate intake.
- Observe for side effects of PN: weight gain greater than 1 kg/day (indicative of fluid overload), elevated temperature or sepsis, high blood glucose levels, shortness of breath, tightness of chest, anemia, nausea and vomiting, jaundice, allergy to protein content of the solutions, pneumothorax, or cardiac arrhythmias.
- Monitor laboratory data and clinical signs to prevent the development of nutrient deficiencies or toxicities.
- Some patients may feel hungry while receiving PN and should be allowed to eat, if possible. If oral intake is contraindicated, give mouth care.
- Begin weaning the client from PN to EN or oral intake as soon as possible. Gradual weaning is necessary to prevent rebound hypoglycemia. PN can be discontinued when enteral intake (an oral diet, tube feeding, or combination of the two) provides at least 60% of estimated calorie requirements.
- Patients who have permanently nonfunctional gastrointestinal tracts require PN indefinitely. For home PN to be successful, clients and their families must be physically and emotionally prepared. Intensive counseling focuses on preparation and administration of the solution, catheter and equipment care, and assessment skills as well as the psychological impact of permanent PN.

hypoglycemia. However, hypoglycemia symptoms have not been reported in studies of abrupt discontinuation of PN in adults (Nirula, Yamanda, and Waxman, 2000).

When the patient is able to begin consuming food enterally (orally or by tube feeding), the amount of PN is gradually reduced to compensate for calories consumed enterally. It is recommended that PN be discontinued when enteral feeding provides more than 60% of calorie goals (McClave et al., 2009).

How Do You Respond?

Why does it seem that "house" diets are not consistent with the *Dietary Guidelines for Americans* for healthy eating (e.g., low in saturated fat, high in fiber)? The purpose of the *Dietary Guidelines for Americans* is to prevent chronic diseases associated with nutritional excesses, such as obesity, heart disease, and high blood pressure. The goal of feeding hospitalized patients is to prevent or treat acute malnutrition associated with illness or hospitalization. Therefore, the focus is not on avoiding excess but on "getting enough."

Is it good practice to color tube feedings? The Academy of Nutrition and Dietetics Evidence Analysis Library (2012) states that blue dye should not be added to EN for the detection of aspiration. The potential risks of using blue dye, such as skin discoloration, contamination of dye, allergic reactions, and association with mortality (exact method unknown), far outweigh any perceived benefit. Furthermore, the presence of blue dye in tracheal secretions is not a sensitive indicator for aspiration.

My patient claims he can taste his tube feeding. Can he? Except for patients who experience gastric reflux, patients cannot truly taste a tube feeding. However, the appearance and aroma of the formula may influence the patient's acceptance and perception of palatability. If the formula's appearance is offensive, cover the feeding reservoir or remove it from the patient's field of vision, if possible.

Case Study

Eugene is a 73-year-old man who weighs 168 pounds and is 5 ft 10 in tall. He has had progressive difficulty swallowing related to supranuclear palsy. He has no other medical history other than hypertension, which is controlled by medication. He denies that the disease interferes with his ability to eat, even though he coughs frequently while eating and has lost 20 pounds over the last 6 months. He is currently hospitalized with pneumonia, and a swallowing evaluation concluded that he should have nothing by mouth (NPO). He has agreed to an NG tube because he believes the "problem" will be short term and he will be able to resume a normal oral diet after he is discharged from the hospital.

- How many calories and how much protein does Eugene need? Is his weight loss classified as "significant"?
- What type of formula would be most appropriate for him? How much formula would he need to meet his calorie requirements? How much formula would he need to meet his vitamin and mineral requirements?
- What type of delivery would you recommend? What would the goal rate be?
- If the doctor convinces him to agree to having a PEG tube placed, what formula and feeding schedule would you recommend for use at home? What does his family need to be taught about tube feedings?

STUDY QUESTIONS

1. Which of the following strategies may help promote an adequate oral intake in hospitalized patients? Select all that apply.
   a. Tell the patient that you wouldn't want to eat the food either but that it is important for the patient's recovery.
   b. Encourage the patient to select his or her own menu.
   c. Offer standby alternatives when the patient cannot find anything on the menu he or she wants to eat.
   d. Advance the diet as quickly as possible, as appropriate.

2. For which of the following situations is a pureed diet most appropriate?
   a. As an initial oral diet after surgery to establish tolerance
   b. As a transition between a full liquid diet and a regular diet
   c. For patients who need a low-fiber diet
   d. For patients who have had their jaw wired

3. Which type of enteral formula would be most appropriate for a patient experiencing malabsorption related to inflammatory bowel disease?
   a. A standard intact formula
   b. A fiber-enriched intact formula
   c. A hydrolyzed formula for malabsorption
   d. A patient with malabsorption cannot receive enteral nutrition

4. Which type of formula may normalize either constipation or diarrhea in tube-fed patients?
   a. A fiber-enriched formula
   b. An isotonic formula
   c. A hydrolyzed formula
   d. A standard, intact formula

5. Which tube-feeding delivery method is most likely to cause dumping syndrome?
   a. Intermittent feedings
   b. Bolus feedings infused into the stomach
   c. Bolus feedings infused into the small intestine
   d. Continuous drip feedings

6. Nausea in a tube-fed patient may be caused by which of the following? Select all that apply.
   a. Malplacement of the feeding tube
   b. A feeding rate that is too rapid
   c. Providing an excessive volume of formula
   d. Feeding too soon after intubation
   e. Anxiety
   f. Using a formula that is low in residue

7. Which of the following are indications for using parenteral nutrition? Select all that apply.
   a. Paralytic ileus
   b. Intractable vomiting
   c. Dysphagia
   d. Coma

8. It is recommended that parenteral nutrition not be used when the patient is adequately nourished and expected to resume oral intake within
   a. 2 to 3 days
   b. 5 to 7 days
   c. 7 to 14 days
   d. 14 to 21 days

KEY CONCEPTS

■ Hospital food is intended to prevent malnutrition and nutrient deficiencies, not to prevent chronic disease. Regular diets may not be consistent with *Dietary Guidelines for Americans,* which recommends limiting intakes of fat, saturated fat, cholesterol, and sodium.

■ Oral diets are classified as "regular," consistency modified, and therapeutic. Combination diets (e.g., a low-sodium, soft diet) are often ordered.

■ Patients with altered appetites or increased needs may benefit from supplements given with or between meals. A variety of supplements are available (clear liquid, milk based, routine, modified routine, puddings, and bars); they vary in nutritional composition, cost, and taste.

■ Although enteral nutrition is defined as any feeding through the gastrointestinal tract, it is most commonly used to refer to tube feedings. Tube feedings are preferred to parenteral nutrition whenever the gastrointestinal tract is at least partially functional, accessible, and safe to use. Tube feedings may be delivered through transnasal tubes or through ostomy sites into the gastrointestinal tract.

■ The choice of tube-feeding method depends on the patient's digestive and absorptive capacities, where the feeding is to be infused, the size of the feeding tube, the patient's nutritional needs, present and past medical history, and tolerance.

■ Standard tube-feeding formulas require normal digestion; they contain intact molecules of protein, carbohydrate, and fat. Intact formulas come in several varieties: high protein, high calorie, fiber added, and disease specific.

■ Hydrolyzed formulas are made from partially or totally predigested nutrients; they are higher in cost and osmolality; and they are used when digestion is impaired. Specially defined formulas are available for specific metabolic disorders (e.g., renal failure, hepatic failure).

■ Routine formulas provide 1.0 to 1.2 cal/mL; high-calorie or "plus" formulas range from 1.5 to 2.0 cal/mL.

■ The volume of formula needed to meet RDIs for vitamins and minerals is available from the manufacturer.

■ Most patients receiving enteral nutrition need additional free water to meet their estimated requirements. Free water includes water used to flush the tube and bolus infusions of water.

■ Most hydrolyzed formulas are low residue or residue free. Intact formulas range from low-residue to fiber-enriched formulas and may help regulate bowel patterns, but study results are conflicting.

■ Osmolality, the concentration of particles in solution, does usually not affect tolerance in most people.

■ Policies for initiating and advancing tube feedings vary among facilities. Generally, enteral feedings are started at full strength. Stable patients may begin an enteral feeding at the goal rate; enteral feedings in critically ill patients may begin at a rate of 10 to 40 mL/hour and increase by 10 to 20 mL/hour every 8 to 12 hours as tolerated. A suggested maximum flow rate for gastric feedings is 125 mL/hour; feedings at 140 to 160 mL/hour are usually well tolerated when infused into the intestines.

■ Continuous drip infusion with a pump is the preferred method for delivering tube feedings to critically ill patients and should be used whenever feedings are infused into the jejunum. Intermittent feedings may be preferable for long-term tube feeding and home enteral nutrition because they more closely resemble a normal intake and allow the client freedom between feedings. Bolus feedings into the intestine are not recommended.

■ Enteral nutrition is safe but not without the risk of various GI, metabolic, and respiratory complications. Aspiration is one of the most serious complications of enteral feedings and may be related to inhibited cough reflex, delayed gastric emptying, or gastroesophageal reflux. Ensuring the tube is properly placed and that it remains in position and elevating the head of the bed at least 30 degrees help reduce the risk of aspiration.

■ Parenteral nutrition (PN) delivers nutrients directly into the bloodstream when the gastrointestinal tract is nonfunctional or when oral or enteral intake is inadequate to meet the patient's needs.

■ PN is usually infused into a central, large-diameter vein, which quickly dilutes the hypertonic solution. Less frequently used is peripheral PN; it must be near-isotonic to avoid collapsing small-diameter veins, so the amount of calories it supplies is limited.

■ Various concentrations of amino acids, dextrose, lipid emulsions, electrolytes, multivitamins, and trace elements may be given by vein. Compounding is the process of combining the formula ingredients; it may be done manually by a hospital pharmacist or by automated compounding equipment.

■ Because parenteral nutrition has numerous potential metabolic, infectious, and mechanical complications, it should be used only when necessary and discontinued as soon as feasible. It is never an emergency procedure.

Check Your Knowledge Answer Key

1. **TRUE** Hospitalized patients are at risk of malnutrition. Some patients are admitted with malnutrition related to acute or chronic illness; others develop malnutrition over the course of hospitalization because intake is poor. Factors leading to poor intake may include fear, pain, or anxiety; culturally or religiously unacceptable food choices; altered meal schedule; inappropriate food texture; failure to advance a diet as tolerated; or tasteless food.

2. **FALSE** There is little evidence to support a slow diet progression after surgery. Most patients can tolerate a regular diet by the first or second postoperative meal. Dietary restrictions are not necessarily helpful in relieving flatulence, nausea, or vomiting that occurs secondary to anesthesia and decreased bowel motility.

3. **TRUE** Modular products, either singly or in combination, can increase the calorie or protein density of food or enteral formulas.

4. **FALSE** For most people, osmolality does not affect tolerance.

5. **FALSE** Although the terms *fiber* and *residue* are often used interchangeably, they are not synonymous. Fiber refers to carbohydrates not digested in the gastrointestinal tract. Residue is composed of fiber along with undigested food, intestinal secretions, bacterial cell bodies, and cells from the intestinal lining.

6. **TRUE** The individual's capability to digest food is a primary consideration when choosing a tube-feeding method for a patient. Intact formulas are appropriate when digestion is normal; hydrolyzed formulas are necessary when digestion is altered.

7. **TRUE** Continuous drip feedings are recommended for critically ill patients because there is a lower risk for aspiration, a decreased risk of diarrhea, and a decrease in the hypermetabolic response to stress when compared to other delivery methods.

8. **TRUE** Parenteral nutrition may be infused into a peripheral or central vein, but because smaller diameter veins cannot handle hypertonic formulas, they are limited in the amount of calories they can provide. Most parenteral nutrition is infused through a central vein.

9. **FALSE** While hyperglycemia commonly occurs in patients receiving PN, it may not be solely related to PN nor it is harmless. An underlying disease state, such as sepsis, diabetes, trauma, or other physiologic stress, may contribute to hyperglycemia. Hyperglycemia is associated with immune function impairments and increased risk of infectious complications, and may complicate weaning from a ventilator.

10. **FALSE** Coloring tube formulas with food dye does not prevent aspiration and is associated with potential complications, such as contamination of the dye, allergy to the dye, and increased mortality from unknown cause.

Websites

American Society for Parenteral and Enteral Nutrition Guidelines and Standards Library at
  www.nutritioncare.org/Library.aspx
Enteral product information at **www.abbottnutrition.com** and **www.nestle-nutrition.com**
The Oley Foundation, a nonprofit organization to help patients, families, and clinicians involved
  with home parenteral or enteral nutrition, at **www.oley.org**

References

Academy of Nutrition and Dietetics Evidence Analysis Library. (2012). *Critical illness evidence-based nutrition practice guidelines.* Available at www.adaevidencelibrary.com/topic .cfm?cat=4800. Accessed on 4/27/12.

American Dietetic Association. (2008). Position of the American Dietetic Association: Health implications of dietary fiber. *Journal of the American Dietetic Association, 108,* 1716–1731.

Bankhead, R., Boullata, J., Brantley, S., Corkins, M., Guenter, P., Krenitsky, J., . . . Wessel, J. (2009). Enteral nutrition practice recommendations. *Journal of Parenteral and Enteral Nutrition, 33,* 122–167.

Dupertuis, Y., Kossovsky, M., Kyle, U., Raguso, C., Genton, L., & Pichard, C. (2003). Food intake in 1707 hospitalised patients: A prospective comprehensive hospital survey. *Clinical Nutrition, 22,* 115–123.

Fitzpatrick, T. (2010). Room service refined. *Food Management, 8,* 52–54.

Koretz, R. (2007). Do data support nutrition support? Part I: Intravenous nutrition. *Journal of the American Dietetic Association, 107,* 988–996.

Kruizenga, H. M., Van Tilde, M. W., Slidell, J. C., Thijs, A., Ader, H. J., & Van Bokhorst-de van der Schueren, M. A. (2005). Effectiveness and cost-effectiveness of early screening and treatment of malnourished patients. *The American Journal of Clinical Nutrition, 82,* 1082–1089.

Lord, L. (2003). Restoring and maintaining patency of enteral feeding tubes. *Nutrition in Clinical Practice, 18,* 422–426.

Marcuard, S., Stegall, K., & Trogdon, S. (1989). Clearing obstructed feeding tubes. *Journal of Parenteral and Enteral Nutrition, 12,* 81–83.

McClave, S., Martindale, R., Vanek, V., McCarthy, M., Roberts, P., Taylor, B., . . . Cresci, G. (2009). Guidelines for the provision and assessment of nutrition support therapy in the adult critically ill patient: Society of Critical Care Medicine (SCCM) and American Society for Parenteral and Enteral Nutrition (ASPEN). *Journal of Parenteral and Enteral Nutrition, 33,* 277–316.

McWhirter, J., & Pennington, C. (1994). Incidence and recognition of malnutrition in hospital. *British Medical Journal, 308,* 945–948.

Metheny, N. (2006). Preventing respiratory complications of tube feedings: Evidence-based practice. *American Journal of Critical Care, 15,* 360–369.

Mueller, C., Compher, C., & Druyan, M. E. (2011). Clinical Guidelines. Nutrition screening, assessment, and intervention. *Journal of Parenteral and Enteral Nutrition, 35,* 16–24.

Nirula, R., Yamanda, K., & Waxman, K. (2000). The effect of abrupt cessation of total parenteral nutrition on serum glucose: A randomized trial. *The American Surgeon, 66,* 866–869.

Palmer, J., & Metheny, N. (2008). How to try this: Preventing aspiration in older adults with dysphagia. *American Journal of Nursing, 108,* 40–48.

Simons, S., & Abdallah, L. (2012). Bedside assessment of enteral tube placement: Aligning practice with evidence. *American Journal of Nursing, 112,* 40–46.

Stout, S., & Cober, M. (2011). Cyclic parenteral nutrition infusion: Considerations for the clinician. *Practical Gastroenterology, Nutrition Issues in Gastroenterology, 97,* 11–24.

Warren, J., Bhalla, V., & Cresci, G. (2011). Postoperative diet advancement: Surgical dogma vs. evidence based medicine. *Nutrition in Clinical Practice, 26,* 115–125.

16 Nutrition for Patients with Metabolic or Respiratory Stress

CHECK YOUR KNOWLEDGE

TRUE	FALSE		
☐	☐	**1**	Aggressive nutrition therapy can reverse the metabolic derangements of severe stress.
☐	☐	**2**	Stress hormones promote the breakdown of stored nutrients and lean body mass.
☐	☐	**3**	The metabolic response to severe stress lasts 2 to 48 hours after injury.
☐	☐	**4**	The acute-phase inflammatory response causes albumin levels to fall.
☐	☐	**5**	In critically ill patients, bowel sounds must be present before enteral nutrition support can begin.
☐	☐	**6**	There are numerous methods for estimating the calorie needs of people who are critically ill.
☐	☐	**7**	In patients with severe stress, it is better to overfeed than underfeed.
☐	☐	**8**	Stressed patients with low serum iron levels should be supplemented with iron to promote healing.
☐	☐	**9**	Extensive burns are the greatest stress a person can experience.
☐	☐	**10**	People with COPD generally need fewer calories than healthy people because they are less physically active.

LEARNING OBJECTIVES

Upon completion of this chapter, you will be able to

1 Explain how the hormonal response to severe acute stress impacts metabolism.
2 Explain why enteral nutrition, when feasible, is a superior to parenteral nutrition in patients who are critically ill.
3 Discuss the cause and signs of refeeding syndrome.
4 Teach a client how to increase protein and calorie intake.
5 Devise a high-calorie, high-protein menu with small frequent meals.
6 Counsel a patient with COPD on how to overcome symptoms that interfere with intake, such as anorexia, dyspnea, and early satiety.

Critical illness generally refers to any acute, life-threatening illness or injury, such as trauma (e.g., gunshot wounds, motor vehicle accidents, severe burns), certain diseases (e.g., pancreatitis, acute renal failure), extensive surgery, or infection. It elicits the stress response, a body-wide emergency reaction designed to reestablish homeostasis. However, if uncontrolled, the once protective stress response ceases to be beneficial and instead can threaten survival through profound changes in metabolism. Early nutrition support, mainly through enteral nutrition (EN), may reduce the severity of the illness, reduce complications, decrease length of stay in the intensive care unit (ICU), and improve outcomes (Martindale et al., 2009).

This chapter discusses the stress response and nutrition therapy for critical illness. Nutrition therapy for burns and respiratory stress is presented.

METABOLIC STRESS

Stress Response: a complex series of hormonal and metabolic changes that occur to enable the body to adapt to stressors.

Metabolic Stress: altered body chemistry related to the body's response to injury or disease.

Shock: a clinical syndrome characterized by varying degrees of decreased tissue oxygenation and impaired flow of blood to the heart.

The **stress response** is the body's attempt to promote healing and resolve inflammation when homeostasis is disrupted. The intensity of the stress response depends to some extent on the cause and/or severity of the initial injury; for instance, the larger the body surface area burned, the greater is the intensity of the stress response that follows (Prins, 2009). Hormonal and inflammatory responses account for the changes in metabolic rate, heart rate, blood pressure, and nutrient metabolism that characterize **metabolic stress.**

Hormonal Response to Stress

The stress response has three phases: the ebb phase, the flow phase, and the recovery or resolution phase. The ebb phase typically lasts for 12 to 24 hours postinjury. It is characterized by **shock** with hypovolemia and diminished tissue oxygenation. Cardiac output, oxygen consumption, urinary output, and body temperature fall, and glucagon and catecholamine levels rise. Treatment goals are to restore blood flow to organs, maintain adequate oxygenation to all tissues, and stop bleeding. This initial phase ends when the patient is hemodynamically stable.

The flow phase, marked by metabolic abnormalities, follows (Box 16.1). A spike in circulating levels of hormones that direct the "fight or flight response" promotes the breakdown of stored nutrients to meet immediate energy needs. Glucagon stimulates the release of glucose from liver glycogen and the synthesis of glucose from amino acids (gluconeogenesis).

Box 16.1	SUMMARY OF METABOLIC ABNORMALITIES CAUSED BY THE STRESS RESPONSE

- Increase in circulating levels of catecholamines (epinephrine, norepinephrine), glucagon, and cortisol
- Glycolysis (breakdown of liver and muscle glycogen)
- Release of amino acids from skeletal muscle protein catabolism
- Negative nitrogen balance, increased urinary nitrogen excretion
- Gluconeogenesis (synthesis of glucose from amino acids)
- Hyperglycemia, insulin resistance
- Hypermetabolism
- Increase in positive acute-phase proteins, such as C-reactive protein
- Decrease in negative acute-phase proteins, such as albumin, prealbumin, and transferrin

Hypercatabolism: higher than normal breakdown of large molecules into smaller ones, such as muscle protein into amino acids.

Hypermetabolism: higher than normal metabolism.

Acute-Phase Response: trauma- or inflammation-induced release of inflammatory mediators that cause changes in the levels of plasma proteins and clinical symptoms of inflammation.

C-reactive Protein: an acute-phase protein that is produced by the liver and released into circulation during acute inflammation.

Cytokines: a group name for more than 100 different proteins involved in immune responses. Prolonged production of proinflammatory cytokines promotes hypercatabolism.

Negative Nitrogen Balance: a state that occurs when nitrogen excretion exceeds nitrogen (protein) intake.

Systemic Inflammatory Response Syndrome (SIRS): a whole-body response to inflammation characterized by elevated heart rate, increased respiratory rate, increased white blood cell counts, and fever.

Sepsis: systemic inflammatory response syndrome caused by infection.

Multiple Organ Failure: impaired organ function, usually of two or more organ systems, resulting from an uncontrolled inflammatory response; also known as multiple organ dysfunction syndrome.

Catecholamines (epinephrine and norepinephrine) have similar effects as they stimulate an increase in metabolic rate. Cortisol promotes insulin resistance, protein catabolism from skeletal muscle tissue, and the release of fatty acids from adipose tissue. As body stores and tissues are catabolized, energy expenditure and metabolic rate increase, creating a state of **hypercatabolism** and **hypermetabolism**. Oxygen consumption, cardiac output, carbon dioxide (CO_2) production, and body temperature increase. The length of this phase depends on the severity of injury or infection and the development of complications (American Dietetic Association, 2008).

Resolution of the stress leads to the recovery phase, which is marked by anabolism and a return to normal metabolic rate.

Systemic Inflammatory Response to Stress

Many critically ill patients experience an **acute-phase response** as the body attempts to destroy infectious agents and prevent further tissue damage. It is characterized by a change of at least 25% in the plasma concentration of certain proteins known as acute-phase proteins. Inflammation causes positive acute-phase proteins, such as **C-reactive protein**, to increase in concentration. Negative acute-phase proteins, such as albumin, prealbumin, and transferrin, decrease in response to inflammation, so they are not valid criteria for assessing nutritional status during inflammation (Martindale et al., 2009). **Cytokines** and other immune system molecules are responsible for regulating acute-phase proteins; they also produce changes in other cells that cause systemic symptoms of inflammation, such as anorexia, fever, lethargy, and weight loss.

The inflammatory response has a greater impact on the patient's metabolic needs than does the cause of critical illness (Academy of Nutrition and Dietetics, 2012). A **negative nitrogen balance** occurs as muscle protein is catabolized to provide amino acids for protein synthesis, immune system proteins, and glucose synthesis. An increased risk of infection, impaired or delayed wound healing, and body wasting may result. Unfortunately, the inflammatory response causes changes in metabolism that are relatively resistant to the supply of nutrients (Academy of Nutrition and Dietetics, 2012).

Systemic inflammatory response syndrome (SIRS) is an acute, life-threatening condition that may occur when severe inflammation lasts longer than a few days. Widespread activation of inflammatory pathways results in critical elevations of heart rate, respiratory rate, white blood cell count, and/or body temperature. When these symptoms are caused by infection, the result is **sepsis**. SIRS and sepsis cause excessive fluid accumulation, low blood pressure, and impaired blood flow. Inadequate oxygenation of tissues can lead to shock, **multiple organ failure**, and death. The patient's prior nutritional status is an important predictor or morbidity and mortality (Biolo, Grinble, and Preiser, 2003).

Nutrition Therapy

Nutrition therapy, via enteral nutrition (EN) (tube feeding) or parenteral nutrition (PN), is recognized as an integral component of critical care. The goals of nutrition therapy are to mitigate the metabolic response to stress, prevent and repair cell damage, and support normal immune system functioning (Martindale et al., 2009). Studies show that appropriate nutrition care can also reduce the risk of complications in critically ill patients (Academy of Nutrition and Dietetics, 2012). Less clear is what and how much is optimal for critically ill patients. Box 16.2 summarizes current guidelines for nutrition support in critically ill patients, which are discussed in the following sections.

Box 16.2   RECOMMENDATION SUMMARY FOR CRITICALLY ILL PATIENTS

Method of Feeding
- EN is strongly recommended over PN when appropriate.
- EN should start within 24 to 48 hours following admission.
- Either gastric or small bowel feedings are appropriate; consider small bowel feedings if patient is at high risk for aspiration or has intolerance to gastric feedings.

Calories
- Calorie needs can be determined by predictive equations or measured by indirect calorimetry. A simple formula is 25 to 30 cal/kg/day.
- ≥50% to 65% of target calories should be achieved over the first week of hospitalization.
- If 100% of target calories is not met after 7 to 10 days, supplemental PN should be considered.
- Permissive underfeeding is recommended in obese patients. For BMI ≥30, the goal is to not exceed 60% to 70% of target calories, or 11 to 14 cal/kg actual body weight/day.

Protein
- In patients with a BMI <30, provide 1.2 to 2.0 g/kg actual body weight/day; burn and multitrauma patients may have higher needs.
- In patients with a BMI of 30 to 40, provide ≥2.0 g/kg ideal body weight/day.
- In patients with a BMI ≥40, provide ≥2.5 g/kg ideal body weight/day.

Other
- Immune-modulating EN formulas (e.g., formulas supplemented with arginine, glutamine, nucleic acid, omega-3 fatty acids, and antioxidants) should be used for patients with major elective surgery, trauma, burns, and head and neck cancer, and critically ill patients on mechanical ventilation; they should be used with caution in patients with severe sepsis.
- Burn, trauma, and mixed ICU patients may benefit from supplemental glutamine if they are not already receiving a glutamine-enriched formula.
- An EN formula with an anti-inflammatory lipid profile (e.g., omega-3 fish oils, borage oil) and antioxidants is appropriate for patients with acute respiratory distress and severe acute lung injury.
- It is not known whether probiotics benefit general ICU patients, but they decrease infection in patients with transplants, major abdominal surgery, and severe trauma.
- Vitamins E and C and selenium, zinc, and copper may improve outcomes for patients with burns, trauma patients, and those requiring mechanical ventilation.
- Soluble fiber may be beneficial in stable patients who develop diarrhea; insoluble fiber should be avoided by all critically ill patients.

Source: McClave, S., Martindale, R., Vanek, V., Cave, M., DeLegge, M., Dibaise, J., . . . Ochoa, J. (2009). Guidelines for the provision and assessment of nutrition support therapy in the adult critically ill patient: Society of Critical Care Medicine and American Society for Parenteral and Enteral Nutrition. *Journal of Parenteral and Enteral Nutrition, 33,* 277–316.

Calories

There is not a universally agreed upon standard for determining calorie needs in critically ill patients. The Academy of Nutrition and Dietetics (AND) evidence-based guideline for critical illness recommends indirect calorimetry for determining resting metabolic rate (AND Critical Care Evidence Analysis Workgroup, 2012). However, **indirect calorimetry** is not commonly done because the equipment is expensive, technical expertise is required to use the equipment and interpret the results, and it cannot be performed on all patients, such as on patients with a chest tube, those using supplemental oxygen, or patients who are uncooperative (Frankenfield et al., 2007).

Calorie needs can be imprecisely estimated by using predictive equations, of which more than 200 have been published. The Penn State equations may be accurate more often than other equations in obese and nonobese critically ill patients (Frankenfield, Schubert, Alam, and Cooney, 2009). They were developed specifically for mechanically ventilated

Indirect Calorimetry: an indirect estimate of resting energy expenditure that measures the ratio of CO_2 expired to the amount of oxygen inspired and uses those values in a mathematical equation.

Resting Metabolic Rate (RMR): the calories expended maintaining basic, involuntary activities needed to sustain life, such as beating the heart, inflating the lungs, and secreting enzymes. Commonly used interchangeably with basal metabolic rate (BMR), except that RMR has less stringent criteria for fasting and activity and thus is slightly higher than BMR.

critically ill patients. However, they are complex formulas that use **resting metabolic rate (RMR)** calculated from the Mifflin formula plus require minute ventilation in liters per minute read from the ventilator and the patient's maximum body temperature in the previous 24 hours in degrees centigrade (Box 16.3). Often a simple formula is used, such as 25 to 30 cal/kg of admission weight for nonobese adults. For obese patients with a body mass index (BMI) greater than 30, calories may be estimated by using 11 to 14 cal/kg of actual body weight/day or 22 to 25 cal/kg of ideal body weight/day (McClave et al., 2011).

Underfeeding. The intended benefit of providing adequate calories is to improve morbidity and mortality by preventing the complication of malnutrition. However, controversy exists over what is the optimal dose of calories for critically ill patients. Some research shows that underfeeding a critically ill patient for a short period of time is associated with better outcomes (Arabi et al., 2010, 2011). Proposed mechanisms by which underfeeding is beneficial include a decrease in hyperglycemia and lower carbon dioxide production from less hypercatabolism. A prospective cohort study showed that underfeeding during critical illness (e.g., 80% of goal calories) is associated with shorter ICU and hospital stays when compared to receiving more nutrition (Hise et al., 2007). It is recommended that critically ill obese patients receive 60% to 70% of calorie requirements to promote a decrease in fat mass while improving insulin sensitivity (McClave et al., 2011). Potential mechanisms by which underfeeding benefits patients include less hyperglycemia; lower production of proinflammatory cytokines; less nutrient oxidation; and less hypermetabolism leading to less carbon dioxide production (Zaloga, 2012). Other research indicates that protocols designed to increase the delivery of EN to close to target range improve outcomes (Barr, Hecht, Flavin, Khorana, and Gould, 2004). Although there is disagreement over whether 100% of target calories is appropriate, it is generally agreed that more than 50% to 65% of goal calories be achieved over the first week of hospitalization (Martindale et al., 2009).

Refeeding Syndrome: a potentially fatal complication that occurs from an abrupt change from a catabolic state to an anabolic state and increase in insulin caused by a dramatic increase in calories.

Refeeding Syndrome. **Refeeding syndrome** is a disorder that may affect as many as 34% of critically ill patients, producing symptoms that range from mild to life threatening

---

Box 16.3   PENN STATE PREDICTIVE EQUATIONS FOR DETERMINING CALORIE NEEDS IN CRITICAL ILLNESS

Modified Penn State Equation
Used for patients with BMI over 30 and older than 60 years old.

$$RMR = \text{Mifflin*}(0.71) + V_E (64) + T_{max} (85) - 3085$$

Penn State Equation
Used for patients of any age with BMI below 30 *or* patients who are younger than 60 years old with BMI over 30.

$$RMR = \text{Mifflin*}(0.96) + V_E (31) + T_{max} (167) - 6212$$

*Mifflin–St. Jeor formula:

Men: $RMR = (9.99 \times weight) + (6.25 \times height) - (4.92 \times age) + 5$

Women: $RMR = (9.99 \times weight) + (6.25 \times height) - (4.92 \times age) - 161$

V_E = minute ventilation in liters per minute read from the ventilator.

T_{max} = maximum body temperature in the previous 24 hours in degrees centigrade.

Source: Academy of Nutrition and Dietetics. (2012). *Nutrition care manual.* Available at http://www.nutritioncaremanual.org. Accessed on 5/21/2012.

Box 16.4   Conditions That Increase the Risk for Refeeding Syndrome

Chronic alcoholism
Chronic undernutrition or malnutrition of calories and/or protein
Morbid obesity with recent massive weight loss
Prolonged fasting
Long-term use of simple intravenous hydration
Cardiac and cancer cachexia

Source: Academy of Nutrition and Dietetics. (2012). *Nutrition care manual. Refeeding syndrome.* Available at http://www.nutritioncaremanual.org/content.cfm?ncm_content_id=92079. Accessed on 5/22/12.

(AND, 2012). While it is important to provide enough calories to promote recovery and support immune function, reintroducing carbohydrates to patients who have adapted to starvation by burning fat increases insulin secretion and the need for thiamin and minerals involved in carbohydrate metabolism. Hypophosphatemia, hypokalemia, and hypomagnesemia can occur as cells rapidly remove these minerals from the bloodstream. Edema and heart failure can result from sodium and fluid retention. Thiamin deficiency can cause acidosis, hyperventilation, and neurologic impairments. For patients at high risk for refeeding syndrome (Box 16.4), daily monitoring of electrolyte levels and more conservative advancement of enteral feeding rates are necessary.

Protein

Protein is the most important macronutrient for wound healing, supporting immune function, and maintaining lean body mass. For most critically ill patients, the increased need for protein is proportionately higher than the increased need for calories (Martindale et al., 2009). Yet as with calories, the recommendations for protein are not universally agreed upon, and there may be more uncertainty over protein requirements than calorie needs (AND, 2012). Recommended amounts range from 1.2 g/kg to more than 2.0 g/kg, or 20% to 25% of total calories, depending on the patient's weight and type of critical illness. There is little evidence to support or refute any of the methods used in determining protein requirements in critically ill patients (AND, 2012).

Besides the total quantity of protein provided, the specific types of amino acids given may influence the stress response and recovery. Arginine and glutamine, two nonessential amino acids, may become conditionally essential during periods of stress. Arginine synthesis may be limited during illness; it plays a role in cellular immunity and promotes proliferation of T lymphocytes. Glutamine appears to be rapidly depleted during stress; it provides fuel for cells of the immune system, especially T lymphocytes (Martindale et al., 2009).

Carbohydrates and Fat

The remaining calories are provided by carbohydrates and fats. There is insufficient evidence to recommend high or low intakes of either of these nutrients in critically ill patients. An enteral formula with anti-inflammatory omega-3 fish oils and antioxidants is recommended in patients with acute lung injury and acute respiratory distress syndrome (Martindale et al., 2009). However, the optimal dose and ratio of omega-3 fatty acids and antioxidants are not known.

Fluid

During periods of acute stress, fluid requirements are highly individualized according to losses that occur through exudates, hemorrhage, emesis, diuresis, diarrhea, and fever. The physician determines the patient's fluid needs based on intake and output, blood pressure, heart rate, respiratory rate, and body temperature. Care is taken to avoid overhydration; decreased renal output is a frequent complication of metabolic stress.

Micronutrients

Vitamin and mineral requirements during stress are unclear. Fluid shifts that occur during the acute-phase response may be responsible for the apparent decrease in plasma concentrations of certain vitamins. When the acute phase is resolved, plasma vitamin concentrations often return to normal. Supplemental vitamins may be needed only when low vitamin concentrations persist beyond the acute-phase response.

The low plasma concentrations of zinc and iron, characteristic of the acute-phase response, may be a protective mechanism by the body to make them unavailable to replicating bacteria. Providing iron during infection may impair the body's ability to resist infection. However, zinc plays an important role in wound healing, and adequate levels are essential to ensure healing.

Trauma and burn patients have been documented to have high urinary and tissue losses of the trace elements selenium, zinc, and copper. When supplements of these three trace elements were given to severely burned patients, they experienced significantly fewer infections as a result of fewer pulmonary infections (Berger et al., 2007). Wound healing was also improved in the supplemented group, with fewer skin grafts required.

Method of Feeding

Evidence suggests EN is superior to PN and that the amount of calories and protein delivered during the early stages of ICU admission impacts patient mortality (Alberda et al., 2009). Early EN helps maintain the integrity of the gastrointestinal (GI) tract, modulate the stress and inflammatory responses, and lessen disease severity (Martindale et al., 2009). To be most efficacious in reducing the risk of infectious complications, EN should be initiated as soon as fluid resuscitation is complete and the patient is hemodynamically stable, preferably within the first 24 to 48 hours. While either a gastric or small bowel feeding is acceptable, studies show that small bowel EN has a lower risk of ventilator-associated pneumonia (VAP) (AND Critical Care Evidence Analysis Workgroup, 2012). Studies support the idea that bowel sounds and passing flatus or stool are not required before EN can begin in critically ill patients, based on the rationale that bowel sounds are only indicative of contractility and do not necessarily relate to mucosal integrity or absorptive capacity. As long as the patient remains hemodynamically stable, feedings into the GI tract are considered safe and appropriate for critically ill patients with mild to moderate ileus (Martindale et al., 2009).

For many reasons, ICU patients typically receive lower amounts of calories and protein than what are prescribed (Cahill, Dhalival, Day, Jiang, and Heyland, 2010), such as the use of low initial feeding rates, slow rate advancement, and frequent interruptions with no provision to "catch up" to the prescribed volume. A study by Heyland et al. (2010) showed that starting EN at the goal rate, setting higher gastric residual volume thresholds, and allowing nurses to make up for lost time in the feeding are some safe and effective strategies to enhance EN delivery. Using a calorie-dense enteral formula (e.g., 2.0 cal/mL) also helps patients to meet their estimated needs (Sheean, Peterson, Zhao, Gurka, and Braunschweig, 2012).

When EN is not feasible or available, PN should be considered

- Only after the first 7 days of hospitalization in a previously well-nourished patient who has not received any nutrition therapy since admission
- As soon as possible after admission and adequate resuscitation in patients who have evidence of malnutrition upon admission
- For 5 to 7 days preoperatively and into the postoperative period in a malnourished patient who is expected to undergo major upper GI surgery. Because it may not influence the outcome when used for a short duration, PN should be initiated only if the anticipated length of PN therapy is 7 days or more.

EN is initiated as soon as possible in patients on PN. As calorie intake from EN increases, the volume of PN is decreased to avoid complications from overfeeding. When patients receive more than 60% of target calorie requirements, PN is discontinued.

Recovery

Patients are typically transitioned to an oral diet as soon as possible, usually following extubation. The goal of nutrition therapy is to maximize intake to preserve lean body mass. However, a recent study on the adequacy of oral intake in the 7 days following extubation revealed that the mean calorie and protein intake for the entire study group never exceeded 55% of daily requirements (Peterson et al., 2010). A number of contributing factors are likely, including residual pain after endotracheal tube removal, delays in writing the diet order, restrictive diets, patient fatigue, anorexia, GI upset, and nothing by mouth (NPO) orders for tests or procedures. Because it is estimated that patients must consume 75% of daily requirements to prevent weight loss (Kondrup, 2001), monitoring oral intake and individualizing nutrition therapy are vital to optimize recovery. A high-calorie, high-protein diet with small frequent meals may help maximize intake (Box 16.5). A nutrient-dense diet provides nutrients important for wound healing and recovery (Table 16.1). Supplemental tube feedings may be necessary when calorie needs are not met through an oral intake.

Box 16.5   A SAMPLE HIGH-CALORIE, HIGH-PROTEIN MENU

Breakfast
Orange juice
Cheese and mushroom omelet
Wheat toast with butter and jelly
Milk
Coffee with whipped cream added

Snack
Smoothie made with yogurt, instant breakfast mix, whole milk, and strawberries

Lunch
New England clam chowder
Chicken salad sandwich on a croissant
Milk
Ice cream with chocolate sauce and whipped cream

Snack
Cottage cheese with fruit
Roll with butter

Dinner
Meat loaf with gravy
Baked potato with sour cream
Broccoli with cheese sauce
Spinach salad with hard cooked eggs, onions, walnuts, and vinaigrette dressing
Milk
Carrot cake with cream cheese frosting

Snack
Tuna salad sandwich
Melon topped with fruited yogurt

Table 16.1   Nutrients Important for Wound Healing and Recovery

Nutrient	Rationale for Increased Need	Possible Deficiency Outcome
Protein	To replace lean body mass lost during the catabolic phase after stress To restore blood volume and plasma proteins lost during exudates, bleeding from the wound, and possible hemorrhage To replace losses resulting from immobility (increased excretion) To meet increased needs for tissue repair and resistance to infection	Significant weight loss Impaired/delayed wound healing Shock related to decreased blood volume Edema related to decreased serum albumin Diarrhea related to decreased albumin Anemia Increased risk of infection related to decreased antibodies, impaired tissue integrity Increased mortality
Calories	To replace losses related to lack of oral intake and hypermetabolism during catabolic phase after stress To spare protein To restore normal weight	Signs and symptoms of protein deficiency due to use of protein to meet energy requirements Extensive weight loss
Water	To replace fluid lost through vomiting, hemorrhage, exudates, fever, drainage, diuresis To maintain homeostasis	Signs, symptoms, and complications of dehydration such as poor skin turgor, dry mucous membranes, oliguria, anuria, weight loss, increased pulse rate, decreased central venous pressure
Vitamin C	Important for capillary formation, tissue synthesis, and wound healing through collagen formation Needed for antibody formation	Impaired/delayed wound healing related to impaired collagen formation and increased capillary fragility and permeability Increased risk of infection related to decreased antibodies
Thiamin, niacin, riboflavin	Requirements increase with increased metabolic rate	Decreased enzymes available for energy metabolism
Folic acid, vitamin B_{12}	Needed for cell proliferation and, therefore, tissue synthesis Important for maturation of red blood cells Impaired folic acid synthesis related to some antibiotics; impaired vitamin B_{12} absorption related to some antibiotics	Decreased or arrested cell division Megaloblastic anemia
Vitamin A	Important for immune function	Decreased immune function and increased risk of infectious morbidity and mortality
Vitamin K	Important for normal blood clotting Impaired intestinal synthesis related to antibiotics	Prolonged prothrombin time
Iron	To replace iron lost through blood loss	Signs, symptoms, and complications of iron deficiency anemia such as fatigue, weakness, pallor, anorexia, dizziness, headaches, stomatitis, glossitis, cardiovascular and respiratory changes, possible cardiac failure
Zinc	Needed for protein synthesis and wound healing Needed for normal lymphocyte and phagocyte response	Impaired/delayed wound healing Impaired immune response

BURNS

Extensive burns are the most severe form of metabolic stress. The extensive inflammatory response causes rapid fluid shifts and large losses of fluid, electrolytes, protein, and other nutrients from the wound. Fluid and electrolyte replacement to maintain adequate blood volume and blood pressure is the priority of the initial postburn period.

The degree of hypermetabolism and hypercatabolism in the metabolic response phase parallels the extent of the burn injury; metabolic rate reaches a maximum of double the normal rate when total body surface area (TBSA) exceeds 60% (Prins, 2009). Loss of lean body mass can be severe. The requirements and/or metabolism of macronutrients are increased or altered. Fluid and electrolyte imbalances, paralytic ileus, anorexia, pain, infection or other complications, emotional trauma, and medical–surgical procedures may complicate nutrition support.

Nutrition Therapy

As with metabolic stress caused by other stressors, the nutrition priority is to meet calorie and protein needs. Similar to other critical illnesses, universal agreement on how to determine calorie and protein needs is lacking. While indirect calorimetry accurately measures energy requirements over the 30 minutes of study, extrapolating the results to a 24-hour period may underestimate actual need, which includes energy spent on activity and increased energy used during the stress of painful procedures (Prins, 2009). Also imprecise are predictive equations, such as the Harris–Benedict equation and the Curreri formula (Box 16.6). General guidelines for increasing protein and calorie density of foods appear in Box 16.7. Calorie and protein needs increase if complications develop or if there were preexisting conditions and lessen as wound healing progresses. However, wound closure

---

Box 16.6   PREDICTIVE EQUATIONS FOR BURNS

HARRIS–BENEDICT EQUATION FOR CALCULATING RESTING METABOLIC RATE (RMR)

Females

$$RMR = 655.1 + (9.6 \times \text{weight in kg}) + (1.9 \times \text{height in cm}) - (4.7 \times \text{age in years})$$

Males

$$RMR = 66.5 + (13.8 \times \text{weight in kg}) + (5.0 \times \text{height in cm}) - (6.8 \times \text{age in years})$$

Total energy requirement = RMR × stress factor × activity factor

(Activity factor = 1.2 in bed, 1.3 if ambulatory, 1.05 if ventilated)

Extent of Burn	Stress Factor	Protein Need
Moderate (15%–30% TBSA)	×1.5	1.5 g/kg
Major (15%–30% TBSA)	×1.5–1.8	1.5–2.0 g/kg
Massive (≥50% TBSA)	×1.8–2.1	2.0–2.3 g/kg

Curreri formula: (25 cal × kg of body weight) + (40 cal × %TBSA)

For burns covering more than 50% of TBSA, use a maximum value of 50%.

Box 16.7   WAYS TO INCREASE PROTEIN AND CALORIE DENSITY OF FOODS

Ways to Increase Protein Density
- Add skim milk powder to milk.
- Substitute milk for water in recipes.
- Melt cheese on sandwiches, casseroles, hot vegetables, or potatoes.
- Spread peanut butter on apples or crackers or mix into hot cereals.
- Sprinkle nuts on cereals, desserts, or salads; mix into casseroles or stir-fry.
- Coat breaded meats with eggs first; add chopped hard-cooked eggs to casseroles.
- Top fruit with yogurt.
- Use plain yogurt in place of sour cream.
- Add commercially available whey protein powder to water, milk, shakes, or smoothies.

Ways to Increase Calorie Density
- Spread cream cheese on hot bread.
- Add butter or margarine to hot foods: potatoes, vegetables, cooked cereal, rice, pasta, pancakes, and soups.
- Use gravy over potatoes, meat, or vegetables.
- Use mayonnaise in place of salad dressing.
- Use whipped cream on desserts and in coffee and tea.
- Add honey to cooked cereals, fruit, coffee, or tea.
- Add marshmallows to hot chocolate.

does not result in an immediate decrease in calorie needs, and elevated requirements may persist for 9 to 12 months after a burn (Pereira, Murphy, and Herndon, 2005).

Nutrition support is necessary when burns cover more than 20% of TBSA. Unless contraindicated, EN is used over PN; PN is used with extreme caution because of the increased risks for infection and sepsis but may be necessary for supplemental nutrition if nutrition needs are extremely high. Early enteral feedings, initiated as soon as 6 hours following burn injury, may help maintain intestinal mucosa (Gottschlich et al., 2002). Early feedings may also reduce episodes of infection and the degree of the hypermetabolic stress response (AND, 2012). Early nasojejunal or jejunostomy feedings are possible because postburn ileus has been shown to be confined to the stomach and colon (Waymack and Herndon, 1992). Immune-modulating formulas supplemented with arginine, glutamine, nucleic acids, omega-3 fatty acids, and antioxidants are recommended for patients with burns (Martindale et al., 2009).

For burns covering less than 20% of TBSA, an oral high-protein, high-calorie diet can adequately meet protein and calorie requirements. Small frequent meals of calorie- and protein-dense foods help maximize intake (see Box 16.7). Daily calorie counts may be used to monitor intake. When intake is less than 75% of estimated need for more than 3 days, EN should be used for total or supplemental nutrition (AND, 2012). Supplemental tube feedings given during the night are useful when nutritional needs are not met through food alone. If oral intake is negligible, EN can provide 100% of need. Frequently, a combination of oral diet and EN is needed to meet patient needs.

Although it is generally agreed that vitamin needs increase in burn patients because of losses from wounds, the need for healing, and changes in metabolism, the exact requirements are not known (AND, 2012). Supplements of vitamin C, vitamin A, and zinc plus a multivitamin are recommended by the Shriners Burn Hospital for patients with burns on more than 20% of TBSA (AND, 2012). The trace elements selenium, zinc, and copper have been shown to promote healing and decrease the risk of infections in burn patients (Berger et al., 2007). Supplements may be needed for patients consuming an oral diet; EN and PN formulas generally provide more than the Dietary Reference

Intakes (DRIs) for vitamins and minerals in the volume necessary to meet the elevated calorie needs.

RESPIRATORY STRESS

Respiratory Stress: impaired gas exchange between the air and blood that leads to lower levels of oxygen in the blood and higher levels of CO_2.

Respiratory stress occurs when gas exchange between the air and blood is impaired, leading to lower levels of oxygen in the blood and higher levels of CO_2. Like metabolic stress, respiratory stress may cause hypermetabolism and a loss of muscle mass and function. When nutritional needs are not met—whether from increased needs related to hypermetabolism or inadequate intake related to anorexia and dyspnea—fewer nutrients are available to maintain respiratory muscle function. Gas exchange and exercise tolerance are further compromised, and a downhill spiral of malnutrition and worsening respiratory status may ensue. Chronic or acute respiratory stress can lead to respiratory failure, multiple organ failure, and death.

Chronic Obstructive Pulmonary Disease

As many as 30% of patients with chronic obstructive pulmonary disease (COPD) have low BMI (≤20), and the risk of COPD-related death doubles with weight loss (AND Critical Care Evidence Analysis Workgroup, 2012). Many patients with COPD are hypermetabolic from increased energy spent on labored breathing. Chronic inflammation also increases metabolism and impairs appetite. Anorexia may occur from fatigue, depression, anxiety, changes in taste, excess mucus production, dyspnea, or decreased peristalsis and digestion secondary to inadequate oxygen to GI cells. Early satiety may be related to flattening of the diaphragm and a decrease in abdominal volume or from bloating related to swallowed air. Steroid therapy increases the risk of GI upset and peptic ulcer disease. Malnourished patients with COPD have a poorer prognosis than well-nourished patients (Norman, Pichard, Lochs, and Pirlich, 2008).

Nutrition Therapy

Correcting or preventing malnutrition—namely, maintaining or restoring body weight, lean body mass, and respiratory muscle function—is a priority for patients with COPD. Generally, a high-calorie, high-protein diet is used. Strategies for improving intake are tailored to the patient's symptoms (Table 16.2). Evidence suggests that a high-calorie intake is most effective when combined with anabolic exercise (Corbridge, Wilken, Kapella, and Gronkiewicz, 2012). Some patients may be overweight or may experience undesirable weight gain from chronic steroid use. Because excess weight poses an additional burden on the respiratory system, a healthy, calorie-restricted diet to promote gradual weight loss is recommended for these patients.

For patients hospitalized with exacerbation of COPD, calorie needs may be 140% above RMR. If indirect calorimetry is not available, a reasonable starting point is to provide 25 to 30 cal/kg. Protein needs may be 1.2 g/kg of body weight (Thorsdottir and Gunnarsdottir, 2002). In patients who require mechanical ventilation, care is taken to avoid overfeeding because it increases CO_2 production, which can complicate ventilation. Specially formulated enteral products are available for patients with respiratory disease. They are higher in fat (and therefore lower in carbohydrates) than routine formulas (e.g., 55% of total calories from fat vs. 33% of total calories in routine formulas) based on the assumption that lesser amounts of carbohydrate yield less CO_2, but these formulas have not been shown to improve clinical outcomes.

Table 16.2 Strategies to Promote Eating in Patients with COPD Based on Symptoms

Symptom	Strategies to Promote Eating
Anorexia	Eat small frequent meals. Eat most nutritionally dense foods first. Drink high-protein, high-calorie nutrition formulas between meals.
Shortness of breath	Eat small frequent meals. Eat a soft diet, avoiding foods that are difficult to chew or swallow. Rest before eating. Use bronchodilators before eating.
Fatigue	Rest before eating.
Early satiety	Limit "empty" liquids with meals (e.g., coffee, tea, water, carbonated beverages). Eat small, frequent, nutritionally dense meals. Avoid "gassy" foods. Try high-calorie, high-protein nutrition formulas.
Dry mouth	Add gravies and sauces to foods. Use artificial saliva before eating. Avoid dry and salty foods.
Constipation/ straining at stool	Increase fiber intake, such as increasing intake of ready-to-eat bran or whole wheat cereals or drinking commercially prepared oral supplements with added fiber such as Promote with Fiber.
Thick mucus	Increase fluid intake.

NURSING PROCESS: *Metabolic Stress*

Yin is a frail, 74-year-old man admitted to the hospital with multiple serious but non–life-threatening injuries resulting from a car accident. He weighs 122 pounds and is 5 ft 6 in tall.

Assessment

Medical–Psychosocial History

- Current diagnoses and medications
- Medical history, including hyperlipidemia, hypertension, cardiovascular disease, renal impairments, diabetes, GI complaints
- Medications that affect nutrition, such as lipid-lowering medications, cardiac drugs, antihypertensives
- Extent of injuries; significance of GI trauma, if appropriate
- Hemodynamic status; signs and symptoms of hemorrhaging
- Neurologic status (e.g., confusion, disorientation); ability to eat, ability to self-feed
- GI functions such as hypoactive bowel sounds, distention, complaints of nausea, anorexia
- Psychosocial and economic issues prior to injury, such as whether finances, loneliness, or isolation impaired his food intake; determine who does food shopping and preparation and whether the client is a candidate for the Meals on Wheels program

(continues on page 436)

NURSING PROCESS: *Metabolic Stress* (continued)

Anthropometric Assessment	• Height, current weight
	• Recent weight history; usual weight
	• Body mass index (BMI)
Biochemical and Physical Assessment	• Complete blood count
	• Blood chemistry, including major electrolytes
	• Serum glucose
	• Input and output
	• Clinical symptoms of malnutrition such as wasted appearance
Dietary Assessment	• Do you have any difficulty chewing or swallowing?
	• Do you have nausea or any other symptoms that interfere with your ability to eat?
	• Are you able to feed yourself?
	• Do you follow a special diet at home?
	• Do you have enough food to eat at home?
	• Do you have any food intolerances or allergies?
	• Do you have any cultural, religious, or ethnic food preferences?
	• Do you take vitamins, minerals, or supplements? If so, what?
	• How much alcohol do you consume?

Diagnosis

Possible Nursing Diagnoses	Altered nutrition: eating less than the body needs r/t low calorie intake and increased requirements related to injuries

Planning

Client Outcomes	The client will
	• Maintain normal fluid and electrolyte balance
	• Meet 75% of his goal calories and protein via oral diet with supplements
	• Describe the principles and rationale of a high-calorie, high-protein diet
	• Avoid complications of undernutrition, such as weight loss, poor wound healing, infections

Nursing Interventions

Nutrition Therapy	• Initially give intravenous fluid and electrolytes as ordered
	• When oral intake begins, encourage the intake of calorie- and protein-dense foods first; encourage intake of between-meal supplements
Client Teaching	Instruct the client on
	• The importance of protein and calories in promoting wound healing and recovery and overall health
	• The eating plan essentials, including
	• How to increase calories and protein in the diet (Box 16.7)
	• To eat small frequent meals to maximize intake

NURSING PROCESS: *Metabolic Stress* (continued)

Evaluation

Evaluate and Monitor

- Monitor fluid and electrolyte balance and other biochemical values.
- Monitor intake and the need for total or supplemental EN.
- Monitor weight.
- Monitor for complications, such as delayed wound healing or infection.
- Observe for tolerance to oral diet.
- Suggest changes in the meal plan as needed.
- Provide periodic feedback and reinforcement.

HOW DO YOU RESPOND?

Do flavored waters marketed to improve immune function really work? There are several flavored waters available on grocery store shelves that feature descriptive terms such as "defend," "protect," or "immunity" on the label. All of these products contain added vitamins and/or minerals, such as vitamins A, C, D, or E, B vitamins, or zinc. Some provide calories from sweeteners, others are calorie free. While certain vitamins and minerals *are* important for normal immune system functioning, it is a huge leap to conclude that any of these products provide health benefits beyond those obtained from a normal mixed diet. Consuming more than required of any nutrients necessary for immune system functioning does not boost immune function—unless the immune system was impaired because of a nutrient deficiency. Manufacturers are free to put in whatever nutrients they desire in whatever amounts they choose; scientific evidence of benefit or need is not required to make a function claim.

CASE STUDY

Samuel was diagnosed with COPD 7 years ago and has had recurrent bronchitis over the past 40 years. He is 68 years old, 5 ft 9 in tall, and weighs 134 pounds. About 3 years ago, he had a normal adult weight of 150 to 155 pounds. He has lost 7 pounds in the last month due to lack of appetite and early satiety. He complains of a dry mouth and that "food has lost its taste." He is currently on multiple medications, including a bronchodilator, an inhaler, and an antibiotic. He uses oxygen as needed. During his recent hospitalization for pneumonia, the dietitian told him he should be eating at least 2000 calories, but he doesn't have the energy to prepare or eat that much food.

His usual intake appears in the box on the left.

Breakfast:	Coffee with creamer 2 Pieces of white toast with jelly
Lunch:	Cheese and crackers Banana Coffee with creamer
Dinner:	Canned soup with oyster crackers Ice cream Coffee with creamer

- Evaluate Samuel's current BMI and normal adult weight. Calculate his percent weight loss over the past month. Is it significant?

(continues on page 438)

CASE STUDY (continued)

- What factors contribute to Samuel's poor appetite and intake? What specific strategies would you recommend he implement to improve his intake?
- Is 2000 calories an appropriate amount of daily calories for him? How much protein should he consume in a day?

  ▶ Devise a sample menu for him that takes into account the calories and protein he needs and his symptoms of anorexia, early satiety, dry mouth, and fatigue.

STUDY QUESTIONS

1. Which of the following strategies would be most appropriate for a patient with COPD who is experiencing early satiety?
   a. Limiting "empty" beverages at meals
   b. Resting before eating
   c. Using bronchodilators before eating
   d. Limiting salt intake

2. When teaching a client diagnosed with COPD about nutritional needs, which of the following types of diet should the nurse discuss?
   a. A high-calorie, high-protein diet
   b. A low-residue diet
   c. A low-fat, low-cholesterol diet
   d. A low-sodium diet

3. In a burned patient with a functional GI tract, why is enteral nutrition preferred over parenteral nutrition?
   a. Because enteral nutrition can provide higher amounts of calories and protein.
   b. Because enteral nutrition is less likely to interfere with oral intake.
   c. Because enteral nutrition is less expensive.
   d. Because enteral nutrition has a lower risk of infectious complications.

4. Why may underfeeding critically ill patients be beneficial?
   a. Because it provides less work for the GI tract to do.
   b. Because all methods of measuring a person's energy expenditure overestimate their needs so a lower calorie load is a prudent approach.
   c. Because it provides fewer substrates for the body to make proinflammatory molecules and has a positive effect on hyperglycemia.
   d. Because it causes stress hormone levels to drop.

5. What is the primary intervention in the initial postburn period?
   a. Parenteral nutrition
   b. Supplements of trace elements
   c. Fluid and electrolytes
   d. A low-carbohydrate diet to decrease CO_2 production

6. What does a spike in C-reactive protein indicate in people with acute metabolic stress?
   a. Protein needs are not being met.
   b. Protein intake is adequate.
   c. An inflammatory response is occurring.
   d. The inflammatory response has ended.

7. What would the maximum daily protein requirement be for a 70-kg person with severe burns?
   a. 56 g
   b. 70 g
   c. 105 g
   d. 140 g

8. If underfeeding is used for critically ill patients, when should the calories begin to be advanced toward 100% of need?
   a. After 3 to 5 days
   b. After 5 to 7 days
   c. After 7 to 10 days
   d. After 10 days

KEY CONCEPTS

- The ebb phase following acute illness or injury lasts approximately 24 hours and is resolved when the patient is hemodynamically stable.
- The flow phase is a metabolic response to acute stress that is characterized by hormonal and inflammatory responses that change the body's chemistry. The duration of this phase varies with the severity of the stress and whether complications develop.
- Stress hormones increase blood glucose levels, metabolism, and body protein catabolism.
- The inflammatory response is mediated by immune system components that alter the concentration of certain plasma proteins. C-reactive protein is a positive acute-phase protein that is used as an indicator of inflammation in acute stress.
- Nutritional needs are considered after the patient is hemodynamically stable. The primary nutritional concern is the breakdown of body protein because protein deficiency increases the risks of infection, delayed or impaired wound healing, and mortality. Nutrition therapy focuses on preserving lean body mass and preventing or alleviating malnutrition.
- Recommendations regarding calorie and protein requirements during critical illness are imprecise. Indirect calorimetry is the gold standard for calculating calorie needs. Predictive equations are less reliable. Calories per kilogram may be used when indirect calorimetry is not available.
- Providing 50% to 65% of actual calorie needs may be initially optimal in critically ill patients, possibly by several different mechanisms. If underfeeding is used, the calories are gradually increased after the first 3 to 5 days and eventually reach 100% over the next 3 to 5 days.
- Protein requirements are generally based on weight and range from 1.0 to 2.0 g/kg or higher, depending on the type and severity of stressors as well as the patient's age and prior nutritional status.
- Fluid needs during metabolic stress are highly variable and are determined by the physician.
- Micronutrient requirements during metabolic stress are not clear. Serum levels of vitamins may decrease because of fluid shifts, not necessarily because of deficiency. Low concentrations of iron and zinc in the blood may be a protective mechanism to make these nutrients unavailable for replicating bacteria.
- EN is preferred over PN whenever the GI tract is functional and the patient is hemodynamically stable.

- PN is required when the GI tract is nonfunctional or when nutritional needs are so high they cannot be met by oral nutrition and/or EN alone. The risk of infection and complications is higher with PN than EN.
- Oral intake is resumed when possible. Small, frequent meals help achieve a high-calorie, high-protein intake.
- Extensive burns are the most severe form of stress that a person can experience. Nutritional support may be complicated by stress ulcers, anorexia, pain, and the consequences of medical–surgical treatments.
- Severe burns dramatically impact calorie, protein, and micronutrient needs. An oral high-calorie, high-protein diet with various vitamin and mineral supplements may be adequate for burns covering less than 20% of TBSA. For more extensive burns, EN support is necessary, and early feedings are recommended. PN support may be needed because nutritional needs are so high. PN is used with caution because of the increased risk of infection.
- Patients with COPD are often underweight and malnourished. Shortness of breath can make eating difficult, and decreased oxygenation of the GI cells can impair peristalsis and digestion. Metabolism may be elevated from increased energy expenditure related to labored breathing and/or from chronic inflammation.
- Nutrition-dense, easy-to-consume foods are preferred for patients with chronic respiratory disorders. Patients on ventilator support may be given restricted carbohydrate enteral formulas to lower CO_2 production, but their efficacy is not known.

Check Your Knowledge Answer Key

1. **FALSE** Aggressive nutrition therapy can improve some of the metabolic derangements of stress, but complete reversal only occurs after the underlying stressor is resolved.

2. **TRUE** Stress hormones have catabolic actions in the body; that is, they stimulate the breakdown of glycogen, adipose tissue, and lean body mass. They function opposite to insulin, which lowers blood glucose levels.

3. **FALSE** The metabolic response to stress begins after the first 2 to 48 hours. Its duration is related to the severity of stress, the number of stressors, and the individual's ability to adapt to stress.

4. **TRUE** The acute-phase inflammatory response causes a decrease in serum albumin and other negative acute-phase proteins. C-reactive protein is a positive acute-phase protein that rises in response to inflammation.

5. **FALSE** Feeding into the GI tract is safe even before bowel sounds or passing of flatus/stool is observed. It is considered safe and appropriate to feed patients with mild to moderate ileus as long as they remain hemodynamically stable.

6. **TRUE** There are numerous predictive equations available that may be used to estimate calorie needs during critical illness. They are all imprecise and may underestimate or overestimate actual calorie requirements. The Penn State equations that were developed specifically for critically ill patients on mechanical ventilation may be accurate more often than other equations. An easier equation is to multiply the patient's weight by a recommended factor, such as 25 to 30 cal/kg.

7. **TRUE** Underfeeding is associated with lower risks than overfeeding, possibly because a lower nutrient and calorie load may lower hyperglycemia, decrease proinflammatory cytokine production, reduce CO_2 production, and lower nutrient oxidation.

8. **FALSE** The drop in serum iron that occurs during the acute-phase response may be a compensatory mechanism to remove iron, so it is not available for use by replicating bacteria. Supplemental iron may impair the body's ability to fight infection.

9. **TRUE** Extensive burns are the most severe form of stress and dramatically increase the need for calories, protein, nutrients, and fluid.

10. **FALSE** COPD actually increases RMR through labored breathing and possibly through chronic inflammation. Weight loss may occur even when intake appears normal.

Student Resources on thePoint

For additional learning materials, activate the code in the front of this book at
http://thePoint.lww.com/activate

Websites

American Association of Critical Care Nurses at **www.aacn.org**
American Burn Association at **www.ameriburn.org**
American Lung Association at **www.lungusa.org**
Burn Survivor Resource Center at **www.burnsurvivor.com**
Society of Critical Care Medicine Surviving Sepsis Campaign at **www.survivingsepsis.org**

References

Academy of Nutrition and Dietetics. (2012). *Nutrition care manual.* Available at www.nutritioncaremanual.org. Accessed 5/17/12.

Academy of Nutrition and Dietetics Critical Care Evidence Analysis Workgroup. (2012). *Critical illness. Evidence-based nutrition practice guidelines.* Available at http://andevidencelibrary.com/topic.cfm?cat=4800&auth=1. Accessed on 5/19/12.

Alberda, C., Gramlich, L., Jones, N., Jeejeebhoy, K., Day, A. G., Dhaliwal, R., & Heyland, D. K. (2009). The relationship between nutritional intake and clinical outcomes in critically ill patients: Results of an international multicenter observation study. *Intensive Care Medicine, 35,* 1728–1737.

American Dietetic Association (2008). *Nutrition care manual.* Available at www.nutritioncaremanual.org. Accessed on 8/25/08.

Arabi, Y., Haddad, S., Tamin, S., Rishu, A. H., Sakkijha M. H., Kahoul, S. H., & Britts, R. J. (2010). Near-target caloric intake in critically ill medical-surgical patients is associated with adverse outcomes. *Journal of Parenteral and Enteral Nutrition, 34,* 280–288.

Arabi, Y., Tamin, H., Dhar, G., Al-Dawood, A., Al-Sultan, M., Sakkijha, M. H., . . . Brits, R. (2011). Permissive underfeeding and intensive insulin therapy in critically ill patients: A randomized controlled trial. *The American Journal of Clinical Nutrition, 93,* 569–577.

Barr, J., Hecht, M., Flavin, K., Khorana, A., & Gould, M. K. (2004). Outcomes in critically ill patients before and after the implementation of an evidence-based nutritional management protocol. *Chest, 125,* 1446–1457.

Berger, M. M., Baines, M., Falloul, W., Benathan, M., Chiolero, R. L., Reeves, C., . . . Shenkin, A. (2007). Trace element supplementation after major burns modulates antioxidant status and clinical course by way of increased tissue trace element concentrations. *The American Journal of Clinical Nutrition, 85,* 1293–1300.

Biolo, G., Grinble, G., & Preiser, J. (2003). Position paper of the ESICM Working Group on Nutrition and Metabolism. Metabolic basis of nutrition in intensive care unit patients: Ten critical questions. *Intensive Care Medicine, 28,* 1512–1520.

Cahill, N., Dhalival, R., Day, A. Jiang, X., & Heyland, D. (2010). Nutrition therapy in the critical care setting: What is "best achievable" practice? An international multicenter observational study. *Critical Care Medicine, 38,* 395–401.

Corbridge, S., Wilken, L., Kapella, M., & Gronkiewicz, C. (2012). An evidence-based approach to COPD: Part 1. *American Journal of Nursing, 112,* 46–57.

Frankenfield, D., Hise, M., Malone, A., Russell, M., Gradwell, E., & Compher, C. (2007). Prediction of resting metabolic rate in critically ill adult patients: Results of a systematic review of the evidence. *Journal of the American Dietetic Association, 107,* 1552–1561.

Frankenfield, D., Schubert, A., Alam, S., & Cooney, R. (2009). An analysis of estimation methods for resting metabolic rate in critically ill adults. *Journal of Parenteral and Enteral Nutrition, 33,* 27–36.

Gottschlich, M., Jenkins, M., Mayes, T., Khoury, J., Kagan, R., & Warden, G. (2002). The 2002 Clinical Research Award. An evaluation of the safety of early vs delayed enteral support and effects on clinical, nutritional, and endocrine outcomes after severe burns. *The Journal of Burn Care & Rehabilitation, 23,* 401–415.

Heyland, D., Cahill, N., Dhaliwal, R., Wang, M., Day, A. G., Alenzi, A., . . . McClave, S. A. (2010). Enhanced protein-energy provision via the enteral route in critically ill patients: A single center feasibility trial of the PEPuP protocol. *Critical Care, 14,* R78.

Hise, M. E., Halterman, K., Gajewski, B. J., Parkhurst, M., Moncure, M., & Brown, J. C. (2007). Feeding practices of severely ill intensive care unit patients: An evaluation of energy sources and clinical outcomes. *Journal of the American Dietetic Association, 107,* 458–465.

Kondrup, J. (2001). Can food in hospitals be improved. *Clinical Nutrition, 20,* 153–160.

Martindale, R., McClave, S., Vanek, V., McCarthy, M., Roberts, P., Taylor, B., . . . Cresci, G. (2009). Guidelines for the provision and assessment of nutrition support therapy in the adult critically ill patient: Society of Critical Care Medicine and American Society for Parenteral and Enteral Nutrition. *Journal of Parenteral and Enteral Nutrition, 33,* 277–316.

McClave, S., Kushner, R., Van Way, C., II, Cave, M., DeLegge, M., Dibaise, J., . . . Ochoa, J. (2011). Nutrition therapy of the severely obese, critically ill patient: Summation of conclusions and recommendations. *Journal of Parenteral and Enteral Nutrition, 35,* 88S–96S.

Norman, K., Pichard, C., Lochs, H., & Pirlich, M. (2008). Prognostic impact of disease-related malnutrition. *Clinical Nutrition, 27,* 5–15.

Pereira, C., Murphy, L., & Herndon, D. (2005). Altering metabolism. *Journal of Burn Care and Rehabilitation, 26,* 194–199.

Peterson, S., Tsai, A., Scala, C., Sowa, D., Sheean, P., & Braunschweig, C. (2010). Adequacy of oral intake in critically ill patients 1 week after extubation. *Journal of the American Dietetic Association, 11,* 427–433.

Prins, A. (2009). Nutritional management of the burn patient. *South African Journal of Clinical Nutrition, 22,* 9–15.

Sheean, P., Peterson, S., Zhao, W., Gurka, D., & Braunschweig, C. (2012). Intensive medical nutrition therapy: Methods to improve nutrition provision in the critical care setting. *Journal of the Academy of Nutrition and Dietetics, 112,* 1073–1079.

Thorsdottir, I., & Gunnarsdottir, I. (2002). Energy intake must be increased among recently hospitalized patients with chronic obstructive pulmonary disease to improve nutritional status. *Journal of the American Dietetic Association, 102,* 247–249.

Waymack, J., & Herndon, D. (1992). Nutritional support of burned patient. *World Journal of Surgery, 16,* 80–86.

Zaloga, P. (2012). *Permissive underfeeding of critically ill patients. Nestle nutrition.* Available at www.nestle-nutrition.com/topics. Accessed 5/22/12.

17 Nutrition for Patients with Upper Gastrointestinal Disorders

CHECK YOUR KNOWLEDGE

TRUE **FALSE**

☐ ☐ **1** People who have nausea should avoid liquids with meals.

☐ ☐ **2** Thin liquids, such as clear juices and clear broths, are usually the easiest items to swallow for patients with dysphagia.

☐ ☐ **3** All patients with dysphagia are given solid foods in pureed form.

☐ ☐ **4** In people with GERD, the severity of the pain reflects the extent of esophageal damage.

☐ ☐ **5** High-fat meals may trigger symptoms of GERD.

☐ ☐ **6** Losing weight, if overweight, helps manage GERD.

☐ ☐ **7** Spicy foods cause ulcers in susceptible people.

☐ ☐ **8** A bland diet promotes healing of peptic ulcers.

☐ ☐ **9** People with dumping syndrome should avoid sweets and sugars.

☐ ☐ **10** Pernicious anemia is a potential complication of gastric surgery.

LEARNING OBJECTIVES

Upon completion of this chapter, you will be able to

1 Give examples of ways to promote eating in people with anorexia.

2 Describe nutrition interventions that may help maximize intake in people who have nausea.

3 Compare the three levels of solid food textures included in the National Dysphagia Diet.

4 Compare the four liquid consistencies included in the National Dysphagia Diet.

5 Plan a menu appropriate for someone with GERD.

6 Teach a patient about the role of nutrition therapy in the treatment of peptic ulcer disease.

7 Give examples of nutrition therapy recommendations for people experiencing dumping syndrome.

Nutrition therapy is used in treating many digestive system disorders. For many disorders, diet merely plays a supportive role in alleviating symptoms rather than altering the course of the disease. For other gastrointestinal (GI) disorders, nutrition therapy is the cornerstone of treatment. Frequently, nutrition therapy is needed to restore nutritional status that has been compromised by dysfunction or disease.

Table 17.1 The Role of the Upper GI Tract in the Mechanical and Chemical Digestion of Food

Site	Mechanical Digestion	Chemical Digestion
Mouth	Chewing breaks down food into smaller particles. Food mixes with saliva for ease in swallowing.	Saliva contains lingual lipase, which has a limited role in the digestion of fat, and salivary amylase, which begins the process of starch digestion. Food is not held in the mouth long enough for significant digestion to occur there.
Esophagus	Propels food downward into the stomach Lower esophageal sphincter relaxes to move food into stomach.	None
Stomach	Churns and mixes food with digestive enzymes to reduce it to a thin liquid called chyme Forward and backward mixing motion at the pyloric sphincter pushes small amounts of chyme into the duodenum.	Secretes pepsin, which begins to break down protein into polypeptides Secretes gastric lipase, which has a limited role in fat digestion Secretes intrinsic factor, necessary for the absorption of vitamin B_{12} Absorbs some water, electrolytes, certain drugs, and alcohol

This chapter begins with disorders that affect eating and covers disorders of the upper GI tract (mouth, esophagus, and stomach) that have nutritional implications. Table 17.1 outlines the roles these sites play in the mechanical and chemical digestion of food. Problems with the upper GI tract impact nutrition mostly by affecting food intake and tolerance to particular foods or textures. Nutrition-focused assessment criteria for upper GI tract disorders are listed in Box 17.1.

Box 17.1 NUTRITION-FOCUSED ASSESSMENT FOR UPPER GI DISORDERS

- GI symptoms that interfere with intake such as anorexia, early satiety, difficulty chewing and swallowing, nausea and vomiting, heartburn
- Changes in eating made in response to symptoms
- Complications that impact nutritional status, such as weight loss, aspiration pneumonia, diarrhea
- Usual pattern of eating and frequency of meals and snacks
- Adequacy of intake according to MyPlate recommendations, including fluid intake
- Use of tobacco, over-the-counter drugs for GI symptoms, alcohol, and caffeine
- Food allergies or intolerances, such as high-fat foods, citrus fruits, spicy food
- Use of nutritional supplements including vitamins, minerals, fiber, and herbs
- Client's willingness to change his or her eating habits

DISORDERS THAT AFFECT EATING

Anorexia

Anorexia: lack of appetite; it differs from anorexia nervosa, a psychological condition characterized by denial of appetite.

Anorexia is a common symptom of many physical conditions and a side effect of certain drugs. Emotional issues, such as fear, anxiety, and depression, frequently cause anorexia. The aim of nutrition therapy is to stimulate the appetite to maintain adequate nutritional intake. The following interventions may help:

- Serve food attractively and season according to individual taste. If decreased ability to taste is contributing to anorexia, enhance food flavors with tart seasonings (e.g., orange juice, lemonade, vinegar, lemon juice) or strong seasonings (e.g., basil, oregano, rosemary, tarragon, mint).
- Schedule procedures and medications when they are least likely to interfere with meals, if possible.
- Control pain, nausea, or depression with medications as ordered.
- Provide small, frequent meals.
- Withhold beverages for 30 minutes before and after meals to avoid displacing the intake of more nutrient-dense foods.
- Offer liquid supplements between meals for additional calories and protein if meal consumption is low.
- Limit fat intake if fat is contributing to early satiety.

Nausea and Vomiting

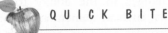 **QUICK BITE**

High-fat foods

- "Fats"—nuts, nut butters, oils, margarine, butter, salad dressings
- Fatty meats, such as many processed meats (bologna, pastrami, hard salami), bacon, sausage
- Milk and milk products containing whole or 2% milk
- Rich desserts, such as cakes, pies, cookies, pastries
- Many savory snacks, such as potato chips, cheese puffs, tortilla chips

Nausea and vomiting may be related to a decrease in gastric acid secretion, a decrease in digestive enzyme activity, a decrease in GI motility, gastric irritation, or acidosis. Other causes include bacterial and viral infection; increased intracranial pressure; equilibrium imbalance; liver, pancreatic, and gallbladder disorders; and pyloric or intestinal obstruction. Drugs and certain medical treatments may also contribute to nausea.

The short-term concern of nausea and vomiting is fluid and electrolyte balance. Intravenous lines can meet

Intractable Vomiting: vomiting that is difficult to manage or cure.

patient needs until an oral intake resumes. With prolonged or **intractable vomiting**, dehydration and weight loss are concerns.

Nutrition intervention for nausea is a commonsense approach. Food is withheld until nausea subsides. When the patient is ready to eat, clear liquids are offered and progressed to a regular diet as tolerated. Small, frequent meals of low-fat, readily digested carbohydrates are usually best tolerated. Other strategies that may help are to

- Encourage the patient to eat slowly and not to eat if he or she feels nauseated.
- Promote good oral hygiene with mouthwash and ice chips.

- Limit liquids with meals because they can cause a full, bloated feeling.
- Encourage a liberal fluid intake between meals with whatever liquids the patient can tolerate, such as clear soup, juice, gelatin, ginger ale, and popsicles.
- Serve foods at room temperature or chilled; hot foods may contribute to nausea.
- Avoid high-fat and spicy foods if they contribute to nausea.

DISORDERS OF THE ESOPHAGUS

Dysphagia: impaired ability to swallow.

Symptoms of esophageal disorders range from difficulty swallowing and the sensation that something is stuck in the throat to heartburn and reflux. **Dysphagia** and gastroesophageal reflux disease are discussed next.

Dysphagia

Swallowing is a complex series of events characterized by three basic phases (Fig. 17.1). Impairments in swallowing can have a profound impact on intake and nutritional status and greatly increase the risk of aspiration and its complications of bacterial pneumonia and bronchial obstruction.

Although aging causes natural changes in the ability to swallow, dysphagia is often related to neurologic impairments, such as dementia, amyotrophic lateral sclerosis (ALS), myasthenia gravis, cerebrovascular accident, traumatic brain injury, cerebral palsy, Parkinson disease, and multiple sclerosis. Mechanical causes include obstruction, inflammation, edema, and surgery of the throat. Refer patients with actual or potential swallowing impairments to the speech pathology department for a thorough swallowing assessment.

Nutrition Therapy

Viscosity: the condition of being resistant to flow; having a heavy, gluey quality.

The goal of nutrition therapy for dysphagia is to modify the texture of foods and/or **viscosity** of liquids to enable the patient to achieve adequate nutrition and hydration while decreasing the risk of aspiration. Solid foods may be minced, mashed, ground, or pureed, and thin liquids may be thickened to facilitate swallowing, but these measures often dilute the nutritional value of the diet and make food and beverages less appealing (Germain, Dufresne, and Gray-Donald, 2006). Emotionally, dysphagia can affect quality of life; patients with dysphagia may feel panic at mealtime, avoid eating with others, and stop eating even when they still feel hungry (Ekberg, Hamdy, Woisard, Wuttge-Hannig, and Ortega, 2002). Meeting nutritional needs is a challenge, and in some instances, enteral nutrition may be necessary.

The American Dietetic Association has published the National Dysphagia Diet, developed by a group of dietitians, speech and language therapists, and a food scientist for the purpose of standardizing dysphagia diets throughout the United States (National Dysphagia Diet Task Force, 2002). It is composed of three levels of solid textures and four liquid consistencies (Table 17.2).

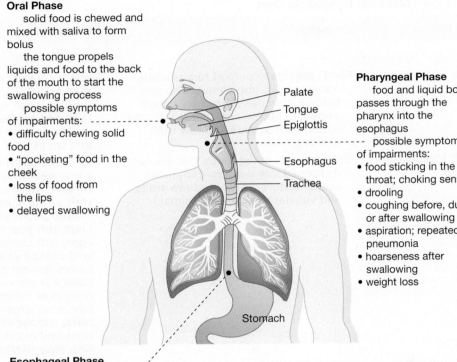

Oral Phase
    solid food is chewed and mixed with saliva to form bolus
    the tongue propels liquids and food to the back of the mouth to start the swallowing process
    possible symptoms of impairments:
- difficulty chewing solid food
- "pocketing" food in the cheek
- loss of food from the lips
- delayed swallowing

Palate
Tongue
Epiglottis

Esophagus

Trachea

Stomach

Pharyngeal Phase
    food and liquid bolus passes through the pharynx into the esophagus
    possible symptoms of impairments:
- food sticking in the throat; choking sensation
- drooling
- coughing before, during, or after swallowing
- aspiration; repeated pneumonia
- hoarseness after swallowing
- weight loss

Esophageal Phase
    bolus passes through esophagus into the stomach via peristaltic movements
    possible symptoms of impairments:
- difficulty with solid food (can handle pureed food)
- heartburn
- vomiting
- burping

■ **FIGURE 17.1**   Swallowing phases and symptoms of impairments.

The levels of solid food and liquids are ordered separately to allow maximum flexibility and safety in meeting the patient's needs. The patient may start at any of the levels. The solid food consistencies include pureed, mechanically altered, and a more advanced consistency of mixed textures. The liquids are described as thin, nectarlike, honeylike, and spoon-thick.

Generally, a speech or language pathologist (SLP) performs a swallowing evaluation on the patient to determine the appropriate consistency of food and liquids and recommends feeding techniques based on the patient's individual status. Changes to the diet prescription are made as the patient's ability to swallow improves or deteriorates.

Generally, moist, semisolid foods are easiest to swallow, such as pudding, custards, scrambled eggs, and yogurt, because they form a cohesive bolus that is more easily controlled. Dry, crumbly, and sticky foods are avoided. Some foods, such as bread, are **slurried** to create a texture easily swallowed while retaining the appearance of "regular" bread. Commercial thickeners added to pureed foods can allow pureed foods to be molded into the appearance of "normal" food, which is more visually appealing than "baby food"

Slurried: a slurry is a thickener dissolved in liquid that is added to dry or pureed foods to produce a texture that is soft and cohesive.

Table 17.2 National Dysphagia Diet

Level of Diet	Description	Foods Allowed
Three levels of solid textures		
Level 1: Pureed	Foods are totally pureed to a smooth, homogenous, and cohesive consistency. Eliminates sticky foods, such as peanut butter, and coarse-textured foods, such as nuts and raw fruits and vegetables	Smooth cooked cereals; slurried or pureed bread products; milk; smooth desserts such as yogurt, pudding, custard, and applesauce; pureed fruits, vegetables, meats, scrambled eggs, and soups
Level 2: Mechanically altered	Soft-textured, moist foods that are easily formed into a bolus. Eliminates coarse textures, nuts, and raw fruits and vegetables (except bananas)	Cooked cereals may have a little texture; some well-moistened, ready-to-eat cereals; well-moistened pancakes with syrup; slurried bread; moist well-cooked potatoes, noodles, and dumplings; soft poached or scrambled eggs; soft canned or cooked fruit; soft, well-cooked vegetables with ½ in pieces (except no corn, peas, and other fibrous vegetables). Moist ground or minced tender meat in pieces no larger than ¼ in, soft casseroles, cottage cheese, tofu; moist cobblers and moist soft cookies; soups with easy-to-chew meat or vegetables
Level 3: Advanced	Near-normal textured foods; excludes crunchy, sticky, or very hard foods. Food is bite-sized and moist.	All breads are allowed except for those that are crusty; moist cereals; most desserts except those with nuts, seeds, coconut, pineapple, or dried fruit; soft, peeled fruit without seeds; moist tender meats or casseroles with small pieces of meat; moist potatoes, rice, and stuffing; all soups except those with chewy meats or vegetables; most cooked, tender vegetables, except corn; shredded lettuce. No nuts, seeds, coconut, and chewy candy
Four liquid consistencies		
Thin	All unthickened beverages and supplements	Clear juices, frozen yogurt, ice cream, milk, water, coffee, tea, soda, broth, plain gelatin, liquidy fruits such as watermelon
Nectarlike	Liquids thicker than water but thin enough to sip through a straw	Nectars, vegetable juices, chocolate milk, buttermilk, thin milkshakes, cream soups, other properly thickened beverages
Honeylike	Liquids that can be eaten with a spoon but do not hold their shape	Honey, tomato sauce, yogurt
Spoon-thick	Liquids thickened to pudding consistency that need to be eaten with a spoon	Pudding, custard, hot cereal

Source: National Dysphagia Diet Task Force. (2002). *National dysphagia diet: Standardization for optimal care.* Chicago, IL: American Dietetic Association.

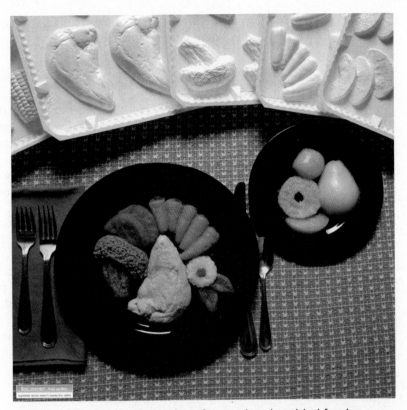

■ **FIGURE 17.2** Examples of pureed and molded foods.

(Fig. 17.2). In studies comparing molded food to standard pureed food, people with dysphagia found the molded food to be more difficult to eat, instead preferring pureed food (Ballou Stahlman, Mertz Garcia, Hakel, and Chambers, 2000). Flavor enhancers, colored plates, and attractive garnishes can improve the appearance of pureed food.

Thickened liquids are more cohesive than thin liquids and are easier to control (Matta, Chambers, Garcia, and McGowan Helverson, 2006). Commercial thickening agents provide instructions on how to mix the product with liquids to achieve the desired consistency, yet wide variations in consistency occur depending on the beverage type, type of thickener (e.g., starch based or gum based), temperature of the liquid, and time between thickened fluid preparation and service to the patient (Adeleye and Rachal, 2007). Commercially prepared thickened beverages are available, but viscosity varies among manufacturers and many product labels do not include viscosity.

Thickened beverages are often poorly accepted, making it difficult to maintain an adequate fluid intake. Many patients would rather risk aspiration than consume thickened liquids (Panther, 2005). Consequently, some facilities have implemented the Frazier Free Water Protocol, which allows patients who are not allowed to consume thin liquids to drink plain water between meals (Garcia and Chambers, 2010). It is based on the assumption that drinking plain water alone is less likely to cause problems if it is aspirated than if it is consumed with food or other liquids. Researchers caution that evidence supporting the use of this protocol is based on data from a single institution (Wagner, 2005).

In addition to modifying the texture of solids and liquids, various feeding techniques may be used to facilitate safe swallowing:

- Serve small, frequent meals to help maximize intake.
- Encourage patients with dysphagia to rest before mealtime. Postpone meals if the patient is fatigued.
- Give mouth care immediately before meals to enhance the sense of taste.
- Instruct the patient to think of a specific food to stimulate salivation. A lemon slice, lemon hard candy, or dill pickles may also help to trigger salivation, as may moderately flavored foods.
- Reduce or eliminate distractions at mealtime so that the patient can focus his or her attention on swallowing. Limit disruptions, if possible, and do not rush the patient; allow at least 30 minutes for eating.
- Place the patient in an upright or high Fowler's position. If the patient has one-sided facial weakness, place the food on the other side of the mouth. Tilt the head forward to facilitate swallowing.
- Use adaptive eating devices, such as built-up utensils and mugs with spouts, if indicated. Syringes should never be used to force liquids into the patient's mouth because this can trigger choking or aspiration. Unless otherwise directed, do not allow the patient to use a straw.
- Encourage small bites and thorough chewing.
- Discourage the patient from consuming alcohol because it reduces cough and gag reflexes.

Gastroesophageal Reflux Disease

Gastroesophageal Reflux Disease (GERD): gastroesophageal reflux is the backflow of gastric acid into the esophagus; gastroesophageal reflux disease occurs when symptoms of reflux happen two or more times a week.

Gastroesophageal reflux disease (GERD) is caused by an abnormal reflux of gastric contents into the esophagus related to an abnormal relaxation of the lower esophageal sphincter (LES) (Vemulapalli, 2008). Factors that lower LES pressure and contribute to gastroesophageal reflux are hiatal hernia, obesity, pregnancy, smoking, and certain medications (e.g., dopamine, morphine). Genetic factors may also play a role. It is a common belief that some foods cause or worsen GERD symptoms, but data are conflicting (Festi et al., 2009).

Although some people may be relatively asymptomatic, complaining only of a "lump" in their throat, indigestion, "heartburn," and regurgitation are common, especially after eating a large or fatty meal. Pain frequently worsens when the person lies down, bends over after eating, or wears tight-fitting clothing. Chronic untreated GERD may cause reflux esophagitis, esophageal ulcers with bleeding, esophageal stricture, dysphagia, pulmonary disease, Barrett esophagus, and esophageal cancer. The amount of acid refluxed, the severity of heartburn, and the damage to the esophagus do not always correlate: severe pain can occur in the absence of esophageal damage and severe damage may occur with minimal heartburn (Stenson, 2006).

Nutrition Therapy

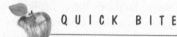

QUICK BITE

Obsolete approaches for GERD and PUD
Bland diet
Increased milk intake

A three-pronged approach is used to treat GERD: lifestyle modification, including nutrition therapy; drug therapy; and surgical intervention, if necessary. Most available evidence shows a link between obesity, especially abdominal obesity, and GERD and that weight

Box 17.2   LIFESTYLE AND NUTRITION THERAPY MODIFICATIONS FOR GERD

Most Likely Effective
Lose weight if overweight.
Engage in moderate physical activity regularly.
Elevate the head of the bed during sleep.
Avoid
- Large meals
- Lying down for 3 hours after meals
- Alcohol
- Heavily spiced food
- Fatty food
Do not smoke.

Possibly Effective
Increase fiber intake.
Eliminate the following to see if symptoms improve:
- Red and black pepper
- Regular and decaffeinated coffee
- Chocolate
- Peppermint and spearmint

loss improves symptoms (Festi et al., 2009). Box 17.2 highlights lifestyle modifications recently proposed by a group of international experts that are most likely to be effective in the management of GERD (Tytgat et al., 2008) as well as other approaches of less certain effectiveness. Patients should always be advised to eliminate individual intolerances. Despite the lack of evidence, lifestyle and diet are considered important adjunct therapies in the treatment of GERD.

DISORDERS OF THE STOMACH

Peptic ulcer disease (PUD) and dumping syndrome from gastric surgery are disorders of the stomach that use nutrition therapy to help control symptoms.

Peptic Ulcer Disease

Peptic Ulcer: erosion of the gastrointestinal mucosal layer caused by an excess secretion of, or decreased mucosal resistance to, hydrochloric acid and pepsin.

The majority of **peptic ulcers** occur in the duodenum; other sites include the lower end of the esophagus, the stomach, and jejunum. *Helicobacter pylori* infection is implicated in an estimated 70% of gastric ulcers and 92% of duodenal ulcers (Makola, Peura, and Crowe, 2007), yet most people infected with *H. pylori* do not develop the disease, which suggests other factors may be involved (Ryan-Harshman and Aldoori, 2004). *H. pylori* appears to secrete an enzyme that depletes gastric mucus, making the mucosal layer more susceptible to erosion. For these patients, destroying the bacteria—typically with a combination of antibiotics and acid-suppressing drugs—generally cures the ulcer. The second leading cause of peptic ulcers is the use of nonsteroidal anti-inflammatory drugs (NSAIDs). Eating spicy food does not cause ulcers.

The most common symptom of ulcers is epigastric pain, which may also be accompanied by bloating, early satiety, and nausea. Pain related to duodenal ulcers typically occurs in the fasting state or during the night and is usually relieved by food. Chronic PUD may be asymptomatic, particularly when ulcers are caused by NSAIDs (Malfertheiner, Chan, and McCall, 2009).

The most common and severe complication of PUD is bleeding. From a nutritional standpoint, pain or early satiety may impair intake and lead to weight loss. Blood loss can lead to iron deficiency. Long-term use of medications to decrease gastric acid production may impair the absorption of calcium, iron, and vitamin B_{12}.

QUICK BITE

Foods high in soluble fiber
Dried peas and beans
Lentils
Oats
Certain fruits and vegetables, such as
    oranges, potatoes, carrots, apples

Although dietary restrictions are commonly used for ulcers, there is no evidence that diet causes PUD or speeds ulcer healing. Patients may be told to avoid coffee, alcohol, and chocolate because these substances stimulate gastric acid secretion, yet consuming moderate amounts of these items has not been shown to impair ulcer healing (Stenson, 2006). Some evidence suggests that a high-fiber diet, especially soluble fiber, may reduce the risk of duodenal ulcer, but other dietary factors, including alcohol and caffeine, have little effect on ulcer risk (Ryan-Harshman and Aldoori, 2004). Nutrition intervention may play a supportive role in treatment by helping to control symptoms. Any of the following strategies may help:

- Avoid items that stimulate gastric acid secretion—namely, coffee (decaffeinated and regular), alcohol, caffeine, and pepper.
- Avoid eating 2 hours before bed.
- Avoid individual intolerances.

Dumping Syndrome

Nutritional complications of gastric surgeries depend on the extent of gastric resection and the type of reconstruction performed. One of the most common complications of gastrectomy and gastric bypass is dumping syndrome, a group of symptoms caused by rapid emptying of stomach contents into the intestine. As the hyperosmolar bolus enters the intestines, fluid shifts from the plasma and extracellular fluid into the intestines to dilute the high particle concentration. The large volume of hypertonic fluid into the jejunum and an increase in peristalsis leads to cramping, diarrhea, and abdominal pain. Weakness, dizziness, and a rapid heartbeat occur as the volume of circulating blood decreases. These symptoms occur within 10 to 20 minutes after eating and characterize the early dumping syndrome.

An intermediate dumping reaction occurs 20 to 30 minutes after eating as undigested food is fermented in the colon, producing gas, abdominal pain, cramping, and diarrhea (Academy of Nutrition and Dietetics, 2012).

Late dumping syndrome occurs 1 to 3 hours after eating and is especially common after consuming simple sugars (Academy of Nutrition and Dietetics, 2012). The rapid absorption of carbohydrate causes a quick spike in blood glucose levels; the body compensates by oversecreting insulin. Blood glucose levels drop rapidly, and symptoms of hypoglycemia develop, such as shakiness, sweating, confusion, and weakness.

A reduced stomach capacity, rapid gastric emptying, and rapid transit time increase the risk of maldigestion, malabsorption, and decreased oral intake. The excretion of calories and nutrients produces weight loss and increases the risk of malnutrition. Other potential nutritional complications are outlined in Table 17.3.

Nutrition Therapy

Nutrition intervention can control or prevent symptoms of dumping syndrome. Unlike most initial postoperative feedings, clear liquids are not used. Patients are started on small, frequent meals consisting of only one or two foods per meal or snack, one of which is a protein. Food must be thoroughly chewed. Liquids are provided 30 minutes to 1 hour after consuming solids, not with meals, because they promote quick movement through the GI tract. Simple sugars and sugar alcohols are avoided to limit the hypertonicity of the mass as it reaches the

Table 17.3 Potential Nutritional Complications of Dumping Syndrome

Potential Complication	Possible Contributing Factors	Possible Treatment
Iron deficiency anemia	Decreased food intake A decrease in hydrochloric acid secretion impairs the conversion of iron to its absorbable form. If the duodenum is bypassed or food moves through it too quickly, iron absorption cannot occur (the duodenum is the site of iron absorption).	Iron supplementation is necessary.
Steatorrhea (excess fat in the stools)	Rapid intestinal time does not allow enough time for fat to be exposed to digestive enzymes. If the duodenum is bypassed, less pancreatic lipase is available to digest fat. Bacterial overgrowth (excessive growth of intestinal bacteria) can develop from low gastric acidity or altered motility; it interferes with the action of bile, which is important for the emulsification of fat.	Supplemental pancreatic enzymes may be necessary. Medium-chain triglycerides may be used for additional calories (but lack the essential fatty acids). Supplements of fat-soluble vitamins may be prescribed; their absorption is dependent on the absorption of fat.
Pernicious anemia	Intrinsic factor, necessary for the absorption of vitamin B_{12} from the intestine, is produced by the stomach. It may be absent after gastric surgery. It may take years for a deficiency to develop.	Injections of vitamin B_{12} may be necessary.
Osteomalacia (softening of the bones)	Calcium is normally absorbed in the duodenum; if it is bypassed or the transit time is too rapid, calcium malabsorption can occur. Fat malabsorption causes calcium and vitamin D to be malabsorbed. Lower calcium intake related to lactose intolerance	Supplements of calcium and vitamin D may be necessary.

jejunum. Lactose may be restricted because lactose intolerance is common. Patients are advised to lie down after eating. **Functional fibers**, such as pectin and guar gum, may be used to delay gastric emptying and treat diarrhea (Academy of Nutrition and Dietetics, 2012). Liquid multivitamin and mineral supplements are recommended, and vitamin B_{12} injections may be necessary depending on the extent of surgery. Over time, the diet is liberalized as the remaining portion of the stomach or duodenum hypertrophies to hold more food and allow for more normal digestion. Box 17.3 features antidumping syndrome diet guidelines (see Chapter 14 for more on bariatric surgery).

Functional Fiber: fiber that has been isolated from food that has beneficial physiologic effects.

QUICK BITE

Sources of sugar alcohols
Dietetic candy
Sugarless gum, cough drops, and mints
Certain fruits: apples, pears, peaches, prunes

Box 17.3   ANTIDUMPING SYNDROME DIET GUIDELINES

Eating strategies

- Eat small, frequent meals.
- Consume beverages between, not with, meals.
- Avoid sugar, honey, syrup, sorbitol, and xylitol and all food and beverages that have any of those listed as one of the first three ingredients on the label.
- Eat a source of protein at each meal because it helps slow gastric emptying.
- Choose low-fiber grains; mostly canned, not fresh fruit; nongassy, well-cooked vegetables without seeds or skins.

Recommended foods

- Breads and cereals: refined plain breads, crackers, rolls, unsweetened cereal, rice, and pasta that provide less than 2 g fiber/serving
- Vegetables: well-cooked or raw vegetables without seeds or skins, strained vegetable juice, lettuce; avoid "gassy" vegetables such as broccoli, cauliflower, cabbage, and corn
- Fruits: banana, soft melons, unsweetened canned fruit
- Milk and milk products: 1% or fat-free milk (if not lactose intolerant); choose yogurt, soy milk, and ice cream without sugar added
- Meat and meat alternatives: tender, well-cooked meat, fish, poultry, egg, and soy without added fat; smooth nut butters. Avoid all of the following: fried meats, fish, and poultry; high-fat luncheon meats, sausage, hot dogs, and bacon; tough or chewy meats; dried peas and beans; nuts
- Fats: oils, butter, margarine, cream cheese, mayonnaise
- Beverages: decaffeinated coffee and tea; sugar-free soft drinks; avoid caffeinated beverages, alcohol
- Other: allowed foods made with artificial sweeteners such as NutraSweet, sucralose, acesulfame potassium

Sample Menu (when recovered enough to eat six times a day)

Breakfast
1 poached egg
1 slice white toast with butter
1 hour later: 1 cup decaffeinated coffee
   with half and half

Midmorning Snack
1 cup yogurt without added sugar
1 hour later: 1 cup plain unsweetened soy milk

Lunch
½ cup cottage cheese with two
   unsweetened, canned peach halves
Dinner roll with butter
1 hour later: 8 oz sugar-free ginger ale

Midafternoon Snack
2 oz cheddar cheese
4 saltine crackers

Dinner
3 oz baked chicken
½ cup white rice with butter
½ cup cooked carrots with butter
1 hour later: caffeine-free tea

Bedtime Snack
1 cup yogurt without added sugar

Source: Academy of Nutrition and Dietetics. (2012). *Nutrition care manual* (online). Copyright 2012. Available at http://www.nutritioncaremanual.org. Accessed on 5/30/12.

NURSING PROCESS: *GERD*

Jason is 28 years old and complains of frequent painful heartburn. He takes antacids on a daily basis and has lost 14 pounds over the last few months. His strategy to avoid pain is to avoid eating. He smokes two packs of cigarettes per day. He is 5 ft 8 in tall, weighs 170 pounds, and has an appointment to see his doctor. In the meantime, he has come to you, the corporate nurse on staff where he works, to see what he can do to help control his heartburn.

Assessment

Medical–Psychosocial History	▪ Medical history that would contribute to GERD, such as hiatal hernia
	▪ Symptoms that may affect nutrition, such as difficulty swallowing or nausea and vomiting
	▪ Use of medications that may decrease lower esophageal sphincter (LES) pressure, such as anticholinergic agents, diazepam, or theophylline
	▪ Use of medications that may damage the mucosa, such as NSAIDs or aspirin
	▪ History of smoking
	▪ Level of activity
Anthropometric Assessment	Body mass index, percent weight loss
Biochemical and Physical Assessment	Abnormal lab values, if available, especially hemoglobin and hematocrit because low values may indicate bleeding
Dietary Assessment	▪ How many meals do you eat daily?
	▪ Would you say your meals are small, medium, or large in size?
	▪ Are there any particular foods that cause indigestion, especially alcohol, coffee, tea, caffeine, pepper, mint, chocolate, or fatty foods?
	▪ What foods do you avoid?
	▪ Can you correlate your symptoms to
	▪ Lying down after eating?
	▪ Wearing tight clothes?
	▪ Eating right before bed?
	▪ Do you take vitamins, minerals, herbs, or other supplements?
	▪ Do you have ethnic, religious, or cultural food preferences?

Diagnosis

Possible Nursing Diagnoses	Altered nutrition: eating less than the body needs as evidenced by weight loss related to inadequate intake secondary to heartburn

Planning

Client Outcomes	The client will
	▪ Report relief from symptoms
	▪ Consume adequate calories and nutrients
	▪ Use less medication to control symptoms
	▪ Explain the role of diet in controlling GERD symptoms
	▪ Exhibit normal laboratory values

(continues on page 456)

NURSING PROCESS: *GERD* (continued)

Nursing Interventions

Nutrition Therapy

- Avoid items that increase gastric acid secretion and/or lower LES pressure:
  - Alcohol
  - Black and red pepper
  - Coffee
  - Chocolate
  - Fatty foods
  - Mint
- Eat small frequent meals to avoid increasing intra-abdominal pressure but avoid eating within 3 hours of bedtime
- Consume liquids between meals instead of with meals to limit distention of the stomach
- Avoid spicy, acidic, or tomato-based foods that may irritate the esophagus
- Eliminate any foods not tolerated

Client Teaching

Instruct the client
- That nutrition interventions may help control symptoms but do not treat the underlying problem
- On lifestyle modifications that may help improve symptoms, such as losing weight, smoking cessation, and regular exercise
- To avoid pressure on the abdomen and LES,
  - Raise the head of the bed
  - Do not bend over or lie down after eating
  - Do not wear tight-fitting clothes

Evaluation

Evaluate and Monitor

- Monitor for improvement in symptoms
- Monitor weight
- Monitor for medication usage

HOW DO YOU RESPOND?

If over-the-counter drugs to combat heartburn are as good as advertised, why should I worry about what to eat if taking a pill can allow me to eat what I want without any pain? Although they work well, relying on medications to stave off pain after eating whatever, whenever, and in any amount is foolhardy. All medications have the potential to cause side effects, and pain is a signal that something is wrong. Encourage clients to implement eating and lifestyle changes to see if those strategies alone can prevent symptoms.

CASE STUDY

Barbara is a 72-year-old woman with a "Type A" personality who was diagnosed with a peptic ulcer more than 40 years ago. At that time, her doctor told her to follow a bland diet and eat three meals per day with three snacks per day of whole milk to "quiet" her stomach. She meticulously complied with the diet to the point of becoming obsessive about eating anything that may not be "allowed." She lost 15 pounds by following the bland diet because her intake was so restricted. She recently began experiencing ulcer symptoms and has put herself back on the bland diet, convinced it is necessary in order to recover from her ulcer.

Yesterday, she ate the following:

Breakfast:	1 poached egg 2 slices dry white toast 1 cup whole milk
Morning Snack:	1 cup whole milk
Lunch:	¾ cup cottage cheese with ½ cup canned peaches
Afternoon snack:	1 cup whole milk
Dinner:	3 oz boiled chicken ½ cup boiled plain potatoes ½ cup boiled green beans ½ cup gelatin
Evening snack:	1 cup whole milk

- Barbara's 1600-calorie MyPlate plan calls for 1.5 cups of fruit, 2 cups of vegetables, 5 grains, 5 oz of meat/beans, 3 cups of milk, and 5 teaspoons of oils. How does her intake compare? What food groups is she undereating? Overeating? What are the potential nutritional consequences of her current diet?
- What other information would be helpful for you to know in dealing with Barbara?
- Barbara clearly wants to be on a bland diet; what would you tell her about diet recommendations for PUD? What recommendations would you make to improve her symptoms and meet her nutritional requirements while respecting her need to follow a "diet"?

STUDY QUESTIONS

1. The patient asks if coffee is bad for his peptic ulcer. Which of the following would be the nurse's best response?
   a. "Coffee does not cause ulcers, and drinking it probably does not interfere with ulcer healing. You may try eliminating it from your diet to see what impact it has on your symptoms and then decide whether or not to avoid it."
   b. "Both caffeinated and decaffeinated coffee can cause ulcers and interfere with ulcer healing. You should eliminate both from your diet."
   c. "You need to eliminate caffeinated coffee from your diet, but it is safe to drink decaffeinated coffee."
   d. "You can drink all the coffee you want; it does not affect ulcers."

2. Which statement indicates the patient needs further instruction about GERD?
   a. "I know a bland diet will help prevent the heartburn I get after eating."
   b. "Lying down after eating can make GERD symptoms worse."
   c. "High-fat meals can make GERD symptoms worse."
   d. "Losing excess weight can help prevent symptoms of GERD."

3. Which of the following snacks would be best for a patient who wants to eat who has nausea?
   a. Cheese
   b. Peanuts
   c. Banana
   d. A milkshake

4. The nurse knows her instructions have been effective when the patient with dumping syndrome verbalizes she should
   a. Avoid lying down after eating.
   b. Drink liquids between, not with, meals.
   c. Eat simple sugars in place of starches.
   d. Avoid protein.

5. A patient with dumping syndrome asks why it is so important to avoid sugars and sweets. Which of the following is the nurse's best response?
   a. "Sugars and sweets provide empty calories, so they should be limited in everyone's diet."
   b. "Sugars draw water into the intestines and cause cramping and diarrhea."
   c. "Sugar makes blood glucose levels increase; hyperglycemia is a complication of dumping syndrome."
   d. "Avoiding sugars and sweets helps ensure that they will not displace the intake of protein, which you need for healing."

6. Which of the following is an appropriate breakfast for a patient on a level 1 dysphagia diet?
   a. Poached egg
   b. Cream of wheat
   c. Granola with milk
   d. Toast cut into small pieces

7. A patient who develops pernicious anemia after gastric surgery needs supplemental
   a. Protein
   b. Iron
   c. Folic acid
   d. Vitamin B_{12}

8. The best dessert for a patient with GERD is
   a. Chocolate cake
   b. Peppermint ice cream
   c. Cheesecake
   d. Applesauce

KEY CONCEPTS

■ Nutrition therapy for GI disorders may help minimize or prevent symptoms. For some GI disorders, nutrition therapy is the cornerstone of treatment.

■ Small, frequent meals may help to maximize intake in patients who have anorexia. Avoiding high-fat foods may lessen the feeling of fullness.

■ After nausea and vomiting subside, low-fat, easily digested carbohydrate foods, such as crackers, toast, oatmeal, and bland fruit, usually are well tolerated. Patients should avoid liquids with meals because liquids can promote the feeling of fullness.

■ The National Dysphagia Diet has three different solid food textures and four different liquid consistencies. A speech and language pathologist recommends the appropriate level for solids and liquids based on a swallowing evaluation.

- Pureed foods are less calorically dense than normal textured foods. They are also less visually appealing. Patients with dysphagia are monitored for poor intakes and weight loss.
- People with GERD should lose weight if overweight; not smoke; avoid large meals and bedtime snacks; eliminate individual intolerances; and avoid alcohol, highly spicy foods, and fatty foods. Other approaches that may be effective include eating a high-fiber diet and eliminating regular and decaffeinated coffee, chocolate, and peppermint and spearmint flavors.
- There is no evidence that diet causes ulcers or promotes their healing. Patients are commonly advised to avoid items that stimulate gastric acid secretion and any foods not tolerated.
- Nutrition therapy for dumping syndrome consists of eating small, frequent meals; eating protein at each meal; and avoiding concentrated sugars and sugar alcohols. Liquids should be consumed 1 hour before or after eating instead of with meals.

Check Your Knowledge Answer Key

1. **TRUE** Drinking liquids with meals may promote a bloated feeling and contribute to nausea. Encourage patients to drink fluids between meals, especially clear liquids such as water, clear juices, gelatin, ginger ale, and popsicles.

2. **FALSE** Thin liquids are the most difficult consistency to control for people who have swallowing difficulties. Thickened liquids have a more cohesive consistency that is easier to manage.

3. **FALSE** The degree of texture modification for dysphagia is determined by the individual's ability to chew and swallow. There are three levels of solid textures: pureed, mechanically altered, and an advanced consistency of mixed textures.

4. **FALSE** The severity of the pain is not correlated to the extent of esophageal damage. Some people have severe damage with only minor symptoms.

5. **TRUE** Fat lowers LES pressure, so high-fat meals may cause symptoms of GERD.

6. **TRUE** Losing weight, if overweight, helps manage GERD.

7. **FALSE** There is no evidence that any particular foods cause ulcers, but avoiding highly spicy food may improve symptoms when a person has GERD.

8. **FALSE** A bland diet is considered obsolete. It does not promote ulcer healing, and eating moderate amounts of nonbland foods has not been shown to irritate peptic ulcers.

9. **TRUE** People with dumping syndrome should avoid sugars and sweets because they contribute to a high osmolar load when the gastric contents enter the intestine. Over time, the diet is liberalized to allow sugars and sweets as the remaining stomach and intestine accommodate to the change in the stomach's holding capacity.

10. **TRUE** Because intrinsic factor is produced in the stomach and is necessary for the intestinal absorption of vitamin B_{12}, people who have had a gastrectomy are at risk of developing pernicious anemia. The symptoms may take years to develop because the body stores vitamin B_{12}.

Student Resources on thePoint

For additional learning materials, activate the code in the front of this book at
http://thePoint.lww.com/activate

Websites

American College of Gastroenterology at **www.acg.gi.org**
American Gastroenterological Association at **www.gastro.org**
Dysphagia Resource Center at **www.dysphagia.com**
Helicobacter Foundation at **www.helico.com**
National Digestive Diseases Information Clearinghouse (NDDIC), a service of the National Institute of Diabetes and Digestive and Kidney Diseases (NIDDK), National Institutes of Health at **http://digestive.niddk.nih.gov**

References

Academy of Nutrition and Dietetics. (2012). *Nutrition care manual.* Available at http://www .nutritioncaremanual.org. Accessed on 5/30/12.

Adeleye, B., & Rachal, C. (2007). Comparison of the rheological properties of ready-to-serve and powdered instant food-thickened beverages at different temperatures for dysphagic patients. *Journal of the American Dietetic Association, 107,* 1176–1182.

Ballou Stahlman, L., Mertz Garcia, J., Hakel, M., & Chambers, E., IV. (2000). Comparison ratings of pureed versus molded fruits: Preliminary results. *Dysphagia, 15,* 2–5.

Ekberg, O., Hamdy, S., Woisard, V., Wuttge-Hannig, A., & Ortega, P. (2002). Social and psychological burden of dysphagia: Its impact on diagnosis and treatment. *Dysphagia, 17,* 139–146.

Festi, D., Scaioli, E., Baldi, F., Vestito, A., Pasqui, F., Di Biase, A. R., & Colecchia, A. (2009). Body weight, lifestyle, dietary habits and gastroesophageal reflux disease. *World Journal of Gastroenterology, 15,* 1690–1701.

Garcia, J., & Chambers, E. (2010). Managing dysphagia through diet modifications. *American Journal of Nursing, 110,* 26–33.

Germain, S., Dufresne, T., & Gray-Donald, K. (2006). A novel dysphagia diet improves the nutrient intake of institutionalized elders. *Journal of the American Dietetic Association, 106,* 1614–1623.

Makola, D., Peura, D., & Crowe, S. (2007). Helicobacter pylori infection and related gastrointestinal diseases [Review]. *Journal of Clinical Gastroenterology, 41,* 548–558.

Malfertheiner, P., Chan, F., & McCall, K. (2009). Peptic ulcer disease. *The Lancet, 374,* 1449–1461.

Matta, Z., Chambers, E., IV, Garcia, J., & McGowan Helverson, J. M. (2006). Sensory characteristics of beverages prepared with commercial thickeners used for dysphagia diets. *Journal of the American Dietetic Association, 106,* 1049–1054.

National Dysphagia Diet Task Force. (2002). *The national dysphagia diet: Standardization for optimal care.* Chicago, IL: American Dietetic Association.

Panther, K. (2005). The Frazier Free Water Protocol. Perspectives on swallowing and swallowing disorders. *Dysphagia, 14,* 4–9.

Ryan-Harshman, M., & Aldoori, W. (2004). How diet and lifestyle affect duodenal ulcers. *Canadian Family Physician, 50,* 727–732.

Stenson, W. (2006). The esophagus and the stomach. In M. E. Shils, M. Shike, A. C. Ross, B. Caballero, & R. J. Cousins (Eds.), *Modern nutrition in health and disease* (10th ed., pp. 1179–1188). Philadelphia, PA: Lippincott Williams & Wilkins.

Tytgat, G., McColl, K., Tack, J., Holtmann, G., Hunt, R. H., Malfertheiner, P., . . . Batchelor, H. K. (2008). New algorithm for the treatment of gastroesophageal reflux disease. *Alimentary Pharmacology and Therapeutics, 27,* 249–256.

Vemulapalli, R. (2008). Diet and lifestyle modifications in the management of gastroesophageal reflux disease. *Nutrition in Clinical Practice, 23,* 293–298.

Wagner, L. C. B. (2005). Ethical and legal implications of the Franzer Free Water Protocol. Perspectives on swallowing and swallowing disorders. *Dysphagia, 14,* 21–24.

18 Nutrition for Patients with Disorders of the Lower GI Tract and Accessory Organs

CHECK YOUR KNOWLEDGE

TRUE	FALSE	
☐	☐	**1** A high-fiber diet can prevent or alleviate constipation in most people.
☐	☐	**2** A clear liquid diet is the best oral diet for a patient with acute diarrhea.
☐	☐	**3** Probiotics are nondigestible fibers that stimulate the growth of intestinal bacteria.
☐	☐	**4** Many people with lactose intolerance can tolerate cheddar cheese.
☐	☐	**5** People with inflammatory bowel disease (IBD) should follow a low-fiber diet to prevent exacerbation of their disease.
☐	☐	**6** People with celiac disease need a gluten-free diet even when they are asymptomatic.
☐	☐	**7** A high-fiber diet has been proven to control symptoms of irritable bowel syndrome.
☐	☐	**8** A low-fiber diet increases the risk of diverticular disease.
☐	☐	**9** Fat is the nutrient most problematic for people with chronic pancreatitis.
☐	☐	**10** Most people with gallstones benefit from a low-fat diet.

LEARNING OBJECTIVES

Upon completion of this chapter, you will be able to

1 Modify a regular diet to be high in fiber.
2 Instruct a patient on the nutrition therapy recommendations for diarrhea.
3 Give examples of appropriate nutrition interventions for various symptoms and complications of malabsorption syndrome.
4 Modify a regular diet to be low in lactose.
5 Identify sources of gluten.
6 Instruct a patient with an ileostomy on appropriate diet modifications.
7 Compare a low-fat diet to a regular diet.

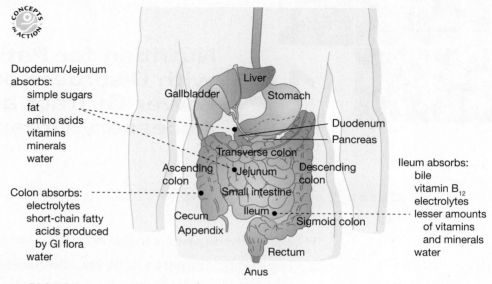

■ FIGURE 18.1   The sites of nutrient absorption.

The lower gastrointestinal (GI) tract consists of the small and large intestines, rectum, and anus. Ninety to 95% of nutrient absorption occurs in the first half of the small intestine (Fig. 18.1). The large intestine absorbs water and electrolytes and promotes the elimination of solid wastes. The accessory organs—liver, gallbladder, and pancreas—play vital roles in nutrient digestion. With many disorders of the lower GI tract and accessory organs, nutrition therapy is used to improve or control symptoms; replenish losses; and promote healing, if applicable. For one GI disorder, celiac disease, nutrition therapy is the sole mode of treatment. This chapter presents nutrition therapy for altered bowel elimination, malabsorption syndromes, disorders of the large intestine, and disorders of the accessory organs. Box 18.1 lists nutrition-focused assessment criteria for lower GI disorders.

Box 18.1   NUTRITION-FOCUSED ASSESSMENT FOR LOWER GI DISORDERS

- GI symptoms that interfere with intake, such as anorexia, early satiety, pain, abdominal distention
- Changes in eating made in response to symptoms
- Complications that impact nutritional status, such as weight loss, diarrhea, blood loss
- Usual pattern of eating and frequency of meals and snacks
- Adequacy of intake according to MyPlate recommendations, including fluid intake
- Use of tobacco, over-the-counter drugs for GI symptoms, alcohol, and caffeine
- Food allergies or intolerances, such as high-fat foods, milk, high-fiber foods
- Use of nutritional supplements including vitamins, minerals, fiber, and herbs
- Client's willingness to change his or her eating habits

ALTERED BOWEL ELIMINATION

Constipation

Constipation is defined as fewer than three bowel movements per week. Usually, the stools are hard, dry, small, and difficult to eliminate. The most common causes are low-fiber or high-fat diets (Academy of Nutrition and Dietetics [AND], 2012). Constipation can also occur secondary to irregular bowel habits, psychogenic factors, lack of activity, chronic laxative use, metabolic and endocrine disorders, and bowel abnormalities (e.g., tumors, hernias, strictures). Certain medications, such as codeine, aluminum hydroxide, iron supplements, and morphine, cause constipation. Contrary to popular belief, daily bowel movements are not necessary provided the stools are not hard and dry.

Nutrition Therapy

Constipation is treated by treating the underlying cause. For most people, increasing fiber and fluid intake effectively relieves and prevents constipation. Fiber is a group name that includes both soluble and insoluble forms; both types are found in all foods that provide fiber and both types impact bowel function. Soluble fibers, such as pectin and psyllium found in oats, legumes, and certain fruits and vegetables, dissolve in water to produce softer, bulkier stools that are more easily passed. Insoluble fiber, such as cellulose found in wheat bran and fruit and vegetable skins, soaks up water in the intestine to increase stool bulk and stimulate peristalsis. An adequate fluid intake is vital; without enough water, a high-fiber diet can worsen constipation, abdominal pain, bloating, and gas (AND, 2012).

The adequate intake (AI) set for fiber is 25 g/day for women and 38 g/day for men, based on amounts needed to protect against coronary heart disease not for optimal bowel function. The amount of fiber needed to alleviate constipation varies among individuals. The average American adult consumes approximately 12 to 18 g of fiber per day (Institute of Medicine, 2005).

A high-fiber diet is a regular diet with fiber-rich foods replacing low-fiber foods, such as whole wheat bread in place of white bread. Fresh fruits, vegetables, and dried peas and beans are encouraged (Box 18.2). However, most fruits, vegetables, and whole wheat breads provide only 1 to 3 g of fiber per serving; without a high-fiber cereal or daily intake of dried peas and beans, many people may require a fiber supplement to meet the Dietary Reference Intake (DRI) for fiber (Timm and Slavin, 2008).

It is common practice to recommend that fiber intake be gradually increased to avoid symptoms of intolerance such as gas, cramping, and diarrhea. If these side effects do occur, they are usually temporary and subside within several days. To achieve maximum benefit, fiber intake should be spread throughout the day.

Other interventions to promote bowel regularity include increasing aerobic exercise; consuming **probiotics** or **prebiotics** daily, such as yogurt containing live bacterial cultures, acidophilus milk, and kefir; and initiating a bowel retraining program when applicable.

Probiotics: live microorganisms found in food that, when consumed in adequate amounts, are beneficial to health.

Prebiotics: nondigestible food components that stimulate the growth of probiotic bacteria within the large intestine.

QUICK BITE

Fiber supplements
Promoted for regularity
Metamucil
Ready Fiber
Citrucel

Diarrhea

Diarrhea is a common symptom of many GI disorders and infectious diseases and is a frequent side effect of chemotherapy and radiation. It is characterized by an increase in the frequency of bowel movements and/or water content of stools, which alters either the consistency or

Box 18.2 HIGH-FIBER DIET

- A high-fiber diet is a regular diet that substitutes whole grains for refined grains and is high in other fiber-rich foods—namely, fresh fruits, vegetables, and dried peas and beans.
- Unprocessed bran may be added as tolerated.
- At least eight 8-oz glasses of fluid are recommended daily.
- A high-fiber diet is used for constipation, diverticulosis, and irritable bowel syndrome. It may also promote weight loss and helps lower serum cholesterol levels and improve glucose tolerance in diabetes. All healthy Americans are urged to increase their intake of fiber.
- The diet should not be used in cases of intestinal inflammation or stenosis, gastroparesis, postgastrectomy, or pseudo-obstruction.

Guidelines to Achieve a High-Fiber Diet
- Substitute whole grains for refined grains.

Use	In place of
Whole wheat bread	White bread
Brown rice	White rice
Whole wheat pasta	White pasta
Bran or whole-grain cereal	Refined cereals
Whole wheat flour	White flour

- Eat more dried peas or beans.
- Eat more fresh fruit; leave the skin on whenever possible. Apples, blackberries, blueberries, figs, dates, kiwifruit, mango, oranges, pears, prunes, strawberries, and raspberries are high in fiber.
- Eat more vegetables. Cooked asparagus, green beans, broccoli, Brussels sprouts, cabbage, carrots, celery, corn, eggplant, parsnips, peas, snowpeas, Swiss chard, and turnips are good choices.
- Other foods with fiber include popcorn, nuts, sunflower seeds, and sesame seeds.

Sample Menu

Breakfast	Lunch	Dinner	Snacks
Prune juice	Split pea soup	Roast chicken	Low-fat popcorn
Bran flakes with milk	Ham sandwich on whole wheat bread with lettuce and tomato	Brown rice	Dried fruit and nuts
Whole wheat toast with jelly	Fresh strawberries	Tossed salad with fresh vegetables	Raw carrots and celery with dip
Fresh orange sections	Date cookie	Steamed broccoli	
	Milk	Whole wheat roll with butter	
		Milk	
		Blueberries over ice cream	

Potential Problems	Recommended Interventions
Flatus, distention, cramping, and osmotic diarrhea related to increasing fiber content of the diet too much or too quickly	Initiate a high-fiber diet gradually to develop the patient's tolerance. If symptoms of intolerance persist, reduce fiber content to maximum amount tolerated by the patient.

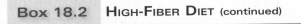

Box 18.2   HIGH-FIBER DIET (continued)

Patient Teaching
Instruct the patient that

- A high-fiber diet increases stool bulk and speeds passage of food through intestines.
- Increasing fiber intake gradually may be better tolerated than increasing fiber intake quickly.
- Fiber intake may be increased by making subtle changes in eating and cooking habits such as eating more fresh fruits and vegetables, especially with the skin on.
- Switching to high-fiber breads and cereals can significantly increase fiber intake; the first ingredient on the label should be "whole wheat" or "100% whole wheat," not just "wheat."
- A variety of foods high in fiber should be eaten; numerous forms of fiber exist, and each performs a different action in the body (see Chapter 2).
- A meatless main dish made with dried peas and beans is a high-fiber alternative to traditional entrées.
- Fresh or dried fruit make high-fiber snacks.
- Although nuts and seeds are high in fiber, they are also high in fat and should be used sparingly.
- Coarse, unprocessed wheat bran is most effective as a laxative; it can be incorporated into the diet by mixing it with juice or milk; by adding it to muffins, quick breads, casseroles, and meat loaves before baking; or by sprinkling it over cereal, applesauce, eggs, or other foods.
- Bran should be added to the diet slowly (up to 3 tbsp/day) to decrease the likelihood of developing flatus and distention.
- Certain foods (in addition to being high in fiber) have laxative effects: prunes and prune juice, figs, and dates.
- At least eight 8-oz glasses of fluid should be consumed daily.

volume of fecal output. A rapid transit time decreases the time available for water, sodium, and potassium to be absorbed through the colon; the result is more water and electrolytes in the stools and the potential for dehydration, hyponatremia, hypokalemia, acid–base imbalance, and metabolic acidosis. Chronic diarrhea can lead to malnutrition related to impaired digestion, absorption, and intake. Diarrhea is a major cause of childhood death worldwide; an estimated 840,000 children died from its complications in 2011 (World Health Organization, 2012).

Osmotic diarrhea occurs when there is an increase in particles in the intestine, which draws water in to dilute the high concentration. The causes of osmotic diarrhea include maldigestion of nutrients (e.g., lactose intolerance), excessive intake of sorbitol or fructose, dumping syndrome, tube feedings, and some laxatives. It is cured by treating the underlying cause.

Secretory diarrhea is related to an excessive secretion of fluid and electrolytes into the intestines. Bacterial, viral, protozoan, and other infections cause secretory diarrhea, as do some medications and some GI disorders, such as Crohn disease and celiac disease. An excessive amount of bile acids or unabsorbed fatty acids in the colon can also cause secretory diarrhea. If the cause is infection, antibiotics are the primary component of treatment. Symptoms may be treated with medications that decrease GI motility or thicken the consistency of stools, such as the soluble fiber psyllium (Metamucil).

Nutrition Therapy

Nutrition therapy for diarrhea is largely supportive and depends on the severity of diarrhea and the underlying cause. Maintaining or restoring fluid and electrolyte balance is the primary

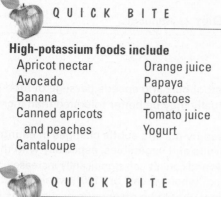

Q U I C K   B I T E

High-potassium foods include

Apricot nectar	Orange juice
Avocado	Papaya
Banana	Potatoes
Canned apricots and peaches	Tomato juice
Cantaloupe	Yogurt

Q U I C K   B I T E

Items that stimulate GI motility
Diarrhea may improve by avoiding foods that stimulate GI motility, such as the following:

- Alcohol
- Caffeine
- Items high in simple sugars, such as milk (lactose), fruit (fructose), and carbonated beverages (sucrose)
- High-fiber and gas-producing foods, such as nuts, beans, corn, broccoli, and cabbage
- Sugar alcohols (e.g., sorbitol in "dietetic" products)

Lactose: the disaccharide (double sugar) in milk composed of glucoses and galactose.

focus. Mild diarrhea lasting 24 to 48 hours usually requires no nutrition intervention other than encouraging a liberal fluid intake to replace losses. High-potassium foods are encouraged. Clear liquids are avoided because they have high osmolality related to their high sugar content, which may promote osmotic diarrhea. For more serious cases, commercial (e.g., Pedialyte, Rehydralyte) or homemade oral rehydration solutions or intravenous (IV) therapy are used to replace fluid and electrolytes.

Probiotics may help lessen diarrhea related to use of antibiotics or lactose intolerance (Douglas and Sanders, 2008). Because it is not known which strains or doses of probiotics may be most beneficial, it may be prudent to obtain probiotics from food sources instead of supplements (Fig. 18.2). On a short-term basis, a low-fiber diet (Box 18.3) that is also low in fat and lactose may help decrease bowel stimulation. This diet may be inadequate in some nutrients depending on the specific foods chosen. Patients with intractable diarrhea may need complete bowel rest (i.e., total parenteral nutrition, or TPN).

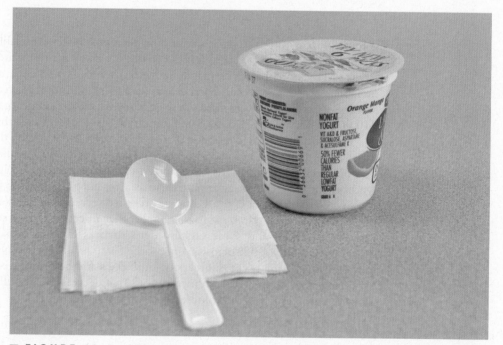

■ **FIGURE 18.2**   Many yogurts now contain beneficial microorganisms called "probiotics."

Box 18.3   LOW-FIBER DIET

- This diet restricts fiber to decrease the volume and frequency of stools.
- This diet is a short-term diet to be used when the bowel is inflamed, such as in the acute stages of diverticulitis, ulcerative colitis, and regional enteritis. It may also be used for esophageal and intestinal stenosis and in preparation for bowel surgery.

General Guidelines to Achieve a Low-Fiber Diet
- Use refined breads and cereals that provide 0 to 1 g fiber/serving, such as white bread and rolls, white pasta, white rice, low-fiber cereals.
- Eat only vegetables that do not have skins or seeds and are well cooked.
- Choose canned or cooked fruit and fruit juices without pulp (except prune juice); ripe bananas, citrus sections without membranes.
- Eat plain desserts made without nuts or coconut, such as plain cakes, puddings (rice, bread, plain), cookies, and ice cream.
- Avoid foods high in fiber.
  - Whole-grain breads and cereals
  - Most raw vegetables, vegetables with seeds, gassy vegetables, cooked greens or spinach
  - Fresh fruit with skins or seeds, dried fruits, prune juice
  - Dried peas and beans
  - Anything containing nuts, seeds, or coconut; popcorn

Additional Recommendations
- Avoid milk and milk products that contain lactose if lactose intolerance is suspected. Low-lactose and lactose-free alternatives include acidophilus milk, yogurt, soy milk, and almond milk.
- Avoid high-fat protein foods (sausage, bacon, many cold cuts) and high-fat dairy products (whole milk, sour cream, ice cream).
- Avoid items that stimulate GI motility: alcohol, caffeine, sorbitol, and xylitol.
- Limit beverages made with high-fructose corn syrup (HFCS) to 12 oz/day.
- Probiotic foods may help, such as yogurt with live bacterial cultures, acidophilus milk, and kefir.

Sample Menu

Breakfast	Lunch	Dinner	Snacks
Strained orange juice Poached egg White toast with jelly	Tomato juice Turkey sandwich on white bread with salad dressing Canned peach halves	Roast chicken White rice Cooked carrots Italian bread with olive oil Gelatin made with ripe bananas Soy milk	Saltine crackers Rice cakes Tomato juice Fresh banana Milk

Potential Problems	Recommended Interventions
Constipation related to low fiber content of diet; insufficient fiber intake causes decrease in stool bulk and slowing of intestinal transit time	Liberalize diet to allow more fiber; this diet is intended to be short-term.
Persistent diarrhea related to poor tolerance of even small amounts of fiber contained in a low-residue diet; tolerance of fiber varies among patients and conditions	Further reduce fiber content by eliminating all fruits and vegetables except strained fruit juice.

(continues on page 468)

Box 18.3   LOW-FIBER DIET (continued)

Patient Teaching
Instruct the patient that

- Reducing fiber slows passage of food through the bowel.
- Fiber is a component of plants and, therefore, is found in fruits, vegetables, whole grains, dried peas and beans, and nuts.
- Diet is intended to be short-term.
- Food preparation techniques to reduce fiber include removing skins, seeds, and membranes of fruits and vegetables that are high in fiber and cooking allowed vegetables until they are very tender.

MALABSORPTION DISORDERS

Malabsorption: a broad term that describes altered or inadequate nutrient absorption from the GI tract.

Malabsorption occurs secondary to nutrient maldigestion or from alterations to the absorptive surface of the intestinal mucosa. Generally, malabsorption related to maldigestion involves one or few nutrients, whereas malabsorption that stems from an altered mucosa is more generalized, resulting in multiple nutrient deficiencies and weight loss.

Symptoms of malabsorption vary with the underlying disorder, ranging from minimal to widespread and serious. Malabsorption may be suspected in patients who have weight loss, growth failure, bloating, and flatulence (Kelly, 2006). Watery diarrhea and distention are symptoms of malabsorption from carbohydrate maldigestion (e.g., lactose intolerance), whereas the passage of less frequent stools that are oily, bulky, and foul-smelling is a symptom of malabsorption related to fat maldigestion (e.g., pancreatitis). The excretion of fat in the stools means that essential fatty acids, fat-soluble vitamins, calcium, and magnesium are also lost through the stools. Deficiencies of these nutrients can cause metabolic complications (Table 18.1). Appetite may be poor and nutrient needs may be elevated for healing. The risk for malnutrition can be high.

Steatorrhea: excess fat in the stools that are loose, foamy, and foul-smelling.

The goal of nutrition therapy for malabsorption syndromes is to control **steatorrhea**, promote normal bowel elimination, restore optimal nutritional status, and promote healing, when applicable. Nutrition therapy is individualized according to symptoms and complications; possible diet modifications appear in Table 18.2. Specific malabsorption syndromes are discussed in the following sections—namely, lactose intolerance, inflammatory bowel disease (IBD), celiac disease, and short bowel syndrome.

Table 18.1 Potential Secondary Nutrient Deficiencies of Malabsorption Syndrome

Potential Secondary Nutrient Deficiencies	Potential Problems
Protein	Hypoalbuminemia, edema, muscle weakness, increased risk of infection, poor wound healing
Potassium	Muscle weakness
Calcium, magnesium, vitamin D	Osteomalacia and bone pain
Calcium, magnesium	Tetany
B-complex vitamins	Stomatitis, cheilosis, glossitis, and dermatitis
Iron, folic acid, vitamin B_{12}	Anemia, fatigue, pallor, weakness, palpitations, anorexia, indigestion, sore mouth
Vitamin K	Purpura and easy bleeding
Vitamin A	Roughening of skin, impaired night vision, increased risk of infections

Table 18.2 Nutrition Therapy for Malabsorption Symptoms

Symptoms	Dietary Interventions	Rationale
Anorexia	Small, frequent meals	To maximize intake
	Commercial supplements	Liquid supplements are easy to consume, are nutritionally dense, and leave the stomach quickly
	Enteral nutrition if anorexia is severe and/or prolonged	To meet calorie and nutrient needs until the patient is able to consume an adequate oral intake
Diarrhea	Low-fiber diet	To minimize stimulation to the bowel
	Ensure adequate fluid and electrolytes.	Increased losses of fluid and electrolytes in the stool
Lactose intolerance	Avoid lactose.	Lactase activity may be lost during acute episodes of malabsorption due to altered integrity and function of intestinal villi cells; lactase deficiency may persist into remission.
Nephrolithiasis (calcium oxalate stones related to increased oxalate absorption secondary to increased fecal excretion of calcium)	Limit high-oxalate foods, such as chocolate, cocoa, certain fruits and vegetables, grits, soy products, peanut butter.	To decrease the amount of oxalate available for absorption
	Adequate fluid	To dilute the urine
Nutrient deficiencies	Nutrient-dense diet	To replenish losses, facilitate healing, and meet increased needs related to the metabolism of a high-calorie, high-protein diet
	Vitamin supplements; may need water-soluble forms of the fat-soluble vitamins	Dietary sources may not be adequate to meet need. Water-soluble forms do not require normal fat absorption to be absorbed, as do fat-soluble vitamins in their natural form.
	Oral or parenteral vitamin B_{12}	Bacterial overgrowth, pancreatic insufficiency, and ileal disease or resection impair B_{12} absorption.
	Calcium supplements	Serum calcium may be low related to low serum albumin or calcium malabsorption related to poor vitamin D absorption or the binding of calcium with unabsorbed fats to form unabsorbable soaps.
	Other mineral supplements	Magnesium levels are often low in some malabsorption syndromes; losses of zinc are high in patients with fistulas.
Steatorrhea	Limit fat.	To avoid aggravating fat malabsorption
	MCT oil may be used for calories.	MCT oil is absorbed without undergoing digestion.

(continues on page 470)

Table 18.2 Nutrition Therapy for Malabsorption Symptoms (continued)

Symptoms	Dietary Interventions	Rationale
Tissue damage (e.g., resulting from inflammation or surgery) and/or weight loss	Increase calories (2000–3500 cal/day) Increase protein (1.0–1.5 g/kg/day)	Calories and protein are needed to facilitate healing and restore weight.
Calcium oxalate kidney stones related to binding of calcium to fat instead of oxalate, leaving increased amount of oxalate available for absorption into the blood	Increase fluids Avoid high-oxalate foods, such as green leafy vegetables, chocolate milk, dried peas and beans, potatoes, and whole wheat products.	To dilute the urine To limit oxalate available for absorption

Lactose Intolerance

Lactose intolerance occurs when lactase, the enzyme that splits lactose into its component simple sugars glucose and galactose, is absent or deficient. Without adequate lactase, lactose digestion is impaired; particles of undigested lactose increase the osmolality of intestinal contents, which may lead to osmotic diarrhea. Lactose is fermented in the colon, which produces bloating, cramping, and flatulence. Symptoms occur between 15 minutes and 2 hours after eating and range from mild to severe, depending on the amount of lactase actually produced and the amount of lactose consumed.

Primary lactose intolerance occurs in "well" people who simply do not secrete adequate lactase. Eighty percent or more of Asians, Native Americans, and Africans are lactose intolerant; lactose intolerance is least common in people of northern European descent (National Institute of Diabetes and Digestive and Kidney Diseases [NIDDK], 2012c). People with primary lactose intolerance may be asymptomatic when they consume doses less than 4 to 12 g of lactose (e.g., ⅓ to 1 cup of milk) or when lactose is consumed as part of a meal. Chocolate milk is usually better tolerated than plain milk, and because much of the lactose in yogurt is digested by its bacteria, it is also usually well tolerated unless milk is added. Simply knowing individual limits (e.g., 8 oz of milk with dinner is tolerated but 8 oz of milk between meals is not) is enough to prevent symptoms. For people who want to consume milk or lactose-containing foods beyond their limit, lactose-reduced milk and lactase enzyme tablets or liquid may be used.

A more problematic lactose intolerance occurs secondary to GI disorders that alter the integrity and function of intestinal villi cells, where lactase is secreted. For instance, people with IBD lose lactase activity when the disease is active and sometimes for a prolonged period afterward. The loss of lactase may also develop secondary to malnutrition because the rapidly growing intestinal cells that produce lactase are reduced in number and function. Secondary lactose intolerance tends to be more severe than primary lactose intolerance, and symptoms occur more quickly after eating lactose.

Nutrition Therapy

Nutrition therapy for lactose intolerance is to reduce lactose to the maximum amount tolerated by the individual (Box 18.4). For patients with GI disorders, a lactose-restricted diet is indicated at least until the disorder is resolved and sometimes for a prolonged period thereafter. Because lactose is used as an ingredient in many foods and drugs, a lactose-free diet is not realistic.

Box 18.4   LOW-LACTOSE DIET

- Lactose is the sugar in milk; limit or avoid milk and foods made with milk.
- Individual tolerance varies; eat dairy foods as tolerance allows.
- Choose nondairy sources of calcium to ensure an adequate intake, such as canned salmon with bones, calcium-fortified tofu, orange juice, and soy milk; shellfish; "greens" such as turnip, collard, and kale; dried peas and beans; broccoli; and almonds.
- Read labels to identify lactose.
  - Lactate, lactic acid, lactalbumin, and casein are lactose free.
  - Kosher foods labeled *pareve* are made without milk.
  - Avoid products whose ingredient list contains butter, cream, milk, milk solids, or whey.

Lactose-Free Milk and Nondairy Foods	Low-Lactose Dairy Foods	Possible Hidden Sources of Lactose
Lactose-free milk	Aged cheese, such as	Bread
Almond, rice, or soy milk	cheddar, Swiss, and parmesan	Baked goods
Soy yogurt, soy cheese	Cream cheese	Breakfast cereals
Soy sour cream	Ricotta cheese	Instant potatoes and soups
	Cottage cheese	Margarine
	Yogurt	Lunch meats
		Salad dressings
		Mixes for pancakes, biscuits and cookies
		Powdered meal replacement supplements

Inflammatory Bowel Disease

Inflammatory bowel disease (IBD) primarily refers to two chronic inflammatory GI diseases: Crohn disease and ulcerative colitis. IBD is believed to be caused by an abnormal immune response to a complex interaction between environmental and genetic factors (Hanauer, 2006). Crohn disease and ulcerative colitis are characterized by periods of exacerbation and remission; they share common symptoms and treatments (Table 18.3).

Nutrition Therapy

Nutrition therapy for IBD depends on the presence and severity of symptoms, the presence of complications, and the nutritional status of the patient. Diet restrictions are kept to a minimum to encourage an adequate intake, and the diet is liberalized during periods of remission. Patients are often reluctant to eat because they associate eating with pain and diarrhea. In general, Crohn disease is more likely to cause nutritional complications than ulcerative colitis.

Glutamine: a nonessential amino acid that maintains the integrity of the intestinal mucosa and helps prevent pathogenic bacteria from crossing the intestinal barrier into the bloodstream, thereby reducing the risk of GI-derived septicemia.

The focus of therapy for acute exacerbation of IBD is to correct deficiencies by providing nutrients in a form the patient can tolerate. In some cases, a hydrolyzed enteral feeding, possibly one fortified with **glutamine**, may be used to minimize fecal volume. Parenteral nutrition (PN) has not been shown to be advantageous over enteral nutrition (EN) but may be necessary in patients who need complete bowel rest due to extreme malabsorption or fistulas (AND, 2012).

Table 18.3 Comparison Between Crohn Disease and Ulcerative Colitis

	Crohn's Disease	Ulcerative Colitis
Area affected	Can occur anywhere along the GI tract but most commonly occurs in the ileum and colon	Confined to the rectum and colon
Disease pattern	Inflammation is discontinuous, with normal tissue between patches of inflamed tissue. All layers of the bowel are affected.	Inflammation is continuous, beginning at rectum and usually extending into the colon. Affects only the mucosal layer
Main symptoms	Diarrhea, abdominal pain, weight loss	Diarrhea, abdominal pain, rectal bleeding Weight loss, fever, and weakness are common when most of the colon is involved.
Complications	Fistulas, abscesses Stricture of the ileum Bowel perforation Bowel obstructions may occur from scar tisssue formation. Toxic megacolon Increased risk of intestinal cancer	Tissue erosin and ulceration Toxic megacolon Greatly increased risk of cancer
Nutritional complications	Impaired bile acid reabsorption may cause malabsorption of fat, fat-soluble vitamins, calcium, magnesium, and zinc. Malnutrition may occur from nutrient malabsorption, decreased intake, or intestinal resections. Anemia related to blood loss or malabsorption Vitamin B_{12} deficiency related to B_{12} malabsorption from the ileum due to inflammation	Anemia related to blood loss Dehydration and electrolyte imbalances related to diarrhea Protein depletion from losses through inflamed tissue
Medical treatment	Antidiarrheals, immunosuppressants, immunomodulators, biologic therapies, and anti-inflammatory agents	Antidiarrheals, immunosuppressants, and anti-inflammatory agents
Surgical intervention	Most common procedure is ileostomy; disease often recurs in the remaining intestine.	Most common procedure is total colectomy; surgery prevents recurrence.

For patients consuming food orally, a low-fiber diet is recommended to minimize bowel stimulation (see Box 18.3). Protein and calories are increased to facilitate healing. Lactose is avoided if lactose intolerance is suspected. Small, frequent meals may help maximize intake. Other diet modifications are made according to symptoms (see Table 18.2).

The diet is liberalized as soon as possible, and a diet as near normal as tolerated is recommended during remission. A pilot study suggests that a low-FODMAP (fermentable oligosaccharides, disaccharides, and monosaccharides and polyols) diet may benefit patients whose IBD is in remission and who do not have strictures but who have irritable bowel syndrome symptoms (Gearry et al., 2009). See the section on irritable bowel syndrome.

Celiac Disease

Celiac disease is a genetic autoimmune disorder characterized by chronic inflammation of the proximal small intestine mucosa related to a permanent intolerance to certain proteins found in wheat, barley, and rye. When ingested, these proteins trigger an immune response that damages the villi that line the mucosa of the small intestine. Malabsorption of carbohydrates, protein, fat, vitamins, and minerals may occur, resulting in diarrhea, flatulence, weight loss, vitamin and mineral deficiencies (e.g., folate, calcium, iron, and vitamin D), iron deficiency anemia, and loss of bone.

Symptoms and their severity vary widely among individuals, depending on the patient's age and the duration and extent of the disease. Children typically exhibit GI symptoms such as chronic diarrhea, abdominal distention, vomiting, constipation, fatty stools, weight loss, irritability, and failure to thrive. Adults may also present with diarrhea, constipation, weight loss, weakness, flatus, abdominal pain, and vomiting or with non-GI symptoms such as unexplained iron deficiency anemia, chronic fatigue, bone or joint pain, infertility, and unexplained neurologic disorders. In 15% to 25% of people with celiac disease, **dermatitis herpetiformis** is the presenting symptom (NIDDK, 2012a). Although these patients do not usually have GI symptoms, results of serology and biopsies are identical to those of people with celiac disease. Symptoms of dermatitis herpetiformis respond to a gluten-free diet (Niewinski, 2008).

Dermatitis Herpetiformis: a chronic inflammatory skin disease characterized by groups of red, raised blisters that itch and burn.

People with subclinical celiac disease have no symptoms, yet they have positive serologic test results, and biopsy of the intestinal villi shows atrophy. These people are identified through screening of at-risk groups or from biopsies obtained for other reasons, such as dyspepsia. People who have a first-degree relative with celiac disease, people with Down syndrome, and those with an autoimmune disease are at risk for celiac disease. Untreated celiac disease is associated with an increased incidence of small bowel cancers and enteropathy-associated T-cell lymphoma (Card, West, and Holmes, 2004).

Nutrition Therapy

Gluten: a general name for the storage proteins gliadin (in wheat), secalin (in rye), and hordein (in barley).

The only scientifically proven treatment for celiac disease is to completely and permanently eliminate **gluten** from the diet. A gluten-free diet (Box 18.5) allows the villi to return toward normal and improvements in diarrhea and weight loss may begin within weeks of starting the diet. A gluten-free diet can restore body weight and nutritional status, although it may take at least 12 months of dietary compliance (American Gastroenterological Association, 2006). However, a gluten-free diet does not guarantee mucosal recovery in all adults. A recent study showed that after 2 years of adherence to a gluten-free diet, only 34% of adults were confirmed to have mucosal recovery (Rubio-Tapio et al., 2010). After 5 years, one out of three adults studied still had intestinal damage, even though the symptoms of diarrhea and weight loss were eliminated.

Gluten is found in wheat, rye, and barley—grains that form the foundation of a healthy diet in most cultures. Pure oats are gluten free and, therefore, not harmful to people with celiac disease. However, there is worldwide concern that the risk of oats being contaminated with gluten is unacceptably high. The Academy of Nutrition and Dietetics Celiac Disease Evidence-Based Nutrition Practice Guidelines recommend that only oats labeled gluten-free be consumed as tolerated, up to 50 g daily, which is approximately ½ cup of dry rolled oats (AND Evidence Analysis Library, 2012).

Box 18.5   GLUTEN-FREE DIET

- Gluten, a protein fraction found in wheat, rye, and barley, is eliminated. Oats are at high risk of gluten contamination, so only oats labeled gluten-free are allowed. All products made from these grains or their flours are eliminated.
- Many foods are naturally gluten free: milk, butter, cheese; fresh, frozen, and canned fruits and vegetables; fresh meat, fish, poultry, eggs; dried peas and beans; nuts; corn; and rice.

Allowed Grains and Related Foods	Grains to Eliminate	Questionable Foods (may contain wheat, barley, or rye)

Amaranth
Arrowroot
Buckwheat
Cassava
Corn, cornstarch
Flax
Gums
  Acacia (gum Arabic)
  Carob bean gum
  Carrageenan
  Cellulose
  Guar
  Locust bean
  Xanthan
Indian rice grass
Job's tears
Legumes, legume flours
Millet
Nut flours
Oats (uncontaminated)
Potatoes, potato flour
Quinoa
Rice, all plain; rice flour
Sago
Seeds
Soy
Sorghum
Tapioca
Teff
Wild rice
Yucca
	Wheat–all forms including
	- Wheat flours, such as bromated flour, durum flour, enriched flour, graham flour, phosphated flour, plain flour, self-rising flour, semolina, white flour
	- Wheat starch, wheat bran, wheat germ, cracked wheat, hydrolyzed wheat protein, farina
	- Einkorn, emmer, spelt, kamut
	Barley
	Rye
	Malt
	Triticale (a cross between wheat and rye)
		Brown rice syrup
		Chips/potato chips
		Candy
		Cold cuts, hot dogs, salami, sausage
		Communion wafer
		Flavored or herbal coffee
		Flavored or herbal tea
		French fries
		Gravy
		Imitation fish
		Meat substitutes
		Matzo
		Rice and corn cereals (may contain barley malt)
		Rice mixes
		Sauces
		Seasoned or dry roasted nuts
		Seasoned tortilla chips
		Self-basting turkey
		Soups
		Soy sauce
		Vegetables in sauce

Sample Menu

Breakfast	Lunch	Dinner	Snacks
Orange juice Cornflakes Milk Coffee	Cuban black beans with rice Pure corn tortilla Milk Trail mix over plain yogurt Coffee/tea	Tomato juice Roast chicken Baked potato with margarine Tossed salad with olive oil and cider vinegar dressing Steamed broccoli Corn bread made without wheat flour Blueberries over ice cream made without gluten stabilizers	Plain nuts Rice cake Banana Apple slices with peanut butter

Box 18.5   GLUTEN-FREE DIET (continued)

Additional Considerations

- Patients may be discouraged and overwhelmed when faced with a lifelong restricted diet. Provide support, encouragement, and thorough diet instructions.
- The patient may be temporarily lactose intolerant and may require a lactose-restricted diet.

Potential Problems	Recommended Interventions
Increased expense related to buying special gluten-free foods	Encourage the patient to use as many "normal" items as possible such as corn cereals, grits, rice, and rice cereals; they are easy to obtain and less expensive than special products.
Inadequate intake of several nutrients (niacin, folate, zinc, and iron) related to the lower content of these nutrients in gluten-free products compared to the enriched and fortified grains and cereals they replace	Encourage a varied diet of allowed foods; recommend a gluten-free, age-appropriate multivitamin and mineral supplement.
Inadequate intake of fiber related to the absence of whole wheat products	Encourage fiber from legumes, nuts, fruit, vegetables, and gluten-free whole grains such as flax seed, millet, uncontaminated oats, quinoa, brown rice, and amaranth.

Patient Teaching

Instruct the patient on the importance of adhering to the diet even when no symptoms are present. "Cheating" on the diet can damage intestinal villi even if no symptoms develop. To permanently eliminate all flours and products containing wheat, rye, barley, triticale, and malt, the patient should

- Read labels. As per the Food Allergen Labeling and Consumer Protection Act of 2004, all food products must be clearly labeled to indicate the presence of wheat. This Act simplifies label reading to identify wheat gluten, but less obvious sources of gluten from barley (e.g., malt flavorings and extracts) require more careful reading. Patients should check with the manufacturer *before* using products of questionable composition.
- Use corn, potato, rice, arrowroot, and soybean flours and their products.
- Use the following as thickening agents: arrowroot starch, cornstarch, tapioca starch, rice starch, and sweet rice flour.
- Eat an otherwise normal, well-balanced diet adequate in nutrients and calories. Lactose is restricted only if not tolerated. Weight gain may be slowly achieved.

Provide the patient with the following aids:

- A detailed list of foods allowed and not allowed
- Information regarding support groups; see websites at the end of this chapter
- Gluten-free recipes

A gluten-free diet requires a major lifestyle change, so compliance is a major challenge. Gluten-free products (e.g., breads, pastry) made with rice, corn, or potato flour have different textures and tastes than "normal" products and are not well accepted. They are also expensive. Even patients who are willing to comply have difficulty following the diet because of the pervasiveness of gluten in processed foods and medications and confusion over identifying sources of gluten on food labels. The diet is very restrictive, requires conscientious label reading, and is difficult to adhere to while eating out.

Many patients with celiac disease eat gluten occasionally or in normal amounts and do not complain of symptoms. Yet even without symptoms, the intestinal mucosa is abnormal in most patients, and the risk of cancer is increased. Conversely, strict adherence to a gluten-free diet usually allows the mucosa to heal, resolves GI symptoms, and helps prevent complications associated with long-term untreated celiac disease, such as non-Hodgkin lymphoma (Thompson, 2005). Patients need to understand that the long-term effects of eating even small amounts of gluten are harmful, even in asymptomatic patients.

Short Bowel Syndrome

Short Bowel Syndrome (SBS): a complex condition resulting from extensive surgical resection of the intestinal tract usually because of inflammatory bowel disease, cancer, or obstruction.

Short bowel syndrome (SBS) occurs when the bowel is surgically shortened to the extent that the remaining bowel is unable to absorb adequate levels of nutrients to meet the individual's needs. Typically a loss of more than 50% to 70% of the small bowel results in SBS (Parrish, 2005). Symptoms include diarrhea, steatorrhea, weight loss, and dehydration. Impaired growth may occur in children. Crohn disease, traumatic abdominal injuries, malignant tumors, and mesenteric infarction are the most common reasons for extensive intestinal resections that result in SBS.

Nutrition complications experienced by people with SBS depend on the amount and location of resected and remaining bowel. Patients who have 150 cm or more of remaining small bowel without a colon, or 60 to 90 cm of remaining small bowel with a colon, initially require PN and may progress to an oral diet over a 1- to 2-year period (Matarese et al., 2005). Adaptation depends on the length of remaining jejunum and/or ileum and whether the colon is present. Other factors that influence adaptation include the patient's age; whether the ileocecal valve remains; the health of the remaining bowel; and the health of the stomach, liver, and pancreas (Fessler, 2007). Patients with less than 100 to 140 cm of small bowel and no colon will likely need either intestinal transplantation or permanent PN.

Nutrition Therapy

In the early months after bowel surgery, PN is the major source of nutrition and hydration until the remaining bowel adapts. However, it is now accepted that patients should consume whole-food diets or, if enterally fed, an intact formula as soon as possible for maximum bowel stimulation and adaptation and to reduce reliance on PN (Parrish, 2005). Nutrition may be provided by several different combinations, such as an oral diet with PN or EN or PN with EN; daytime feedings may be by one route, nocturnal by another. When the patient can consume oral nutrition without excessive stool or ostomy output and can maintain or gain weight, the amount of PN is gradually decreased (Fessler, 2007). During the weaning process, PN may be infused every other day.

Consuming intact nutrients promotes bowel adaptation because they stimulate blood flow to the intestine and the secretion of pancreatic enzymes and bile acids (Fessler, 2007). However, because of malabsorption and steatorrhea, patients may need to consume 200%

to 400% more than their estimated needs to compensate for losses (Parrish, 2005). Other considerations are as follows:

- If the patient's colon is intact, a lower fat intake is recommended to avoid steatorrhea and increased fluid losses: approximately 50% to 60% carbohydrates, 20% to 30% protein, and 20% to 30% fat (Parrish, 2005). The intake of complex carbohydrates is encouraged because colonic bacteria ferment them to short-chain fatty acids, an important source of energy.
- When the colon is absent (e.g., patients with jejunostomies or ileostomies), a higher fat diet is preferable: approximately 20% to 30% carbohydrate, 20% to 30% protein, and 50% to 60% fat (Parrish, 2005).
- Medium-chain triglyceride (MCT) oil is often recommended as a source of calories because it is absorbed directly through the mucosa. However, MCT is less effective than long-chain triglycerides at promoting bowel adaptation and is costly and unpalatable. Commercial beverages that contain MCT oil, such as Promote or Nutren 2.0, may be a more acceptable option.
- Six to eight small meals per day are recommended. Food should be thoroughly chewed to increase the surface area for enzymes and bile to work.
- Liquids should be consumed after meals and snacks, not with food. Solids leave the stomach more slowly than liquids.
- Simple sugars are avoided to limit the osmolar load to the intestine and osmotic diarrhea.
- Salty foods are encouraged when the colon is removed.
- Lactose intolerance may occur, although small amounts of lactose may be tolerated if spread out over the day (Parrish, 2005).
- Other diet modifications are made according to the patient's symptoms/complications (see Table 18.2). A sample menu appears in Box 18.6.

Box 18.6   SAMPLE MENU FOR PATIENT WITH SHORT BOWEL SYNDROME (APPROXIMATELY 2400 CALORIES, 50% CARBOHYDRATE, 20% PROTEIN, 30% FAT; LOW LACTOSE, LOW SUGAR)

Breakfast
1 cup Rice Krispies
2 oz Lactaid milk
Poached egg
2 slices toast with diet jelly

Snack
6 oz artificially sweetened low-fat yogurt
½ bagel with margarine
½ banana

Snack
8 oz Promote (low-fat, lactose-free, high-protein oral formula)

Lunch
3 oz deli turkey with mayonnaise on a hamburger roll
½ cup canned peaches
8 oz artificially sweetened low-fat yogurt

Snack
2 slices zucchini bread
1 oz cheese

Snack
1 oz pretzels
½ banana

Dinner
3 oz lean roast beef
Roasted potatoes
½ cup green beans
Dinner roll with 1 tsp butter
½ cup unsweetened applesauce

Snack
8 oz Promote

Note: Throughout the day in between meals: 1.5 to 2.0 L of fluid or more as needed.

CONDITIONS OF THE LARGE INTESTINE

Irritable Bowel Syndrome

Functional Bowel Disorder: functional GI disease with symptoms attributed to the middle or lower GI tract. Diagnosis is based on established criteria and the exclusion of organic causes.

Irritable bowel syndrome (IBS), one of the most frequently diagnosed digestive disorders in the United States, is a **functional bowel disorder**. It affects as many as 20% of American adults, predominately women (NIDDK, 2012b). Although it is commonly categorized as a motility disorder, there are likely many factors involved in its etiology, including genetics, environmental factors, alterations in gut flora, nervous system alterations, and psychosocial stressors (Clark and DeLegge, 2008). Symptoms include lower abdominal pain; excessive flatus; bloating; and altered GI motility, which may be constipation, diarrhea, or alternating periods of each. IBS can significantly impair quality of life.

IBS may be treated with a variety of therapies aimed at controlling symptoms. Antidiarrheals, antispasmodics, and antidepressants are pharmacologic options that meet with limited success. Complementary therapies include psychotherapy, hypnotherapy, acupuncture, and herbal therapies. Bulking agents and laxatives may be prescribed when constipation is the predominate symptom. Current treatments are largely inadequate and not supported by research data.

Nutrition Therapy

Traditional nutrition therapy for IBS is also less than ideal. A high-fiber diet has been studied extensively in IBS with mixed results (Wald and Rakel, 2008). Although it increases stool volume and frequency, a high-fiber intake may worsen the symptom of bloating. Lactose intolerance may affect a third of patients with IBS, although many are not truly deficient in the enzyme lactase. It may be that proteins or other substances in milk with immunogenic properties stimulate the GI tract in susceptible individuals (Sanjeevi and Kirby, 2008). Peppermint oil relaxes the smooth muscle of the GI tract and relieves IBS symptoms more effectively than placebo (Heizer, Southern, and McGovern, 2009). Emerging evidence suggests that probiotics, such as yogurt, kefir, and acidophilus milk, improve IBS symptoms by increasing beneficial bacteria in the large bowel, decreasing bacterial overgrowth in the small bowel, and promoting a balance of pro- and anti-inflammatory factors (Meier, 2010). It is not known what species, strains, or doses of probiotics are most beneficial. Other anecdotal nutritional approaches are to eat small meals, avoid caffeine, eat less fat, and follow an **elimination diet** to identify potential food intolerances or allergies.

Elimination Diet: a diet that eliminates foods suspected of producing symptoms of intolerance or allergies; suspected foods are added back to the diet individually to identify offending foods.

The malabsorption of fructose is gaining attention as a major dietary trigger for IBS (Barrett and Gibson, 2007). Incomplete digestion of fructose and other short-chain carbohydrates distends the bowel via osmotic effects and rapid fermentation. The result is gas, pain, and diarrhea in sensitive people. Interestingly, fructose malabsorption is probably a normal phenomenon, occurring in varying degrees in about 80% of people who consume fructose without other food (Barrett and Gibson, 2007). Although eating free fructose causes symptoms, consuming fructose with a near equal concentration of glucose is likely to be well tolerated because glucose promotes its absorption. That is why fructose from white sugar (composed of equal parts of glucose and fructose) is generally completely absorbed, but fructose from a pear, which contains approximately four times more fructose than glucose, is poorly absorbed.

The low-FODMAP diet has been shown to improve symptoms in 86% of participants compared to 49% improvement in the standard diet group (Staudacher, Whelan, Irving, and Lomer, 2011). Another study confirmed sustained and substantial relief of all IBS symptoms in 74% of patients treated with a low-FODMAP diet (Sheperd and Gibson, 2006). The diet restricts

- Honey and certain fruits (high in free fructose)
- Wheat, onions, garlic, and inulin (fructans)
- Milk and ice cream (lactose)
- Legumes (galacto-oligosaccharides)
- Sugarless gums, mints, and dietetic foods containing sugar alcohols such as sorbitol, mannitol, isomalt, or xylitol

Tolerance to FODMAPs is dose related; although small amounts of FODMAPs may be tolerated, eating beyond a person's threshold causes symptoms to develop. Research also supports the use of a low-FODMAP diet for patients in remission from IBD but who have IBS symptoms (Gearry et al., 2009). Box 18.7 outlines a low-FODMAP diet. More research is needed to determine the FODMAP content of foods.

Diverticular Disease

Diverticula: pouches that protrude outward from the muscular wall of the intestine usually in the sigmoid colon.

Diverticulitis: inflammation and infection that occurs when fecal matter gets trapped in the diverticula.

Bacterial Overgrowth: excessive bacterial growth in the stomach or small intestine that impairs digestion and absorption; may be caused by low gastric acidity, altered GI motility, mucosal damage, or contamination.

Diverticulosis: an asymptomatic condition characterized by diverticula.

Although diverticular disease is thought to be related to interactions of colon structure, intestinal motility, diet, and genetics, its exact cause is poorly understood. Diverticulosis is the condition in which **diverticula** form within the intestinal lumen, most commonly in the sigmoid colon. **Diverticulitis** occurs when diverticula become inflamed, possibly from trapped stool or bacteria. Symptoms of diverticulitis include cramping, alternating periods of diarrhea and constipation, flatus, abdominal distention, and low-grade fever. Potential complications include occult blood loss and acute rectal bleeding, leading to iron deficiency anemia; abscesses and bowel perforation, leading to peritonitis; fistula formation causing bowel obstruction; and **bacterial overgrowth** (in small bowel diverticula) that leads to malabsorption of fat and vitamin B_{12}.

The long-held theory that diverticular disease is caused by a low-fiber diet has been challenged. A cross-sectional study of more than 2100 participants showed that a high-fiber diet and increased frequency of bowel moments are associated with a greater, not lower, prevalence of **diverticulosis** and that diverticulosis is not related to low physical activity, fat intake, or red meat intake (Peery et al., 2012).

Nutrition Therapy

Despite the lack of proven efficacy, a high-fiber diet is recommended to prevent and improve symptoms of diverticulosis and prevent diverticulitis based on the theory that soft, bulky stools that are easily passed decrease pressure within the colon. Once the diverticula develop, a high-fiber diet cannot make them disappear. It is common practice for patients to be told to avoid nuts, seeds, and popcorn based on the theory that these can become trapped in diverticula and cause inflammation; yet there is no scientific evidence to support this practice (Strate, Liu, Syngal, Aldoori, and Giovannucci, 2008).

During an acute phase of diverticulitis, patients are given nothing by mouth (NPO) until bleeding and diarrhea subside. Oral intake resumes with clear liquids and progresses to a low-fiber diet until inflammation and bleeding are no longer a risk (AND, 2012). A high-fiber diet is recommended unless symptoms of diverticulitis recur. Patients who are treated with a low-fiber diet in the hospital may be reluctant to switch to a high-fiber diet on discharge. Diet compliance depends on the patient's understanding of the rationale and benefits of a high-fiber diet for long-term treatment of diverticulosis and prevention of diverticulitis.

Box 18.7 Low-FODMAP Diet

- A low-FODMAP diet limits fruits and fruit juices with high levels of fructose. Fruits and juices that have more glucose and less fructose may be tolerated in measured amounts.
- Because high-fructose corn syrup (HFCS) is half glucose and half fructose, it may be tolerated by some people when consumed in limited amounts.
- Sugar alcohols (polyols) are sorbitol, mannitol, xylitol, and maltitol. Sorbitol is found naturally in fruits and fruit juices; this and other sugar alcohols are used as artificial sweeteners in sugar-free gums, mints, and other "diet" foods.

Guidelines to Achieve a Low-FODMAP Diet

- Avoid products that list fructose, crystalline fructose (not HFCS), honey, and sorbitol on the label.
- Avoid sugar alcohols found in "diet" or "dietetic" foods.
- Limit beverages with HFCS to 12 oz or less per day. Consume with food for improved tolerance.
- Fresh or frozen fruit may be better tolerated than canned fruit.
- Cooked vegetables may be better tolerated than raw.
- Fructose and sorbitol may be ingredients in medications. Check with the pharmacist.
- Tolerance is impacted by the dose eaten at any one time.
- Avoid lactose if lactose intolerant.

	Foods Low in FODMAP	High-FODMAP Foods to Avoid	Questionable Foods/Foods to Limit
Fruit	Bananas, blackberries, blueberry, grapefruit, honeydew, kiwifruit, lemons, limes, mandarin orange, melons (except watermelon), oranges, passion fruit, pineapple, raspberries, rhubarb, strawberries, tangelos	Fruit: apples, pear, guava, honeydew melon, mango, Asian pear, papaya, quince, star fruit, watermelon Stone fruit: apricots, peaches, cherries, plums, nectarines Fruits high in sugar: grapes, persimmon, lychee Dried fruit Fruit juice Dried fruit bars Fruit pastes and sauces: tomato paste, chutney, plum sauce, sweet and sour sauce, barbecue sauce Fruit juice concentrate	Fruit canned in heavy syrup, other fruits
Vegetables	Bamboo shoots, bok choy, carrots, cauliflower*, celery, cucumber*, eggplant*, green beans*, green peppers*, leafy greens, parsnip, pumpkin, spinach, sweet potatoes, white potatoes, other root vegetables	Onion, leek, asparagus, artichokes, cabbage, Brussels sprouts, beans Legumes	Avocado, corn, mushrooms, tomatoes, other beans

Box 18.7   Low-FODMAP Diet (continued)

	Foods Low in FODMAP	High-FODMAP Foods to Avoid	Questionable Foods/ Foods to Limit
Other	All meats All fats Yogurt and hard cheeses Eggs Aspartame (Equal, NutraSweet) Saccharin (Sweet'N Low) Sugar Glucose Maple syrup	Wheat and wheat products Rye and rye products Pasta made from wheat Cereal made from wheat Cakes, cookies, crackers made from wheat Fortified wines: sherry, port, etc. Chicory-based coffee substitute Honey Certain additives identified on food labels, such as inulin (often labeled as chicory root extract), fructo-oligosaccharides, sorbitol, mannitol, xylitol, maltitol, isomalt Desserts sweetened with fructose or sorbitol (e.g., ice cream, cookies, popsicles)	Items containing HFCS if not tolerated Milk and other sources of lactose if not tolerated

*Possible gas-forming foods that may need to be avoided.

Source: University of Virginia (UVA) Nutrition Services, UVA Digestive Health Center. (n.d.). *Low FODMAP diet*. Available at www.medicine.virginia.edu/clinical/departments/medicine/divisions/igestive-heatlh/nutrition-support-team/patient-education/Low_FODMAP_Diet_9-12-11.pdf. Accessed on 6/5/12.

Ileostomies and Colostomies

Ileostomy: a surgically created opening (stoma) on the surface of the abdomen from the ileum.

Colostomy: a surgically created opening on the surface of the abdomen from the colon.

Effluent: flowing discharge.

An **ileostomy** and a **colostomy** are performed after part or all of the colon, anus, and rectum are removed, usually for treatment of severe IBD, intestinal lesions, obstructions, or colon cancer.

Potential nutritional problems arise because large amounts of fluid, sodium, and potassium are normally absorbed in the colon. The smaller the length of remaining colon, the greater is the potential for nutritional problems. For that reason, ileostomies create more problems than colostomies, in which some of the colon is retained. **Effluent** from an ileostomy is liquidy; fluid and electrolyte losses are considerable, and the absorption of fat, fat-soluble vitamins, bile acid, and vitamin B_{12} is decreased. Effluent through a colostomy varies from liquid to formed stools, depending on the length of colon that remains. Over time, adaptation occurs.

Nutrition Therapy

The goals of nutrition therapy for ileostomies and colostomies are to promote healing postoperatively; minimize symptoms; and prevent nutrient deficiencies, dehydration, and electrolyte imbalances. Initially, only clear liquids that are low in simple sugars (e.g., diluted fruit juice, broth, tea) are given to reduce the risk of osmotic diarrhea. The diet is advanced to a low-fiber diet (see Box 18.3) to reduce stool output. Patients need extra protein and calories to promote healing and may have experienced weight loss prior to surgery related to diarrhea or the underlying disease. Fear of eating is common. Within 6 weeks after surgery, the patient should be consuming a near-regular diet. Nutrition therapy guidelines focus on minimizing symptoms (Box 18.8.) Foods not tolerated initially can be reintroduced in a few months.

Obtaining adequate fluid and electrolytes is a major concern. A high fluid intake (8–10 cups daily) is needed to replenish losses. A high fluid intake is especially important for ileostomy patients to maintain a normal urine output and minimize the risk of renal calculi. Many patients inaccurately assume that a high fluid intake contributes to diarrhea. Reassure the patient that excess fluid is excreted through the kidneys, not the stoma.

Box 18.8 NUTRITION THERAPY GUIDELINES FOR COLOSTOMIES AND ILEOSTOMIES

Colostomies
- Begin with a clear liquid diet; progress to a low-fiber diet. A near-normal diet is generally achieved within 6 weeks
- Avoid any food not tolerated; reintroduce item after a couple of weeks
- Consume adequate fluid: 8–10 cups/day or more
- Avoid practices that may contribute to swallowed air and gas formation
  Chewing gum, using a straw, carbonated beverages, smoking, chewing tobacco, eating quickly
- Avoid odor and/or gas-causing foods
  Alcohol, asparagus, dried peas and beans, broccoli, Brussels sprouts, cabbage, cauliflower, eggs, fish
- Avoid foods that may cause blockage
  Apple skin, cabbage, celery, coconut, corn, dried fruit, grapes, nuts
- Add foods that may thicken stool
  Applesauce, bananas, banana flakes, cheese, pasta, pectin, potatoes, rice
- Add foods that may decrease odor
  Buttermilk, parsley, yogurt, kefir, cranberry juice

Ileostomies: All of the Above Plus
- Eat meals on a schedule to help promote a regular bowel pattern. Eating the largest meal in the middle of the day and a small evening meal helps to reduce nighttime stool output.
- Initially eat small, frequent meals.
- Chew food thoroughly because improperly chewed food can cause a stomal blockage.
- Avoid beverages with meals if experiencing high output; consume before or after eating.
- Encourage higher salt intake to replenish losses.
- Use oral rehydration beverages to help maintain fluid and electrolyte balance.
- Limit fat if the patient has steatorrhea or diarrhea from a significant ileal resection. MCT oil may be used for calories because it is absorbed without the aid of bile salts.
- Provide supplemental nutrients as needed. Because vitamin B_{12} is normally absorbed in the distal ileum, anemia related to vitamin B_{12} malabsorption can occur in patients with ileostomies, necessitating lifelong parenteral injections or nasal sprays of vitamin B_{12}.

DISORDERS OF THE ACCESSORY GI ORGANS

The liver, pancreas, and gallbladder are known as accessory organs of the GI tract. Although food does not come in direct contact with these organs, they play vital roles in the digestion of macronutrients. Liver disease, pancreatitis, and gallbladder disease are discussed next.

Liver Disease

Steatohepatitis: fat accumulation in the liver with inflammation.

Hepatitis: inflammation of the liver that may be caused by viral infections, alcohol abuse, and hepatotoxic chemicals such as chloroform and carbon tetrachloride.

Cirrhosis: liver disease that occurs when damaged liver cells are replaced by functionless scar tissue, seriously impairing liver function and disrupting normal blood circulation through the liver.

Hepatic Encephalopathy: the central nervous system (CNS) manifestations of advanced liver disease characterized by irritability, short-term memory loss, and impaired ability to concentrate.

Hepatic Coma: unconsciousness caused by severe liver disease.

The liver is a highly active organ involved in the metabolism of almost all nutrients. After absorption, almost all nutrients are transported to the liver, where they are "processed" before being distributed to other tissues. The liver synthesizes plasma proteins, blood clotting factors, and nonessential amino acids and forms urea from the nitrogenous wastes of protein. Triglycerides, phospholipids, and cholesterol are synthesized in the liver, as is bile, an important factor in the digestion of fat. Glucose is synthesized, and glycogen is formed, stored, and broken down as needed. Vitamins and minerals are metabolized, and many are stored in the liver. Finally, the liver is vital for detoxifying drugs, alcohol, ammonia, and other poisonous substances.

Liver damage can have profound and devastating effects on the metabolism of almost all nutrients. It can range from mild and reversible (e.g., fatty liver) to severe and terminal (e.g., hepatic coma). Liver failure can occur from chronic liver disease or secondary to critical illnesses.

Fatty liver disease is abnormal fat deposition in the liver. Fatty liver occurs in the majority of patients with alcoholic liver disease. Nonalcoholic fatty liver disease (NAFLD) is the most common cause of chronic liver disease in developed nations and may affect 20% or more of American adults (Naniwadekar, 2010). It is generally found as a component of metabolic syndrome—a cluster of symptoms that include abdominal obesity, insulin resistance, hypertension, and abnormal blood lipid levels. Other causes include exposure to drugs and toxic metals, long-term PN, and GI bypass surgery. Fatty liver can range in severity, from uncomplicated steatosis, which is often asymptomatic and benign, to **steatohepatitis**, literally fatty liver with inflammation.

Although fatty liver can cause **hepatitis**, the most frequent causes are infection from hepatitis viruses A, B, and C. Early symptoms of hepatitis include anorexia, nausea and vomiting, fever, fatigue, headache, and weight loss. Later, symptoms such as dark-colored urine, jaundice, liver tenderness, and, possibly, liver enlargement may develop. In many cases, particularly those caused by hepatitis A, liver cell damage that occurs from acute hepatitis is reversible with proper rest and adequate nutrition.

Sometimes, acute hepatitis advances to chronic hepatitis, especially when hepatitis is caused by hepatitis C. Scarring from chronic hepatitis can lead to **cirrhosis**. Liver damage progresses slowly, and some patients are asymptomatic. Early nonspecific symptoms include fever, anorexia, weight loss, and fatigue. Glucose intolerance is common. Later, portal hypertension, dyspepsia, diarrhea or constipation, jaundice, esophageal varices, hemorrhoids, ascites, edema, bleeding tendencies, anemia, hepatomegaly, and splenomegaly may develop. Malnutrition is common and a major risk factor for mortality (Bajaj, 2010). Cirrhosis can progress to **hepatic encephalopathy** and **hepatic coma**.

The liver "fails" when liver cell loss is extensive. Ominous changes in mental function, such as impaired memory and concentration, slow response time, drowsiness, irritability, flapping tremor, and fecal odor of the breath, signal hepatic encephalopathy, which may progress to hepatic coma. Although the exact cause of these central nervous system changes is unknown, a high serum ammonia level plays a major role because it affects cerebral edema and neurotransmitter function (Caruana and Shah, 2011).

Nutrition Therapy

The objectives of nutrition therapy for liver disease are to avoid or minimize permanent liver damage, restore optimal nutritional status, alleviate symptoms, and avoid complications. Adequate protein and calories are needed to promote liver cell regeneration. However, regeneration may not be possible if liver damage is extensive.

NAFLD may be best treated with weight loss and exercise. Studies show that even a modest weight loss of 5% to 10% of body weight can be enough to improve NAFLD and metabolic syndrome (Naniwadekar, 2010). Rapid weight loss (generally more than 3½ pounds/week) should be avoided: rapid breakdown of adipose tissue can deliver an excessive load of fatty acids to the liver. Studies suggest that omega-3 fatty acids may reduce fat content in the liver and decrease inflammation (Zhu, Liu, Chen, Huang, and Zhang, 2008). Nutrition interventions should include management of metabolic syndrome, if appropriate (see Chapter 20).

Patients with acute hepatitis may have difficulty consuming an adequate diet because of anorexia, early satiety, and fatigue. Generally, patients need 30 to 35 cal/kg of body weight and 1.0 to 1.2 g protein/kg body weight (AND, 2012). A balanced diet with between-meal feedings of commercial supplements may help ensure an adequate intake. Sodium is restricted for patients with ascites, and fat is limited to <30% of total calories if steatorrhea is present. For people with chronic hepatitis, dietary restrictions are usually not necessary unless symptoms interfere with nutrient intake or utilization.

Malnutrition is common among patients with cirrhosis and may be related to impaired intake, impaired absorption, altered metabolism, or iatrogenic causes. Nutrition therapy guidelines based on those alterations are outlined in Table 18.4. Generally, a high-calorie, high-protein diet is provided; fat is limited if not tolerated. Sodium and fluid are restricted, depending on the amount of fluid accumulation and serum sodium levels. Adjustments in

Table 18.4 Nutrition Therapy Recommendations for Cirrhosis Based on Factors Related to Malnutrition

Factors Related to Malnutrition	Nutrition Therapy Recommendations
Altered metabolism • Increased or decreased metabolic rate • Increased protein requirements • Glucose intolerance	Adjust calories as needed. Generally, calorie needs are higher than normal due to weight loss and an increased protein requirement. Vitamin supplements may be ordered. Protein requirement may be 0.8–1.2 g/kg. If glucose intolerant, encourage complex carbohydrates and consistent meal timing.
Impaired intake • Anorexia • Early satiety • Fatigue • Esophageal varices	Small, frequent meals and in between meal supplements may help maximize intake. Modify texture (soft, low-fiber, or liquids), as needed, if patient has esophageal varices.
Impaired absorption • Inadequate bile flow • Bacterial overgrowth • Pancreatic insufficiency	Limit fat to <30% of calories if patient has steatorrhea. MCT oil can provide additional calories. Water-miscible forms of vitamins A, D, and E plus calcium and zinc may be needed to compensate for increased excretion.
Iatrogenic factors • Frequent paracentesis • Diuresis	Limit sodium to <2000 mg/day if patient as ascites or edema. Limit fluid to 1200–1500 mL/day if serum sodium is 128 mEq/L.

food texture and the frequency and timing of meals may help promote intake. Vitamin and mineral supplements are needed. Meeting nutrient and calorie needs is difficult, and EN support may be necessary.

Nutrition Therapy for Liver Transplantation

Liver transplantation is a treatment option for patients with severe and irreversible liver disease. Many patients awaiting a transplant are malnourished. Moderate to severe malnutrition increases the risk of complications and death after transplantation. Whenever possible, nutrient deficiencies and imbalances are corrected before the transplantation to promote a positive outcome.

There is not one specific posttransplant diet. Nutrient recommendations vary with the posttransplant stage and are individualized according to the patient's nutritional status, weight, tolerance, and laboratory values. Eating resumes as soon as possible after surgery, usually within 2 to 4 days. Calorie and protein needs are increased from the stress of surgery. Small, frequent meals and commercial supplements may help maximize intake. Vitamin and mineral supplements are ordered. Although oral nutrition is the preferred route, EN support is used if the patient is unable to consume adequate nutrition for 5 to 7 days.

After the initial hypermetabolic period, the patient's calorie and protein needs return toward normal. Long-term complications associated with immunosuppressive therapy, such as excessive weight gain, hypertension, hyperlipidemia, osteopenic bone disease, and diabetes, may require nutrition therapy. The use of immunosuppressant drugs elevates the importance of safe food handling practices to avoid foodborne illness.

Pancreatitis

The pancreas is responsible for secreting enzymes needed to digest dietary carbohydrates, protein, and fat. Until they are needed, these enzymes are held in the pancreas in their inactive form. Inflammation of the pancreas causes digestive enzymes to be retained in the pancreas and converted to their active form so they literally begin to digest the pancreas. Because the pancreas also produces insulin, people with **pancreatitis** may also develop hyperglycemia related to insufficient insulin secretion.

Pancreatitis: inflammation of the pancreas.

Alcohol abuse and gallstones account for more than 70% of cases of acute pancreatitis (Owyang, 2008). Other causes include hypertriglyceridemia ($\geq$1000 mg/dL), cystic fibrosis, renal failure, and the use of certain medications. Patients present with acute abdominal pain in the upper quadrant, nausea, and vomiting. Levels of serum **amylase** and **lipase** are elevated. Mild acute pancreatitis usually resolves in a few days without permanent damage. Moderate to severe forms often require prolonged hospitalization that may preclude patients from eating.

Amylase: a class of enzymes that split starch molecules.

Lipase: an enzyme that splits fat molecules.

Acute pancreatitis that is not resolved or recurs frequently can lead to chronic pancreatitis (CP). Alcohol abuse and cigarette smoking are independent risk factors for CP; genetics may also play a role (Yadav et al., 2009). The hallmark feature of CP is severe, intermittent epigastric pain that is often made worse by eating. Nausea and vomiting accompany severe pain. Scarring and fibrosis can lead to impaired endocrine and exocrine function, resulting in diabetes and malabsorption, especially of fat. An inadequate intake related to pain combined with malabsorption can lead to malnutrition and weight loss.

Nutrition Therapy

Acute pancreatitis is treated by reducing pancreatic stimulation. In mild cases, the patient is given pain medications, IV therapy, and NPO. Generally, when pain subsides, amylase levels begin to subside and there are no complications; patients are given a clear liquid diet and advanced to a low-fat diet as tolerated. Small, frequent meals may be better tolerated initially because they help to reduce the amount of pancreatic stimulation at each meal. A prospective, randomized trial by Jacobson et al. (2008) showed that initiating a solid low-fat diet after mild acute pancreatitis was safe and provided more calories than a clear liquid diet, although the length of hospitalization did not improve. Likewise, Sathiaraj et al. (2008) showed no difference in symptom relapse in patients who were given a solid food diet compared to those who were started on a clear liquid diet.

Patients with moderate to severe acute pancreatitis are ordered NPO, and a nasogastric tube is inserted to suction gastric contents. Appropriate measures are taken to correct fluid and electrolyte imbalance, to control pain, and to treat or prevent symptoms. Hypermetabolism and hypercatabolism increase protein and calorie needs. EN is recommended within 24 to 48 hours of admission and after fluid resuscitation in patients who are not expected to tolerate an oral diet within 5 to 7 days (McClave et al., 2009). Although feedings into the jejunum do not cause fewer complications than those into the stomach or duodenum, they are preferred because they are associated with the lowest level of pancreatic secretions. The choice of formula (e.g., standard versus hydrolyzed) does not seem to affect tolerance (McClave et al., 2009). PN is recommended only if EN fails and the patient has had no nutritional support for more than 5 days (McClave et al., 2009).

The goals of nutrition therapy for chronic pancreatitis are to maintain weight, reduce steatorrhea, minimize pain, and avoid acute attacks while meeting the patient's nutrient needs. A mildly low-fat diet (Box 18.9) that is high in protein is recommended. Fat is restricted further for patients with steatorrhea. Patients whose insulin secretion is impaired may need a carbohydrate-controlled diet to help control hyperglycemia. Supplements of antioxidants may help reduce pancreatic inflammation and pain in patients with either acute or chronic pancreatitis, but the best mixture and doses are not known (Chauhan, Pannu, and Forsmark, 2012). Taking pancreatic enzyme replacement pills at the beginning, end, and during each meal is crucial for maximum effectiveness.

Gallbladder Disease

The gallbladder's role in digestion is to store and release bile, which prepares fat for digestion. Bile, which is made in the liver, consists of cholesterol, bile salts, bile pigments, and water. As it is held in the gallbladder, water is slowly removed from bile, making it more concentrated and increasing the likelihood that solids (either cholesterol crystals or pigment material) will precipitate out into clumps known as gallstones. Incomplete emptying of the gallbladder may also be involved in gallstone formation.

Cholelithiasis: formation of gallstones.

A large majority of people with **cholelithiasis** are asymptomatic, but some experience episodic, upper GI pain that spreads to the chest and shoulders in a manner similar to the symptoms of a heart attack. For some people, eating a fatty meal precipitates symptoms; for others, symptoms develop during sleep. Gallstones that obstruct the cystic duct can lead to **cholecystitis**, causing abdominal pain, nausea and vomiting, jaundice, fever, fat intolerance, and flatulence. Surgical removal of the gallbladder may be used to treat symptomatic gallstones. After the gallbladder is removed, the common bile duct collects and holds bile until mealtime when it is released into the duodenum.

Cholecystitis: inflammation of the gallbladder.

No diet modifications are necessary for healthy people with asymptomatic gallstones. Patients with symptomatic gallstones may be told to limit their intake of fat based on the rationale that limiting fat intake reduces stimulation to the gallbladder and minimizes pain. However, it is not known if patients with gallstones are any more intolerant of fat than the general population. Other practices, based more on popular belief than on scientific data, include limiting spicy foods, high-fiber foods, and foods that cause gas. Most patients do not experience problems after recovery from surgery.

Box 18.9 LOW-FAT DIET

- Total fat is limited to reduce symptoms of steatorrhea and pain in patients who are intolerant to fat, such as for people with chronic pancreatitis, Crohn disease, radiation enteritis, and short bowel syndrome.

Guidelines to Achieve a Low-Fat Diet
- Eat nonfat or low-fat food to meet appropriate MyPlate amounts.
- Select only very lean meats, fish, and skinless poultry; egg whites; and low-fat egg substitutes.
- Bake, broil, or boil foods instead of frying.
- Use milk and dairy products that provide less than 1 g fat per serving and use low-fat cheese with 3 g or less of fat per serving.
- Enjoy all fruits and vegetables that are prepared without added fat except avocado and coconut.
- Choose grain products that are prepared without added fat (e.g., avoid muffins, waffles, biscuits, pastries, other baked goods).
- Choose low-fat desserts: sherbet, fruit ices, gelatin, angel food cake, vanilla wafers, graham crackers, nonfat ice cream and frozen yogurt, and fruit whips with gelatin.
- Limit fats to less than eight equivalents per day. Each of the following constitutes one serving (one "equivalent"):

1 tsp butter, margarine, shortening, oil, or mayonnaise	1 tbsp heavy cream
1 tbsp diet margarine, diet mayonnaise, or reduced-calorie cream salad dressing	2 tsp regular creamy salad dressing
	2 tsp peanut butter
	2 tsp light cream
1 strip crisp bacon	6 small nuts
1 tbsp sesame, sunflower, or pumpkin seeds	8–10 olives
	⅛ medium avocado
2 tbsp sour cream, cream cheese, half-and-half, or coffee whitener	

Sample Menu

Breakfast	Lunch	Dinner	Snacks
Orange juice Oatmeal with fat-free milk Whole wheat toast with jelly	Fat-free vegetable soup 2 oz of fat-free ham on whole wheat bread with lettuce and fat-free mayonnaise Fresh strawberries Fat-free milk	2 oz broiled lean chicken Brown rice Tossed salad with vegetables and fat-free dressing Steamed broccoli Whole wheat roll with 1 tsp butter Blueberries Fat-free milk	Fat-free popcorn Carrots and celery with fat-free dressing Tomato juice

Potential Problems	Recommended Interventions
Noncompliance related to decreased palatability and satiety from the reduction in fat intake	Encourage the patient to eat a variety of foods and to use nonfat and fat-free versions of familiar foods. Encourage use of butter-flavored sprinkles and sprays to season hot vegetables and potatoes.

(continues on page 488)

Box 18.9   LOW-FAT DIET (continued)

Potential Problems	Recommended Interventions
Persistent symptoms of steatorrhea or pain after eating that are related to fat intolerance	Decrease fat content by eliminating fat equivalents and limiting the amount of low-fat meat allowed.
Inadequate intake of iron related to the limited allowance of meat (red meat is the best absorbed source of iron in the diet)	Monitor hemoglobin and hematocrit; recommend iron supplements as needed.
	Encourage a liberal intake of high-iron foods such as fortified cereals and grains and dried peas and beans; advise the patient to consume a rich source of vitamin C at each meal to maximize iron absorption.

Patient Teaching
Ensure the patient understands that

- The total amount of dietary fat must be reduced regardless of the source.
- Sources of fat may be visible (e.g., butter, margarine, shortening, fat on meat, salad dressings) or invisible (e.g., marbled meat, whole milk and whole-milk products, egg yolks, nuts).
- Substitutions can be made to individualize the diet.
- Oil-packed tuna and salmon may be used if thoroughly rinsed.
- Fat-free salad dressings may be used as desired.

Tips for reducing fat content when eating out
- Choose juice or broth-based soup instead of cream soup as an appetizer.
- Use lemon, vinegar, low-calorie dressing (if available), or fresh ground pepper on salad, or request that the dressing be brought on the side.
- Order plain baked or broiled foods.
- Avoid warm bread and rolls, which absorb more butter than those at room temperature.
- Order fresh fruit, gelatin, or sherbet for dessert.
- Request milk for coffee or tea in place of cream and nondairy creamers.

Food preparation techniques to reduce fat content
- Trim fat from meat and remove skin from chicken before cooking.
- Place meats to be baked or roasted on a rack to allow the fat to drain.
- Bake, broil, steam, or sauté foods in a vegetable cooking spray or allowed fats.
- Cook with bouillon, lemon, vinegar, wine, herbs, and spices instead of adding fat.
- Make fat-free soup stock by preparing the stock a day ahead and refrigerating it overnight. The fat will harden and can easily be removed from the surface. Make fat-free gravies also by this method.
- Purchase "select" grade meats because they are lower in fat than "choice" and "prime" grades.

NURSING PROCESS: *Crohn Disease*

Andrew is a 20-year-old man who is admitted to the hospital for suspected Crohn disease. His chief complaints are crampy abdominal pain, diarrhea, weight loss, fatigue, and anorexia. He has lost 15 pounds since his symptoms began 2 weeks ago. He is prescribed intravenous fluids, sulfasalazine, prednisone, an antidiarrheal medication, and a diet as tolerated.

Assessment

Medical–Psychosocial History	▪ Medical and surgical history
	▪ Use of prescribed and over-the-counter medications
	▪ Support system
Anthropometric Assessment	▪ Height, current weight, usual weight; percent weight loss; body mass index (BMI)
Biochemical and Physical Assessment	▪ Hemoglobin (Hgb), hematocrit (Hct)
	▪ Serum electrolyte levels
	▪ Prealbumin, if available
	▪ Blood pressure
	▪ Signs of dehydration (poor skin turgor, dry mucous membranes, etc.)
Dietary Assessment	▪ How has your intake changed since you began experiencing symptoms?
	▪ Do you know if any particular foods cause problems? Did you have any food intolerances or allergies before your symptoms began?
	▪ How many meals per day are you eating?
	▪ How much fluid are you drinking in a day?
	▪ Have you ever followed any kind of diet before?
	▪ Do you take vitamins, minerals, or other supplements?
	▪ Do you use alcohol?
	▪ Who prepares your meals?

Diagnosis

Possible Nursing Diagnoses	Altered nutrition: eating less than the body needs related to diarrhea and altered ability to digest and absorb nutrients.

Planning

Client Outcomes	The client will
	▪ Consume adequate calories and protein to restore normal weight.
	▪ Experience improvement in symptoms (diarrhea, abdominal pain, fatigue, anorexia).
	▪ Restore normal fluid balance.
	▪ Describe the principles and rationale of nutrition therapy for Crohn disease and implement the appropriate interventions.

(continues on page 490)

NURSING PROCESS: *Crohn Disease* (continued)

Nursing Interventions

Nutrition Therapy	▪ Provide a low-fat, low-fiber, high-protein, lactose-restricted diet as tolerated
	▪ Provide lactose-free commercial supplements between meals to enhance protein and calorie intake
	▪ Encourage high fluid intake, especially of fluids high in potassium such as tomato juice, apricot nectar, and orange juice
	▪ Promote gradual return to normal diet as tolerated
Client Teaching	Instruct the client
	▪ On the purpose and rationale of a low-fat, low-fiber, lactose-restricted diet; advise the patient that he may be able to tolerate fiber and milk after the disease goes into remission
	▪ On the importance of consuming adequate protein, calories, and fluid to promote healing and recovery
	▪ To maximize intake by eating small, frequent meals
	▪ To avoid colas and other sources of caffeine because they stimulate peristalsis
	▪ To eliminate individual intolerances
	▪ To chew food thoroughly and avoid swallowing air
	▪ On the importance of consuming adequate fluid while taking sulfasalazine
	▪ That prednisone should improve his appetite but may cause fluid retention and gastrointestinal upset
	▪ To communicate any side effects he experiences from the medications and that, during remission, symptoms may improve by following a low-FODMAP diet

Evaluation

Evaluate and Monitor	▪ Intake and output; fluid and electrolyte status
	▪ Appetite
	▪ Tolerance to fat (may need to reduce fat level)
	▪ Diarrhea (if patient does not tolerate an oral diet, determine whether a defined formula feeding or TPN is appropriate) and other symptoms
	▪ Weight changes and BMI

HOW DO YOU RESPOND?

Are probiotics safe? Probiotics that contain *Lactobacillus, Bifidobacterium, Streptococcus thermophilus*, and *Saccharomyces* strains are safe for use in generally healthy people (Douglas and Sanders, 2008). Other types of probiotics (e.g., *Enterococcus*) should be reserved for specific individuals. People who are immunocompromised, are recovering from surgery, or have altered GI integrity are at increased risk for infection from any source and should not take probiotics without their physician's approval.

Are "live active cultures" the same thing as probiotics? Live cultures are associated with foods; they are often added to ferment foods. Probiotics are live microorganisms that have been shown to benefit health. Some probiotics are not normally found in foods, such as *Escherichia coli*, and so they are not synonymous with "live culture."

CASE STUDY

Brittany is a 33-year-old woman who was recently diagnosed with IBS. She alternates between episodes of diarrhea and constipation and complains of distention and abdominal pain. Her doctor suggested she eat more fiber and take Metamucil. She dislikes whole wheat bread. She is reluctant to take a fiber supplement; she knows fiber helps people with constipation, and because she also has diarrhea, she believes it will only make her problem worse. She is thinking about adding yogurt to her usual diet to see if that helps. She drinks an "irritable bowel syndrome–friendly tea" that is supposed to help, but she hasn't noticed any improvement.

Her usual intake is as follows:

Breakfast:	Orange juice
	White toast with peanut butter
	Coffee
Snacks:	Small bag of chips from the vending machine
Lunch:	Fast-food hamburger on a bun
	Small French fries
	Diet coke
Snacks:	Cheese and crackers
	Glass of wine
Dinner:	Beef or chicken
	Mashed potatoes
	Broccoli
	Tossed salad with Italian dressing
	Ice cream
	Coffee
Snacks:	Milk and cookies, apples

- What does Brittany need to know about fiber and bowel function? What would you say to her about eating more fiber? About taking a fiber supplement? About yogurt? And about "irritable bowel syndrome–friendly tea"?
- What else do you need to know about Brittany to help relieve her symptoms?
- What other diet interventions could she implement to try to improve her symptoms?
- What elimination diet items is she consuming? What alternatives to those foods would you suggest?

STUDY QUESTIONS

1. When developing a teaching plan for a patient who has chronic diarrhea, which of the following foods would the nurse suggest as an appropriate source of potassium?
   a. Tomato juice
   b. Pinto beans
   c. Milk
   d. Broccoli

2. Which statement indicates the patient with an ileostomy needs further instruction about what to eat?
   a. "Drinking lots of water increases the output from my ileostomy."
   b. "It is best to eat a small evening meal."
   c. "Oatmeal and bananas may help control diarrhea."
   d. "A regular eating schedule will help regulate my bowel pattern."

3. The client asks if yogurt with probiotics will relieve her symptoms of irritable bowel syndrome. Which of the following would be the nurse's best response?
   a. "Unfortunately, there isn't anything that will help relieve irritable bowel syndrome."
   b. "Although it is not guaranteed to help, probiotics may help and do not pose a health risk in healthy people."
   c. "Because little is known about the effects of probiotics on health, you should avoid consuming them."
   d. "Probiotics are the only dietary intervention known to help irritable bowel syndrome."

4. The nurse knows his or her instructions have been effective when the client with celiac disease verbalizes that an appropriate breakfast is
   a. Eggs and toast
   b. Grits with berries
   c. Bran flakes cereal with milk
   d. Buttermilk pancakes with syrup

5. Which of the following would be most appropriate in modifying a regular diet to a high-fiber diet?
   a. Ice cream in place of gelatin
   b. Apple in place of apple juice
   c. Rice in place of mashed potatoes
   d. Cream of wheat in place of cream of rice

6. Which of the following may be an appropriate source of calcium for a client who is lactose intolerant?
   a. Aged cheddar cheese
   b. Pudding
   c. Lean meats
   d. Refined breads and cereals

7. A client with fat malabsorption is at risk for which of the following?
   a. Oxalate kidney stones
   b. Constipation
   c. Deficiencies of essential amino acids
   d. Type 2 diabetes

8. Which of the following strategies would help a client achieve a low-fat diet?
   a. Substitute margarine for butter.
   b. Limit portion sizes of meat.
   c. Substitute whole wheat bread for white bread.
   d. Eat more fruit in place of vegetables.

KEY CONCEPTS

- The first half of the small intestine is the site where most nutrients are absorbed. Conditions that affect the small intestine can impair the absorption of one or many nutrients.

- The large intestine absorbs water and electrolytes. Disorders of the colon can cause major problems with fluid and electrolyte balance.

- Most cases of constipation can be alleviated or prevented by increasing fiber and fluid intake. Most Americans consume approximately half the amount of fiber recommended daily.

- To achieve a high-fiber diet, high-fiber foods are eaten in place of those low in fiber, such as whole wheat bread for white bread, high-fiber cereal for refined cereal, and whole fruits for fruit juices. High-fiber foods to add to a usual diet include dried peas and beans, more vegetables, nuts, and seeds.

- Other than encouraging fluids and foods high in potassium, nutrition therapy usually is not necessary for acute diarrhea of short-term duration. Because many clear liquids are hyperosmolar and may contribute to osmotic diarrhea, they should be avoided until diarrhea subsides. Foods that help thicken stools, such as bananas and oatmeal, are encouraged. Patients should avoid items that stimulate peristalsis, such as caffeine; alcohol; and high-fiber, gassy foods.

- A low-fiber diet is appropriate only for short-term use. Its effect is to decrease stimulation to the bowel and slow intestinal transit time.

- Primary lactose intolerance is common in much of the world's adult population; tolerance varies considerably among individuals. Some people tolerate milk with food; others tolerate only lactose-reduced milk. Lactose intolerance that occurs secondary to intestinal disorders is usually more symptomatic than primary lactose intolerance and requires a more restrictive intake.

- During exacerbation of inflammatory bowel diseases, patients need increased amounts of calories and protein and may not tolerate fiber and lactose. Patients are often reluctant to eat, fearing that food will cause pain and diarrhea. Some patients require EN or PN for bowel rest. During remission, the diet is liberalized as tolerated.

- A gluten-free diet prevents intestinal villi changes, steatorrhea, and other symptoms in patients with celiac disease. All forms and sources of wheat, rye, and barley must be permanently eliminated from the diet, even in patients who are asymptomatic. A gluten-free diet requires major lifestyle changes and is difficult to follow.

- Short bowel syndrome occurs in patients who have had more than 50% to 70% of the small intestine removed. Maldigestion and malabsorption may lead to malnutrition. PN is usually used until adaptation begins, although some patients need PN permanently. Patients need to eat as soon as possible to stimulate the bowel and promote adaptation. Tolerance to fat, lactose, and sugar is impaired.

- Irritable bowel syndrome (IBS) is a common but not serious disorder. A high-fiber and/or low-lactose diet may help relieve symptoms in some people. Research on the benefits of probiotics and prebiotics is encouraging but not conclusive. A low-FODMAP diet may offer the most significant and sustained improvement in IBS symptoms.

- During acute diverticulitis, patients may be given a low-fiber diet to reduce bowel stimulation. A recent study showed that a high-fiber diet, traditionally used to prevent diverticular disease, may actually increase, not decrease, the risk of diverticulosis.

- Fluid and electrolytes are of primary concern for patients with ileostomies and colostomies. Low-fiber foods may help to reduce stoma discharge and irritation. Additional calories and protein are needed to promote healing.

■ Adequate calories and protein promote liver cell regeneration in patients with hepatitis and cirrhosis. Sodium and fluid may be restricted if ascites develop. A liquid or soft diet is recommended if regular textured foods irritate esophageal varices.

■ People who have undergone liver transplantation have high protein and calorie needs. Glucose intolerance may occur, and sodium and potassium intakes may be restricted depending on the individual's profile. Immunosuppressant drugs may interfere with intake and appetite.

■ Chronic pancreatitis is treated with a low-fat diet. Patients who develop glucose intolerance may benefit from a carbohydrate-controlled diet.

■ A common practice is to recommend a low-fat diet for patients with symptomatic gallstones and for people who have had a cholecystectomy. Evidence is lacking on the benefits of restricting fat.

Check Your Knowledge Answer Key

1. **TRUE** For most people, consuming more fiber and fluid prevents or alleviates constipation.

2. **FALSE** A clear liquid diet contains items that are hyperosmolar, such as sweetened carbonated beverages, fruit juice, and flavored ices; consuming them may contribute to osmotic diarrhea.

3. **FALSE** Probiotics are living organisms in food that are beneficial to health when consumed in adequate amounts. Prebiotics are nondigestible fibers that promote the growth of intestinal bacteria.

4. **TRUE** Because most of the lactose in cheddar and other natural, aged cheeses has been converted to lactic acid in the cheese-making process, most people who are lactose intolerant can tolerate cheddar cheese.

5. **FALSE** Eating a low-fiber diet is not necessary for people with IBD except during acute exacerbation or if there are strictures. A low-residue diet does not prevent exacerbation of the disease.

6. **TRUE** For a patient with celiac disease, the long-term effects of eating even small amounts of gluten are harmful, even when patients are asymptomatic.

7. **FALSE** Although a high-fiber diet may help relieve symptoms of IBS in some people, it is not guaranteed to help all people with IBS.

8. **FALSE** Although it has commonly been believed that a low-fiber diet increases the risk of diverticular disease, a recent study showed that people who consume a high-fiber diet have a higher prevalence of diverticular disease. The exact mechanism of diverticular disease is not known.

9. **TRUE** Extensive pancreatic damage impairs digestion, especially fat digestion. A low-fat diet is used when pancreatitis causes steatorrhea.

10. **FALSE** Dietary intervention is not necessary for cholelithiasis or cholecystitis.

Websites

Celiac Disease Awareness Campaign of the National Institutes of Health at
   http://www.celiac.nih.gov/
Celiac Disease Foundation at **www.celiac.org**
Celiac Sprue Association/USA at **http://csaceliacs.org**
Crohn's and Colitis Foundation of America at **www.ccfa.org**
Gluten Intolerance Group at **www.gluten.net**
Information on prebiotics and probiotics is available at **www.usprobiotics.org**, a nonprofit
   research and educational website made possible by the California Dairy Research Foundation
   and Dairy & Food Culture Technologies.
National Digestive Disease Information Clearinghouse at **http://digestive.niddk.nih.gov**
United Ostomy Associations of America, Inc. at **www.uoa.org**

References

Academy of Nutrition and Dietetics. (2012). *Nutrition care manual*. Available at
   www.nutritioncaremanual.org. Accessed on 6/11/12.
Academy of Nutrition and Dietetics Evidence Analysis Library. *Academy of Nutrition and Dietetics
   celiac disease evidence-based nutrition practice guidelines.* (2012). Available at (members only)
   http://www.adaevidencelibrary.com/conclusion.cfm?conclusion_statement_id=250229.
   Accessed on 6/8/12.
American Gastroenterological Association, Clinical Practice and Economics Committee. (2006).
   AGA Institute medical position statement on the diagnosis and management of celiac disease.
   Gastroenterology, 131, 1977–1980.
Bajaj, J. (2010). Review article: The modern management of hepatic encephalopathy. *Alimentary
   Pharmacology and Therapeutics, 31,* 537–547.
Barrett, J., & Gibson, P. (2007). Clinical ramifications of malabsorption and fructose and other
   short-chain carbohydrates. *Practical Gastroenterology.* Available at http://www.medicine
   .virginia.edu/clinical/departments/medicine/divisions/digestive-health/nutrition-support-
   team/nutrition-articles/BarrettArticle.pdf. Accessed on 6/8/2012.
Card, T., West, J., & Holmes, G. (2004). Risk of malignancy in diagnosed coeliac disease:
   A 24-year prospective, population-based, cohort study. *Alimentary Pharmacology and
   Therapeutics, 20,* 769–775.
Caruana, P., & Shah, N. (2011, May). Hepatic encephalopathy: Are NH_4 levels and protein restric-
   tion obsolete? *Practical Gastroenterology,* 6–18.
Chauhan, S., Pannu, D., & Forsmark, C. (2012, March). Antioxidants as adjunctive therapy for
   pain in chronic pancreatitis. *Practical Gastroenterology,* 42–49.
Clark, C., & DeLegge, M. (2008). Irritable bowel syndrome: A practical approach. *Nutrition in
   Clinical Practice, 23,* 263–267.
Douglas, L., & Sanders, M. (2008). Probiotics and prebiotics in dietetics practice. *Journal of the
   American Dietetic Association, 108,* 510–521.
Fessler, T. (2007). A dietary challenge: Maximizing bowel adaptation in short bowel syndrome.
   Today's Dietitian, 9, 40–45.
Gearry, R., Irving, P., Barrett, J., Nathan, D., Shepherd, S., & Gibson, R. (2009). Reduction of
   dietary poorly absorbed short-chain carbohydrates (FODMAPs) improves abdominal symptoms in
   patients with inflammatory bowel disease—A pilot study. *Journal of Crohn's and Colitis, 3,* 8–14.
Hanauer, S. (2006). Inflammatory bowel disease: Epidemiology, pathogenesis, and therapeutic
   opportunities. *Inflammatory Bowel Diseases, 12,* S3–S9.
Heizer, W., Southern, S., & McGovern, S. (2009). The role of diet in symptoms of irritable
   bowel syndrome in adults: A narrative review. *Journal of the American Dietetic Association,
   109,* 1204–1214.
Institute of Medicine. (2005). *Dietary reference intakes for energy, carbohydrates, fiber, fat, fatty
   acids, cholesterol, protein, and amino acids.* Washington, DC: National Academies Press.
Jacobson, B. C., VanderVliet, M. B., Hughes, M. D., Maurer, R., McManus, K., & Banks, P. A.
   (2008). A prospective, randomized trial of clear liquids versus low-fat solid diet as the initial
   meal in mild acute pancreatitis. *Nutrition in Clinical Practice, 23,* 341–342.
Kelly, D. (2006). Assessment of malabsorption. In M. Shils, M. Shike, A. Ross, B. Caballero, &
   R. Cousins (Eds.), *Modern nutrition in health and disease* (10th ed.). Philadelphia, PA:
   Lippincott Williams & Wilkins.
Matarese, L. E., O'Keefe, S. J., Kandil, H. M., Bond, G., Costa, G., & Abu-Elmagd, K. (2005).
   Short bowel syndrome: Clinical guidelines for nutrition management. *Nutrition in Clinical
   Practice, 20,* 493–502.

McClave, S., Martindale, R., Vanek, V., McCarthy, M., Roberts, P., Taylor, B., . . . Cresci, G. (2009). Guidelines for the provision and assessment of nutrition support therapy in the adult critically ill patient. *Journal of Parenteral and Enteral Nutrition, 33,* 277–316.

Meier, R. (2010). Probiotics in irritable bowel syndrome. *Annals of Nutrition and Metabolism, 57*(Suppl. 1), 12–13.

Naniwadekar, A. (2010, February). Nutritional recommendations for patients with non-alcoholic fatty liver disease: An evidence based review. *Practical Gastroenterology,* 16.

National Institute of Diabetes and Digestive and Kidney Diseases. (2012a). *Celiac disease.* Available at http://digestive.niddk.nih.gov/ddiseases/pubs/celiac/index.aspx. Accessed on 6/8/12.

National Institute of Diabetes and Digestive and Kidney Disease. (2012b). *Irritable bowel syndrome.* Available at: http://digestive.niddk.nih.gov/ddiseases/pubs/ibs/index.aspx Accessed on 6/8/12.

National Institute of Diabetes and Digestive and Kidney Diseases. (2012c). *Lactose intolerance.* Available at http://digestive.niddk.nih.gov/ddiseases/pubs/lactoseintolerance/index.aspx. Accessed on 6/9/12.

Niewinski, M. (2008). Advances in celiac disease and gluten-free diet. *Journal of the American Dietetic Association, 108,* 661–672.

Owyang, C. (2008). Pancreatitis. In L. Goldman & D. Ausiello (Eds.), *Cecil medicine.* Philadelphia, PA: Saunders.

Parrish, C. (2005, September). The clinician's guide to short bowel syndrome. *Practical Gastroenterology,* 67–106.

Peery, A., Barrett, P., Park, D., Rogers, A. J., Galanko, J. A., Martin, C. F., & Sandler, R. S. (2012). A high-fiber diet does not protect against asymptomatic diverticulosis. *Gastroenterology, 142,* 266–272.

Rubio-Tapio, A., Rahim, M., See, J., Lahr, B., Wu, T., & Murray, T. (2010). Mucosal recovery and mortality in adults with celiac disease after treatment with a gluten free diet. *American Journal of Gastroenterology, 105,* 1412–1420.

Sanjeevi, A., & Kirby, D. (2008). The role of food and dietary intervention in the irritable bowel syndrome. *Practical Gastroenterology.* Available at www.medicine.virginia.edu/clinical/departments/medicine/divisions/digestive-health/nutrition-support-team/nutrition-articles/SanjeeviArticle2.pdf. Accessed 6/8/2012.

Sathiaraj, E., Murthy, S., Mansard, M. J., Rao, G. V., Mahukar, S., & Reddy, D. N. (2008). Clinical trial: Oral feeding with a soft diet compared with clear liquid diet as initial meal in mild acute pancreatitis. *Alimentary Pharmacology and Therapeutics, 28,* 777–781.

Sheperd, S., & Gibson, P. (2006). Fructose malabsorption and symptoms of irritable bowel syndrome: Guidelines for effective dietary management. *Journal of the American Dietetic Association, 106,* 1631–1639.

Staudacher, H., Whelan, K., Irving, P., & Lomer, M. (2011). Comparison of symptom response following advice for a diet low in fermentable carbohydrates (FODMAPs) versus standard dietary advice in patients with irritable bowel syndrome. *Journal of Human Nutrition and Dietetics, 24,* 487–495.

Strate, L., Liu, R., Syngal, S., Aldoori, W., & Giovannucci, E. (2008). Nut, corn, and popcorn consumption and the incidence of diverticular disease. *JAMA, 300,* 907–914.

Thompson, T. (2005). National Institutes of Health consensus statement on celiac disease. *Journal of the American Dietetic Association, 105,* 194–195.

Timm, D., & Slavin, J. (2008). Dietary fiber and the relationship to chronic disease. *American Journal of Lifestyle Medicine, 2,* 233–240.

Wald, A., & Rakel, D. (2008). Behavioral and complementary approaches for the treatment of irritable bowel syndrome. *Nutrition in Clinical Practice, 23,* 284–292.

World Health Organization. (2012). *Child health epidemiology.* Available at www.wholint/maternal/child/adolescent/epidemiology/child/en. Accessed on 6/8/2012.

Yadav, D., Hawes, R., Brand, R., Anderson, M. A., Money, M. E., Banks, P. A., . . . Whitcomb, D. (2009). Alcohol consumption, cigarette smoking, and the risk of recurrent acute and chronic pancreatitis. *Archives of Internal Medicine, 169,* 1035–1045.

Zhu, F., Liu, S, Chen, X., Huang, Z., & Zhang, D. (2008). Effects of n-3 polyunsaturated fatty acids from seal oils on non-alcoholic fatty liver disease associated with hyperlipidemia. *World Journal of Gastroenterology, 14,* 6395–6400.

19 Nutrition for Patients with Diabetes Mellitus

CHECK YOUR KNOWLEDGE

TRUE FALSE

☐ ☐ **1** The progression of prediabetes to diabetes is inevitable.

☐ ☐ **2** The cornerstone of nutrition therapy for diabetes is to eat a low-carbohydrate diet.

☐ ☐ **3** Weight loss lowers the risk of type 2 diabetes only when it achieves a weight within an individual's healthy BMI range.

☐ ☐ **4** Alcohol is more likely to cause hypoglycemia when consumed without food rather than with food.

☐ ☐ **5** People with diabetes should avoid fruit because fructose produces a higher postprandial rise in glucose than sucrose.

☐ ☐ **6** People with diabetes should eat more fiber than the general population.

☐ ☐ **7** All people with diabetes should consume a bedtime snack to avoid hypoglycemia.

☐ ☐ **8** People who practice carbohydrate counting do not have to pay attention to protein or fat intake.

☐ ☐ **9** A chocolate candy bar is a good choice for treating mild hypoglycemia.

☐ ☐ **10** People with diabetes should limit their intake of saturated fat and cholesterol.

LEARNING OBJECTIVES

Upon completion of this chapter, you will be able to

1 Summarize nutrition recommendations for the primary prevention of diabetes.

2 Describe the nutrition recommendations for managing diabetes.

3 Explain nutrition recommendations for managing the complications of diabetes.

4 Compare the use of exchange lists to carbohydrate counting as a means of tracking carbohydrate intake.

5 Compose a 2000-calorie diet using the carbohydrate counting method of meal planning.

6 Determine the number of carbohydrate choices a serving of food provides by using the Nutrition Facts label.

7 Discuss diabetes nutrition therapy in childhood, pregnancy, and older adults.

G lucose circulating in the blood is a source of ready fuel for body cells. It comes primarily from recently absorbed dietary carbohydrates and liver glycogen, although glucose is available from some amino acids and the glycerol portion of fatty acids. All body cells use glucose for energy to some extent; under normal conditions, cells of the brain and the rest of the nervous system rely solely on glucose for energy.

The amount of carbohydrate and, to a lesser extent, the type of carbohydrate consumed are the primary determinants of how quickly and how high blood glucose levels rise after eating. A rise in postprandial blood glucose levels stimulates the pancreas to secrete insulin. As an anabolic hormone, insulin promotes the formation of glycogen, the storage of fat, and protein synthesis; conversely, it inhibits the breakdown of stored macronutrients. Its most well-known role is facilitating glucose uptake from the blood into the cells. The amount and effectiveness of circulating insulin determines how quickly blood glucose levels return to normal after eating.

When insulin secretion is absent or deficient, or circulating insulin is ineffective, glucose levels remain high after eating. Fasting blood glucose levels ≥126 mg/dL indicate diabetes. This chapter presents nutrition therapy aimed at preventing diabetes, managing existing diabetes, and preventing or forestalling diabetes complications.

DIABETES

Diabetes Mellitus: a chronic heterogeneous disorder characterized by elevated blood glucose levels (hyperglycemia) related to a relative or absolute deficiency of insulin.

Diabetes mellitus is a group of metabolic diseases characterized by hyperglycemia related to inadequate insulin secretion, diminished insulin effectiveness, or both. Over time, hyperglycemia damages blood vessels, nerves, and tissues. Diabetes also alters protein and fat metabolism, resulting in muscle wasting and elevated serum triglyceride levels, respectively. Table 19.1 summarizes the actions of insulin and effects of its insufficiency.

Diabetes is one of the most costly and burdensome chronic diseases of our time and is increasing in epidemic proportions. Every 17 seconds, an American is diagnosed with diabetes; if the current trend continues, one in three Americans will have diabetes by 2050

Table 19.1 Actions of Insulin and Effects of Its Insufficiency

Nutrient	Action of Insulin	Results of Insulin Insufficiency
Glucose	Promotes uptake of glucose into cells Promotes formation of glycogen in the liver and muscle Promotes conversion of excess glucose into triglycerides for storage	Decreases uptake of glucose into muscle and adipose Decreases glycogen formation in liver and muscle Increases glycogen breakdown in liver and muscle Increases gluconeogenesis (the formation of glucose from a noncarbohydrate source, such as amino acids or glycerol) Hyperglycemia
Protein	Promotes uptake of amino acids into tissue protein	Decreases uptake of amino acids into muscle Decreases protein synthesis Increases protein breakdown
Fat	Promotes formation of adipose from excess fat	Increases production of ketones in the liver Decreases formation of triglycerides in adipose Increases triglyceride breakdown in adipose Increases serum triglyceride and fatty acid levels

(Anderson, Riley, and Everette, 2012). The statistics are staggering (Centers for Disease Control and Prevention [CDC], 2011).

- In 2010, an estimated 25.8 million Americans, or 8.3% of the population, had diabetes. Of those cases, 7 million were undiagnosed.
- More than 35% of American adults have prediabetes based on fasting glucose or hemoglobin A1c levels.
- In 2010, an estimated 1.9 million Americans aged 20 years or older were newly diagnosed with diabetes.
- Diabetes is the seventh leading cause of death in the United States.
- The estimated direct and indirect cost associated with diabetes in 2010 was $174 billion. This estimate does not include the economic cost of undiagnosed diabetes or the immeasurable costs of pain and suffering related to diabetes (Fowler, 2010).

Type 1 Diabetes

Type 1 Diabetes: diabetes characterized by the absence of insulin secretion.

Polyuria: excessive urine excretion.

Polydipsia: excessive thirst.

Polyphagia: excessive appetite.

Ketoacidosis: the accumulation of ketone bodies leading to acidosis related to incomplete breakdown of fatty acids from carbohydrate deficiency or inadequate carbohydrate utilization.

Insulin Resistance: decreased cellular response to insulin.

Impaired Glucose Tolerance: 2-hour values in the oral glucose tolerance test of 140 to 199 mg/dL.

Impaired Fasting Glucose: fasting plasma glucose levels of 100 to 125 mg/dL.

Prediabetes: fasting plasma glucose of 100 to 126 mg/dL or an oral glucose tolerance test of 140 to 199 mg/dL.

Hyperinsulinemia: elevated blood levels of insulin.

Type 1 diabetes, formerly known as insulin-dependent diabetes mellitus or juvenile diabetes, is characterized by the absence of insulin. It occurs from an autoimmune response that damages or destroys pancreatic beta cells, leaving them unable to produce insulin. Interaction between genetic susceptibility and environmental factors, such as viral infection, is thought to be responsible for type 1 diabetes (Fowler, 2010). There is no known way to prevent type 1 diabetes. All people with type 1 diabetes require exogenous insulin for survival.

Although it can occur at any age, type 1 diabetes is most often detected in children and adolescents. The classic symptoms of **polyuria**, **polydipsia**, and **polyphagia** appear abruptly. Sometimes, the first sign of the disease is **ketoacidosis**. Type 1 diabetes accounts for 5% to 10% of all diagnosed diabetes cases.

Type 2 Diabetes

Type 2 diabetes, previously referred to as non–insulin-dependent diabetes or adult-onset diabetes, can occur at any age and accounts for 90% to 95% of diagnosed cases of diabetes. Unlike type 1 diabetes, in which there is a relatively abrupt and absolute end to insulin production, type 2 diabetes is a slowly progressive disease characterized by a combination of **insulin resistance** and relative insulin deficiency (Fowler, 2010). When cells do not respond to insulin as they should, the pancreas compensates by secreting higher than normal levels of insulin. This period of **impaired glucose tolerance/impaired fasting glucose** is known as **prediabetes**: glucose levels are normal or slightly elevated to levels below the criteria for diabetes and insulin levels are increased. Over time, chronic **hyperinsulinemia** leads to a decrease in the number of insulin receptors on the cells and a further reduction in tissue sensitivity to insulin. Insulin production progressively falls to a deficient level, and frank type 2 diabetes develops. Because hyperglycemia develops gradually in type 2 diabetes and is often not severe enough for patients to recognize any of the classic diabetes symptoms, type 2 diabetes may go undiagnosed for years. Many patients will have already developed complications by the time of diagnosis (Ahmad and Crandall, 2010).

Risk factors for type 2 diabetes appear is Box 19.1. Overweight and obesity are strongly correlated with the development of type 2 diabetes and may be responsible for the growing epidemic (Fowler, 2010). Other risks are increasing age, lack of physical activity, and race/ethnicity. Abdominal obesity, abnormal serum lipid levels (low high-density lipoprotein cholesterol and/or high triglycerides), and hypertension are additional risks that are shared

Box 19.1 RISK FACTORS FOR TYPE 2 DIABETES

- ≥45 years of age
- Overweight (BMI ≥23 kg/m² in Asian Americans; ≥26 kg/m² in Pacific Islanders, ≥25 kg/m² all others)
- First-degree relative with diabetes
- Physically inactive or exercises less than three times per week
- Member of high-risk ethnic group: African American, Latino, Native American, Asian American, Pacific Islander
- Previously identified with prediabetes such as impaired fasting glucose or impaired glucose tolerance
- History of gestational diabetes or giving birth to a baby weighing >9 pounds
- Hypertensive
- HDL <35 mg/dL and/or triglyceride level ≥250 mg/dL
- Acanthosis nigricans

Source: National Diabetes Education Program. (n.d.). *Diabetes risk factors.* Available at http://ndep.nih.gov/am-i-at-risk/DiabetesRiskFactors.aspx. Accessed 6/18/2012.

Metabolic Syndrome: a clustering of inter-related risk factors that include hypertension, low high-density lipoprotein (HDL) cholesterol, high triglycerides levels, and elevated serum glucose; central or abdominal obesity, as indicated by waist circumference, is often an additional criterion.

with the risk of cardiovascular disease. This cluster of risk factors is known as the **metabolic syndrome** (MetS). People with MetS are approximately five times as likely to develop diabetes as those without MetS, and their risk of heart disease is doubled (Alberti et al., 2009; Grundy, 2008). The progression of prediabetes to diabetes is not inevitable. Recent clinical trials have demonstrated that lifestyle modification—namely, modest weight loss, moderate physical activity, and a healthy diet—is the most effective tool in preventing or delaying type 2 diabetes (Ahmad and Crandall, 2010). Interventions that can reverse impaired glucose tolerance early in its course may be the key to preventing long-term complications of diabetes.

Gestational Diabetes

Gestational diabetes mellitus (GDM) is hyperglycemia that develops during pregnancy, usually around the 24th week of gestation. Women who meet the standard criteria for diabetes at their first prenatal visit are diagnosed with overt diabetes, not GDM. Approximately 7% of pregnancies are complicated by GDM (Bantle et al., 2008).

Diabetes increases risks in mother and infant. It increases the risk of preeclampsia, caesarean delivery, and fetal macrosomia and also the risk of hypertension and diabetes after pregnancy (Catalano, Huston, Amini, and Kalhan, 1999). Some studies show that as many as 70% of women who develop GDM will develop type 2 diabetes within 10 years after delivery (Fowler, 2010). GDM increases the risk of newborn death, stillbirth, and infant hypoglycemia in the days after delivery.

Women who fulfill *all* of the following criteria for low GDM risk do not need to be screened for GDM (American Diabetes Association [ADA], 2010):

- Age younger than 25 years old
- Normal body weight
- No first-degree relative with diabetes
- No personal history of abnormal glucose metabolism
- No history of poor obstetric outcome

- Not a member of en ethnic/racial group with a high prevalence of diabetes, such as Native Americans, Hispanic Americans, Mexican Americans, African Americans, Asian Americans, and Pacific Islanders

Women at average risk of GDM should be tested at 24 to 28 weeks of gestation; those at high risk should be tested as soon as feasible and retested at 24 to 28 weeks if not diagnosed at screening. For more on GDM, see Chapter 11.

Long-Term Complications

Sorbitol: the alcohol counterpart of glucose. High glucose levels can lead to an accumulation of sorbitol in cells, which exerts osmotic pressure.

Glycoproteins: compounds containing glucose or glucose fragments and proteins; high glucose levels can promote their formation.

Oxidative Stress: the state in which the production of oxidants (e.g., oxygen and other substances that oxidize other compounds) and free radicals exceeds the body's ability to neutralize their damaging effects.

Sustained hyperglycemia alters glucose metabolism in virtually every tissue. Damage to small vessels (microvascular) can lead to retinopathy, nephropathy, and neuropathy. Large blood vessel (macrovascular) damage increases the risk of cardiovascular disease and stroke. Other complications include impaired wound healing, gangrene, periodontal disease, and increased susceptibility to other illnesses. Although the precise mechanisms by which diabetes causes long-term complications are not completely understood, damage is likely to arise from several different mechanisms, such as an accumulation of **sorbitol**, injury from **glycoproteins**, and **oxidative stress** (Fowler, 2011).

Studies show that improved glycemic control can reduce the risk of complications in both type 1 and type 2 diabetes. According to the CDC (2011),

- Every percentage point drop in hemoglobin A1c can reduce the risk of microvascular complications (retinopathy, nephropathy, neuropathy) by 40%. Actual percentage improvement varies among subgroups.
- Controlling blood pressure lowers the risk of cardiovascular disease in people with diabetes by 33% to 50% and the risk of microvascular complications by approximately 33%.
- Lowering low-density lipoprotein (LDL) cholesterol can reduce cardiovascular complications by 20% to 50%.

DIABETES MANAGEMENT

For both type 1 and type 2 diabetes, nutrition therapy, physical activity, and blood glucose monitoring are integral components of management. Additionally, type 1 diabetes is treated with insulin. If lifestyle interventions fail to achieve glycemic control in people with type 2 diabetes, oral medications and often insulin are added to the regimen. Regardless of the type of diabetes, nutrient recommendations are the same; only issues of body weight and meal timing may differ between the two types of diabetes.

The ADA's position statement on nutrition recommendations and interventions for diabetes are highlighted in the following sections. Goals and interventions are specified for three levels of prevention: the primary prevention of diabetes among people with prediabetes or at high-risk of diabetes; the secondary prevention of managing existing diabetes; and the tertiary prevention of preventing or slowing the rate of diabetes complications (Bantle et al., 2008).

Preventing Diabetes

Because of the strong link between excess weight and insulin resistance/type 2 diabetes, weight loss, through a combination of healthy eating and exercise, is the primary focus of diabetes prevention (Box 19.2). A major, multicenter clinical trial called the Diabetes Prevention Program (DPP) found that in a diverse group of overweight people with impaired glucose tolerance, diet, exercise, and behavior modification decreased the incidence

Box 19.2 LIFESTYLE RECOMMENDATIONS TO PREVENT TYPE 2 DIABETES

- Make lifestyle changes to produce a moderate weight loss of 5% to 15% of initial weight, with a target of 1 to 2 pounds/week.
- Engage in moderate physical activity (e.g., brisk walking) for at least 30 minutes per day, 5 days per week.
- Limit fat to <30% of total calories.
- Reduce portion sizes and daily calorie intake.
- Increase intake of fruit, vegetables, and fiber.

Source: Ahmad, L., & Crandall, J. (2010). Type 2 diabetes prevention: A review. *Clinical Diabetes, 28*, 53–59.

of diabetes by 58% (DPP Research Group, 2002). Study participants walked at moderate intensity, an average of 150 minutes/week, and decreased their intake of fat and calories. Average weight loss was a modest 5% to 7% of initial weight, or about 15 pounds. Participants also benefited from improvements in their lipid profiles, blood pressure, and markers of inflammation (Haffner et al., 2005; Ratner et al., 2005). The DPP results were so quick and convincing that the program was halted a year early. A 10-year follow-up on the original participants showed that the lifestyle intervention group maintained a decreased risk of diabetes over time (DPP Research Group, 2009). Clearly, millions of overweight Americans at high risk for type 2 diabetes can delay and possibly prevent the disease with a modest weight loss brought about by a moderate diet and regular exercise.

There is no one proven strategy that can be uniformly recommended to promote weight loss in all clients. Although standard weight loss diets that provide 500 to 1000 fewer calories than usual daily intake can promote a weight loss of as much as 10% in 6 months, most people regain weight without continued support and follow-up (Bantle et al., 2008). Very-low-calorie diets (~800 cal/day) produce substantial weight loss and rapid improvements in blood glucose and lipid levels in people with type 2 diabetes, but weight gain is common after the diet stops. For some patients, weight loss is achieved by a more flexible strategy using MyPlate as a guide for increasing fruits, vegetables, and whole grains while limiting fats and sweets (see Chapter 8). An individualized approach takes into account the client's treatment goals and his or her ability and willingness to change.

The type of fat consumed may also influence diabetes risk (Bantle et al., 2008). Specifically, a low saturated fat intake may reduce the risk for diabetes by improving insulin resistance and promoting weight loss. Beyond its potential beneficial effects on diabetes risk, a low saturated fat diet is well established as a strategy to lower the risk of heart disease (National Cholesterol Education Program, 2001).

Several studies show that an increased intake of whole grains and fiber lowers the risk of diabetes (Bantle et al., 2008). Whole grains correlate to improved insulin sensitivity, regardless of body weight. Fiber has been associated with improved insulin sensitivity and improved ability to secrete insulin to overcome insulin resistance (Liese et al., 2003).

Managing Diabetes

The primary goal of diabetes management is to keep blood glucose levels as near normal as possible. Additional goals are to

- Attain and maintain reasonable weight
- Attain and maintain control of blood lipid levels and blood pressure
- Prevent or delay the development of acute and chronic complications

- Meet the individual's cultural and personal needs while respecting preferences and willingness to change
- Maintain the pleasure of eating by not limiting any foods unless indicated by scientific evidence

Nutrition therapy is an essential component of diabetes management regardless of the client's weight, blood glucose levels, or use of medication. People with diabetes generally have the same nutritional requirements as the general population; therefore, dietary recommendations to promote health and well-being in the general public—lose weight if overweight, eat less saturated fat and cholesterol, eat more fiber and less sodium—are also appropriate for people with diabetes. Because coronary heart disease (CHD) is the leading cause of death among people with diabetes, it makes sense that nutrition recommendations issued by the ADA to prevent and treat diabetes are remarkably similar to recommendations put forth by the American Heart Association (AHA) for the primary and secondary prevention of CHD (Chapter 20). Nutrition recommendations for diabetes management are summarized in Table 19.2.

Calories and Weight Loss

Body Mass Index (BMI): an index of weight status determined by dividing weight in kilograms by height in meters squared. Current standard for "normal" BMI is 18.5 to 24.9; overweight is 25.0 to 29.9; and obesity begins at 30.0, with ≥40.0 considered extreme obesity.

Consistent with interventions to *prevent* diabetes, recommendations to *manage* type 2 diabetes in overweight and obese people focus on lifestyle modifications that lead to weight loss—namely, a lower calorie intake, healthy food choices, and increased physical activity. Short-term studies show that moderate weight loss (5% of body weight) in people with type 2 diabetes improves insulin resistance, glycemic control, lipid levels, and blood pressure. However, many patients have unsuccessfully tried to lose weight even before being diagnosed with diabetes, and achieving long-term weight loss is difficult for most people. If lifestyle modifications fail to produce weight loss, additional weight loss strategies may be considered. Weight loss medications, when combined with a healthy diet and exercise, can promote a 5% to 10% weight loss. Drug labels state that the medications should only be used in people with diabetes who have a **body mass index (BMI)** >27 (Bantle et al., 2008).

Table 19.2 Nutrition Recommendations for Managing Diabetes

	Recommendations Based on Strong Evidence	Recommendations Based on Limited or Conflicting Evidence
Calories	Lose weight if overweight or obese. Restricted-calorie diets that are either low-carbohydrate or low-fat diets may be effective for up to a year. Physical activity and behavior modification are important for weight loss and vital for maintaining weight loss.	For patients on low-carbohydrate diets, monitor lipid levels, renal function, and protein intake (in patients with nephropathy) and adjust hypoglycemic therapy, as needed.
Carbohydrates	Carbohydrates from fruits, vegetables, whole grains, legumes, and low-fat milk are part of a healthy diet. Monitoring carbohydrate intake is essential to achieve glycemic control. Attention to glycemic index may provide a modest additional benefit above simply consuming a consistent carbohydrate intake.	

(continues on page 504)

Table 19.2 Nutrition Recommendations for Managing Diabetes (continued)

	Recommendations Based on Strong Evidence	Recommendations Based on Limited or Conflicting Evidence
Sweeteners	Foods containing sucrose can be substituted for other carbohydrate foods; if they are eaten as "extras" to the meal plan, they should be covered with insulin or other glucose-lowering medications. Be mindful of the "empty calories" provided by high-sugar foods to avoid consuming excess calories. Sugar alcohols and nonnutritive sweeteners are safe when used within daily intake levels set by the FDA.	
Fiber	Eat an adequate intake of fiber from a wide variety of sources. People with diabetes do not need more fiber than the general population.	
Fat	Limit saturated fat to 7% of total calories. Consume two or more servings of fatty fish per week (excluding commercially fried fish fillets).	Minimize trans fat intake. Limit dietary cholesterol to 200 mg/day.
Protein	In people with type 2 diabetes, protein does not increase plasma glucose levels, so it should not be used to treat acute hypoglycemia or prevent nighttime hypoglycemia.	There is not enough evidence to recommend that protein intake should differ from the usual intake of 15%–20% of total calories consumed for people with type 2 diabetes and normal renal function. High-protein diets (>20% of total calories) are not recommended for weight loss because the long-term effects on diabetes management and complications are unknown.
Alcohol	Alcoholic beverages that contain carbohydrates may raise blood glucose levels.	People with diabetes who choose to drink should limit their intake to one drink per day or less for women and two drinks per day or less for men. Alcohol should be consumed with food to reduce the risk of nighttime hypoglycemia in people who use insulin or drugs that stimulate insulin secretion.
Micronutrients	In the absence of underlying deficiencies, vitamin and mineral supplements do not provide any benefit. Routine supplements of antioxidants (vitamins C and E and beta-carotene) are not recommended due to lack of evidence that they are effective or safe for long-term use.	Chromium supplements are not recommended because no clear benefit has been observed.

Source: American Diabetes Association. (2008). Nutrition recommendations and interventions for diabetes. A position statement of the American Diabetes Association. *Diabetes Care, 31*(Suppl. 1), S61–S78.

Bariatric surgery can dramatically improve type 2 diabetes, resulting in normal blood glucose and hemoglobin A1c levels with discontinuation of all diabetes medications (Rubino, 2008). The return of normal glucose and insulin levels is observed within days after the surgery, suggesting that other factors besides weight loss are involved. Buchwald et al. (2004) found that gastric bypass surgery resolved diabetes in approximately 84% of postsurgery patients and that laparoscopic adjustable gastric banding resolved diabetes in approximately 48% of post-surgery patients. Bariatric surgery is currently reserved for people with a BMI ≥35.

Total Carbohydrates

As previously stated, the nutritional needs of people with diabetes do not differ from the general population, including the need for carbohydrates. For most Americans, carbohydrates provide approximately 50% of total calories consumed, a figure safely within the Acceptable Macronutrient Distribution Range (AMDR) of 45% to 65% of total calories. It is reasonable that people with diabetes follow these guidelines.

At intakes below 45% of total calories, intake of fat is too high and the intake of fiber and vitamins and minerals may be inadequate. At intakes above 65% of total calories, protein needs may not be met. Because consistency in carbohydrate has been shown to improve glycemic control, meal and snack carbohydrate intake should be consistently distributed through the day on a day-to-day basis (Franz et al., 2010). The exception to this recommendation is for people who adjust their mealtime insulin doses or who use an insulin pump because insulin doses are adjusted according to carbohydrate intake.

Consistent with recommendations for the general population, "good carbs" are emphasized over "bad carbs." The majority of carbohydrate calories should come from nutritionally dense foods, such as fruit, vegetables, whole grains, legumes, and low-fat milk. Nutritionally inferior carbohydrates include refined grains (e.g., white bread, white rice, white pasta, foods made with white flour) and foods high in added sugars. It is important to note that these foods are not eliminated, but their intake should be limited so as not to displace the intake of other more nutrient-dense foods.

Glycemic control is dependent on matching carbohydrate intake with the action of insulin or other medication. Carbohydrate monitoring can be achieved by using exchange lists, carbohydrate counting, or experience-based estimation. No single method of estimating carbohydrate intake has been proven superior to the others (Bantle et al., 2008). Several randomized clinical trials have shown that low **glycemic index** diets improve glycemic control, but other trials have not confirmed this (Sheard et al., 2004). The ADA states that a low glycemic index diet may provide a modest benefit in controlling postprandial hyperglycemia when used in place of a high glycemic index diet (Bantle et al., 2008). For more on glycemic index, see Chapter 2.

Glycemic Index: the incremental rise in blood glucose (above baseline) compared to that induced by a standard, usually 50 g of glucose or a white bread challenge.

Sweeteners

Isocalorically: of the same calorie level.

Substantial evidence from clinical studies demonstrates that when sucrose is **isocalorically** substituted for starch, there is no difference in glycemic control in either type 1 or type 2 diabetes (Franz et al., 2002). Sucrose and sucrose-containing foods are not restricted but should be substituted for other carbohydrates in the meal plan, not eaten as "extras." Many people with long-standing diabetes resist accepting this shift in thinking because sugar was once taboo. Others find the freedom to choose sweetened foods difficult not to abuse. Even though foods high in sugar do not aggravate glycemic control, they are usually nutrient poor and may be high in fat. Care should be taken to avoid an excess calorie intake.

The use of fructose as an added sweetener is not recommended because even though it produces a lower postprandial response than sucrose, it may adversely affect serum lipid levels by raising LDL and triglyceride levels (Bantle et al., 2008). There is no reason for people with diabetes to avoid naturally occurring fructose in fruits and vegetables.

Sugar Alcohols: natural sweeteners derived from monosaccharides; these are considered low-calorie sweeteners because they are incompletely absorbed. They produce a smaller rise in postprandial glucose levels and insulin secretion than sucrose.

Nonnutritive Sweeteners: synthetically made sweeteners that do not provide calories.

Plant Sterols/Stanols: naturally occurring substances in plants that help block the absorption of cholesterol from the gastrointestinal tract. Some margarines have plant sterols added for therapeutic benefit.

Sugar alcohols (sorbitol, mannitol, and xylitol) provide fewer calories and cause a smaller increase in glucose than sucrose or glucose. They do not contribute to dental cavities, yet using them is not likely to produce weight loss or improve glycemic control (Bantle et al., 2008). They appear safe to use but may cause diarrhea when consumed in large amounts, especially in children.

The **nonnutritive sweeteners**, saccharin, aspartame, acesulfame potassium, and sucralose, are approved for use by the U.S. Food and Drug Administration (FDA) and may safely be used by people with diabetes. There is no indication that these will promote weight loss or gain (Bantle et al., 2008).

Fiber

The recommendations for fiber are the same as for the general population—that is, 14 g/1000 cal consumed, or approximately 25 g/day for women and 38 g/day for men. Evidence is lacking that amounts greater than this are beneficial for people with diabetes (Wheeler and Pi-Sunyer, 2008). However, foods rich in fiber provide other benefits such as increasing satiety (a plus for weight management); providing vitamins, minerals, and phytochemicals; and lowering serum cholesterol levels (Wheeler and Pi-Sunyer, 2008). People with diabetes are encouraged to eat more fiber than the typical American consumes, but they do not need to eat more than what is recommended for the general population. A variety of sources is recommended.

Fat

People with diabetes appear to have the same cardiovascular risk as people with preexisting cardiovascular disease (CVD), so recommendations concerning fat intake are generally the same for both groups (Bantle et al., 2008). Specifically, people with diabetes are advised to limit their intake of saturated fat to less than 7% of total calories, minimize their intake of trans fat, and consume less than 200 mg of cholesterol daily. Two or more servings of fish per week are recommended for their omega-3 fatty acid content; omega-3 fatty acids have been shown to lower adverse CVD outcomes (Bantle et al., 2008). **Plant sterols/stanols** lower LDL cholesterol by up to 15%, with maximum effects at ~2 g/day, and are another option for lowering CVD risk (Lichtenstein et al., 2006). The difference between these recommendations and those made by the AHA for people with or at risk for CVD is slight; the AHA recommends trans fat be limited to less than 1% of total calories and suggests cholesterol be restricted to less than 300 mg/day (Lichtenstein et al., 2006). Box 19.3 lists tips for achieving a low–saturated fat, low–trans fat, low-cholesterol intake.

Box 19.3 TIPS TO ACHIEVE A LOW–SATURATED FAT, LOW–TRANS FAT, LOW-CHOLESTEROL DIET

- Eat chicken, fish, and beans more often than other types of meat.
- Eat two 3½ oz servings of fish weekly.
- Use lean cuts of meat; remove skin from poultry before eating.
- Limit processed meats that are high in saturated fat.
- Grill, bake, broil, or roast meat, fish, and poultry.
- Limit organ meats.
- Use only nonfat or low-fat milk, cheese, and yogurt.
- Use liquid oils in place of solid fats.
- Use a soft, trans fat–free spread in place of margarine.
- Avoid processed foods such as frozen French fries, frozen chicken fingers, and potato chips.
- Avoid fried fast food.
- Avoid high-fat baked products such as cakes, cookies, crackers, and doughnuts.

Protein

In the typical American diet, including the diets of people with diabetes, protein provides 15% of total calories, a value within the AMDR of 10% to 35% of total calories. There is insufficient evidence to suggest that people with diabetes who have normal renal function should alter their usual intake of protein.

Alcohol

Moderate use of alcohol (1 drink/day or less in women and 2 drinks/day or less in men) by people who have well-controlled diabetes has minimal effects on blood glucose and insulin levels, as long as it is not mixed with another liquid that provides carbohydrates (e.g., mixed drinks). For people who take insulin, alcohol should be consumed with food to avoid hypoglycemia. People with type 1 diabetes should not reduce their food intake to compensate for alcohol calories. Light to moderate use of alcohol by people with diabetes is associated with a lower risk of CVD regardless of the type of beverage consumed (Bantle et al., 2008).

Vitamins and Minerals

The vitamin and mineral requirements of people with diabetes are not different from those of the general population. Supplements provide no proven benefit in managing diabetes unless underlying nutrient deficiencies exist. Uncontrolled diabetes is often associated with micronutrient deficiencies; when deficiencies are diagnosed, the approach should be a balanced diet that supplies natural sources of nutrients.

 QUICK BITE

Sources of chromium

Whole grains	Some dried peas and beans
Nuts	Yeast
Mushrooms	Organ meats
Broccoli	Pork
Egg yolks	

The essential mineral chromium has been studied for its possible role in the prevention and treatment of diabetes. It promotes glucose uptake by cells, possibly by increasing the number and activity of insulin receptors on the cells (Melanson, 2007). Some studies show that chromium supplementation improves glucose tolerance (Anderson, 2000). Although the ADA states that there is currently insufficient evidence to recommend chromium supplementation, an ample dietary intake is advised. Studies are also needed to determine if magnesium and antioxidant supplements are beneficial to type 2 diabetes management (Bantle et al., 2008).

Controlling Diabetes Complications

The progression of microvascular diabetes complications may be modified by improving glycemic control and lowering blood pressure (Bantle et al., 2008). The Diabetes Control and Complications Trial/Epidemiology of Diabetes Interventions and Complications Study showed that during 17 years of prospective analysis, intensive treatment of type 1 diabetes was associated with a 42% risk reduction in all cardiovascular events and a 57% decrease in the risk of nonfatal myocardial infarction, stroke, or death from CVD (Nathan et al., 2005). Table 19.3 highlights the ADA's recommendations for treating and controlling microvascular and cardiovascular complications.

Table 19.3 Nutrition Recommendations for Controlling Diabetes Complications

	Recommendations Based on Strong Evidence	Recommendations Based on Limited or Conflicting Evidence
For microvascular complications	Reduce protein intake to 0.8–1.0 g/kg for people with early-stage chronic kidney disease; lower to 0.8 g/kg for later stages of diabetic kidney disease.	Nutrition therapy used for cardiovascular disease (CVD) risk factors may benefit microvascular complications, such as retinopathy and nephropathy.
Treatment and management of CVD risk	Control hemoglobin A1c as close to normal as possible without significant hypoglycemia. Whether normotensive or hypertensive, lower sodium intake to 2300 mg/day and eat a diet rich in fruits, vegetables, and low-fat dairy products.	For people at risk of CVD, a diet rich in fruit, vegetables, whole grains, and nuts may lower risk. For people with symptomatic heart failure, a sodium intake of <2000 mg/day may improve symptoms. In most people, modest weight loss improves blood pressure.

Source: American Diabetes Association. (2008). Nutrition recommendations and interventions for diabetes. A position statement of the American Diabetes Association. *Diabetes Care, 31*(Suppl. 1), S61–S78.

MEAL PLANNING

Monitoring carbohydrate intake, either by exchange lists, carbohydrate counting, or experience-based estimation, is key to controlling blood glucose levels (Wheeler et al., 2008). Regardless of the strategy used, meal plans are based on the individual's total calorie requirements, usual eating pattern, preferences, and willingness/ability to make dietary changes. Typically, food is spread out over three meals; snacks are necessary for some people, depending on their calorie needs and insulin/medication regime. Snacks are not necessary for obese people with type 2 diabetes who are diet controlled or who take insulin sensitizer oral medications but may be incorporated into the meal plan based on the individual's preference.

Both the exchange lists and carbohydrate counting meal planning approaches specify how many carbohydrate servings should be consumed at each meal and snack and encourage users to do the following:

- Eat a variety of foods.
- Choose fruits, vegetables, whole grains, and low-fat or nonfat milk, cheese, or yogurt for the majority of carbohydrate servings.
- Eat more fiber than usual.
- Limit foods high in sodium.
- Eat 4 to 6 oz (or more, depending on calorie needs) of protein foods spread out over the day.
- Use healthy fats, such as olive oil, canola oil, and nuts.
- Avoid foods high in saturated fat, such as butter, cream, and high-fat meats.
- Avoid foods containing trans fats, such as processed foods made with "partially hydrogenated oils."

Exchange Lists for Meal Planning

Devised by the ADA and the American Dietetic Association, the *Choose Your Foods: Exchange Lists for Meal Planning* is a framework for choosing a healthy diet that groups foods into lists that, per serving size given, are similar in carbohydrate, protein, fat, and calories based on rounded averages (Box 19.4) (ADA and American Dietetic Association, 2008). Its three

Box 19.4   EXCHANGE LISTS FOR DIABETES

Carbohydrate Group

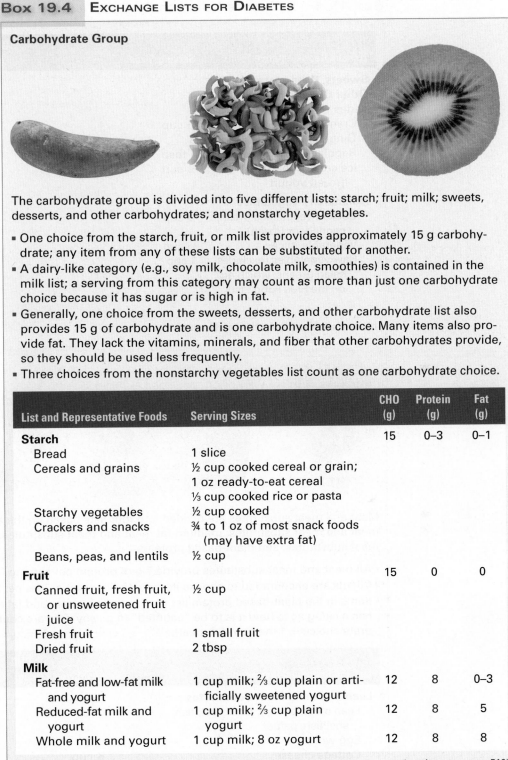

The carbohydrate group is divided into five different lists: starch; fruit; milk; sweets, desserts, and other carbohydrates; and nonstarchy vegetables.

- One choice from the starch, fruit, or milk list provides approximately 15 g carbohydrate; any item from any of these lists can be substituted for another.
- A dairy-like category (e.g., soy milk, chocolate milk, smoothies) is contained in the milk list; a serving from this category may count as more than just one carbohydrate choice because it has sugar or is high in fat.
- Generally, one choice from the sweets, desserts, and other carbohydrate list also provides 15 g of carbohydrate and is one carbohydrate choice. Many items also provide fat. They lack the vitamins, minerals, and fiber that other carbohydrates provide, so they should be used less frequently.
- Three choices from the nonstarchy vegetables list count as one carbohydrate choice.

List and Representative Foods	Serving Sizes	CHO (g)	Protein (g)	Fat (g)
Starch		15	0–3	0–1
Bread	1 slice			
Cereals and grains	½ cup cooked cereal or grain; 1 oz ready-to-eat cereal ⅓ cup cooked rice or pasta			
Starchy vegetables	½ cup cooked			
Crackers and snacks	¾ to 1 oz of most snack foods (may have extra fat)			
Beans, peas, and lentils	½ cup			
Fruit		15	0	0
Canned fruit, fresh fruit, or unsweetened fruit juice	½ cup			
Fresh fruit	1 small fruit			
Dried fruit	2 tbsp			
Milk				
Fat-free and low-fat milk and yogurt	1 cup milk; ⅔ cup plain or artificially sweetened yogurt	12	8	0–3
Reduced-fat milk and yogurt	1 cup milk; ⅔ cup plain yogurt	12	8	5
Whole milk and yogurt	1 cup milk; 8 oz yogurt	12	8	8

(continues on page 510)

Box 19.4 EXCHANGE LISTS FOR DIABETES (continued)

List and Representative Foods	Serving Sizes	CHO (g)	Protein (g)	Fat (g)
Sweets, Desserts, and Other Carbohydrates		15	Varies	Varies
Varies				
Cranberry juice cocktail	½ cup			
Gingersnap cookies	3			
Regular pancake syrup	1 tbsp			
Ice cream, sherbet, or frozen yogurt	½ cup			
Nonstarchy Vegetables		5	2	0
Cooked vegetables (fresh, canned, or frozen)	½ cup			
Vegetable juice	½ cup			
Raw vegetables (excludes salad greens, which are on the Free Food List)	1 cup			

Meat and Meat Substitutes Group

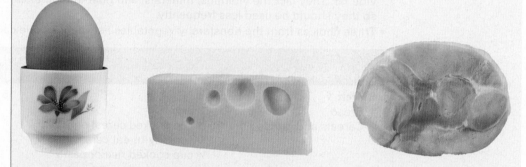

Meat and meat substitutes are divided into four lists based on the amount of fat: lean meat and meat substitutes; medium-fat meat and meat substitutes; high-fat meat and meat substitutes; and plant-based proteins.

- All meat and meat substitutes provide 7 g of protein per serving.
- Clients are encouraged to choose items with 5 g of fat or less per ounce.
- Items in the plant-based protein list vary in carbohydrate and fat content, and so each has a citing as to how it is to be "counted" (e.g., soy nuts are counted as ½ carbohydrate choice + 1 medium-fat meat).

List and Representative Foods	Serving Sizes	CHO (g)	Protein (g)	Fat (g)
Lean Meat and Meat Substitutes		—	7	0–3
Lean meat, poultry, pork, veal; fish, shellfish, game	1 oz			
Egg whites	2			
Cottage cheese	¼ cup			

Box 19.4   EXCHANGE LISTS FOR DIABETES (continued)

List and Representative Foods	Serving Sizes	CHO (g)	Protein (g)	Fat (g)
Medium-Fat Meat and Meat Substitutes		—	7	4–7
Cheese with 4–7 g fat per ounce	1 oz			
Egg	1			
Fried fish	1 oz			
Prime grades of beef, chicken with skin, veal cutlet	1 oz			
High-Fat Meat and Meat Substitutes		—	7	8+
Pork bacon	2 slices			
Regular cheese	1 oz			
Hot dogs	1			
Processed sandwich meats and sausage with 8 g of fat or more per ounce	1 oz			
Plant-Based Proteins		Varies	7	Varies
Soy bacon	3 strips			
Nut butters (e.g., almond butter, cashew butter, peanut butter)	1 tbsp			
Refried beans, canned	½ cup			
Hummus	⅓ cup			

Fats

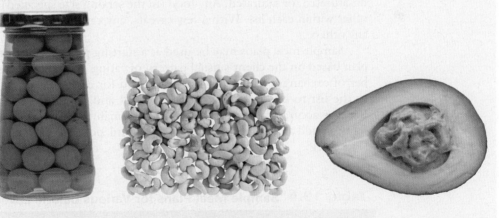

Fats are divided into three lists based on the type of fat they contain: monounsaturated, polyunsaturated, and saturated.

- All items on the fats list provide 5 g of fat per serving.

List and Representative Foods	Serving Sizes	CHO (g)	Protein (g)	Fat (g)
Monounsaturated Fats		—	—	5
Avocado	2 tbsp			
Nut butters	1½ tsp			
Nuts	2–16, depending on the type			
Canola, olive, and peanut oil	1 tsp			
Olives	8–10			

(continues on page 512)

Box 19.4   EXCHANGE LISTS FOR DIABETES (continued)

List and Representative Foods	Serving Sizes	CHO (g)	Protein (g)	Fat (g)
Polyunsaturated Fats		—	—	5
Low-fat margarine	1 tbsp			
Regular mayonnaise	1 tsp			
Corn, soybean, sunflower oil	1 tsp			
Reduced-fat salad dressing	2 tbsp			
Saturated Fats		—	—	5
Bacon	1 slice			
Chitterlings, boiled	2 tbsp			
Half and half cream	2 tbsp			
Salt pork	1/4 oz			
Regular sour cream	2 tbsp			

major categories are carbohydrates, meat and meat substitutes, and fats. Supplemental lists provide guidance on free foods, combination foods, fast foods, and alcohol. Within each of the major groupings are subgroups that form the exchange lists. For instance, the Meat and Substitutes List has separate categories for lean, medium-fat, high-fat, and plant-based proteins; high-sodium foods are identified; and fats are grouped as monounsaturated, polyunsaturated, or saturated. Any food (in the serving size specified) can be exchanged for any other within each list. With a few caveats, any carbohydrate choices can be exchanged for any others.

Sample meal plans may be used as a starting point for creating an individualized meal plan based on the client's usual pattern of eating and preferences (Table 19.4). The number of exchanges from each list is specified for each meal and snack; clients simply refer to the list to choose the appropriate types and amounts of food allowed (Table 19.5). Because accurate portion sizes are vital to maintaining a consistent carbohydrate intake, food should be weighed or measured until portion sizes can be accurately estimated (Fig. 19.1).

Table 19.4   Sample Meal Plans for Various Calorie Levels*

	Calories per Day					
	1200	1600	1800	2000	2200	2400
Carbohydrates						
Starches	5	7	8	9	10	11
Fruits	3	3	3	4	4	4
Milk	2	3	3	3	3	3
Nonstarchy vegetables	3	4	5	6	6	6
Meat and meat substitutes	4 oz	6 oz	6 oz	7 oz	8 oz	8 oz
Fat	3	5	6	6	7	7

*Numbers in the table represent a suggested number of servings per day from each food list based on fat-free milk and lean meats. Actual number of servings may differ based on the client's usual pattern of eating and preferences.

Table 19.5 Sample 1800-Calorie Meal Plan*

	Breakfast	Lunch	Dinner	Bedtime Snack
Carbohydrates				
Starches	2	2	3	1
Fruits	1	1	1	
Milk	1	1	½	½
Nonstarchy vegetables		2	3	
Meat and meat substitutes	1	2	3	
Fat	2	2	2	

*Numbers in the table represent a suggested number of servings per meal from each food list based on fat-free milk and lean meats.

The advantages of using the exchange list system are that it eliminates the need for daily calculations, ensures a relatively consistent intake, and emphasizes important nutrition principles such as using healthy fat and controlling sodium intake. Yet there are several drawbacks. The terminology may be confusing, such as carbohydrate choice versus grams of carbohydrates. Some items on some lists are counted as more than just one choice or

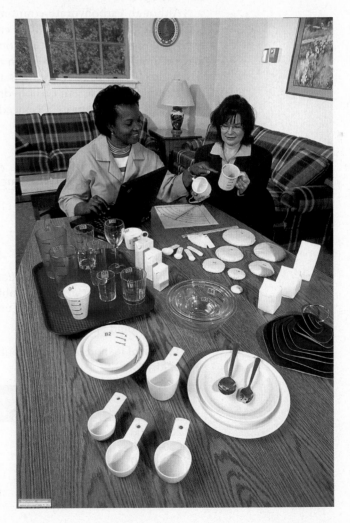

■ FIGURE 19.1 Serving size aids help clients learn appropriate serving sizes. (Photo by Stephen Ausmus. U.S. Department of Agriculture, Agricultural Research Service.)

one exchange, such as black-eyed peas, which are counted as one starch plus one lean meat. Some items appear on more than one list and in different amounts, such as 1 tbsp of peanut butter on the plant-based protein list and 1½ tsp of peanut butter on the monounsaturated fat list. In addition, the exchange system is less flexible than carbohydrate counting and may not be appropriate or acceptable for all age, ethnic, and cultural groups. The exchange list approach is best suited to people who want or need structured meal-planning guidance and are able to understand complex details.

Carbohydrate Counting

Carbohydrate counting is gaining in popularity as an easier and more flexible alternative to using the exchange system. Clients are given an individualized meal pattern that specifies the number of carbohydrate "choices" (one choice = 15 g carbohydrate) for each meal and snack (Box 19.5). Most adults are allowed three to five carbohydrate choices per meal and one to two for each snack, depending on their calorie needs. Sample 1800-calorie menus using carbohydrate counting are featured in Box 19.6. To assist people with identifying sources of carbohydrates and the appropriate portion sizes, clients are given carbohydrate choice lists, similar to the exchange lists but generally focused specifically on carbohydrates. Clients also need to know how to read the Nutrition Facts label to accurately count carbohydrates (Fig. 19.2).

Although carbohydrate counting has the advantage of focusing on a single nutrient (carbohydrates) rather than all the energy-yielding nutrients, protein and fat cannot be disregarded, especially if weight is a concern. The goals of weight control and healthful eating may be forgotten or forsaken when the emphasis is placed solely on carbohydrate.

Basic carbohydrate counting is appropriate for people who understand the importance of consuming a consistent carbohydrate intake to match insulin or medication peaks. Some people progress to a more advanced level of carbohydrate counting that allows clients to

Box 19.5	THE NUMBER OF CARBOHYDRATE CHOICES AT VARIOUS CALORIE LEVELS

One carbohydrate choice equals (15 g carbohydrate)

- 1 serving of starch
- 1 serving of fruit
- 1 serving from the Milk group
- 1 serving from the sweets and desserts group
- 3 servings of nonstarchy vegetables (because they are so low in carbohydrates and are "healthy," often people are encouraged to eat these as desired)

The diet should also include

- 4 to 6 oz of lean meat or meat substitutes per day
- Healthy fats

Total Calories	Carbohydrate Choices for Each Meal	Carbohydrate Choices for Snacks per Day
1200–1500	3	1
1600–2000	4	2–3
2100–2400	5	4–6

Box 19.6 CARBOHYDRATE COUNTING: SAMPLE 1800-CALORIE MENUS

Sample Menu	Carbohydrate Choices	Sample Menu	Carbohydrate Choices
Breakfast			
½ cup orange juice	1	A parfait consisting of	
1 low-fat waffle topped	1	1¼ cup strawberries	1
with ¾ cup blueberries		½ cup low-fat granola	2
1 cup nonfat milk	1	6 oz plain yogurt	1
1 tsp light margarine	1	Coffee	
Lunch			
6-in submarine with	3	Hamburger on a bun	2
2 oz meat and light		1 cup oven-baked French	1
mayonnaise		fries	
1 apple	1	Lettuce and tomato	
Diet soft drink		Light mayonnaise	
		1 cup nonfat milk	1
Dinner			
1 taco shell	2	1 cup spaghetti noodles	3
3 oz taco meat		2 meatballs	
1½ cups combined	1	1 cup spaghetti sauce	1
lettuce, tomato, onion		Tossed salad	
⅓ cup rice	1	1 slice Italian bread	1
1 cup cubed papaya	1	1 tsp butter	
		Diet soft drink	
Bedtime Snack			
½ cup shredded wheat	1	3 cups no fat added popcorn	1
1 cup nonfat milk	1	1 cup nonfat milk	1
Total carbohydrate choices/day	15		15

adjust their mealtime insulin dosage based on the grams of carbohydrate they want to eat and their premeal blood glucose level. Clients feel more in control and benefit from improved glucose control. On the minus side, carbohydrate counting requires clients to be diligent to the plan and prudent in their food choices. Keeping records of blood glucose tests and food intake helps to identify sources of problems.

Changing Behaviors

The diagnosis of diabetes often triggers anxiety and uncertainty. People often see "diet" as the most difficult part of treatment. Even people with healthy eating styles may need to make changes in their intake to improve glycemic control. Giving someone a preprinted list of do's and don'ts can add to a resentful client's frustration. Before recommending dietary changes, it may be useful to ask

- What are your goals for nutrition counseling?
- What behaviors do you want to change?
- What changes can you make in your present lifestyle?

Step 1: Identify the serving size. The nutrition content is based on this serving size.

Example: 1 serving = 3/4 c

Step 2: Find the grams of total carbohydrates. 1 carbohydrate choice = 15 g CHO, with a range of 11–20 counted as 1 choice.

g total carbohydrate	# CHO choices
6–10	1/2
11–20	1
21–25	1 1/2
26–35	2
36–40	2 1/2
41–50	3

The grams of sugar are part of the total carbohydrate and do not require special attention.

Example: 1 serving = 1 1/2 carbohydrate choices

Step 3: Check on the grams of total fiber per serving. If a serving provides >5 g total fiber, subtract 1/2 the total grams of fiber from the grams of carbohydrates (because fiber is relatively nondigestable and provides less than 4 cal/g) to get the total carbohydrate grams.

Example: 1 serving has 10 g fiber
10 g ÷ 2 = 5 g fiber
25 g total carbohydrate − 5 g fiber = 20 g carbohydrate
This counts as 1 carbohydrate choice.

Step 4: If a serving provides more than 5 g of sugar alcohols, subtract 1/2 the grams of sugar alcohol from the carbohydrate grams to get the total carbohydrate grams.

Example: Sugar alcohols are not listed on this nutrition facts label therefore this product does not contain any. No further adjustment in total carbohydrate grams is needed.

Nutrition Facts

Serving Size   3/4 cup (33 g/1.2 oz.)
Servings Per Container   About 11

Amount Per Serving

Calories 110   Calories from Fat 15

% Daily Value**

Total Fat 1.5 g*	**2%**
Saturated Fat 0 g	**0%**
Trans Fat 0 g	
Cholesterol 0 mg	**0%**
Sodium 90 mg	**4%**
Potassium 100 mg	**3%**
Total Carbohydrate 25 g	**8%**
Dietary Fiber 10 g	**18%**
Soluble Fiber 2 g	
Insoluble Fiber 5 g	
Sugars 5 g	
Other Carbohydrate 10 g	
Protein 4 g	

Vitamin A 25% (25% DV as beta carotene)			
Vitamin C 50%	*	Calcium 0%	
Iron 10%	*	Vitamin E 100%	
Vitamin B_6 100%	*	Folic Acid 100%	
Vitamin B_{12} 100%	*	Zinc 10%	

* Amount in cereal. One half cup of fat free milk contributes and additional 40 calories, 65 mg sodium, 6 g total carbohydrates (6 g sugars), and 4 g protein.
** Percent Daily Values are based on a 2,000 calorie diet. Your daily values may be higher or lower depending on your calorie needs.

	Calories:	2,000	2,500
Total Fat	Less than	65 g	80 g
Sat.Fat	Less than	20 g	25 g
Cholesterol	Less than	300 mg	300 mg
Sodium	Less than	2,400 mg	2,400 mg
Potassium		3,500 mg	3,500 mg
Total Carbohydrate		300 g	300 g
Dietary Fiber		25 g	25 g

Calories per gram:
Fat 9   *   Carbohydrate 4   *   Protein 4

■ FIGURE 19.2   Label reading for carbohydrate counting.

- What obstacles may prevent you from making changes?
- What changes are you willing to make right now?
- What changes would be difficult for you to make?

Mastering the intricacies of eating for diabetes—what, when, and why—occurs over a continuum from learning basic facts to assimilating and implementing information. Individuals differ in how much information they want or need to know and in how motivated they are to improve their eating behaviors. Ideally, positive changes occur progressively over time

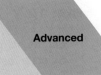

Advanced

Insulin-to-carbohydrate ratios

Limiting saturated fat
Using monounsaturated fat
Label reading
Eating out
Food preparation
Increasing fiber
Limiting sodium

Consistent meal timing
Consistent calorie intake via portion control
Limiting fat and sweets
Estimating portion sizes
Record keeping

Basic
Sources of carbohydrates
Portion sizes of carbohydrates within a meal
Number of carbohydrate servings appropriate for each meal and snack
Sick day management
How to treat hypoglycemia

■ **FIGURE 19.3** An illustration of knowledge and skills attained in stepwise fashion. Actual progression and concepts learned vary among individuals

in stepwise fashion with the client actively involved in goal setting, self-monitoring, and record keeping (Fig. 19.3). In reality, motivation to follow a meal plan may be initially high, but commitment and diligence may dwindle when clients realize that "cheating" does not cause immediate illness. Periodic and ongoing follow-up improves compliance. Arming the client with behavior skills, such as tips for eating out (Box 19.7), provides them with the tools to make better choices. Basic label reading skills are vital (see Fig. 19.2). For more on label reading, see Chapter 9.

Dietary Supplements

The rising incidence of diabetes and chronic nature of the disease contribute to the popularity of using dietary supplements to help treat diabetes or its complications. Several commonly used dietary supplements are highlighted in Table 19.6. Many people do not know that supplement manufacturers do not have to prove safety and efficacy before marketing their products. They may believe that "natural" is synonymous with healthy and that

Box 19.7 Tips for Eating Out

- Eat the same size portion you would at home. Order only what you need and want.
- Select a restaurant with a variety of choices.
- Eat slowly.
- Choose tomato juice, unsweetened fruit juice, clear broth, bouillon, consommé, or shrimp cocktail as an appetizer instead of sweetened juices, fried vegetables, or creamed or thick soups.
- Choose fresh vegetable salads, and use oil and vinegar or fresh lemon instead of regular salad dressings or request that the dressing be put on the side. Avoid coleslaw and other salads with the dressing already added.
- Order plain (without gravy or sauce) roasted, baked, or broiled meat, fish, and poultry instead of fried, sautéed, or breaded entrées. Avoid stews and casseroles. Request a doggie bag if the portion exceeds the meal plan allowance.
- Order steamed, boiled, or broiled vegetables.
- Choose plain, baked, mashed, boiled, or steamed potatoes, rice, or noodles.
- Select fresh fruit for dessert.
- Request a sugar substitute for coffee or tea, if desired.

Table 19.6 Common Supplements Used in Diabetes Management

Supplement	Intended Use/Benefits	Potential Side Effects
Alpha lipoic acid (or lipoic acid)	Used to treat peripheral neuropathy; there is no evidence that it prevents neuropathy, and it is not known whether it slows neuropathy progression or just improves symptoms Lowers blood glucose levels	Rare; may cause hypoglycemia if taken with insulin or secretagogues
Bitter melon (also called bitter gourd or bitter cucumber)	Believed to lower blood glucose levels and hemoglobin A1c, although not always significantly	Gastrointestinal (GI) upset, hemolytic anemia; may cause hypoglycemia if taken with insulin or secretagogues Should not be used by pregnant women due to the risk of possible birth defects and miscarriage
Cassia cinnamon (the type used for baking)	Appears to lower fasting glucose levels but not hemoglobin A1c levels Improves cholesterol and triglyceride levels	Rare and few May cause hypoglycemia if taken with insulin or secretagogues Coumarin, a naturally occurring substance in cassia cinnamon, may lead to or worsen liver damage; some cassia cinnamon supplements are made with water-extracted cinnamon, which may contain less coumarin
Fenugreek	May help lower blood glucose, possibly by stimulating insulin secretion Fenugreek seeds contain fiber that may slow gastric emptying; may also lower serum lipid levels	May cause GI distress Use with caution with anticoagulants May cause hypoglycemia if taken with insulin or secretagogues
Gymnema (also called gurmar, which means "sugar destroyer")	Lowers hemoglobin A1c and fasting glucose levels in type 1 and type 2 diabetes, possibly by promoting glucose uptake by cells and stimulating insulin secretion May lower serum lipid levels	May cause hypoglycemia if taken with insulin or secretagogues Impairs ability to taste sweet or bitter flavors

Source: Campbell, A. (2010). Diabetes and dietary supplements. *Clinical Diabetes, 28*, 35–39.

products used for hundreds of years must be valid and reliable. Before starting a supplement, urge clients to ask the following questions (Campbell, 2010).

- Is there any evidence this supplement may improve diabetes or overall health?
- Is this supplement proven to be safe?
- Could this supplement interact with my other medication?
- Could this supplement interact with other supplements?
- What is the proper form, dose, and concentration of this supplement for me?
- What are the potential side effects of this supplement?
- Under what circumstances should I not take this supplement?
- How long should I use it before judging its effectiveness?

PHARMACOLOGIC MANAGEMENT OF DIABETES

People with type 1 diabetes rely on exogenous insulin for survival—delivered by injection or pump. In contrast, nutrition therapy and exercise are capable of controlling glucose levels for the majority of people with type 2 diabetes. However, because of the progressive nature of the disease, most people with type 2 diabetes eventually require oral agents, insulin, or a combination of both to manage blood glucose levels.

Insulin Therapy for People with Type 1 Diabetes

Insulin preparations vary in how quickly they act, when their peak action occurs, and how long their effects last. They are classified as rapid acting, short acting, intermediate acting, and long acting (Table 19.7). Varying ratios of insulin mixtures may be used to achieve glycemic control.

Usually, intermediate- or long-acting insulin is used to meet basal needs, and a rapid- or short-acting insulin is used before each meal so that the total number of daily injections is three to four. This regimen most closely resembles how insulin is normally secreted, does not require a rigid eating schedule, and decreases the risk of hypoglycemia. Although multiple injections allow for a more flexible lifestyle and better glycemic control, they require frequent and consistent blood glucose testing.

Table 19.7 Insulin: Types, Onset of Action, Peak Activity, and Duration of Activity

Insulin	Onset of Action	Peak Activity	Duration of Activity
Rapid acting lispro aspart glulisine	15 minutes	30 minutes to 2 hours	3–5 hours
Short acting regular	30 minutes	3–4 hours	6–8 hours
Intermediate acting NPH	1–1.5 hours	5–12 hours	10–16 hours
Very long acting glargine detemir	2–4 hours	Flat	24 hours

Sometimes, twice-daily injections of NPH (neutral protamine Hagedorn) and regular insulin are used for a simplified insulin regimen. This approach requires that meals and snacks be consumed at specified times and in consistent amounts to prevent hypoglycemia. For optimum effect, regular insulin should be injected 30 minutes prior to eating, which can be inconvenient. Nighttime hypoglycemia can be a problem with NPH peaking during the night.

Intensive Insulin Therapy for People with Type 1 Diabetes

Intensive insulin therapy is a popular and dynamic insulin regimen for type 1 diabetes. Clients vary their mealtime insulin dose based on the carbohydrate content and timing of the food; they are also able to change their insulin dose for stress or exercise and to change their bolus insulin dose as needed. The regimen may use a long-acting insulin once or twice a day (usually at bedtime) and an injection of rapid-acting insulin before meals and snacks and to correct for high glucose readings. Another option is to have rapid-acting insulin delivered through an insulin pump. An algorithm gives formulas for clients to calculate the **carbohydrate-to-insulin ratio** for the anticipated carbohydrate content of a meal/snack, to correct for a high blood glucose reading, and to determine the amount of basal insulin needed.

Carbohydrate-to-Insulin Ratio: the amount of carbohydrate that can be handled per unit of insulin, usually 15 g CHO requires about one unit of rapid- or short-acting insulin.

Intensive insulin therapy requires more calculations at each meal but allows greater flexibility in when meals are eaten and how much carbohydrate is consumed. An accurate insulin dose also helps clients achieve better glycemic control in that corrections can be made as needed.

Insulin Therapy for People with Type 2 Diabetes

Approximately 30% of people with type 2 diabetes eventually require insulin—either alone or in combination with glucose-lowering medications. Insulin therapy for people with type 2 diabetes often begins with a single injection of intermediate- or long-acting insulin at bedtime when fasting glucose levels are high; oral agents are taken during the day. Another regimen uses a morning injection of rapid- and intermediate-acting insulin with an intermediate- or long-acting insulin at dinner or before bedtime. Self-monitoring of blood glucose levels is needed to optimize doses and timing.

Medications for Type 2 Diabetes

Medications specific for type 2 diabetes vary in their mechanism of action and food concerns (Box 19.8). Medications may be used singly or in combination. They are considered adjunct to nutrition therapy and exercise, not a sole mode of therapy.

EXERCISE

Exercise is an important aspect of treatment for both types of diabetes regardless of weight status unless it is contraindicated for other medical reasons.

Exercise in Insulin Users

Exercise has not been shown to improve glycemic control among people with type 1 diabetes, but it imparts other important benefits such as improving cardiovascular fitness, promoting bone strength, and enhancing the sense of well-being. When diabetes is poorly controlled, exercise may worsen hyperglycemia; without sufficient insulin, the muscle cannot adequately use glucose, so the liver compensates by producing or releasing stored glucose.

Box 19.8   MEDICATIONS FOR TYPE 2 DIABETES

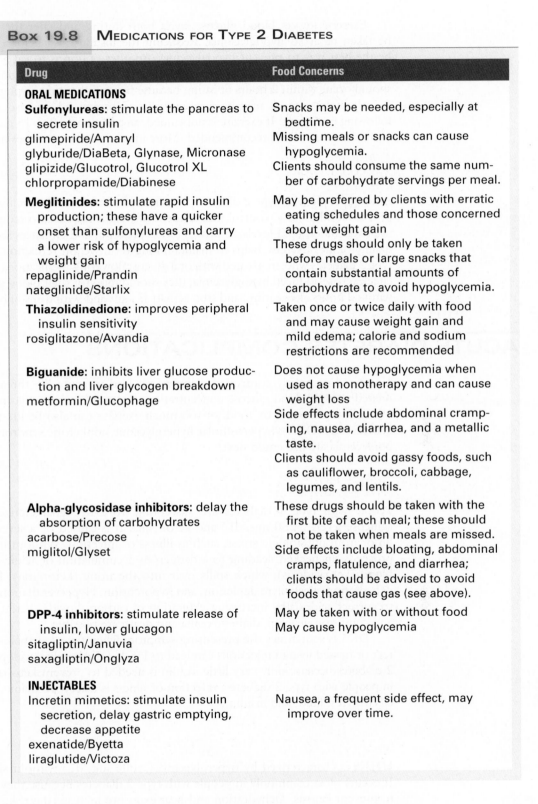

Drug	Food Concerns
ORAL MEDICATIONS	
Sulfonylureas: stimulate the pancreas to secrete insulin glimepiride/Amaryl glyburide/DiaBeta, Glynase, Micronase glipizide/Glucotrol, Glucotrol XL chlorpropamide/Diabinese	Snacks may be needed, especially at bedtime. Missing meals or snacks can cause hypoglycemia. Clients should consume the same number of carbohydrate servings per meal.
Meglitinides: stimulate rapid insulin production; these have a quicker onset than sulfonylureas and carry a lower risk of hypoglycemia and weight gain repaglinide/Prandin nateglinide/Starlix	May be preferred by clients with erratic eating schedules and those concerned about weight gain These drugs should only be taken before meals or large snacks that contain substantial amounts of carbohydrate to avoid hypoglycemia.
Thiazolidinedione: improves peripheral insulin sensitivity rosiglitazone/Avandia	Taken once or twice daily with food and may cause weight gain and mild edema; calorie and sodium restrictions are recommended
Biguanide: inhibits liver glucose production and liver glycogen breakdown metformin/Glucophage	Does not cause hypoglycemia when used as monotherapy and can cause weight loss Side effects include abdominal cramping, nausea, diarrhea, and a metallic taste. Clients should avoid gassy foods, such as cauliflower, broccoli, cabbage, legumes, and lentils.
Alpha-glycosidase inhibitors: delay the absorption of carbohydrates acarbose/Precose miglitol/Glyset	These drugs should be taken with the first bite of each meal; these should not be taken when meals are missed. Side effects include bloating, abdominal cramps, flatulence, and diarrhea; clients should be advised to avoid foods that cause gas (see above).
DPP-4 inhibitors: stimulate release of insulin, lower glucagon sitagliptin/Januvia saxagliptin/Onglyza	May be taken with or without food May cause hypoglycemia
INJECTABLES	
Incretin mimetics: stimulate insulin secretion, delay gastric emptying, decrease appetite exenatide/Byetta liraglutide/Victoza	Nausea, a frequent side effect, may improve over time.

Exercise lowers blood glucose levels both during and after the activity, so care must be taken to avoid hypoglycemia. Reducing the insulin dose before planned exercise may be the best way to prevent hypoglycemia. Another option is to eat a carbohydrate snack if the blood glucose level is less than 100 mg/dL before exercise begins. If possible, exercise should occur within 2 hours of eating because beyond that time hypoglycemia is more likely. A carbohydrate snack may be necessary during prolonged exercise and during the hours following exercising. If exercise is unplanned, an additional 10 to 15 g carbohydrate per hour of moderate activity is recommended. More intense exercise requires more carbohydrate.

Exercise in Type 2 Diabetes

Among people with type 2 diabetes, exercise offers substantial benefits. Regular exercise improves blood glucose control independent of weight loss. It also reduces insulin resistance, improves blood lipid levels, improves blood pressure, and enhances sense of well-being and quality of life. Exercise helps to maintain long-term weight reduction. Because people with type 2 diabetes who are treated with oral glucose-lowering medications or insulin may experience exercise-induced hypoglycemia, they should monitor their blood glucose levels, exercise within 2 hours after eating, and stop activity if signs and symptoms of hypoglycemia develop.

ACUTE DIABETES COMPLICATIONS

Untreated or poorly controlled diabetes can lead to acute life-threatening complications related to high blood glucose concentrations. Conversely, hypoglycemia caused by overuse of medication, too little food, or too much exercise can also be life-threatening. Diabetic ketoacidosis (DKA), hyperosmolar hyperglycemic nonketotic syndrome (HHNS), and hypoglycemia are presented next.

Diabetic Ketoacidosis

People with type 1 diabetes are susceptible to DKA, characterized by hyperglycemia (glucose levels >250 mg/dL) and ketonemia. It is caused by a severe deficiency of insulin or from physiologic stress, such as illness or infection. Without insulin, fat catabolism proceeds unchecked, leading to a dangerous accumulation of acidic ketone bodies in the blood (ketoacidosis), which spills over into the urine (ketonuria). Polyuria may lead to dehydration, electrolyte depletion, and hypotension. Hyperventilation occurs in an attempt to correct acidosis by increasing expiration of carbon dioxide. Fatigue, nausea, vomiting, and confusion develop; diabetic coma and death are possible.

DKA is sometimes the presenting symptom when type 1 diabetes is diagnosed. Incorrect or missed insulin injections can lead to DKA. DKA rarely develops in people with type 2 diabetes because only very little insulin is needed to prevent ketosis. If DKA does occur in people with type 2 diabetes, infection or illness is usually to blame. DKA is treated with electrolytes, fluid, and insulin.

Hyperosmolar Hyperglycemic Nonketotic Syndrome

HHNS is characterized by hyperglycemia (>600 mg/dL) without significant ketonemia. It occurs most commonly in people with type 2 diabetes because they have enough insulin to prevent ketosis. Dehydration and heat exposure increase the risk; illness or infection is usually the precipitating factor. Older people may be particularly vulnerable because they have a diminished sense of thirst or may be unable to replenish fluid losses due to illness or physical impairments. HHNS develops relatively slowly over a period of days to weeks. Symptoms include dehydration, hypotension, decreased mental acuity, confusion, seizures, and coma. The best protection against HHNS is regular glucose monitoring. Treatment includes insulin and fluid and electrolyte replacement.

Hypoglycemia

Hypoglycemia (blood glucose level <70 mg/dL) is often referred to as insulin reaction. It occurs from taking too much insulin (or sulfonylureas but less frequently), inadequate food intake, delayed or skipped meals, extra physical activity, or consumption of alcohol without food. Symptoms include weakness, shakiness, dizziness, cold sweat, clammy feeling, headache, confusion, irritability, and seizure.

Mild hypoglycemia is treated with 15 to 20 g of glucose, although any carbohydrate that contains glucose may be used. Pure sugars are better than items like candy bars, which contain fat that slows the gastric emptying time and delays the rise in blood glucose. After eating a dose of sugar, symptoms normally improve in 10 to 20 minutes. A blood glucose test is repeated in 15 minutes, and another dose of fast-acting sugar is consumed if the glucose level is still low. A meal should be eaten within the next hour.

All clients should carry a readily absorbable source of carbohydrate with them at all times to treat hypoglycemia. Likewise, an appropriate source of carbohydrate should be on the nightstand in case hypoglycemia develops during the night. Frequent bouts of hypoglycemia may mean the care plan needs to be revised or the client needs to be counseled to ensure better compliance.

Patients with long-standing diabetes may develop hypoglycemic unawareness. This occurs because the body no longer signals hypoglycemia. Consistent monitoring of blood glucose is especially important for people who are not cognizant of hypoglycemic symptoms.

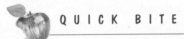

QUICK BITE

To counter mild hypoglycemia
Each of the following contains approximately 15 g of readily absorbable sugar

- 3 to 4 glucose tablets
- 1 individual tube of glucose gel
- 8 to 10 Life Savers
- 4 to 6 oz regular soft drink
- 4 to 6 oz fruit juice

SICK-DAY MANAGEMENT

Acute illnesses, even mild ones such as a cold or flu, can significantly raise blood glucose levels. Unless otherwise instructed by the physician, clients should maintain their normal medication schedule, monitor their blood glucose levels every 2 to 4 hours, and maintain an adequate fluid intake. Urine or blood should be checked for ketones at least twice a day. Unless blood glucose levels are higher than 250 mg/dL, clients should eat the usual amount of carbohydrate, divided into smaller meals and snacks if necessary. Sweetened liquids are generally a well-tolerated source of carbohydrates and fluid. A daily intake of 150 to 200 g of carbohydrates, approximately 45 to 50 g every 3 to 4 hours, is recommended. Examples of items that may be best tolerated during illness is as follows (each serving specified provides approximately one carbohydrate choice [15 g of carbohydrate]):

- 6 oz regularly sweetened ginger ale
- 8 oz sports drink

- ½ cup ice cream
- ½ cup apple juice
- 1 frozen 100% juice bar
- ¼ cup sherbet or sorbet
- ½ cup gelatin
- 1 cup cream soup made with water

LIFE CYCLE CONSIDERATIONS

Diabetes nutrition therapy can influence growth and development in children and adolescents and the quality of life in older adults. Special considerations for these groups are presented in the following sections; diabetes in pregnancy is covered in Chapter 11.

Children and Adolescents

Children with diabetes appear to have the same nutrient needs as their age-matched peers. However, managing diabetes in children and adolescents is complicated by the impact of growth on nutrient needs, irregular eating patterns, and erratic activity levels. More frequent adjustments in insulin and food intake are necessary to compensate for growth and activity needs. Failure to provide adequate calories and nutrients results in poor growth, as does poor glycemic control and inadequate insulin administration. Conversely, excessive weight gain occurs from excessive calorie intake, overtreatment of hypoglycemia, or excess insulin administration. Neither withholding food nor having a child eat when not hungry is an appropriate strategy to manage glucose levels. Rather, individualized meal plans and intensive insulin regimens can provide flexibility for erratic eating, activity, and growth. Box 19.9 lists questions to consider when dealing with children with diabetes.

Although type 2 diabetes is most often diagnosed after 45 years of age, 2002–2005 data show that 3600 American youth are diagnosed with type 2 diabetes annually. For Asian, Pacific Islander, and American Indian youth 10 to 19 years old, the rate of new cases of type 2 diabetes exceeds that of type 1 diabetes (CDC, 2011). Weight control is key to preventing type 2 diabetes in children.

Diabetes in Later Life

There are unique considerations related to aging that affect glycemic control. First, blood glucose levels rise with age for reasons that are unclear. Treatment may not be instituted for glucose elevations that are considered "high" in younger populations but may be "normal" for the elderly. Cognitive impairments, such as memory loss, impaired concentration,

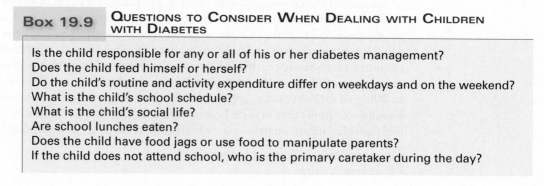

Box 19.9	QUESTIONS TO CONSIDER WHEN DEALING WITH CHILDREN WITH DIABETES

Is the child responsible for any or all of his or her diabetes management?
Does the child feed himself or herself?
Do the child's routine and activity expenditure differ on weekdays and on the weekend?
What is the child's school schedule?
What is the child's social life?
Are school lunches eaten?
Does the child have food jags or use food to manipulate parents?
If the child does not attend school, who is the primary caretaker during the day?

dementia, and depression, may preclude self-management. Physical impairments may impede exercise. Sensory impairments, such as decreased hearing, poor eyesight, and decreased senses of taste and smell, may complicate teaching and self-management. For instance, older clients who could clinically benefit from insulin may be treated instead with oral agents if poor eyesight or decreased manual dexterity precludes self-injection. Older adults may be at greater nutritional risk for a variety of reasons, including poor dentition, physical impairments that make shopping or cooking difficult, poor appetite related to lack of socialization, and an inadequate food budget. For many, a strict calorie-controlled diet is more harmful than beneficial. Because older adults are more susceptible to severe hypoglycemia, a fasting target level of 120 to 150 mg/dL may be considered appropriate.

DIABETIC DIETS IN THE HOSPITAL

Traditionally, standardized calorie-level meal plans based on the exchange lists were used to provide "diabetic" diets to hospitalized diabetics. The physician would order a specific calorie-level "ADA diet" that was composed of specific percentages of carbohydrate, protein, and fat. Because the ADA no longer endorses any single meal plan or specified nutrient composition, it is recommended that this term and approach no longer be used.

Also considered obsolete are "no concentrated sweets," "no sugar added," "low sugar," and "liberal diabetic" diets. They do not reflect the diabetes nutrient recommendations and are unnecessarily restrictive in sugar. These diets may give patients the false impression that glycemic control is achieved by limiting sugar.

An alternative to the traditional "ADA diet" is a consistent carbohydrate diet. In this approach, calories are not specified, but carbohydrate intake is consistent, such as four carbohydrates for every meal with one to two for an evening snack. A typical day's intake from meals and snacks may range from 1500 to 2000 calories, with adjustments made for individual patients as needed. Appropriate modifications in fat intake are made, and consistent timing of meals and snacks is stressed. However, just as there is no longer one diabetic diet, neither is there one correct way to provide nutrition therapy to hospitalized people with diabetes. See Box 19.10 for additional considerations when people with diabetes are hospitalized.

Box 19.10	ADDITIONAL CONSIDERATIONS WHEN PEOPLE WITH DIABETES ARE HOSPITALIZED

- Patients given clear or full liquid diets should receive approximately 200 g of carbohydrate per day in equally divided amounts at meals and snacks. Sugar-free items should not be used. Adjustments in diabetes medication may be needed to achieve glycemic control.
- Sometimes, people with diabetes are given a regular diet based on the rationale that a sliding scale insulin regimen will take care of hyperglycemia related to the stress of hospitalization, acute illness, and changes in diet. While that is true, the risk is that patients may not understand that a "regular" diet is not appropriate after discharge.
- The diet should be progressed as soon as possible after surgery with the goal of providing adequate carbohydrates and calories.
- Continuous monitoring is needed during catabolic illnesses to ensure that nutritional needs are met and hyperglycemia is prevented. Overfeeding exacerbates hyperglycemia.
- For tube feedings, standard enteral formulas (50% of calories from carbohydrate) or a lower carbohydrate content formula (33%–40% carbohydrate) may be used. Medication adjustments are made according to the results of blood glucose monitoring.

NURSING PROCESS: *Type 2 Diabetes*

Mark is 52 years old and is sedentary. His doctor monitored his fasting blood glucose and cholesterol levels for several years, urging Mark to eat better and exercise or he would eventually need medications to bring down both his glucose and cholesterol levels. Mark was unmotivated to change until he was recently diagnosed with type 2 diabetes. His mother went blind from type 2 diabetes, and he is scared the same thing may happen to him. He is 5 ft 9 in tall and weighs 190 pounds. He is hoping the doctor will prescribe medication to control his blood glucose so he won't have to "worry about a diet."

Assessment	
Medical–Psychosocial History	▪ Medical history and comorbidities, including hyperlipidemia, hypertension, CVD, renal impairments, neuropathy, and gastrointestinal complaints
	▪ Use of prescribed and over-the-counter medications
	▪ Psychosocial and economic issues such as the living situation, cooking facilities, adequacy of food budget, education, need for food assistance, and level of family and social support
	▪ Usual activity patterns
Anthropometric Assessment	▪ Height, current weight, usual weight; recent weight history
	▪ BMI
	▪ Waist circumference to identify abdominal obesity
Biochemical and Physical Assessment	▪ Hemoglobin A1c, fasting glucose levels
	▪ Lipid profile
	▪ Measures of renal function, if available
	▪ Blood pressure
	▪ Record of self-monitored blood glucose (SMBG) levels
Dietary Assessment	▪ How many meals and snacks do you usually eat in a day? Do you ever skip meals? Do you eat at regular intervals? When do you eat snacks?
	▪ What is a typical day's intake?
	▪ Have you ever tried to follow a diet or improve your eating habits?
	▪ What questions do you have about nutrition for diabetes?
	▪ How is your appetite?
	▪ Do you have any food intolerances or allergies? Do you ever have gastrointestinal (GI) symptoms that impact what you eat?
	▪ Do you ever experience symptoms of low blood glucose? What do you do to raise your blood glucose when you are feeling low?
	▪ What do you know about how your medication and exercise impact blood glucose levels?
	▪ Are you willing/able to change your eating habits if necessary?
	▪ How do you feel about your weight?
	▪ Do you have any cultural, religious, or ethnic food preferences?
	▪ Who prepares your meals?
	▪ Do you take vitamins, minerals, or other supplements?
	▪ Do you use alcohol?

Diagnosis	
Possible Nursing Diagnoses	Knowledge deficits of nutrition therapy for diabetes mellitus

NURSING PROCESS: *Type 2 Diabetes* (continued)

Planning	

Client Outcomes	**Short term**
	The client will
	■ State three signs/symptoms of hypoglycemia
	■ State three emergency foods to use during hypoglycemic episodes
	■ Eat three meals plus a bedtime snack at approximately the same times every day
	■ Begin strategies to shift toward a nutritionally adequate, balanced, and varied diet that has
	  Four carbohydrate choices at each meal and two at a bedtime snack that are composed of a variety of fruits, vegetables, whole grains, and low-fat or nonfat milk
	  4–6 oz of protein/day
	  Healthy fats
	  Little saturated fat and minimal trans fats
	■ Monitor his blood glucose level daily
	■ Keep periodic food records that include the timing of meals and snacks and type and amount of food eaten
	■ Walk 10 minutes 3 times/day at least 3 days/week
	
	Long term
	The client will
	■ Lose 9 pounds in 6 months (5% of initial weight)
	■ Achieve hemoglobin A1c and preprandial and postprandial blood glucose levels within target levels established by his physician
	■ Avoid hypoglycemia
	■ Improve lipid profile
	■ Prevent or delay chronic complications
	■ Increase physical activity to at least 30 minutes daily five times per week

Nursing Interventions	
Nutrition Therapy	Introduce basic concepts: which foods contain carbohydrates, appropriate serving sizes for carbohydrates, and how many carbohydrate choices are appropriate for each meal and snack
Client Teaching	Instruct the client On the role of nutrition therapy in managing blood glucose levels, including that ■ Nutrition therapy is essential and that nutrition is important even when no symptoms are apparent ■ Medication is used in addition to nutrition therapy not as a substitute ■ Ongoing or follow-up counseling is necessary to make adjustments and expand skills and knowledge to optimize diabetes management

(continues on page 528)

NURSING PROCESS: *Type 2 Diabetes* (continued)

On eating plan essentials, including the importance of

- Eating meals and snacks at regular times every day
- Eating approximately the same amount of food every day, especially the same amount of carbohydrates
- Eating enough high-fiber foods such as whole wheat bread, whole-grain ready-to-eat cereals, whole wheat pasta, brown rice, oats, vegetables, fruit, and dried peas and beans
- Using less fat, sugar, and salt

On behavioral matters, including

- How to read labels to determine the amount of carbohydrate choices a serving of food provides
- Making healthy choices overall, such as lean meats, fat-free milk, soft spread margarines
- Not skipping meals or snacks
- Physical activity goals
- Having a source of glucose handy at all times
- The importance of monitoring food intake and blood glucose levels
- Where to get additional information

Evaluation

Evaluate and Monitor

- Food intake records for consistency in meal timing, the number of carbohydrate choices per meals and snacks, and overall quality and adequacy of food choices made
- Appetite/satiety
- Self-monitoring blood glucose records to determine if 50% are within target range
- Laboratory data as available
- Weight
- Need for nutritional counseling
- Progress toward physical activity goals

How Do You Respond?

How can I follow a diabetic diet with my relentless "sweet tooth"? Small amounts of sweet foods are permitted, especially if weight is not a problem, as long as they are counted as part of the meal plan, not added as "extras." Diabetic recipes are helpful in incorporating sweet foods into the eating pattern. Calorie-free foods sweetened with nonnutritive sweeteners (e.g., saccharin, aspartame) add sweetness and interest without calories. Encourage the client to use artificially sweetened soft drinks and gelatin.

Are "dietetic" products like candy and cookies worth the added expense? Dietetic products are not necessarily calorie-free or specifically intended for diabetics. Foods that are labeled "dietetic" may be made without sugar, without salt, with a particular type of fat, or for special food allergies. Read the ingredient label and check with a diet counselor before adding a dietetic food to the diet—or avoid dietetic foods altogether because they are expensive and usually do not taste as good as the foods they are intended to replace.

CASE STUDY

Keisha is a 42-year-old black female with a BMI of 29. She was recently diagnosed with diabetes and hypertension. Her mother and two sisters also have type 2 diabetes. She is the mother of three children, who each weighed more than 10 pounds at birth. Although she knows she should exercise, she doesn't have time in her busy schedule.

The doctor gave her a 1500-calorie diet and told her if her glucose does not improve, she will have to go on medication and, possibly, insulin. She has tried the "diet" but finds it too restrictive: it tells her to eat things she doesn't like (such as milk) and won't let her eat the things she loves (like sweetened tea and fast foods). She is scared of the potential for needing insulin and the complications associated with diabetes.

- What risk factors does Keisha have for type 2 diabetes?
- Is a 1500-calorie diet appropriate for her? Should it promote weight loss or maintain her current weight?
- What would you tell Keisha about weight and diabetes management?
- What would you tell her about drinking milk? What about sweetened tea and fast foods?
- What approaches would you take to improve compliance yet increase her satisfaction with eating?
- What other lifestyle changes would you propose to Keisha to manage diabetes and reduce the risk of complications?

STUDY QUESTIONS

1. Which statement indicates the patient understands nutrition recommendations regarding carbohydrate intake?
   a. "People with diabetes should avoid sugars and foods that contain sugars."
   b. "It is important to consume the proper balance of starch, sugar, and fiber at each meal."
   c. "It is important to consume the correct amount of carbohydrate at each meal and snack."
   d. "Carbohydrates must be balanced in relation to the amount of protein and fat consumed."

2. The client with type 1 diabetes asks if she can have a glass of wine with dinner on the weekends. Which of the following would be the nurse's best response?
   a. "It is better to have wine between meals than with meals so that it doesn't interfere with your normal food intake."
   b. "People with diabetes cannot have alcohol because it raises blood glucose levels very quickly."
   c. "A mixed drink would be better than wine because the mixer will help slow the absorption of the alcohol."
   d. "An occasional glass of wine with dinner will not cause any problems. Be sure to limit yourself to one serving."

3. When developing a teaching plan for a client who is taking insulin, which of the following foods would the nurse suggest the client carry with him to treat mild hypoglycemia?
   a. Crackers
   b. Peanuts
   c. Chocolate drops
   d. Life Savers

4. The best approach for monitoring carbohydrate intake is to use
   a. The exchange system
   b. Carbohydrate counting
   c. Sample menus
   d. The approach that best helps the individual control blood glucose levels

5. How many carbohydrate choices are provided in a serving of food that supplies 19 grams of carbohydrate?
   a. 1
   b. 2
   c. 3
   d. 4

6. The nurse knows her instructions about label reading have been effective when the client verbalizes that to determine the amount of carbohydrate choices, you must
   a. Add the grams of total carbohydrate and grams of sugars together to determine total carbohydrates provided.
   b. Adjust total carbohydrates for foods that provide more than 5 g of fiber or more than 5 g of sugar alcohols per serving.
   c. Add grams of total carbohydrate, fiber, and sugars to determine total carbohydrate grams.
   d. Use only the grams of total carbohydrate to determine carbohydrate choices.

7. What is the priority for preventing diabetes in people who are at high risk?
   a. Eat a low-carbohydrate diet.
   b. Consume a consistent amount of carbohydrate at every meal.
   c. Achieve moderate weight loss through increased activity and lowered calorie and fat intake.
   d. Eat a low-sugar diet.

8. Which food groups provide carbohydrates? (Select all that apply.)
   a. Vegetables
   b. Fruit
   c. Milk
   d. Meat

KEY CONCEPTS

■ Diabetes is a group of diseases characterized by hyperglycemia. It is increasing in epidemic proportions.

■ Type 1 diabetes is characterized by the lack of insulin secretion. It is usually diagnosed in children and adolescents and is related to genetic and environmental factors.

■ Ninety percent to 95% of diabetes cases are type 2 diabetes. It begins with pre-diabetes that is characterized by insulin resistance and relative insulin deficiency.

Hyperglycemia provides constant stimulation for insulin secretion, leading to hyperinsulinemia.

■ Gestational diabetes is diabetes that develops during pregnancy. It presents numerous risks to mother and infant. Some women enter pregnancy with diabetes that was previously undiagnosed.

■ Long-term diabetes complications include damage to both small and large vessels in the body. Tight glycemic control delays or prevents the onset of long-term microvascular complications and probably macrovascular complications as well.

■ Nutrition therapy is the cornerstone of treatment for all people with diabetes, regardless of weight status, use of medication, blood glucose levels, and presence or absence of symptoms. The goals of nutrition therapy are to achieve optimal blood glucose and lipid levels, attain or maintain reasonable weight, and avoid acute and chronic complications.

■ Lifestyle changes that include moderate weight loss, regular physical activity, and a lowered calorie and fat intake can reduce the risk of developing diabetes.

■ Nutrient needs of people with diabetes are not different than the general population. Dietary recommendations to promote health and well-being, such as eating less saturated fat, trans fat, and cholesterol and more fiber and whole grains, are also appropriate for people with diabetes.

■ The ADA recommends that people with diabetes limit saturated fat intake to less than 7% of total calories and minimize their intake of trans fat. Cholesterol should be limited to less than 200 mg/day, and two servings of fatty fish are recommended per week. These suggestions are relatively consistent with the AHA's dietary recommendations for people at high risk of heart disease.

■ Sucrose ("sugar") is no longer considered detrimental to glucose control so long as it is eaten as part of the meal plan and not as an "extra." However, if weight loss is a goal, high-sugar foods should be limited.

■ Diets for people with diabetes are not "one size fits all." Dietary changes should be made sequentially and restrictions kept to a minimum to maximize compliance.

■ There is not one superior method of monitoring carbohydrate intake. The method used should be determined by the individual's lifestyle, preferences, and willingness/ability to make dietary changes.

■ Exchange lists for diabetes group foods into lists based on their macronutrient content. A meal plan shows the client how many exchanges from each list he or she should have for every meal and snack. Any item in a list can be exchanged for any other. The exchange lists are complex and very structured.

■ Carbohydrate counting focuses mainly on the carbohydrate content of foods; protein and fat are not tightly controlled. Clients select foods for each meal based on how many grams of carbohydrate or carbohydrate choices their meal plan allows. It provides more flexibility than the exchange system and is easier to use.

■ People with type 1 diabetes must take exogenous insulin. Intensive insulin therapy allows clients to determine their premeal insulin dosage based on their glucose level and the amount of carbohydrate they anticipate eating.

■ Although most people with type 2 diabetes have the potential to achieve glycemic control through diet and exercise, the progressive nature of the disease causes most people to eventually need oral medications and/or insulin. Oral medications vary in their mode of action, side effects, and food concerns.

■ Exercise benefits all people with diabetes, regardless of weight status. For people with type 1 diabetes, exercise can improve cardiac risk factors and sense of well-being. For people with type 2 diabetes, exercise can improve glucose control, blood lipid levels, and blood pressure and helps maintain weight loss. For all people with diabetes, care must be taken to avoid exercise induced hypoglycemia.

■ Acute diabetes complications include DKA, HHNS, and hypoglycemia. Acute complications are more likely during illness. Frequent blood glucose monitoring can help avoid acute complications.

■ During acute illness, people with diabetes are urged to keep their normal medication schedule, monitor their blood glucose levels closely, and consume adequate fluids. Clients should eat their usual amount of carbohydrate unless their blood glucose levels are higher than 250 mg/dL. Acceptable sick-day carbohydrates include sugar-sweetened carbonated beverages, fruit juice, sweetened gelatin, ice cream, and cream soups.

■ Children and adolescents have a greater variation in their daily calorie needs than adults do because of their nutritional needs for growth and their more erratic activity and eating patterns. Managing diabetes is more challenging in young people.

■ Older people with diabetes may need to be treated more conservatively than younger people because they are more susceptible to severe hypoglycemia, are at greater nutritional risk, and may have physical or sensory impairments that complicate self-management.

■ Diabetic diets in the hospital were traditionally identified as "ADA diets." Because there is no one diabetic diet recommended for all people with diabetes, this term should be discontinued. Consistent carbohydrate diets are recommended.

Check Your Knowledge Answer Key

1. **FALSE** Diabetes is not an inevitable consequence of prediabetes. Weight loss and exercise can prevent or delay diabetes and normalize blood glucose levels.

2. **FALSE** People with diabetes should consume a "normal" carbohydrate intake of 45% to 65% of total calories (within the Acceptable Macronutrient Distribution Range), just like the general population. Low-carbohydrate diets tend to be high in fat; high saturated fat diets increase the risk of cardiovascular disease.

3. **FALSE** Modest weight loss, such as 5% to 7%, has been shown to dramatically reduce the risk of type 2 diabetes even when healthy BMI is not attained.

4. **TRUE** Alcohol is more likely to cause hypoglycemia when consumed without food rather than with food.

5. **FALSE** People with diabetes should avoid the use of fructose as an added sweetener because it causes adverse effects on serum triglycerides and LDL cholesterol but do not need to avoid natural fructose found in fruit.

6. **FALSE** People with diabetes do not need more fiber than the general population.

7. **FALSE** Hypoglycemia is a risk with insulin and certain oral medications but not with all medications, so the use of snacks should be tailored to the individual's insulin and/or medication regimen. People with type 2 diabetes who are controlled by diet alone do not need snacks, and snacks may be counterproductive in people trying to lose weight.

8. **FALSE** People who practice carbohydrate counting cannot ignore protein and fat intake; they are urged to eat 4 to 6 oz of lean protein/day and choose healthy fats.

9. **FALSE** Although a chocolate candy bar does provide ample sugar, it also provides substantial amounts of fat that delay the absorption of glucose. The best choice for treating mild hypoglycemia is readily absorbable pure sugars, such as glucose tablets, fruit juice, soft drinks, or Life Savers.

10. **TRUE** People with diabetes should limit their intake of saturated fat and cholesterol because their risk of CHD is very high.

Websites

American Diabetes Association at **www.diabetes.org**
Joslin Diabetes Center at **www.joslin.org**
National Institute of Diabetes and Digestive and Kidney Diseases at **www.niddk.nih.gov**

References

Ahmad, L., & Crandall, J. (2010). Type 2 diabetes prevention: A review. *Clinical Diabetes, 28,* 53–59.

Alberti, K., Eckel, R., Grundy, S., Zimmet, P. Z., Cleeman, J. I., Donato, K. A., . . . Smith, S. C., Jr. (2009). Harmonizing the metabolic syndrome. *Circulation, 120,* 1640–1645.

American Diabetes Association. (2010). Diagnosis and classification of diabetes mellitus. *Diabetes Care, 33*(Suppl. 1), S62–S69.

American Diabetes Association & American Dietetic Association. (2008). *Choose your foods: Exchange lists for diabetes.* Alexandria, VA: American Diabetes Association; Chicago, IL: American Dietetic Association.

Anderson, F. (2000). Chromium in the prevention and control of diabetes. *Diabetes & Metabolism, 26,* 22–27.

Anderson, J., Riley, M., & Everette, T. (2012). How proven primary prevention can stop diabetes. *Clinical Diabetes, 30,* 76–79.

Bantle, J., Wylie-Rosett, J., Albright, A. L., Apovian, C. M., Clark, N. G., Franz, M. J., . . . Wheeler, M. L. (2008). Nutrition recommendations and interventions for diabetes. A position statement of the American Diabetes Association. *Diabetes Care, 31*(Suppl. 1), S61–S78.

Buchwald, H., Avidor, Y., Braunwald, E., Jensen, M. D., Pories, W., Fahrbach, K., & Schoelles, K. (2004). Bariatric surgery: A systemic review and meta-analysis. *Journal of the American Medical Association, 292,* 1724–1737.

Campbell, A. (2010). Diabetes and dietary supplements. *Clinical Diabetes, 28,* 35–39.

Catalano, P., Huston, L., Amini, S., & Kalhan, S. (1999). Longitudinal changes in glucose metabolism during pregnancy in obese women with normal glucose tolerance and gestational diabetes mellitus. *American Journal of Obstetrics and Gynecology, 180,* 903–916.

Centers for Disease Control and Prevention. (2011). *National diabetes fact sheet, 2011.* Available at http://www.cdc.gov/diabetes/pubs/pdf/ndfs_2011.pdf. Accessed on 6/18/2012.

Diabetes Prevention Program Research Group. (2002). Reduction in the evidence of type 2 diabetes with lifestyle intervention or metformin. *The New England Journal of Medicine, 346,* 393–403.

Diabetes Prevention Program Research Group. (2009). 10-Year follow-up of diabetes incidence and weight loss in the Diabetes Prevention Program outcomes study. *The Lancet, 374,* 1677–1686.

Fowler, M. (2010). Diabetes: Magnitude and mechanisms. *Clinical Diabetes, 28,* 42–46.

Fowler, M. (2011). Microvascular and macrovascular complications of diabetes. *Clinical Diabetes, 29,* 116–122,

Franz, M. J., Bantle, J. P., Beebe, C. A., Brunzell, J. D., Chiasson, J. L., Garg, A., . . . Wheeler, M. (2002). Evidence-based nutrition principles and recommendations for the treatment and prevention of diabetes and related complications. *Diabetes Care, 25,* 148–198.

Franz, M., Powers, M., Leontos, C., Holzmeister, L. A., Kulkarni, K., Monk, A., . . . Gradwell, E. (2010). The evidence for medical nutrition therapy for type 1 and type 2 diabetes in adults. *Journal of the American Dietetic Association, 110,* 1852–1889.

Grundy, S. (2008). Metabolic syndrome pandemic. *Arteriosclerosis, Thrombosis, and Vascular Biology, 28,* 629–636.

Haffner, S., Temprosa, M., Crandall, J., Fowler, S., Goldberg, R., Horton, E., . . . Barrett-Connor, E. (2005). Intensive lifestyle intervention or metformin on inflammation and coagulation in participants with impaired glucose tolerance. *Diabetes, 54,* 1566–1572.

Lichtenstein, A. H., Appel, L. J., Brands, M., Carnethon, M., Daniels, S., Franch, H. A., . . . Wylie-Rosett, J. (2006). Diet and lifestyle recommendations revision 2006. A scientific statement from the American Heart Association Nutrition Committee. *Circulation, 114,* 82–96.

Liese, A. D., Roach, A. K., Sparks, K. C., Marquart, L., D'Agostino, R. B., Jr., & Mayer-Davis, E. J. (2003). Whole-grain intake and insulin sensitivity: The Insulin Resistance Atherosclerosis Study. *The American Journal of Clinical Nutrition, 78,* 965–971.

Melanson, K. (2007). Diet and nutrients in the prevention and treatment of type 2 diabetes. *American Journal of Lifestyle Medicine, 1,* 339–343.

Nathan, D. M., Cleary, P. A., Backlund, J. Y., Genuth, S. M., Lachin, J. M., Orchard, T. J., . . . Zinman, B. (2005). Intensive diabetes treatment and cardiovascular disease in patients with type 1 diabetes. *The New England Journal of Medicine, 353,* 2643–2653.

National Cholesterol Education Program. (2001). *Third report of the expert panel on detection, evaluation, and treatment of high blood cholesterol in adults (Adult Treatment Panel III). Executive summary* (NIH Publication No. 01-3670). Bethesda, MD: U.S. Department of Health and Human Services, Public Health Service, National Institutes of Health.

Ratner, R., Goldberg, R., Haffner, S., Marcovina, S., Orchard, T., Fowler, S., & Temprosa, M. (2005). Impact of intensive lifestyle and metformin therapy on cardiovascular disease risk factors in the Diabetes Prevention Program. *Diabetes Care, 28,* 888–894.

Rubino, F. (2008). Is type 2 diabetes an operable intestinal disease? A provocative yet reasonable hypothesis. *Diabetes Care, 31*(Suppl. 2), S290–S296.

Sheard, N. F., Clark, N. G., Brand-Miller, J. C., Franz, M. J., Pi-Sunyer, F. X., Mayer-Davis, E., . . . Geil, P. (2004). Dietary carbohydrate (amount and type) in the prevention and management of diabetes: A statement of the American Diabetes Association. *Diabetes Care, 27,* 2266–2271.

Wheeler, M., Daly, A., Evert, A., Franz, M. J., Geil, P., Holzmeister, L., . . . Woolf, P. (2008). Choose your foods: Exchange lists for diabetes (6th ed.). Description and guidelines for use. *Journal of the American Dietetic Association, 108,* 883–888.

Wheeler, M., & Pi-Sunyer, X. (2008). Carbohydrate issues: Type and amount. *Journal of the American Dietetic Association, 108*(Suppl. 1), S34–S39.

20 Nutrition for Patients with Cardiovascular Disorders

CHECK YOUR KNOWLEDGE

TRUE FALSE

☐ ☐ **1** The only diet modifications known to improve blood pressure are lowering sodium intake and losing weight, if overweight.

☐ ☐ **2** The majority of sodium in the typical American diet comes from salt added during cooking and at the table.

☐ ☐ **3** The major emphasis of the DASH diet is to reduce total fat and saturated fat intake.

☐ ☐ **4** High triglyceride levels are a component of metabolic syndrome (MetS) but are not considered to be directly atherogenic. Rather, they are considered a biomarker of cardiovascular disease.

☐ ☐ **5** A traditional Mediterranean diet is a low-fat diet.

☐ ☐ **6** Foods with components that provide cardiometabolic benefits include dairy products and nuts.

☐ ☐ **7** People who do not like whole grains can reap the same cardiometabolic benefits from adding supplemental fiber or bran to their diets.

☐ ☐ **8** Alcohol has both positive and negative effects on heart health.

☐ ☐ **9** Only people with blood pressure greater than 120/80 mmHg need to lower their sodium intake.

☐ ☐ **10** A low-sodium diet for heart failure is based on expert consensus, not randomized study evidence.

LEARNING OBJECTIVES

Upon completion of this chapter, you will be able to

1 Discuss diet and lifestyle interventions for lowering blood pressure.

2 Explain why a food group approach may be better at improving health than focusing on individual nutrients.

3 Compare the DASH diet with the traditional Mediterranean diet.

4 Plan a 2000-calorie DASH eating plan menu.

5 Name foods associated with cardiometabolic benefits.

6 Name foods associated with cardiometabolic risks.

7 Counsel a client on ways to lower sodium intake.

D iseases of the heart accounted for 24.4% of all American deaths in 2010—more than any other single cause or group of causes of death in the United States (National Center for Health Statistics, Centers for Disease Control and Prevention, 2010). Approximately every 25 seconds, an American will have a coronary event, and approximately every minute, someone will die of one (Roger et al., 2012). Suboptimal lifestyle is implicated in many instances of cardiovascular disease (CVD) and its risks (Mozaffarian, Appel, and Van Horn, 2011). This chapter addresses nutrition for preventing and treating CVD.

CARDIOVASCULAR DISEASES

Cardiovascular disease (CVD) is an umbrella term for diseases that affect the heart and blood vessels, such as coronary heart disease (CHD), stroke, heart failure (HF), hypertension, and arterial diseases. Atherosclerotic CVD is caused by atherosclerosis, a progressive narrowing and hardening of blood vessels. CHD, which makes up more than half of all cardiovascular events in men and women younger than 75 years of age (Roger et al., 2012), occurs when atherosclerosis affects coronary arteries. Atherosclerotic CVD may lead to blocked blood flow to the heart (myocardial infarction), brain (cerebrovascular accident), or legs (peripheral arterial disease). Atherosclerosis can also cause a ballooning out of blood vessel walls (aneurysm).

The American Heart Association Strategic Planning Task Force has developed the following impact goals: "By 2020, to improve the cardiovascular health of all Americans by 20% while reducing deaths from CVD and stroke by 20%" (Lloyd-Jones et al., 2010). Part of the process of formulating those goals was to define cardiovascular health and the metrics to be used to monitor cardiovascular health over time. Ideal cardiovascular health is defined by various behaviors and health factors (Table 20.1).

Hypertension

Hypertension is a symptom, not a disease, arbitrarily defined as sustained elevated blood pressure greater than or equal to 140/90 mmHg ("arbitrarily defined" because problems associated with high blood pressure occur on a continuum with no obvious threshold of where risk begins, including the prehypertension range of 120–139/80–89 mmHg) (Lichtenstein et al., 2006). Hypertension is one of the most important modifiable risk factors for heart disease, stroke, kidney disease, and peripheral arterial disease (PAD). Hypertension is associated with shorter overall life expectancy, shorter life expectancy free of CVD, and more years lived with CVD (Franco, Peeters, Bonneux, and de Laet, 2005). People in middle age who experience increases or decreases in blood pressure have higher and lower remaining lifetime risks for CVD, respectively (Allen et al., 2012). Prevention efforts should emphasize the importance of lowering blood pressure and avoiding or delaying hypertension to reduce the lifetime risk of CVD.

Hypertension is one of the most common chronic conditions in the United States. An estimated 28.67% of American adults have hypertension (Yoon, Burt, Louis, and Carroll, 2012), and another 29.7% are estimated to have prehypertension (Ogunniyi, Croft, Greenlund, Giles, and Mensah, 2010). The prevalence of hypertension in blacks in the United States is among the highest in the world (Roger et al., 2012). Compared to nonblacks, blacks develop hypertension earlier in life, have much higher average blood pressures, and have higher rates of hypertension-related complications, especially fatal stroke and end-stage kidney disease (Roger et al., 2012).

Hypertension is the result of environmental factors (obesity, physical inactivity, sodium intake, and alcohol intake), genetic factors, and interactions among these factors (Appel et al., 2006). Diet is a prominent, and likely predominant, environmental factor.

Table 20.1 Definitions of Poor and Ideal Cardiovascular Health Among Adults 20 Years and Older

Metric	Poor Health	Ideal Health
Smoking	Yes	Never or quit more than 12 months ago
Body mass index	≥30	<25
Physical activity	None	150 or more min/week of moderate intensity or moderate + vigorous intensity or 75 or more min/week of vigorous intensity
Healthy diet	0–1 components	4–5 components
Appropriate calories within a DASH-type eating plan that includes but is not limited to*		
1. 4.5 or more cups of fruits and vegetables daily		
2. Two or more 3½ oz servings of fish/week, preferably oily fish		
3. Three or more 1 oz equivalent servings of whole grains daily		
4. Less than 1500 mg sodium per day		
5. Less than 36 oz/week of sugar-sweetened beverages		
Secondary metrics include Four or more servings of nuts, legumes, and seeds per week Two or fewer servings of processed meats per week Less than 7% of total calories from saturated fat		
Total cholesterol	≥240 mg/dL	<200 mg/dL
Blood pressure	Systolic ≥140 mmHg or diastolic ≥90 mmHg	<120/<80 mmHg
Fasting plasma glucose level	≥126 mg/dL	<100 mg/dL

*Intake goals are based on a 2000-calorie diet and should be adjusted accordingly for other calorie levels.

Source: Lloyd-Jones, D., Hong, Y., Labarthe, D., Mozaffarian, D., Appel, L. J., Van Horn, L., . . . Rosamond, W. D. (2010). Defining and setting national goals for cardiovascular health promotion and disease reduction: The American Heart Association's Strategic Impact Goal through 2020 and beyond. *Circulation, 121,* 586–613.

Nutrition Therapy

Nutrition therapy has the potential to

- Lower blood pressure and prevent hypertension in people who are normotensive or prehypertensive.
- Eliminate the need for medication in people with stage 1 hypertension. Diet is the initial treatment before drug therapy is introduced.
- Lower blood pressure and reduce the dose of medication needed in people who have hypertension and are treated with medication (Appel et al., 2006).

Historically, nutrition interventions to prevent or treat hypertension included weight loss, a sodium-restricted diet, and decreased alcohol intake (Joint National Committee, 2004). Today, those approaches are combined with or part of the DASH diet.

The DASH Diet. Dietary Approaches to Stop Hypertension (DASH) was a multicenter feeding study funded by the National Heart, Lung, and Blood Institute (NHLBI) that set out to test whether eating whole "real" foods rather than individual nutrients would lower blood pressure as a result of some combination of nutrients, interactions among individual nutrients, or other food factors (Appel et al., 1997). The results clearly showed that eating a diet rich in fruit, vegetables, low-fat dairy products, and whole grains; moderate in poultry, fish, and nuts; and low in fat, red meat, and added sugar substantially lowers both systolic and diastolic blood pressures as well as low-density lipoprotein (LDL) cholesterol. Reductions in blood pressure were similar in men and women and similar in magnitude to the effects seen with drug monotherapy for mild hypertension.

The DASH eating plan was rich in potassium, magnesium, calcium, and fiber and low in total fat, saturated fat, and cholesterol. Protein content was slightly increased. It is likely that several aspects of the diet, not just one nutrient or food, lowered blood pressure (Appel et al., 2006). Especially noteworthy is that the decrease in blood pressure occurred without lowering sodium intake and without lowering calories to produce weight loss.

A second study, DASH-sodium, was designed to test whether limiting sodium on a DASH diet would yield even better results (Sacks et al., 2001). The results showed the following:

- Lowering sodium with either the control diet or DASH diet lowers blood pressure; the lower the sodium intake, the lower the blood pressure.
- At each sodium level, blood pressure was lower on the DASH diet than on the control diet.
- The greatest reduction in blood pressure occurred at 1500 mg of sodium.
- The greatest blood pressure reductions occurred in blacks; middle-aged and older people; and people with hypertension, diabetes, or chronic kidney disease.

The DASH diet is promoted by the NHLBI and American Heart Association as a healthy dietary pattern to prevent and treat hypertension (Appel et al., 2006; U.S. Department of Health and Human Services [USDHHS], National Institutes of Health, NHLBI, 2006). Food group recommendations are designed to meet macronutrient and micronutrient needs based on a person's total calorie intake. Table 20.2 features the number of servings from each food group recommended at various calorie levels of the DASH diet.

Reduce Sodium Intake. Lowering sodium intake to lower blood pressure is a recommendation in almost every country that has issued guidelines for preventing and treating CVD (Whelton et al., 2012). Based on the strength of evidence that shows excess sodium intake is related to

QUICK BITE

Sodium content of selected foods

	Sodium (mg)
1 packet dry onion soup mix	3132
1 tsp salt	2325
1 fast-food single cheeseburger with condiments and bacon	1314
1 6-in, fast-food tuna salad sub	1293
1 large fast-food taco	1233
2 fast-food pancakes with syrup	1104
1 cup canned macaroni and cheese	1061
1 fast-food beef chimichanga	910

Source: *U.S. Department of Agriculture National Nutrient Database for Stand Reference, Release 25.* Available at https://www.ars.usda.gov/SP2UserFiles/Place/12354500/Data/SR25/nutrlist/sr25w307.pdf. Accessed on 12/20/12.

Table 20.2 The DASH Eating Plan at Various Calorie Levels

Food Group and Representative Serving Sizes	1200 Calories	1400 Calories	1600 Calories	1800 Calories	2000 Calories	2600 Calories	Types of Foods Recommended
Grains 1 slice bread; ½ cup cooked rice, pasta, or cereal	4–5	5–6	6	6	6–8	10–11	Whole grains are recommended for most grain servings, such as whole wheat bread, whole-grain cereals, whole wheat pasta, and brown rice. Commercial products, such as crackers, cookies, chips, and cakes, should be trans fat free and low in fat
Vegetables 1 cup raw leafy vegetable ½ cup cut-up raw or cooked vegetable ½ cup vegetable juice	3–4	3–4	3–4	4–5	4–5	5–6	All fresh, plain frozen, and low-sodium canned vegetables Use preparation methods to retain the fiber content, such as leaving skins on potatoes.
Fruits 1 medium fruit ¼ cup dried fruit ½ cup fresh, frozen, or canned fruit ½ cup fruit juice	3–4	4	4	4–5	4–5	5–6	All; eat skins and seeds for fiber whenever possible Whole fruits are better choices than fruit juice.
Fat-free or low-fat milk and milk products 1 cup milk or yogurt 1½ oz natural cheese	2–3	2–3	2–3	2–3	2–3	3	Nonfat or low-fat milk, yogurt, and cheese
Lean meats, poultry, and fish 1 oz lean meat, poultry, or fish 1 egg	3 or less	3–4 or less	3–4 or less	6 or less	6 or less	6 or less	Broil, roast, or poach meats; trim away visible fat Lean cuts of beef (sirloin tip, round steak, arm roast), lean cuts of pork (center-cut ham, loin chops, tenderloin) Ground beef that is at least "90% lean"

(continues on page 540)

Table 20.2 The DASH Eating Plan at Various Calorie Levels (continued)

Food Group and Representative Serving Sizes	1200 Calories	1400 Calories	1600 Calories	1800 Calories	2000 Calories	2600 Calories	Types of Foods Recommended
							Skinless poultry (chicken breast and turkey cutlets are the leanest poultry choices) Fish and seafood that are not fried Limit egg yolks to 4 per week; egg whites or egg substitutes as desired
Nuts, seeds, and legumes ⅓ cup or 1½ oz nuts 2 tbsp peanut butter 2 tbsp or ½ oz seeds ½ cup cooked legumes	3 per week	3 per week	3–4 per week	4 per week	4–5 per week	1	Any unsalted nuts and seeds Any dried peas and beans (drain and rinse canned varieties)
Fats and oils 1 tsp soft margarine 1 tsp oil	1	1	2	2–3	2–3	3	Canola, olive, corn, and safflower oils Soft trans fat–free margarines in tubs or spray form Low-fat mayonnaise Light salad dressing
Sweets and added sugars 1 tbsp sugar 1 tbsp jelly or jam ½ cup sorbet and ices	3 or less per week	3 or less per week	3 or less per week	5 or less per week	5 or less per week	Less than 2	Sweets that are low in fat, such as low-fat ice cream, low-fat pudding, sorbets, ices, fruit bars, angel food cake, fig bars
Maximum sodium limit	2300 mg/day	2300 mg/day	2300 mg/day	2300 mg/day	2300 mg/day	2300 mg/day	

Source: U.S. Department of Agriculture, U.S. Department of Health and Human Services. (2010). *Dietary guidelines for Americans, 2010* (7th ed.). Available at www.health.gov/dietaryguidelines. Accessed on 12/17/12.

hypertension, CVD, and stroke and that lowering sodium intake has the potential to prevent hypertension and reduce the risk of CVD and stroke events, the American Heart Association recommends the entire U.S. population consume less than 1500 mg of sodium per day (Lloyd-Jones et al., 2010). The DASH diet guidelines recommend that sodium intake initially be gradually lowered to 2300 mg and gradually decreased to 1500 mg for maximum benefit. Table 20.3 shows a DASH diet menu at two different sodium levels.

Food consumption data from 2003 to 2008 show that 97% of American adults consume more than 1500 mg of sodium daily (Cogswell et al., 2012). A drastic reduction in sodium intake is not easily achieved in the context of the typical American diet that relies heavily on commercially processed foods with high levels of "hidden" sodium (Whelton et al., 2012). Approximately 77% of the sodium in a typical American diet comes from processed foods (Box 20.1). Tips for lowering sodium intake appear in Box 20.2.

Increase Potassium. One factor that may contribute to the effectiveness of the DASH diet in lowering blood pressure is its potassium content (Hu, 2003). As potassium intake increases, blood pressure decreases in hypertensive and nonhypertensive people (Appel et al., 2006). Foods emphasized in the DASH diet—namely, fruits, vegetables, whole grains, and dairy products—provide significant amounts of potassium. The Adequate

Table 20.3 2000-Calorie DASH Menus at Two Sodium Levels

2400-mg Sodium Menu	Sodium (mg)	Substitutions to ↓ Sodium to 1500 mg	Sodium (mg)
Breakfast		The same as the 2400-mg sodium menu except	
¾ cup wheat flakes cereal	199	2 cups puffed wheat cereal	1
1 slice whole wheat bread	149		149
1 medium banana	1		1
1 cup nonfat milk	126		126
1 cup orange juice	5		5
1 tsp soft margarine	51	1 tsp soft margarine, unsalted	1
Lunch			
Beef sandwich			
2 oz ham, low sodium	101	2 oz beef, eye of round	35
1 tbsp Dijon mustard	360	1 tbsp low-fat mayonnaise	101
2 slices cheddar cheese, reduced fat	260	2 slices Swiss cheese, natural	109
1 sesame roll	319		319
1 large leaf romaine lettuce	1		1
2 slices tomato	22		22
1 cup low-fat, low-sodium potato salad	12		12
1 medium orange	0		0
Dinner			
3 oz cod with lemon juice	90		90
½ cup brown rice	5		5
½ cup cooked spinach	88		88
1 small corn bread muffin	363	1 small dinner roll	146
1 tsp soft margarine	51	1 tsp soft margarine, unsalted	1
Snacks			
1 cup fruit yogurt, fat free, no added sugar	107		107
¼ cup dried fruit	6		6
2 large graham cracker rectangles	156		156
1 tbsp peanut butter, reduced fat	101	1 tbsp peanut butter, unsalted	3
Total sodium (mg)	**2228**		**1539**

Box 20.1   THE EFFECT OF FOOD PROCESSING ON SODIUM CONTENT

Food Groups	Sodium (mg)
Whole and other grains and grain products*	
Cooked cereal, rice, pasta, unsalted, ½ cup	0–5
Ready-to-eat cereal, 1 cup	0–360
Bread, 1 slice	110–175
Vegetables	
Fresh or frozen, cooked without salt, ½ cup	1–70
Canned or frozen with sauce, ½ cup	140–460
Tomato juice, canned, ½ cup	330
Fruit	
Fresh, frozen, canned, ½ cup	0–5
Low-fat or fat-free milk and milk products	
Milk, 1 cup	107
Yogurt, 1 cup	175
Natural cheeses, 1½ oz	110–450
Processed cheeses, 2 oz	600
Nuts, seeds, and legumes	
Peanuts, salted, ½ cup	120
Peanuts, unsalted, ½ cup	0–5
Beans, cooked from dried or frozen, without salt, ½ cup	0–5
Beans, canned, ½ cup	400
Lean meats, fish, and poultry	
Fresh meat, fish, poultry, 3 oz	30–90
Tuna canned, water pack, no salt added, 3 oz	35–45
Tuna canned, water pack, 3 oz	230–350
Ham, lean, roasted, 3 oz	1020

*Whole grains are recommended for most grain servings.

Source: U.S. Department of Health and Human Services, National Institutes of Health, National Heart, Lung, and Blood Institute. (2006). *Your guide to lowering your blood pressure with DASH* (NIH Publication No. 06-4082). Available at http://www.nhlbi.nih.gov/health/public/heart/hbp/dash/new_dash.pdf. Accessed on 7/16/08.

Intake (AI) for potassium is 4700 mg, an amount not usually met in a typical American diet but one that can be easily consumed on a DASH diet.

Lose Weight. Observational and clinical studies consistently show that weight is directly related to blood pressure and weight loss lowers blood pressure, even if **healthy weight** is not attained (Appel et al., 2006). The greater the weight loss, the greater is the reduction in blood pressure in both hypertensive and nonhypertensive people (Stevens et al., 2001). Although it is not known whether weight loss can blunt age-related increases in blood pressure, evidence shows that achieving a healthy weight is an effective intervention to prevent and treat hypertension (Appel et al., 2006). Because maintaining weight loss is so difficult, preventing weight gain is critical in people of normal weight.

Low-calorie DASH diet meal patterns are available (see Table 20.2). Blood pressure improves when weight loss occurs whether the low-calorie diet is low in fat or low in carbohydrates (Brinkworth, Noakes, Buckley, Keogh, and Clifton, 2009). However, both low-fat and low-carbohydrate diets may provide low levels of food components important for

Healthy Weight: body mass index of 18.5 to 24.9.

Box 20.2   Tips to Lower Sodium Intake

In General
- Eat more meals at home. Cook in batches and freeze for use on busy days.
- Avoid or limit convenience foods, such as boxes mixes, frozen dinners, and canned goods.
- Read labels to find items lowest in sodium.
- Don't add salt when cooking.

Grains
- Use less bread.
- Cook rice and pasta without adding salt.
- Eat cereals without added salt, such as oatmeal, shredded wheat, and puffed whole-grain cereal.
- Avoid instant flavored rice, pasta, and cereal mixes.

Vegetables
- Eat more fresh or frozen vegetables without salt added.
- Rinse canned vegetables before using.
- Switch to pasta sauce without added salt or dilute regular bottled pasta sauce with equal parts of no-salt-added tomato sauce.
- Substitute fresh vegetables for pickles and other pickled foods.

Fruits
- Fresh, frozen, and canned fruits are salt free; enjoy.

Milk and Milk Products
- Use cheese sparingly, especially processed cheeses.

Protein Foods
- Choose fresh poultry, fish, and lean meat instead of canned, smoked, deli, or other processed varieties.
- Limit frozen dinners.
- Limit cured meat intake, such as sausages and hot dogs.
- Limit imitation crab and lobster products.
- Limit soy substitutes, such as imitation ground beef or chicken.
- Use no-salt-added nut butters.

Fats and Oils
- Use homemade vinegar and oil dressings instead of bottled salad dressings.

Miscellaneous
- Use herbs and spices instead of salt to season foods.
- Replace garlic and onion salts with garlic and onion powders.
- Use reduced-salt or no-salt-added condiments such as ketchup, soy sauce, and mayonnaise.
- Use no-salt-added broth to make soup instead of using canned soup.

When Eating Out
- Request that food not be salted, if possible.
- Choose fruit juice instead of soup for an appetizer.

(continues on page 544)

Box 20.2   Tips to Lower Sodium Intake (continued)

- Use oil and vinegar or fresh lemon instead of regular salad dressing.
- Choose foods that are grilled, baked, or roasted.
- Order plain meat and vegetables without gravy or sauce, or order them "on the side" and use sparingly.
- Choose plain baked potatoes and season sparingly with sour cream, butter, or pepper.
- Select fresh fruit for dessert. If the client is going to splurge, ice cream or sherbet is a better choice than pie, cake, cookies, or other desserts.
- Avoid fast-food restaurant meals, which usually are high in sodium. If you have to go, order a child-sized meal.
- Order sandwiches without mayonnaise, sauces, or condiments; load with lettuce, tomato, and onion.

cardiac and overall health. For instance, very-low-carbohydrate diets are inadequate in fiber and very-low-fat diets may be deficient in vitamin E or B_{12} (see Table 20.1).

Limit Alcohol. Observational studies and clinical trials show a direct dose-dependent relationship between alcohol and blood pressure, especially when alcohol intake is more than 2 drinks/day (Xin et al., 2001). If people choose to drink, alcohol intake should be limited to 2 drinks or less per day for men and 1 drink or less per day for women (Appel et al., 2006). One drink is equivalent to 12 oz of beer, 5 oz of wine, or 1.5 oz of 80-proof distilled spirits.

Atherosclerosis

Atherosclerosis: the formation of plaque along the smooth inner walls of arteries, which results in progressive narrowing and diminished blood flow to the tissue they supply.

Coronary Heart Disease: damage to the heart resulting from inadequate supply of blood to the heart.

Plaque: deposits of fatty material, cholesterol, calcium, and other blood components that are covered with connective tissue and embedded in the artery wall.

Atherosclerosis is the underlying cause of most CVDs, such as **coronary heart disease** (CHD), ischemic stroke, and PAD. It is a progressive process that begins in childhood or adolescence and may continue for decades before symptoms occur.

Initially, a microscopic but chronic injury to the artery wall—such as that from smoking, hypertension, or hyperglycemia—causes an immune response that attracts monocytes and platelets to the injured area. These cells trap LDL cholesterol and grow to become fatty streaks (Fig. 20.1). Over time, deposits of smooth muscle cells, connective tissue cells, calcium, and cholesterol cause the fatty streak to enlarge and harden into **plaque**. Narrowing inside the arterial lumen restricts blood flow to the surrounding tissue. Figure 20.2 illustrates the relationship between hypertension and atherosclerosis.

Elevated levels of LDL cholesterol promote atherosclerosis, particularly if the LDLs are oxidized; oxidation may occur from free radicals generated by macrophages, by endothelial cells, or from various enzymatic reactions. Oxidized LDLs are actively retained in the artery wall, contributing to plaque formation. As the level of LDL increases, so does the risk of developing CVD (Expert Panel on Detection, Evaluation, and Treatment of High Blood Cholesterol in Adults, 2002). Because high-density lipoprotein (HDL) cholesterol helps prevent oxidation of LDL and removes cholesterol from circulation, low levels of HDL are a risk factor for atherosclerosis. Table 20.4 outlines classification of cholesterol levels.

Complications of atherosclerosis depend on the size, stability, and location of the plaque. Plaques can grow large enough to completely block an artery. More often, complications are from an unstable plaque rupturing, which triggers the formation of a blood clot (thrombus) that may break away (embolus) and travel to a smaller artery where it can cause a myocardial infarction (coronary arteries) or stroke (brain).

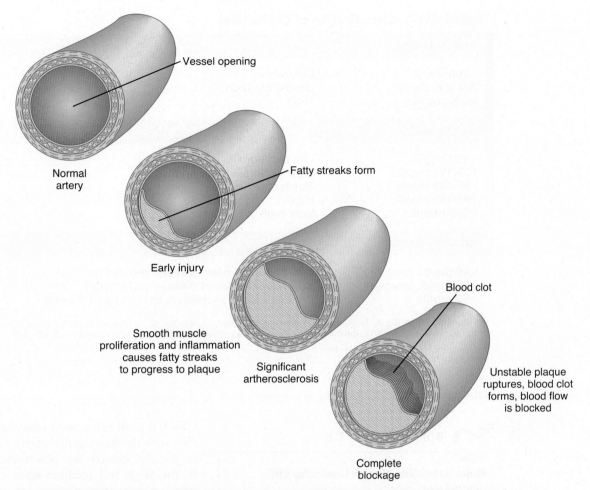

Vessel opening

Normal artery

Fatty streaks form

Early injury

Smooth muscle proliferation and inflammation causes fatty streaks to progress to plaque

Significant artherosclerosis

Blood clot

Unstable plaque ruptures, blood clot forms, blood flow is blocked

Complete blockage

■ FIGURE 20.1   Schematic of atherosclerosis. The plaque develops by a series of events that begins with microscopic injury to the artery lining. The arteries narrow down and the condition is exacerbated by the propensity of clots to form on unstable ruptured plaques.

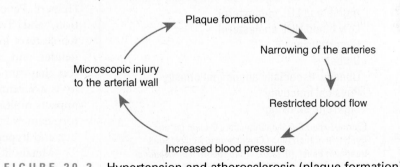

Plaque formation

Narrowing of the arteries

Restricted blood flow

Increased blood pressure

Microscopic injury to the arterial wall

■ FIGURE 20.2   Hypertension and atherosclerosis (plaque formation) are intertwined.

Table 20.4 Classification of Cholesterol

Total Cholesterol	
<200 mg/dL	Desirable
200–239 mg/dL	Borderline high
≥240 mg/dL	High

LDL Cholesterol	
<100 mg/dL	Optimal (ideal)
100–129 mg/dL	Near optimal/above optimal
130–159 mg/dL	Borderline high
160–189 mg/dL	High
≥190 mg/dL	Very high

HDL Cholesterol	
<40 mg/dL men	Risk factor for heart disease and stroke
<50 mg/dL women	Risk factor for heart disease and stroke
≥60 mg/dL	Provides some protection against heart disease

Source: Roger, V., Go, A., Lloyd-Jones, D., Benjamin, E., Berry, J., Borden, W., . . . Turner, M. (2012). Heart disease and stroke statistics—2012 update: A report from the American Heart Association. *Circulation, 125,* e2–e220.

Coronary Heart Disease

QUICK BITE

Major nonmodifiable risk factors for CHD
Increasing age
Male gender
Family history of premature heart disease

Major modifiable risk factors for CHD
An atherogenic diet (high in saturated fat and
   low in fruits, vegetables, and whole grains)
High blood LDL cholesterol
Low blood HDL cholesterol
Hypertension
Diabetes
Obesity, especially abdominal obesity
Physical inactivity
Cigarette smoking

Source: Expert Panel on Detection, Evaluation, and Treatment of High Blood Cholesterol in Adults (Adult Treatment Panel III). (2002). *Third report of the National Cholesterol Education Program (NCEP)* (NIH Publication No. 02-5215). Bethesda, MD: National Heart, Lung, and Blood Institute.

Hypercholesterolemia: generic term to describe high levels of cholesterol in the blood.

CHD, a term often used interchangeably with the more generic term CVD, is usually caused by atherosclerosis in the large and medium-sized coronary arteries. Most plaques are unstable; blood clots that form after these plaques rupture are responsible for causing ischemia and tissue damage.

Numerous risk factors have been identified in the development of CHD (Expert Panel on Detection, Evaluation, and Treatment of High Blood Cholesterol in Adults, 2002). Genetics, gender, and advancing age are risk factors that cannot be modified; diet quality is a modifiable risk factor. Diet also impacts multiple cardiovascular risk factors, namely hypertension, diabetes, obesity, and **hypercholesterolemia**.

Metabolic syndrome (MetS) is a risk factor for CVD and type 2 diabetes. It consists of a cluster of metabolic abnormalities—namely, elevated triglycerides, low HDL cholesterol, high blood pressure, high fasting blood glucose levels, and central obesity (Alberti et al., 2009). Physical inactivity and obesity are major contributors to

Table 20.5 Diagnostic Criteria for Metabolic Syndrome

Risk Factor	Defining Level
Metabolic syndrome is confirmed by the presence of three of the following five risks:	
Abdominal obesity*	
Men	≥40-in waist (>35 in for Asian men)
Women	≥35-in waist (>31 in for Asian women)
	Or population- and country-specific definitions
Elevated triglycerides	≥150 mg/dL, or taking medication for high triglyceride levels
Low HDL	
Men	≤40 mg/dL in men
Women	≤50 mg/dL in women
	Or taking medication for low HDL
Elevated blood pressure	≥130 mmHg systolic blood pressure
	≥85 mmHg diastolic blood pressure
	Or drug treatment in a patient with a history of hypertension
Elevated fasting glucose	≥100 mg/dL or taking medication to control blood sugar level

Source: Miller, M., Stone, N., Ballantyne, C., Bittner, V., Criqui, M. H., Ginsberg, H. N., . . . Pennathur, S. (2011). Triglycerides and cardiovascular disease. A scientific statement from the American Heart Association. *Circulation, 123,* 2292–2333.

Atherogenic: able to cause or promote atherosclerosis.

Biomarker: an indicator of a biologic state.

Trans Fats: fatty acids with hydrogen atoms on opposite sides of the double bond. Most trans fats in the diet come from partially hydrogenated fats.

Omega-3 Fatty Acids: a polyunsaturated fatty acid in which the first double bond is three carbon atoms away from the methyl (CH_3) end of the carbon chain. Eicosapentaenoic acid (EPA) and docosahexaenoic acid (DHA) are omega-3 fatty acids found in oily fish.

MetS, but metabolic susceptibility is usually needed for MetS to manifest (Grundy, 2008). People with MetS have double the risk of developing CVD over the following 5 to 10 years compared with people without the syndrome, and risk of type 2 diabetes increases fivefold (Alberti et al., 2009). Although there is disagreement over the diagnostic criteria used to define MetS, three abnormal findings out of five qualify a person for MetS (Table 20.5). Management consists of treating the abnormalities, such as controlling blood pressure and losing weight.

Of the five possible components of MetS, high triglycerides are the second most common finding after high blood pressure (Kasai et al., 2006). Although longitudinal and cross-sectional studies suggest that high triglyceride levels may be a predictor of CVD risk, clinical studies have failed to demonstrate the prognostic value of triglyceride levels in MetS. According to the American Heart Association, triglycerides are not directly **atherogenic** but are an important **biomarker** of CVD risk because they are associated with other atherogenic particles (Miller et al., 2011). Triglyceride levels can decrease 20% to 50% as a result of healthy lifestyle changes, such as weight loss, substituting grains with fiber for simple carbohydrates, eliminating **trans fats**, restricting fructose and saturated fatty acids, choosing a Mediterranean diet, and consuming **omega-3 fatty acids** from fish oil (Miller et al., 2011). Very high triglyceride levels, which increase the risk of pancreatitis, are additionally treated with abstinence from alcohol and possibly triglyceride-lowering medication.

DIET IN CARDIOVASCULAR HEALTH PROMOTION

The relationship between diet and CVD has been a major focus of health research for almost half a century (Mente, de Koning, Shannon, and Anand, 2009). Diet modification is a critical part of population-based strategies to prevent CHD (Maruthur, Wang, and Appel, 2009) and is also associated with secondary prevention of recurrent CVD events in who have CVD or diabetes (Dehghan et al., 2012)

Overall Food Patterns

The American Heart Association's position is that a healthy diet should focus on food patterns rather than individual nutrients, although nutrient (e.g., trans fat, sodium) intakes should be consistent with already established recommendations (Appel et al., 2006; Lichtenstein et al., 2006). Evidence increasingly supports the idea that a nutrient-based approach may be less helpful or even misleading for establishing dietary guidelines to prevent chronic diseases because nutrients are not consumed in isolation (Dehghan et al., 2012). The health effects of food, unlike the effects of single nutrients, are likely to occur from a synergy of interactions between multiple food components, such as fiber, specific fatty acids, and potassium (Mozaffarian and Ludwig, 2010). For instance, a single focus on avoiding saturated fat may make some people forgo nuts even though randomized controlled trials show that eating nuts has several cardioprotective benefits, including lowering total cholesterol and LDL cholesterol (Banel and Hu, 2009; Kendall, Josse, Esfahani, and Jenkins, 2010). New advances provide substantial evidence on the positive and negative cardiometabolic effects of foods (Tables 20.6 and 20.7) (Mozaffarian, Appel, et al., 2011). A food pattern approach, compared to single nutrients, is easier to communicate and implement for practitioners, individuals, and policy makers.

A DASH-Style Diet

The American Heart Association's diet metric for ideal cardiovascular health is to consume appropriate calories within a DASH-style diet (Lloyd-Jones et al., 2010) that includes but is not limited to the following:

- 4.5 or more cups of fruits and vegetables daily
- Two or more 3½ oz servings of fish per week, preferably oily fish
- Three or more 1 oz equivalent servings of whole grains daily
- Fewer than 1500 mg sodium per day
- Less than 36 oz/week of sugar-sweetened beverages

Secondary metrics include the following:

- Four or more servings of nuts, legumes, and seeds per week
- Two or fewer servings of processed meats per week
- Less than 7% of total calories from saturated fat

The amounts listed are based on a 2000-calorie diet and will vary depending on the calorie content of the diet. The standards for evaluating diet quality for poor and ideal health appear in Table 20.1.

A food group approach that emphasizes fruits, vegetables, beans, nuts, and whole grains and limits red or processed meats, refined carbohydrates, and other processed foods—such as the DASH diet—not only improves hypertension but also other cardiovascular risk factors, such as hypercholesterolemia and obesity (Mozaffarian, Appel, et al., 2011). The DASH diet also may potentially prevent type 2 diabetes (Liese, Nichols, Sun, D'Agostino, and Haffner, 2009), and in people who have type 2 diabetes, the DASH diet has been shown to improve numerous cardiac risk factors, including waist circumference, systolic and diastolic blood pressure, fasting blood glucose, hemoglobin A1c, triglyceride levels, LDL cholesterol, HDL cholesterol, and total cholesterol (Azadbakht et al., 2011). The DASH diet is even recommended by the *Dietary Guidelines for Americans, 2010* as a healthy eating pattern for *all* Americans (U.S. Department of Agriculture, USDHHS, 2010).

Table 20.6   Foods Associated with Cardiometabolic Benefits

Food	Components Implicated in Benefits	Possible Cardiometabolic Benefits
Fruits and vegetables	Antioxidant vitamins, potassium, magnesium, fiber, phytochemicals	Improvements in blood pressure, lipid levels, insulin resistance, weight control Lower incidence of CHD Lower incidence of stroke (fruit) Benefits are not replicated with equivalent amounts of mineral or fiber supplements.
Whole grains	B vitamins, vitamin E, fiber, folate, minerals, phytochemicals, fatty acids	Improvements in glucose-insulin homeostasis; may reduce inflammation and promote weight loss Whole-grain oats decrease LDL cholesterol without lowering HDL cholesterol. Higher fiber content contributes to the lower incidence of CHD, diabetes, and possibly stroke from whole grains; the effect of whole grains is not replicated from equivalent amounts of supplemental fiber bran, or isolated micronutrients.
Fish	Specific proteins, unsaturated fats, vitamin D, selenium, omega-3 fatty acids	In human trials, fish oil lowers triglyceride levels, systolic and diastolic blood pressure, and resting heart rate. May reduce inflammation and limit platelet aggregation Lower incidence of CHD, ischemic stroke, cardiac death
Nuts	Unsaturated fatty acids, vegetable proteins, fiber, folate, minerals, antioxidants, phytochemicals	Lower total cholesterol, LDL cholesterol, and postprandial hyperglycemia from high-carbohydrate meals When added to weight loss diets, weight loss is either unchanged or greater. Lower incidence of CHD
Dairy products	It is not known which constituents of dairy products offer cardiometabolic benefits; possibly specific fatty acids, proteins, vitamins, and other nutrients may be responsible	May improve satiety and weight loss May contribute to improvements in blood pressure, lipid levels, and insulin resistance regardless of changes in weight Lower risk of stroke and diabetes
Vegetable oils	Polyunsaturated fatty acids (PUFAs), monounsaturated fatty acids, plant-derived omega-3 fatty acids	Improvements in blood lipids and lipoproteins and lower CVD events when PUFAs replace saturated fatty acids Monounsaturated fats from vegetable oils (e.g., olive oil) may lower CVD risk.
Legumes	Micronutrients, phytochemicals, fiber	Nutrient package may reduce cardiometabolic risk.

Source: Mozaffarian, D., Appel, L., & Van Horn, L. (2011). Components of a cardioprotective diet. New insights. *Circulation, 123,* 2870–2891.

Table 20.7 Foods Associated with Cardiometabolic Risks

Food	Components Implicated in Adverse Effects	Possible Cardiometabolic Risks
Foods and fats containing partially hydrogenated vegetable oils	Trans fatty acids	Strongest link to CHD risk of all types of fat
Red and processed meats such as bacon, sausage, hot dogs	Heme iron, saturated fatty acids, dietary cholesterol; sodium and preservatives (in processed meats)	Consumption of processed meats but not unprocessed red meats associated with higher incidence of CHD and diabetes mellitus. Red meat and processed meat may increase risk of CHD when they are eaten in place of poultry, fish, and plant proteins.
Sugar-sweetened beverages, sweets, and grain-based desserts and bakery foods	Sugars, refined grains	Sugar-sweetened beverages are linked to obesity; lack of satiety from liquid sugar may contribute to positive calorie balance. Sugar-sweetened beverages may displace the intake of more healthful beverages. High sugar-sweetened beverage consumption associated with higher incidence of diabetes, MetS, and possibly CHD. Refined carbohydrates are devoid of beneficial nutrients and may displace more healthful foods.

Source: Mozaffarian, D., Appel, L., & Van Horn, L. (2011). Components of a cardioprotective diet. New insights. *Circulation, 123,* 2870–2891.

Traditional Mediterranean Diet

Another heart healthy food group approach is the traditional Mediterranean diet (Fig. 20.3). Like the DASH diet, it is characterized by a high intake of vegetables, fruits, whole grains, plant proteins (e.g., nuts and legumes), and fish. It includes a moderate intake of alcohol, normally with meals, and a low intake of refined grains, sweets, and red meat (approximately twice per month) (Kastorini et al., 2011). It is not a low-fat diet but is low in animal fat and therefore low in saturated fat and cholesterol. Olives and olive oil contribute to high monounsaturated fat content.

The health-enhancing benefits of a Mediterranean diet may be due to its anti-inflammatory and antioxidant effects as well as the effects of its individual components, especially olive oil, fruits and vegetables, whole grains, and fish (Giugliano and Esposito, 2008). Studies link a traditional Mediterranean diet with the following:

- A decreased risk of CHD, cancer, and total mortality (Sofi, Abbate, Gensini, and Casini, 2010)
- Improvements in obesity and type 2 diabetes (Buckland, Bach, and Serra-Majem, 2008; Giugliano and Esposito, 2008)

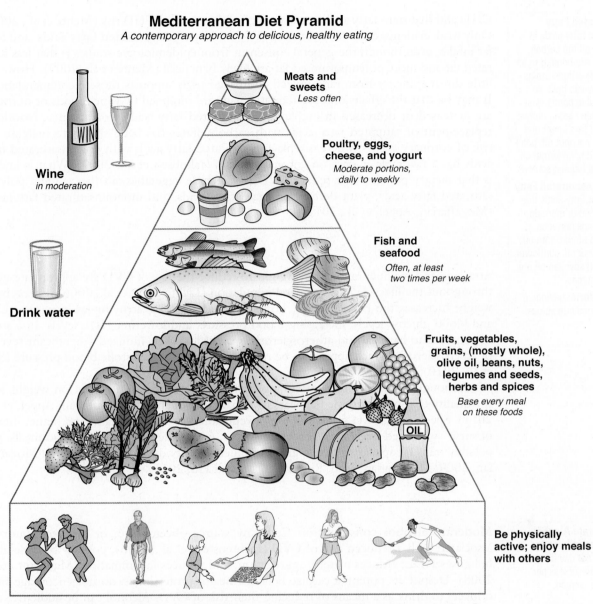

Mediterranean Diet Pyramid
A contemporary approach to delicious, healthy eating

Meats and sweets
Less often

Poultry, eggs, cheese, and yogurt
Moderate portions, daily to weekly

Fish and seafood
Often, at least two times per week

Fruits, vegetables, grains, (mostly whole), olive oil, beans, nuts, legumes and seeds, herbs and spices
Base every meal on these foods

Wine
in moderation

Drink water

Be physically active; enjoy meals with others

■ **FIGURE 20.3** Mediterranean diet pyramid. (© 2009 Oldways Preservation & Exchange Trust • www.oldwayspt.org)

- Improvements in MetS components, including abdominal obesity, lipid levels, glucose metabolism, and blood pressure (Kastorini et al., 2011)
- A lower risk of incident CHD and stroke in women (Fung et al., 2009)

Monounsaturated Fatty Acids: fatty acids that have only one double bond between two carbon atoms; olive oil, canola oil, and poultry are rich sources.

Quality of Fat

Traditionally, a low-fat diet has been recommended to decrease the risk of CVD. However, it now appears that the type of fat consumed is far more relevant than the percentage of calories consumed from fat (Mente et al., 2009). There is strong evidence that nuts, **monounsaturated fatty acids**, and a Mediterranean diet pattern are protective against

Saturated Fatty Acids: fatty acids in which all the carbon atoms are bonded to as many hydrogen atoms as they can hold, so no double bonds exist between carbon atoms; animal fats (meat and dairy), coconut oil, palm oil, and palm kernel oil are the biggest sources.

Polyunsaturated Fatty Acids: fatty acids that have two or more double bonds between carbon atoms; corn oil, safflower oil, sunflower oil, and soybean oil are rich sources.

Isocaloric: having similar calorie values.

CHD and that trans fatty acids are associated with increased CHD risk (Mente et al., 2009). Only weak evidence exists for **saturated fatty acids, polyunsaturated fatty acids,** and total fat intake, even though the general consensus from epidemiologic studies is that less saturated fat and more polyunsaturated fat are likely beneficial (Mente et al., 2009). However, little direct evidence from randomized controlled trials supports those recommendations. It may be that the effects of saturated fatty acids are modified by which foods or nutrients are increased or decreased in exchange for saturated fatty acids. For instance, **isocaloric** replacement of saturated fatty acids with carbohydrates has been shown to increase the risk of coronary events, whereas replacing saturated fatty acids with polyunsaturated fatty acids has a favorable impact on coronary events (Jakobsen et al., 2009). What is known is that dietary patterns that reduce CVD risk include vegetable oils that contain polyunsaturated fatty acids, plant-derived omega-3 fatty acids, and monounsaturated fatty acids (Mozaffarian, Appel, et al., 2011).

Healthy Weight

Attaining and maintaining healthy weight to reduce the risk of CVD are appropriate goals throughout the lifecycle in the general population (Lichtenstein et al., 2006). Excess body weight increases the risk of CHD, HF, stroke, and cardiac arrhythmias by raising LDL and blood glucose levels; increasing blood pressure; and lowering HDL levels. In a study of people who have carotid atherosclerosis, weight loss diets induced a significant reversal of atherosclerosis, which appears to be related to decreases in systolic blood pressure (Shai et al., 2010).

Although the macronutrient composition of the diet has little effect on weight loss, the quality of foods consumed appears to impact diet quantity (Mozaffarian, Appel, et al., 2011). Specifically, lower intakes of fruits, vegetables, and whole grains and higher intakes of sugar-sweetened beverages, processed snacks, energy-dense foods, fast-food meals, and possibly trans fat appear to have a greater influence on body weight (Micha and Mozaffarian, 2009; Mozaffarian, Hao, Rimm, Willett, and Hu, 2011).

Alcohol

Moderate Alcohol Consumption: two drinks per day for men; one drink or less per day for women.

Moderate alcohol consumption from any source—beer, wine, or distilled liquor—is associated with a reduced risk of CVD (Lichtenstein et al., 2006), possibly because alcohol raises HDL, reduces platelet aggregation, and reduces inflammation (Merchant et al., 2008). Despite its potential cardiac benefits, health professionals do not encourage nondrinkers to drink as a means of reducing their risk of CVD. Alcohol can be addictive, and high intakes are associated with high triglyceride levels, hypertension, liver damage, physical abuse, vehicular and work accidents, and increased risk of breast cancer (Lichtenstein et al., 2006). People who do drink should do so in moderation.

Dietary Supplements

There is a lack of convincing evidence to support the use of supplements to lower CVD risk. Results of the Physician's Health Study II showed that taking a daily multivitamin did not reduce major cardiovascular events, myocardial infarction, stroke, or CVD mortality in male physicians after more than a decade of treatment and follow-up (Sesso et al., 2012). Certain supplements, including beta-carotene, calcium, and vitamin E, can even be harmful (Mozaffarian, Appel, et al., 2011).

Currently, only omega-3 fatty acids can be recommended as a supplement to prevent CVD, but optimal doses and target populations have not been determined (Mozaffarian,

Appel, et al., 2011). Observational studies, randomized clinical trials, and experimental studies provide strong evidence that modest consumption of fish (one to two servings per week of oily fish) or fish oil supplements (approximately 250 mg/day of eicosapentaenoic acid [EPA] and docosahexaenoic acid [DHA]) substantially lowers the risk of CHD death (Mozaffarian, 2008).

Is a "Heart Healthy" Diet and Lifestyle for Everyone?

For "healthy" people, the DASH style diet and traditional Mediterranean style diet may help prevent hypertension, CHD, stroke, type 2 diabetes, and obesity if calories are appropriate. These diets are consistent with the *Dietary Guidelines for Americans, 2010* and MyPlate eating plans. There are few situations in which this "diet" and the recommendations to lose weight, if overweight, and exercise more are inappropriate. Smoking cessation is *always* an appropriate lifestyle choice.

For people who are not "healthy" (e.g., those who are being treated for CHD, hypertension, or diabetes), these diets and lifestyle changes are an integral part of management. Even among people who have had complications of CVD, such as a heart attack or stroke, these diet and lifestyle changes are recommended to prevent subsequent cardiac events. With attention to cultural considerations, as appropriate (Box 20.3), these diet and lifestyle recommendations come close to being "one size fits all." Tips for making heart healthy food choices appear in Box 20.4.

HEART FAILURE

Heart failure (HF) is a major and growing public health problem in the United States and is one of the most common reasons for hospital admission and readmission among people age 65 years and older (Hall, DeFrances, Williams, Golosinskiy, and Schwartzman, 2010). An estimated 5.8 million people in the United States have HF (NHLBI, 2012). Advances in treatment options have led to improvements in outcomes over the past decade; however, the 1-year mortality rate remains high at 29.6% (Chen, Normand, Wang, and Krumholz, 2011).

HF is a syndrome characterized by specific symptoms—namely, shortness of breath, fatigue, and edema. Neurohormonal abnormalities and elevated levels of inflammatory markers and oxidative stress are involved in this systemic illness (von Haehling, Doehner, and Anker, 2007). CHD, hypertension, and diabetes are prevalent causes; arrhythmias and valve disorders may also cause HF. Obesity, MetS, and previous heart attack increase the risk for HF.

Nutrition Therapy

Sodium restriction is recommended in all patients with HF (Lindenfeld et al., 2010). Despite the theoretical basis for limiting sodium intake, the American Heart Association acknowledges that the recommendation to limit sodium is based on expert consensus only, not empirical evidence (Hunt et al., 2005). In fact, two randomized trials suggest that a normal sodium intake, combined with appropriate medications and fluid restriction, could restore intravascular volume and renal blood flow and facilitate renal excretion of sodium and water (Paterna, Gaspare, Fasullo, Sarullo, and Di Pasquale, 2008; Paterna, Parrinello, et al., 2008). In both studies, patients consuming the higher amounts of sodium (e.g., 2800 mg) had better outcomes (fewer readmissions and improved creatinine clearance, respectively) than participants consuming a low-sodium diet (e.g., 1800 mg). Conversely, Arcand et al. (2011) showed that ambulatory HF patients who consume higher amounts of sodium are at greater risk of acute decompensated HF exacerbation. Although the optimal

Box 20.3   Cultural Considerations

For all cultural groups, emphasize the positive aspects of their eating styles and suggest modifications to lower the fat and sodium content of traditional foods.

African American Tradition
Traditional soul foods tend to be high in saturated fat, cholesterol, and sodium. On the positive side, there is a heavy emphasis on vegetables and complex carbohydrates. Changes in cooking techniques can improve fat, cholesterol, and sodium content, such as

- Using nonstick skillets sprayed with cooking spray when pan-frying eggs, fish, and vegetables
- Using small amounts of liquid smoke flavoring in place of bacon, salt pork, or ham
- Using more seasonings, such as onion, garlic, and pepper, in place of some of the salt
- Using turkey ham or turkey sausage in place of bacon
- Using "lite" or sugar-free syrups
- Using egg substitutes or egg whites in pancakes and biscuits

Mexican American Tradition
The traditional diet is primarily vegetarian with a heavy emphasis on fruits, vegetables, rice, and dried peas and beans. Processed foods are used infrequently.
Cooking techniques rely on frying and stewing with liberal amounts of oil or lard. An alternative is to sauté or stew with small amounts of canola or olive oil. High-fat meats and lard are commonly used. Using less meat, choosing lower fat, varieties, trimming visible fat, and substituting oil for lard are heart healthy alternatives.

Chinese American Tradition
Traditional Chinese cooking relies heavily on vegetables and rice with plants providing the majority of calories. Meat is used more as a condiment than an entrée. Cooking techniques tend to preserve nutrients. Sauces add little fat.
Sodium intake is high related to heavy use of soy sauce, MSG, and salted pickles. Reduced-sodium soy sauce is available, but it is still high in sodium. Because of the difficulty in eliminating the use of soy sauce, a more practical approach is to gradually use less.

Native American/Alaska Native Traditions
Widely diverse eating styles make useful generalizations difficult.
In general,

- Encourage traditional cooking methods such as baking, roasting, boiling, and broiling.
- Encourage the use of traditional meats, such as fish, deer, and caribou.
- Remove fat from canned meats.
- Use vegetable oil for frying instead of lard or shortening.

Jewish Tradition
Many traditional foods are high in sodium such as *kosher* meats (salt is used in the koshering process), herring, lox, pickles, canned chicken broth or soups, and delicatessen meats (e.g., corned beef, pickled tongue, pastrami).
Pareve (neutral) nondairy creamers are often used as a dairy substitute in meals containing meat, but they are high in fat. Encourage light and fat-free versions.
Encourage methods to lower fat in traditional recipes such as

- Baking instead of frying potato pancakes
- Limiting the amount of schmaltz (chicken fat) used in cooking
- Using reduced-fat or fat-free cream cheese on bagels
- Using low-fat or nonfat cottage cheese, sour cream, and yogurt in kugels and blintzes

Box 20.4   Tips for Eating a Heart Healthy Diet

- Use the Nutrition Facts panel on food products to comparison shop.
- Replace white enriched breads and cereals with whole grains, such as whole wheat, oats, barley, corn, popcorn, brown rice, wild rice, buckwheat, triticale, bulgur, millet, quinoa, and sorghum.
- Limit high-calorie bakery products—they usually contain white flour, added sugars, and hydrogenated fats.
- Eat a variety of fresh, frozen, and canned fruits and vegetables without added sugars, salt, or high-calorie sauces
- Eat occasional meatless meals that feature legumes, tofu, or vegetables.
- Use herbs and spices, lemon juice, and flavored vinegars to flavor vegetables and other foods without fat.
- Choose fat-free or low-fat milk and dairy products.
- Choose lean meats and poultry, and remove skin from poultry before eating.
- Eat oily fish, such as mackerel, salmon, herring, lake trout, tuna, and white fish, twice a week.
- Limit processed meats.
- Trim away visible fat from meats before cooking; drain ground beef after browning.
- Bake, broil, grill, or poach meat, poultry, or fish instead of frying.
- Skip high-fat sauces and gravies.
- Prepare foods from "scratch" instead of purchasing convenience foods and mixes, which tend to be high in saturated fat.
- Use liquid oils in place of solid fats.
- Make fat-free soup stock by preparing the stock a day ahead and refrigerating it overnight. The fat will harden and can be removed easily from the surface. Also use this method to make fat-free gravies thickened with cornstarch.
- Use these low-fat snack ideas: low-fat yogurt, fresh fruits and vegetables, dried fruit, unbuttered popcorn, unsalted pretzels, bread sticks, melba toast, frozen juice bars, and low-fat crackers.
- Avoid sugar-sweetened beverages.

sodium intake for HF is not known, the Heart Failure Society of America recommends that sodium be limited to between 2000 and 3000 mg/day for patients with the clinical syndrome of HF and to less than 2000 mg/day for people in moderate to severe HF (Lindenfeld et al., 2010) (Box 20.5).

Other diet modifications are made as appropriate, such as

- A fluid restriction of less than 2 L/day for patients with severe hyponatremia (serum sodium <130 mEq/L) and for all patients with fluid retention that is difficult to control despite high doses of diuretic medication and sodium restriction.
- Appropriate nutrition therapy counseling if comorbidities, such as diabetes, renal disease, or hyperlipidemia, are present.
- Protein fortification, because patients with HF have protein needs higher than normal (1.12 g/kg not the Recommended Dietary Allowance of 0.8 g/kg), even when they are not malnourished (Nutrition Care Manual, 2012). Patients who are malnourished require more.
- Small, frequent meals to limit gastric distention and pressure on the heart.
- Soft, easy-to-chew foods for patient with fatigue.

Box 20.5   2000-mg, SODIUM-RESTRICTED DIET

Although a 2000-mg sodium diet is considered "restricted," it is more than the Adequate Intake (AI) of 1500 mg, the level that may be optimal for preventing and treating hypertension. It is a restriction when compared to the typical American intake. Sometimes, sodium is more severely restricted (e.g., to 1000 mg), and diets that are severely restricted in sodium are unpalatable, extremely difficult to follow, and likely have inadequate concentrations of some nutrients. To promote compliance and allow greater flexibility, exchange lists featuring the sodium content of high- and low-sodium foods may be used.

General Guidelines

- Eliminate processed and prepared foods and beverages high in sodium; use fresh, frozen, and canned low-sodium products.
- Do not use salt in cooking or at the table.
- Read Nutrition Facts labels; most foods eaten should provide less than 300 mg sodium per serving. Foods that fall under these guidelines include the following:

Most breads; many ready-to-eat cereals, cooked cereals, pasta, rice, and other starches cooked without salt

Fresh and frozen vegetables; low-sodium or sodium-free canned vegetables and soups

Fresh and canned fruit

Low-fat and nonfat milk and yogurt; small amounts of low-fat natural cheese

Fresh and frozen meats; low-sodium canned tuna, dried peas and beans, eggs

Baked goods made without baking soda, angel food cake

Tub or liquid margarine; vegetable oils

Patient Teaching

Provide general information:

- Reducing sodium intake will help the body rid itself of excess fluid and help lower high blood pressure.
- Sodium appears in the diet in the form of salt and, to some degree, in almost all foods and beverages. Most unprocessed, unsalted foods are low in sodium; they account for approximately 12% of usual sodium intake.
- Approximately 77% of the sodium in a typical American diet comes from processed foods. Sodium-containing compounds are used extensively as preservatives (sodium propionate, sodium sulfite, and sodium benzoate), leavening agents (sodium bicarbonate, baking soda, and baking powder), and flavor enhancers (e.g., salt, monosodium glutamate [MSG]) and are found in foods that may not taste salty.
- Salt substitutes replace sodium with potassium or other minerals. "Low-sodium" salt substitutes are not sodium free and may contain half as much sodium as regular table salt. Use neither type without a physician's approval.
- The preference for salty taste eventually will decrease.
- When an occasional food containing more than 300 mg/serving is eaten, balance it out with low-sodium foods the rest of the day.
- Try to make low-sodium choices while dining out (see Box 20.2).

Teach the client food preparation techniques to minimize sodium intake:

- Prepare foods from "scratch" whenever possible.
- Experiment with sodium-free seasonings, such as herbs, spices, lemon juice, vinegar, and wine. Fresh ingredients are more flavorful than dried ones.
- Try a commercial "salt alternative" for sodium-free flavor enhancement.
- Consult a low-sodium cookbook.

Box 20.5   2000-mg, SODIUM-RESTRICTED DIET (continued)

Teach the client how to read labels:

- Salt, MSG, baking soda, and baking powder contain significant amounts of sodium. Other sodium compounds such as sodium nitrite, benzoate of soda, sodium saccharin, and sodium propionate add less sodium to the diet.
- "Sodium free," "low sodium," "very low sodium," and "reduced" or "less" sodium are reliable terms.
- A variety of low- and reduced-sodium products are available, such as bread and bread products, cereal, crackers, cakes, cookies, pastries, soups, bouillon, canned vegetables, tomato products, meats, entrées, processed meats, hard and soft cheeses, condiments, nuts and peanut butter, butter, margarine, salad dressings, and snack foods. The difference in flavor between some low-sodium products and their high-sodium counterparts is barely noticeable; others taste flat and may need to have herbs or spices added.

- Nutritional supplements for additional protein and calories for patients with weight loss or muscle wasting (cardiac cachexia).
- Potassium and thiamin supplements, as needed, to compensate for losses in patients on diuretics.

Malnutrition among patients with congestive heart failure, known as cardiac cachexia, may occur from decreased sensation of hunger, diet restrictions, fatigue, shortness of breath, nausea, or anxiety. Patients with cardiac cachexia need a high-calorie, high-protein, high-nutrient diet while maintaining a low-sodium diet. Caloric density and nutrient density are important to maximize intake. If enteral feedings are necessary, a concentrated formula is used to limit fluid intake.

Micronutrient deficiencies may occur from poor intake, inflammation, oxidative stress, and increased urinary losses secondary to drug therapy (McKeag, McKinley, Woodside, Harbinson, and McKeown, 2012). Although observational studies suggest a relationship between HF and altered micronutrient intake and status, research is limited, and more studies are needed to determine whether micronutrient supplements are appropriate.

NURSING PROCESS: *Heart Failure*

Mrs. Gigante is a 79-year-old widow admitted with moderate to severe HF, with a long-standing history of hypertension and one previous myocardial infarction. She lives alone. She relies heavily on convenience foods, such as canned and packaged soups, frozen dinners, canned pasta, and tuna fish sandwiches, because she is too tired to cook. She appears frail and has significant lower extremity edema.

Assessment

Medical–Psychosocial History	
	■ Medical history and comorbidities including diabetes, hypertension, myocardial infarction, alcohol abuse, and other CHD risk factors
	■ Use of medications that affect nutrition, such as diuretics, antihypertensives, antidiabetics, and lipid-lowering medications; adherence to prescribed drug therapy

(continues on page 558)

NURSING PROCESS: *Heart Failure* (continued)

	▪ Complaints including activity intolerance, fatigue, and shortness of breath
	▪ Behaviors suggesting restlessness, anxiety, or confusion
	▪ Psychosocial and economic issues, such as living situation, cooking facilities, financial status, education, and eligibility for the Meals on Wheels program
	▪ Understanding of the relationship between sodium, fluid accumulation, and symptoms of congestive heart failure
	▪ Motivation to change eating style
Anthropometric Assessment	▪ Height, weight; body mass index (BMI)
	▪ Recent weight history, especially rapid weight gain
Biochemical and Physical Assessment	▪ Blood pressure
	▪ Measure of edema
	▪ Laboratory values related to comorbidities, such as total cholesterol, LDL, HDL, and triglyceride levels
	▪ Serum osmolality, serum sodium, blood urea nitrogen (BUN)/creatinine ratio, and hematocrit
	▪ Intake and output
	▪ Lung sounds for crackles
	▪ Respirations for breathing effort
Dietary Assessment	▪ How many meals and snacks do you usually eat?
	▪ What is your usual 24-hour food intake like?
	▪ What cooking methods do you use to prepare your food?
	▪ How is your appetite?
	▪ Do you feel full quickly after you start to eat?
	▪ Have you ever been advised to follow a certain kind of diet in the past? If so, how did you change your eating habits?
	▪ Do you watch the kind of fats you eat?
	▪ Do you try to limit your intake of salt?
	▪ How many glasses of fluid do you drink in a day?
	▪ Do you have health impairments that impact your ability to shop, cook, or eat?
	▪ Do you have any cultural, religious, or ethnic influences on your food preferences or eating habits?
	▪ Do you take any vitamins, minerals, and nutritional supplements? If so, what are the reasons?
	▪ Do you use alcohol or caffeine?

Diagnosis

Possible Nursing Diagnoses	Excess fluid volume related to impaired excretion of sodium and water as evidenced by 3+ peripheral edema

NURSING PROCESS: *Heart Failure* (continued)

Planning	
Client Outcomes	The client will • Attain and maintain normal fluid balance • Consume a varied and nutritious diet with adequate calories to attain healthy body weight • Limit sodium intake • Explain how and why sodium is limited in her diet

Nursing Interventions	
Nutrition Therapy	• Provide a 2-g sodium diet as ordered • Provide five to six small meals to limit gastric distention and pressure on the heart • Monitor input and output for need for fluid restriction
Client Teaching	Instruct the client On the roles of sodium, fluid, and medication in managing HF On the availability of a Meals on Wheels–type program. Explain that Meals on Wheels can provide her with the appropriate diet after discharge to ensure that she gets the proper foods even on days when she feels short of breath or too tired to cook. (Notify the discharge planner that the client may be a candidate for Meals on Wheels.) On eating plan essentials, such as • Eliminating the use of salt in cooking and at the table • Using low-sodium canned foods when available • Avoiding other high-sodium foods • Limiting milk intake to 2 cups daily • Increasing intake of high-potassium foods • Avoiding alcohol • Adhering to fluid restriction if appropriate On behavioral matters, including the following: • How to read labels to identify and avoid foods that provide more than 300 mg sodium per serving • Trying for a gradual reduction in sodium intake, which may be easier to comply with than an abrupt withdrawal of sodium. Because the preference for salt gradually diminishes when intake is limited, following a low-sodium diet tends to get easier with time. • Timing meals and snacks to avoid shortness of breath and fatigue • Identifying physical activity goals, if applicable and appropriate

Evaluation	
Evaluate and Monitor	• Monitor weight daily for rapid weight gain • Monitor edema and other signs and symptoms of fluid retention • Assess tolerance to small meals • Determine need for additional diet counseling

HOW DO YOU RESPOND?

My doctor put me on a pill to lower my cholesterol. Do I still need to change what I eat now that my cholesterol level is normal? Cholesterol-lowering medications like Lipitor, Zocor, Mevacor, and Pravachol are not meant to be used in place of healthful eating and other lifestyle modifications. Although these drugs are very powerful, their effectiveness can be undermined by a "bad" diet. Urge clients to commit to lifestyle changes to give their medication the greatest chance of success.

I do everything right and still my LDL cholesterol is sky high. Why? People with a genetic form of hypercholesterolemia generally have an LDL of 190 mg/dL or higher. For them, diet will not effectively lower LDL to acceptable levels. Still, diet, exercise, and weight loss are important—maybe even more important than for other people—because of the potential beneficial effects on other risks, such as blood pressure and insulin sensitivity.

CASE STUDY

Matt is 34 years old. His BMI is 28 and has steadily increased over the last few years when he accepted a position with his company that requires frequent travel. It is hard for him to exercise, and he eats out often. He is a "steak and potatoes" kind of guy who wouldn't dream of eating lunch or dinner without meat as the centerpiece of the meal. At his most recent annual employee physical, Matt's total cholesterol level was 245 mg/dL, his HDL level was 50, fasting glucose level was 92, and his blood pressure was 154/85. His father died of a heart attack at age 49. Matt feels doomed by genetics and is resistant to going on medication because of the potential side effects. He is willing to try to change his diet and lifestyle but is skeptical that it will help.

- What risks does Matt have for heart disease?
- Knowing that he is willing to change his diet and lifestyle, what additional information would you ask of Matt before devising a teaching plan?
- What diet recommendations would you prioritize in helping Matt initiate a heart healthy diet? What suggestions could you offer him to help him meet these recommendations?
- How would you respond to Matt's skepticism that diet and lifestyle factors will probably not lower his risk of heart disease?

STUDY QUESTIONS

1. Which statement indicates the patient understands the instruction about a DASH-style diet?
   a. "The most important thing about a DASH diet is to eat less cholesterol. No egg yolks for me."
   b. "I need to eat more fruits, vegetables, and whole grains."
   c. "As long as I don't add salt to my food while cooking or at the table, I will be able to achieve a low-sodium diet."
   d. "I had given up sugar-sweetened soft drinks but now I am going to go back to drinking them because they are allowed on my diet."

2. The client asks if he can continue using butter on his DASH-style healthy diet. Which of the following would be the nurse's best response?
   a. "No, butter does not fit into a heart healthy diet."
   b. "Butter is not limited in a heart healthy diet because most people only use small amounts."
   c. "You can use small amounts of butter if you are willing to compromise on other foods, such as eating meatless meals occasionally."
   d. "You can use small amounts of butter if you give up meat entirely."

3. When developing a teaching plan for a client on a low-sodium diet, which of the following foods would the nurse advise the client to limit?
   a. Processed cheese
   b. Canned fruit
   c. Eggs
   d. Milk

4. The nurse knows that instructions for a healthy diet have been effective when the client expresses a need to eat more
   a. Oily fish and nuts
   b. Lean red and deli meats
   c. Diet soda and diet desserts
   d. Italian bread and cornflakes

5. Which of the following recommendations would be most appropriate to limit trans fats?
   a. Avoid red meats.
   b. Avoid egg yolks and shellfish.
   c. Avoid corn oil.
   d. Avoid commercially made baked goods and stick margarines.

6. A client asks how to alter a diet to lower high triglyceride levels. Which of the following is the nurse's best response?
   a. "Alcohol lowers triglycerides, but don't drink more than 2 drinks daily."
   b. "Lower your cholesterol intake by eliminating egg yolks and butter."
   c. "Eat less sodium by avoiding processed foods and don't salt your food at the table."
   d. "Eat more fish and substitute whole grains for refined grains."

7. The client understands that losing weight will help lower blood pressure. What does the client need to know about weight loss diets?
   a. For overall health and weight, it doesn't matter what kind of diet you choose.
   b. A very-low-carbohydrate diet is best because it promotes quick weight loss and is nutritionally adequate in all food components known to provide cardiometabolic benefits.
   c. The appropriate calorie level DASH diet can promote weight loss while providing adequate amounts of food components that have cardiometabolic benefits.
   d. Low-fat, low-calorie diets are the best for overweight cardiac clients because benefits are achieved from reducing all types of fat in the diet.

8. The number of 3½ oz servings of oily fish recommended is
   a. 2/month
   b. 1/week
   c. 2/week
   d. 3 to 4/week

KEY CONCEPTS

- The American Heart Association's metric for a healthy diet for "ideal" cardiovascular health is to achieve four to five of the following components within the context of a calorie-appropriate, DASH-style diet: 4.5 cups or more of fruits and vegetables daily; two 3½ oz servings of fish per week, preferably oily fish; three or more 1-oz equivalent servings of whole grains daily; less than 1500 mg sodium per day; and less than 36 oz/week of sugar-sweetened beverages. Secondary metrics are to consume four or more servings of nuts, legumes, and seeds per week; two or fewer servings of processed meats per week; and less than 7% of total calories from saturated fat.

- Dietary factors play a prominent role in blood pressure regulation. The DASH-sodium diet effectively lowers blood pressure and cholesterol levels. It is low in sodium; rich in fruits, vegetables, and whole grains; moderate in poultry, fish, and nuts; and limited in fat, red meat, and added sugar.

- The DASH diet is rich in potassium, a nutrient known to help control blood pressure. Other lifestyle factors that help control blood pressure include losing weight if overweight and using alcohol moderately, if at all.

- Atherosclerosis is a progressive disease that may begin in childhood or adolescence and continue for decades before symptoms develop. CHD is the most common atherosclerotic CVD and the leading cause of death in the United States.

- An atherogenic diet is a risk factor for CHD. Diet also impacts other risk factors for CHD, such as hypertension, diabetes, obesity, and hypercholesterolemia.

- Metabolic syndrome (MetS) is a risk factor for CVD and type 2 diabetes. Diagnosis is made when three of the following are present: hypertension, high triglycerides, low HDL cholesterol, abdominal obesity, and elevated fasting glucose.

- High triglycerides are a biomarker for CVD risk, not independently atherogenic. Nutrition interventions to lower triglycerides include weight loss, replacing refined grains with whole grains, eliminating trans fats, lowering saturated fat and fructose intake, and eating omega-3 fatty acids from fish. A Mediterranean-style diet is recommended.

- Focusing on eating patterns, not individual nutrients, may be more effective in achieving better health. Both the DASH diet and Mediterranean diet have been shown to lower the risk of CVD as well as improve other health risks.

- Traditionally, low-fat diets have been recommended for cardiac health. It now appears that the type of fat is more important than the total amount of fat. Particular types of fat may have a positive or negative impact on cardiac risks depending on their source. For instance, monounsaturated fats in red meats may have a negative effect, whereas monounsaturated fats from olive oil have a positive impact.

- Attaining and maintaining healthy weight reduces the risk of CVD, hypertension, diabetes, and heart failure.

- People who choose to drink alcohol should limit their intake to 2 drinks per day (males) or 1 drink per day (females). Alcohol has positive health benefits, such as raising HDL cholesterol and reducing platelet aggregation, but it also raises blood pressure and other health risks.

- With the exception of fish oil supplements, supplements have not been shown to reduce cardiac risks, and some may even increase risk.

- A 2000-mg, sodium-restricted diet is often used to manage heart failure (HF). It is not known whether a low-sodium diet can prevent HF in high-risk people. Fluid restriction may be necessary for patients with hyponatremia.

Check Your Knowledge Answer Key

1. **FALSE** While lowering sodium intake and losing weight are effective strategies for lowering blood pressure, the total diet is important. It is likely that multiple components of food interact synergistically to lower blood pressure.

2. **FALSE** The majority of sodium in the typical American diet comes from the sodium added during food processing.

3. **FALSE** The DASH diet is a food group approach that emphasizes fruits, vegetables, and whole grains; is moderate in fish, poultry, and nuts; and low in fat, red meat, and added sugars.

4. **TRUE** High triglyceride levels are a component of MetS but are not considered to be directly atherogenic. However, they are an important biomarker of CVD risk.

5. **FALSE** A traditional Mediterranean diet is not a low-fat diet, but it is low in animal fat, which means it is low in saturated fat and cholesterol. Its relatively high fat content, mostly in the form of monounsaturated fats, comes from olives and olive oil.

6. **TRUE** Foods with components that provide cardiometabolic benefits include dairy products and nuts as well as fruits, vegetables, whole grains, vegetable oils, fish, and legumes.

7. **FALSE** The cardiometabolic benefits of whole grains are not replicated by simply adding supplemental fiber or bran to the diet. It is likely that a combination of factors and their interactions are responsible for the health benefits obtained from eating whole grains.

8. **TRUE** Alcohol increases HDL cholesterol, lowers systemic inflammation, and reduces platelet aggregation. However, high intakes increase blood pressure and triglyceride levels and are associated with liver damage, physical abuse, and vehicular and work accidents.

9. **FALSE** All Americans, whether normotensive or hypertensive, are urged to lower their sodium intake to lower blood pressure.

10. **TRUE** A low-sodium diet for HF is based on expert consensus, not randomized study evidence. The theoretical basis is that lowering sodium lowers fluid retention; however, some studies suggest that lowering sodium actually worsens fluid retention.

Student Resources on thePoint

For additional learning materials, activate the code in the front of this book at
http://thePoint.lww.com/activate

Websites

American Heart Association at **www.americanheart.org**
Heart and Stroke Foundation of Canada at **www.hsf.ca**
Mediterranean Diet Pyramid at **www.oldways.org**
National Heart, Lung and Blood Institute at **www.nhlbi.nih.gov**; to estimate your risk of heart disease, go to **www.nhlbi.nih.gov/guidelines/cholesterol/index.htm** and click on 10-year risk calculator—online version

References

Alberti, K., Eckel, R., Grundy, S., Zimmet, P. Z., Cleeman, J. I., Donato, K. A., . . . Smith, S. C., Jr. (2009). Harmonizing the metabolic syndrome. *Circulation, 120,* 1640–1645.
Allen, N., Berry, J., Nihg, H., Van Horn, L., Dyer, A., & Lloyd-Jones, D. M. (2012). Impact of blood pressure and blood pressure change during middle age on the remaining lifetime risk for cardiovascular disease. The Cardiovascular Lifetime Risk Pooling Project. *Circulation, 125,* 37–44.

Appel, L. J., Brands, M. W., Daniels, S. R., Karanja, N., Elmer, P. J., & Sacks, F. M. (2006). Dietary approaches to prevent and treat hypertension. A scientific statement from the American Heart Association. *Hypertension, 47*, 296–308.

Appel, L., Moore, T., Obarzanek, E., Vollmer, W. M., Svetkey, L. P., Sacks, F. M., . . . Karanja N. (1997). A clinical trial of the effects of dietary patterns on blood pressure. *New England Journal of Medicine, 336*, 1117–1124.

Arcand, J., Ivanov, J., Sasson, A., Floras, V., Al-Hesayen, A., Azevedo, E. R., . . . Newton, G. E. (2011). A high-sodium diet is associated with acute decompensated heart failure in ambulatory heart failure patients: A prospective follow-up study. *American Journal of Clinical Nutrition, 93*, 332–337.

Azadbakht, L., Fard, N., Karimi, M., Baghaei, M. H., Surkan, P. J., Rahimi, M., . . . Willett, W. C. (2011). Effects of the Dietary Approaches to Stop Hypertension (DASH) eating plan on cardiovascular risks among type 2 diabetic patients. *Diabetes Care, 34*, 55–57.

Banel, D., & Hu, F. (2009). Effects of walnut consumption on blood lipids and other cardiovascular risk factors: A meta-analysis and systematic review. *American Journal of Clinical Nutrition, 90*, 56–63.

Brinkworth, G., Noakes, M., Buckley, J., Keogh, J., & Clifton, P. (2009). Long-term effects of a very-low-carbohydrate weight loss diet compared with an isocaloric low-fat diet after 12 months. *American Journal of Clinical Nutrition, 90*, 23–32.

Buckland, G., Bach, A., & Serra-Majem, L. (2008). Obesity and the Mediterranean diet: A systematic review of observational and intervention studies. *Obesity Reviews, 9*, 582–593.

Chen, J., Normand, S., Wang, Y., & Krumholz, H. (2011). National and regional trends in heart failure hospitalization and mortality rates for Medicare beneficiaries, 1998-2008. *Journal of the American Medical Association, 306*, 1669–1678.

Cogswell, M., Zhang, Z., Carriquiry, A., Gunn, J. P., Kuklina, E. V., Saydah, S. H., . . . Moshfegh, A. J. (2012). Sodium and potassium intakes among US adults: NHANES 2003-2008. *American Journal of Clinical Nutrition, 96*, 647–657.

Dehghan, M., Mente, A., Teo, K., Gao, P., Sleight, P., Dagenais, G., . . . Yusuf, S. (2012). Relationship between healthy diet and risk of cardiovascular disease among patients on drug therapies for secondary prevention. *Circulation, 126*, 2705–2712.

Expert Panel on Detection, Evaluation, and Treatment of High Blood Cholesterol in Adults (Adult Treatment Panel III). (2002). *Third report of the National Cholesterol Education Program (NCD)* (NIH Publication No. 02-5215). Bethesda, MD: National Heart, Lung, and Blood Institute.

Franco, O., Peeters, A., Bonneux, L., & de Laet, C. (2005). Blood pressure in adulthood and life expectancy with cardiovascular disease in men and women: Life course analysis. *Hypertension, 46*, 280–286.

Fung, T., Rexrode, K., Mantzoros, C., Manson, J. E., Willett, W. C., & Hu, F. B. (2009). Mediterranean diet and incidence of and mortality from coronary heart disease and stroke in women. *Circulation, 119*, 1093–1100.

Giugliano, D., & Esposito, K. (2008). Mediterranean diet and metabolic diseases. *Current Opinion in Lipidology, 19*, 63–68.

Grundy, S. (2008). Metabolic syndrome pandemic. *Arteriosclerosis, Thrombosis, and Vascular Biology, 28*, 629–636.

Hall, M., DeFrances, C., Williams, S., Golosinskiy, A., & Schwartzman, A. (2010). *National Hospital Discharge Survey: 2007 summary* (National Health Statistics Reports, No. 29). Hyattsville, MD, National Center for Health Statistics.

Hu, F. (2003). Plant-based foods and prevention of cardiovascular disease: *An overview. American Journal of Clinical Nutrition, 78*, 544S–551S.

Hunt, S. A., Abraham, W. T., Chin, M. H., Feldman, A., Francis, G., Ganiats, T., . . . Riegel, B. (2005). ACC/AHA 2005 Guidelines update for the diagnosis and management of chronic heart failure in the adult. *Circulation, 112*, 1825–1852.

Jakobsen, M., O'Reilly, E., Heitmann, B., Pereira, M. A., Bälter, K., Fraser, G. E., . . . Ascherio, A. (2009). Major types of dietary fat and risk of coronary heart disease: A pooled analysis of 11 cohort studies. *American Journal of Clinical Nutrition, 89*, 1425–1432.

Joint National Committee. (2004). *The seventh report of the joint national committee on prevention, detection, evaluation, and treatment of high blood pressure: Complete report* (NIH Publication No. 04-5230). Bethesda, MD: National Institutes of Health.

Kasai, T., Miyauchi, K., Kurata, T., Ohta, H., Okazaki, S., Miyazaki, T., . . . Daida, H. (2006). Prognostic value of the metabolic syndrome for long-term outcomes in patients undergoing percutaneous coronary intervention. *Circulation Journal, 70*, 1531–1537.

Kastorini, C., Milionis, H., Esposito, K., Giugliano, D., Goudevenos, J. A., & Panagiotakos, D. B. (2011). The effect of Mediterranean diet on metabolic syndrome and its components. *Journal of the American College of Cardiology, 57*, 1299–1313.

Kendall, C., Josse, A., Esfahani, A., & Jenkins, D. (2010). Nuts, metabolic syndrome and diabetes. *British Journal of Nutrition, 104*, 465–473.

Lichtenstein, A. H., Appel, L. J., Brands, M., Carnethon, M., Daniels, S., Franch, H. A., . . . Wylie-Rosett, J. (2006). Diet and lifestyle recommendations revision 2006. A scientific statement from the American Heart Association Nutrition Committee. *Circulation, 114*, 82–96.

Liese, A., Nichols, M., Sun, X., D'Agostino, R. B., Jr., & Haffner, S. M. (2009). Adherence to the DASH diet is inversely associated with incidence of type 2 diabetes: The insulin resistance atherosclerosis study. *Diabetes Care, 32*, 1434–1436.

Lindenfeld, J. J., Albert, N., Boehmer, J., Collins, S. P., Ezekowitz, J. A., Givertz, M. M., . . . Walsh, M. N. (2010). Executive summary: Heart Failure Society of America 2010 comprehensive heart failure practice guideline. *Journal of Cardiac Failure, 16*, 475–539.

Lloyd-Jones, D., Hong, Y., Labarthe, D., Mozaffarian, D., Appel, L. J., Van Horn, L., . . . Rosamond, W. D. (2010). Defining and setting national goals for cardiovascular health promotion and disease reduction: The American Heart Association's Strategic Impact Goal through 2020 and beyond. *Circulation, 121*, 586–613.

Maruthur, N., Wang, N., & Appel, L. (2009). Lifestyle interventions reduce coronary heart disease risk. Results from the PREMIER trial. *Circulation, 119*, 2026–2031.

McKeag, N., McKinley, M., Woodside, J., Harbinson, M. T., & McKeown, P. P. (2012). The role of micronutrients in heart failure. *Journal of the Academy of Nutrition and Dietetics, 112*, 870–886.

Mente, A., de Koning, L., Shannon, H., & Anand, S. (2009). A systematic review of the evidence supporting a causal link between dietary factors and coronary heart disease. *Archives of Internal Medicine, 169*, 659–669.

Merchant, A. T., Kelemen, L. E., de Koning, L., Lonn, E., Vuksan, V., Jacobs, R., . . . Anand, S. S. (2008). Interrelation of saturated fat, trans fat, alcohol intake, and subclinical atherosclerosis. *American Journal of Clinical Nutrition, 87*, 168–174.

Micha, R., & Mozaffarian, D. (2009). Trans fatty acids: Effect on metabolic syndrome, heart disease and diabetes. *Nature Reviews: Endocrinology, 5*, 335–344.

Miller, M., Stone, N., Ballantyne, C., Bittner, V., Criqui, M. H., Ginsberg, H. N., . . . Pennathur, S. (2011). Triglycerides and cardiovascular disease. A scientific statement from the American Heart Association. *Circulation, 123*, 2292–2333.

Mozaffarian, D. (2008). Fish and n-3 fatty acids for the prevention of fatal coronary heart disease and sudden cardiac death. *American Journal of Clinical Nutrition, 87*(Suppl.), 1991S–1996S.

Mozaffarian, D., Appel, L., & Van Horn, L. (2011). Components of a cardioprotective diet. New insights. *Circulation, 123*, 2870–2891.

Mozaffarian, D., Hao, T., Rimm, E., Willett, W. C., & Hu, F. B. (2011). Changes in diet and lifestyle and long-term weight gain in women and men. *New England Journal of Medicine, 364*, 2392–2404.

Mozaffarian, D., & Ludwig, D. (2010). Dietary guidelines in the 21st century: A time for food. *Journal of the American Medical Association, 304*, 681–682.

National Center for Health Statistics, Centers for Disease Control and Prevention. (2010). *Deaths, percent of total deaths, and death rates for the 15 leading causes of death: United States and each state, 2010.* Available at http://www.cdc.gov/nchs/data/dvs/LCWK9_2010.pdf. Accessed on 12/13/12.

National Heart Lung and Blood Institute. (2012). *What is heart failure?* Available at http://www.nhlbi.nih.gov/health/health-topics/topics/hf/. Accessed on 12/18/12.

Nutrition Care Manual. (2012). *Heart failure.* Nutrition prescription. Available at www.nutritioncaremanual.org. Accessed on 12/19/12.

Ogunniyi, M., Croft, J., Greenlund, K., Giles, W., & Mensah, G. (2010). Racial/ethnic differences in microalbuminuria among adults with prehypertension and hypertension. NHANES, 1999-2006. *American Journal of Hypertension, 23*, 859–864.

Paterna, S., Gaspare, P., Fasullo, S., Sarullo, F., & Di Pasquale, P. (2008). Normal-sodium diet compared with low-sodium diet in compensated congestive heart failure: Is sodium an old enemy or a new friend? *Clinical Science (London), 114*, 221–230.

Paterna, S., Parrinello, G., Cannizzaro, S., Fasullo, S., Torres, D., . . . Di Pasquale, P. (2008). Medium term effects of different dosage of diuretic, sodium, and fluid administration on neurohormonal and clinical outcome in patients with recently compensated heart failure. *American Journal of Cardiology, 103*, 93–102.

Roger, V., Go, A., Lloyd-Jones, D., Benjamin, E., Berry, J., Borden, W., . . . Turner, M. (2012). Heart disease and stroke statistics—2012 update: A report from the American Heart Association. *Circulation, 125,* e2–e220.

Sacks, F., Svetkey, L., Vollmer, W., Appel, L. J., Bray, G. A., Harsha, D., . . . Lin., P. H. (2001). Effects on blood pressure of reduced dietary sodium and the Dietary Approaches to Stop Hypertension (DASH) diet. *New England Journal of Medicine, 344,* 3–10.

Sesso, H., Christen, W., Bubes, V., Smith, J. P., MacFadyen, J., Schvartz, M., . . . Gaziano, J. M. (2012). Multivitamins in the prevention of cardiovascular disease in med. The Physicians' Health Study II randomized controlled trial. *Journal of the American Medical Association, 308,* 1751–1760.

Shai, I., Spence, J., Schwarzfuchs, D., Henkin, Y., Parraga, G., Rudich, A., . . . Stampfer, M. J. (2010). Dietary intervention to reverse carotid atherosclerosis. *Circulation, 121,* 1200–1208.

Sofi, F., Abbate, R., Gensini, D., & Casini, A. (2010). Accruing evidence about benefits of adherence to the Mediterranean diet on health: An updated systematic review and meta-analysis. *American Journal of Clinical Nutrition, 92,* 1189–1196.

Stevens, V. J., Obarzanek, E., Cook, N. R., Lee, I., Appel, L., West, D., . . . Cohen, J. (2001). Long-term weight loss and changes in blood pressure: Results of the Trials of Hypertension Prevention, phase II. *Annals of Internal Medicine, 134,* 1–11.

U.S. Department of Agriculture, U.S. Department of Health and Human Services. (2010). *Dietary guidelines for Americans, 2010* (7th ed.). Available at www.health.gov/dietaryguidelines. Accessed 12/12/12.

U.S. Department of Health and Human Services, National Institutes of Health, National Heart, Lung, and Blood Institute. (2006). *Your guide to lowering your blood pressure with DASH* (NIH Publication No. 06-4082). Available at http://www.nhlbi.nih.gov/health/public/heart/hbp/dash/new_dash.pdf. Accessed on 7/16/08.

von Haehling, S., Doehner, W., & Anker, S. (2007). Nutrition metabolism, and the complex pathophysiology of cachexia in chronic heart failure. *Cardiovascular Research, 73,* 298–309.

Whelton, P., Appel, L., Sacco, R., Anderson, C. A., Antman, E. M., Campbell, N., . . . Van Horn, L. V. (2012). Sodium, blood pressure, and cardiovascular disease. Further evidence supporting the American Heart Association sodium reduction recommendations. *Circulation, 126,* 2880–2889.

Xin, X., He, J., Frontini, M. G., Ogden, L. G., Motsamai, O. I., & Whelton, P. K. (2001). Effects of alcohol reduction on blood pressure: A meta-analysis of randomized controlled trials. *Hypertension, 38,* 1112–1117.

Yoon, S., Burt, V., Louis, T., & Carroll, M. (2012). *Hypertension among adults in the United States, 2009-1020* (NCHS Data Brief, No. 107). Hyattsville, MD: National Center for Health Statistics.

21 Nutrition for Patients with Kidney Disorders

CHECK YOUR KNOWLEDGE

TRUE   FALSE

☐ ☐ **1** Early in the course of chronic kidney disease, limiting protein may help to preserve kidney function.

☐ ☐ **2** Foods high in protein tend to be high in phosphorus.

☐ ☐ **3** Milk is the best source of protein for people with chronic kidney disease.

☐ ☐ **4** All people with chronic kidney disease need to limit their potassium intake.

☐ ☐ **5** People with chronic renal disease tend to have accelerated atherosclerosis and may benefit from eating a heart healthy diet.

☐ ☐ **6** Dialysis causes protein requirements to increase about 50% above normal.

☐ ☐ **7** People receiving peritoneal dialysis absorb calories from the dialysate.

☐ ☐ **8** People who have gained more than 2 pounds between dialysis treatments have eaten too many calories.

☐ ☐ **9** People with calcium oxalate renal stones should avoid calcium.

☐ ☐ **10** Increasing fluid intake can effectively prevent kidney stones from forming, eliminating the need for any other nutrition or medical interventions.

LEARNING OBJECTIVES

Upon completion of this chapter, you will be able to

1 Explain nutrition therapy recommendations for nephrotic syndrome.

2 Describe the impact chronic kidney disease (CKD) has on nutritional status and requirements.

3 Compare nutrient recommendations for CKD to the Dietary Reference Intake (DRI) for healthy people.

4 Develop a teaching plan to help a client with CKD adhere to nutrient recommendations.

5 Compare nutrient recommendations for predialysis to those for patients on dialysis.

6 Compare nutrient recommendations for dialysis to those for posttransplant patients.

7 Describe the challenges in providing adequate nutrition to people with acute kidney injury.

8 Teach nutrition therapy recommendations to a client with a history of calcium oxalate kidney stones.

Nitrogenous Wastes: wastes produced from nitrogen—namely, ammonia, urea, uric acid, and creatinine.

Renin: an enzyme secreted by the kidneys that activates the precursor of angiotensin, a hormone involved in blood pressure regulation.

Erythropoietin: a hormone secreted by the kidneys that stimulates the bone marrow to produce red blood cells.

The kidneys perform many vital functions. They maintain normal blood volume and composition by reabsorbing needed nutrients and excreting wastes through urine; urinary excretion is the primary method by which the body rids itself of excess water, **nitrogenous wastes**, electrolytes, sulfates, organic acids, toxic substances, and drugs. The kidneys help to regulate acid–base balance by secreting hydrogen ions to increase pH and excreting bicarbonate to lower pH. The kidneys are involved in blood pressure regulation through the action of **renin** and in red blood cell production through the action of **erythropoietin**. Because vitamin D is converted to its active form in the kidneys, it has an important role in maintaining normal metabolism of calcium and phosphorus.

Kidney diseases can have a profound impact on metabolism, nutritional status, and nutritional requirements. In 2010, kidney diseases (nephritis, nephrotic syndrome, and nephrosis) were the eighth leading cause of death in the United States (Murphy, Xu, and Kochanek, 2012). This chapter presents nutrition therapy for nephrotic syndrome, chronic kidney disease (CKD), acute kidney injury (AKI), and urolithiasis.

NEPHROTIC SYNDROME

Nephrotic Syndrome: a collection of symptoms that occurs when increased capillary permeability in the glomeruli allows serum proteins to leak into the urine.

Proteinuria: protein in the urine; also known as albuminuria.

Hypoalbuminemia: low blood levels of albumin, the most abundant plasma protein.

Hyperlipidemia: abnormally high level of lipids in the blood, such as LDL cholesterol and triglycerides.

High Biologic Value (HBV): refers to protein sources that contain all the essential amino acids in relatively the same proportions as needed by humans to support growth and health. They also contain nonessential amino acids.

Nephrotic syndrome is a generic term that refers to a kidney disorder characterized by urinary protein losses greater than 3.5 g/day. **Proteinuria, hypoalbuminemia, hyperlipidemia,** and edema are major symptoms. Increased urinary losses of proteins such as albumin, transferrin, immunoglobulins, vitamin D–binding protein, and anti–blood clotting proteins may lead to protein–calorie malnutrition, anemia, increased risk of infection, vitamin D deficiency, and increased clotting, respectively. Hyperlipidemia increases the risk of cardiovascular disease and progressive renal damage.

Causes of nephrotic syndrome include diabetes, autoimmune diseases (e.g., lupus, IgA nephropathy), infection, and certain chemicals and medications. In some cases, treating the underlying disorder corrects nephrotic syndrome. In others, especially diabetes, nephrotic syndrome may be the beginning of CKD.

Nutrition Therapy

The main goal of nutrition therapy is to reduce proteinuria to prevent complications, protect kidney function, reduce the risk of atherosclerosis, and maintain good nutritional status (Kalista-Richards, 2011).

Although nephrotic syndrome is characterized by increased urinary losses of albumin and other proteins, a high-protein diet is contraindicated because it exacerbates urinary protein losses, promoting further kidney damage. A protein intake of 0.7 to 0.8 g/kg/day is suggested with at least half of the protein from **high biologic value (HBV)** sources, such as meat, fish, poultry, milk, eggs, and soy (Kalista-Richards, 2011). Soy protein may be better than other HBV protein sources at decreasing proteinuria and lipid levels (Velasquez and Bhathena, 2001). To spare protein and maintain weight, calorie intake should be increased to approximately 35 cal/kg/day. Other nutrition therapy recommendations for nephrotic syndrome are featured in Table 21.1.

CHRONIC KIDNEY DISEASE

Chronic kidney disease (CKD) is characterized by a gradual decline in renal function related to progressive irreversible nephron damage. Early in the course of CKD, functioning nephrons enlarge to compensate for those that have been destroyed. Patients

Table 21.1   Nutrition Therapy for Nephrotic Syndrome

Dietary Component	Recommendation	Rationale
Protein	0.7–0.8 g/kg/day; soy protein may be more beneficial than animal proteins	To minimize proteinuria; soy protein may decrease proteinuria and blood lipid levels more than beef and pork
Calories	35 cal/kg	To maintain weight and spare protein A lower calorie intake to promote weight loss is recommended if blood pressure or hyperlipidemia is a problem.
Sodium	2–3 g	To help control edema; fluid restriction is generally not necessary
Fat and cholesterol	<30% of calories from total fat, low–saturated fat, low cholesterol, and low trans fats 12 g of fish oil per day may be useful for IgA nephropathy	To improve hyperlipidemia
Vitamins and minerals	Dietary Reference Intake (DRI) amounts unless otherwise indicated	A multiple vitamin may be used to prevent nutrient deficiencies because many vitamins are bound to protein and are lost through proteinuria. Vitamin D and calcium are given if vitamin D is deficient. Iron and zinc are given if deficient.

Source: American Academy of Nutrition and Dietetics. (2012). *Nutrition care manual.* Available at www.nutritioncaremanual.org. Accessed on 6/27/2012; and Kalista-Richards, M. (2011). The kidney: Medical nutrition therapy—Yesterday and today. *Nutrition in Clinical Practice, 26,* 143–150.

Chronic Kidney Disease (CKD): a decrease in kidney function defined as an estimated glomerular filtration rate <60 mL/min/1.73 m^2 and/or evidence of kidney damage, including persistent albuminuria, defined as >30 mg of urine albumin per gram of urine creatinine.

Glomerular Filtration Rate (GFR): the rate at which the kidneys form filtrate estimated from the amount of creatinine excreted per 24 hours. Normal GFR is about 120 to 130 mL/min.

Estimated Glomerular Filtration Rate (eGFR): determined through an equation that takes into account serum creatinine level, age, gender, and race.

Urine Albumin-to-Creatinine Ratio (UACR): an estimate of 24-hour urinary albumin excretion.

are asymptomatic, and urine volume may be normal despite the decrease in **glomerular filtration rate (GFR)**. Nephron destruction may go on for months or years before CKD is diagnosed. When CKD progresses to kidney failure, also known as end-stage renal disease (ESRD), dialysis or kidney transplantation is necessary for survival. **Estimated glomerular filtration rate (eGFR)** and **urine albumin-to-creatinine ratio (UACR)** are used to diagnose and monitor CKD (Table 21.2).

Diabetes and hypertension are the leading causes of CKD, accounting for approximately 70% of new cases in the United States in 2006 (Centers for Disease Control and Prevention [CDC], 2010). Diabetic kidney disease (DKD), formerly known as diabetic nephropathy, refers to CKD believed to arise from diabetes. Other risk factors for CKD include cardiovascular disease, obesity, hypercholesterolemia, and a family history of CKD (CDC, 2010) as well as recurrent urinary tract infections, HIV infection, and immunologic diseases (National Kidney Disease Education Program [NKDEP], 2011). Compared with whites, African Americans, Native Americans, and Hispanics are at increased risk for CKD.

Symptoms and Complications of CKD

In the early stages of CKD, patients may experience anorexia, fatigue, headache, hypertension, nausea, vomiting, proteinuria, and hematuria. Electrolyte balance is maintained as functioning nephrons work harder to compensate for those destroyed. Likewise, hormonal

Table 21.2   Criteria for Diagnosing and Monitoring Kidney Function

Criteria	Significance	Values	Assessment
Estimated glomerular filtration rate (eGFR): estimated from an equation that uses creatinine, age, gender, and race	Measures filtration rate of the functioning nephrons Declining values increase the likelihood and severity of complications.	**Measured in mL/ min/1.73 m^2** Normal young adult, 120–130; decreases with aging CKD, 15–59 Kidney failure, <15	Monitored to determine effectiveness of nutrition therapy Stable values may indicate therapy is effective; declining values signal a deterioration of kidney function
Urine albumin-to-creatinine ratio: an estimate of 24-hour urine albumin excretion	Albuminuria usually signals nephron damage. Albuminuria is an independent risk factor for CKD progression and is a marker for cardiovascular disease mortality in hypertension.	**Measured in mg/g** Normal, 0–30 Albuminuria, >30	Change in albuminuria may reflect effectiveness of therapy and risk of progression. A decrease in albuminuria may be associated with improved renal and cardiovascular risks.

Source: National Kidney Disease Education Program. (2011). *Chronic kidney disease and diet: Assessment, management, and treatment. Treating CKD patients who are not on dialysis* (NIH Publication No. 11-7406). Washington, DC: USDHHS, NIDDK, NKDEP.

changes occur to offset metabolic alterations but may increase the risk of other complications. For instance, aldosterone secretion increases to prevent hyperkalemia but may lead to hypertension. Parathyroid hormone secretion increases to help prevent hyperphosphatemia but promotes bone loss and the risk of renal osteodystrophy. Eventually, electrolyte imbalances develop when eGFR is extremely low, when hormones fail to compensate for metabolic alterations, or when the intake of fluid and electrolytes is either too high or too low.

As kidney disease progresses, the likelihood and severity of metabolic complications increase. Complications are interrelated and multifactorial, and the disruption to homeostasis is profound. For instance, malnutrition and protein–energy wasting may occur from poor intake related to dietary restrictions, anorexia, alterations in taste, nausea, vomiting, stomatitis, depression, or anxiety. Nutrient deficiencies may also occur from impaired gastrointestinal (GI) absorption or from increased urinary excretion. Malnutrition has far-reaching effects, such as impairments in immunity, wound healing, and GI function. Other complications include

Uremic Syndrome: a cluster of symptoms related to the retention of nitrogenous substances in the blood such as uremia, anemia, bone disease, hormonal imbalances, bleeding impairment, impaired immunity, fatigue, decreased mental acuity, muscle twitches, cramps, anorexia, unpleasant nausea, vomiting, diarrhea, itchy skin, and gastritis.

Active Form of Vitamin D: 1,25-dihydroxycholecalciferol.

- Fluid retention as evidenced by increased blood pressure, weight gain, edema, shortness of breath, and lung crackles
- **Uremic syndrome** related to the retention of nitrogenous wastes
- Metabolic acidosis because the kidneys are unable to excrete hydrogen ions produced through normal metabolic processes
- Anemia related to impaired synthesis of erythropoietin; GI absorption of iron is also impaired, and iron intake may be inadequate.
- Renal osteodystrophy related to impaired synthesis of the **active form of vitamin D,** increased secretion of parathyroid hormone, and acidosis
- Impaired synthesis of renin contributes to hypertension.

- Metabolism is altered from impaired inactivation of certain peptide hormones, such as insulin, parathyroid hormone, and glucagon.
- Accelerated atherosclerosis increases the risk of coronary heart disease, myocardial infarction, and further renal damage.

Predialysis Nutrition Therapy

The goals of nutrition therapy are to

- Slow the progression of CKD
- Treat complications

The interventions needed to meet these objectives vary among individuals and according to the nature and stage of the disease. Table 21.3 highlights predialysis nutrition therapy recommendations including selection details.

To slow the progression of CKD, sodium is restricted to control blood pressure and excessive protein intake is avoided to limit proteinuria. A heart-healthy diet is recommended to decrease the risk of cardiovascular disease. Good glucose control in people newly diagnosed with diabetes may slow the progression of CKD (NKDEP, 2011).

As renal function deteriorates, diet modifications are made in response to symptoms and laboratory values and require frequent monitoring and adjustment. Eventually, alterations in the intake of protein, calories, potassium, phosphorus, calcium, and other vitamins and minerals are necessary and add to the complexity of the diet.

Protein

Traditionally, protein was restricted to 0.6 to 0.75 g/kg/day or less, supported by results from the Modification of Diet in Renal Disease (MDRD) study that showed that tight control of blood pressure and a restricted protein intake of 0.3 to 0.6 g/kg/day helped delay the progression of kidney disease (Levey et al., 1996). However low-protein diets are difficult to implement, and compliance is poor. Kopple (2008) states that in his experience, only approximately 15% of CKD patients are able to follow a low-protein diet comfortably. Severe protein-restricted diets also increase the risk that not enough protein is consumed to meet protein requirements, which can result in increases in body protein catabolism, serum creatinine levels, and the risk of protein malnutrition.

Although the optimal level of protein intake for people with CKD is not known, it is agreed that excessive protein intakes should be avoided to decrease proteinuria and further decline in kidney function. Currently the recommended protein intake for people with nondiabetic CKD is 0.8 g/kg/day, which is the Recommended Dietary Allowance (RDA) for protein (NKDEP, 2011). The Kidney Disease Outcomes Quality Initiative (KDOQI) guidelines are slightly more restrictive at 0.75 g/kg when eGFR is ≥30 and 0.6 g/kg with 50% as HBV when eGFR is <25 (National Kidney Foundation, 2002). HBV proteins are emphasized because they provide a higher percentage of essential amino acids, which may promote reuse of circulating nonessential amino acids for protein synthesis, and by doing so minimizes urea production.

While clinical studies show that a low-protein diet is potentially beneficial for patients with nondiabetic renal disease, a meta-analysis of randomized controlled trials showed that a low-protein diet was not associated with

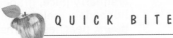

QUICK BITE

Sources of HBV protein
  Eggs
  Meat, fish, poultry
  Milk, yogurt, cheese
  Soy

Table 21.3 Predialysis Nutrition Therapy Recommendations

Nutrient/Rationale	Nutrition Intervention	Selection Details
Recommendations for all people with CKD		
Protein: limiting protein may reduce albuminuria and improve blood glucose control, hyperlipidemia, blood pressure, renal bone disease, and metabolic acidosis (de Zeeuw et al., 2004)	Avoid excessive protein intake. Diabetic: 0.8–1.0 g/kg/day Nondiabetic: 0.8 g/kg/day In nondiabetic patients, 0.6 g/kg/day may be even more beneficial but is difficult to achieve. Avoiding excessive protein also reduces intake of phosphorus and potassium.	Keep meat, fish, and poultry servings to 2–3 oz and milk and yogurt to ½ cup. Spread sources of protein over the day. Choose more animal sources of protein (meat, fish, poultry, milk, yogurt) and less plant sources (beans, nuts, grains).
Sodium: limiting sodium helps control blood pressure to slow the progression of CKD and may lower cardiovascular disease (CVD) risk	Limit to 1500 mg/day.	Choose fresh or plain frozen vegetables over canned and fresh meat over processed meat. Avoid convenience items such as canned or dried soups, bottled salad dressings, and frozen dinners. Use herbs and spices as alternatives to salt to season food. Read Nutrition Facts labels and compare brands to choose lower sodium items.
Heart healthy: to lower CVD risks	Limit saturated fat, cholesterol, and trans fat.	Cook with nonstick spray or olive oil instead of butter. Grill, bake, roast, or broil meats instead of cooking with added fat. Trim visible fat from meat and remove poultry skin before eating. Buy lean cuts of meat and drain fat when possible.
Additional restrictions that may be necessary as CKD progresses		
Potassium	Limit potassium when serum value is >5 mEq/L.	Unlike sodium, potassium cannot be tasted and rarely appears on the Nutrition Facts label, making it difficult to comply with a potassium-restricted eating plan. Protein foods (meat, fish, poultry, beans, dairy, nuts) provide potassium. Choose refined grains over whole grains, such as white bread, pasta, cereals, and rice instead of whole wheat bread, whole-grain cereal, whole wheat pasta, and brown rice. The potassium content of fruits and vegetables varies. Choose Fruit: apples, canned apricots, berries, cranberry juice, grapes, grapefruit, honeydew melon, mangoes, papayas, pears, peaches, plums, pineapple, tangerines, and watermelon Vegetables: bell peppers, canned bamboo shoots, fresh broccoli, cabbage, carrots, cauliflower, raw celery, raw onions, corn, cucumber, eggplant, green beans, kale, lettuce, fresh mushrooms, okra, cooked summer squash

Table 21.3 Predialysis Nutrition Therapy Recommendations (continued)

Nutrient/Rationale	Nutrition Intervention	Selection Details

		Avoid
		   Fruit: fresh apricots, bananas, cantaloupe, dates, nectarines, kiwi, prunes, prune juice, oranges, orange juice, raisins
		   Vegetables: winter squash, avocado, baked beans, beet and other greens, cooked broccoli, cooked Brussels sprouts, chard, chili peppers, cooked mushrooms, potatoes, pumpkin, cooked spinach, split peas, lentils, legumes, sweet potatoes, yams, vegetable juice, tomatoes, tomato products
		The potassium content of most vegetables can be leached by soaking sliced vegetables in water overnight, draining the water, and then boiling them in fresh water.
		Drain canned fruit and vegetables before eating.
		Avoid salt substitutes that contain potassium.
		Limit foods that contain potassium chloride on the ingredient list; it may be used in place of salt in some packaged foods.
		For people with diabetes, use apple, grape, or cranberry juice instead of orange juice for hypoglycemia.

Phosphorus	Restriction may not be necessary until CKD is advanced; optimal allowance is not known.	Phosphorus intake is decreased when protein (meat, fish, poultry, dairy, legumes, nuts) intake is restricted. To lower intake even more, limit foods with phosphorus additives (e.g., "phos" identified on the ingredient list). Avoiding whole grains also lowers phosphorus intake. Beverages packaged in glass usually do not contain phosphate additives, but the same product packaged in plastic does (Gutekunst, 2010). The Nutrition Facts label does not include information on phosphorus content, so identifying high-phosphorus items can be difficult; some, but not all, companies post nutrition information that includes phosphorus content on their websites.

Source: National Kidney Disease Education Program. (2011). *Chronic kidney disease and diet: Assessment, management, and treatment. Treating CKD patients who are not on dialysis* (NIH Publication No. 11-7406). Washington, DC: USDHHS, NIDDK, NKDEP.

significant improvement in renal function in patients with either type 1 or type 2 diabetes (Pan, Guo, and Jin, 2008). Thus, one notable difference between guidelines for diabetic kidney disease and nondiabetic guidelines is that protein allowance is slightly higher at 0.8 to 1.0 g/kg/day based on studies that show this level of protein stabilizes or reduces albuminuria, slows the deterioration of GFR, and may possibly prevent kidney failure (Burrowes, 2008). Also, when protein decreases, the amount of carbohydrate and/or fat increases, which may not be ideal for diabetic control or managing the risk of heart disease, respectively.

Calories

Whenever protein intake is marginal or restricted, it is vital that calorie intake is adequate so that protein can be used for protein synthesis instead of as an energy source. The KDOQI nutrition guidelines recommend 35 cal/kg/day for people younger than 60 years and 30 to 35 cal/kg/day for people 60 years and older, with an individual's weight status and needs considered (National Kidney Foundation, 2002). Clients may be advised to increase their intake of pure sugars (e.g., Fruit Roll-Ups, jelly beans, marshmallows, honey, jam, cotton candy) and pure fats (e.g., butter, margarine, mayonnaise, oils) to meet their calorie requirements while keeping protein intake low, even though they are not considered "nutritious." In this population in whom diabetes and hyperlipidemia are common, an increased intake of pure sugars and pure fats is seemingly contraindicated. The best protein-free calorie option is to choose foods rich in monounsaturated fats such as canola oil, olive oil, and trans fat–free margarines.

Sodium

Hypertension increases the risk of CKD; CKD causes hypertension. In clinical trials and epidemiologic studies, limiting sodium in people with hypertension has been shown to improve blood pressure control (NKDEP, 2011). To decrease the risk of CKD or slow its progression, it is recommended that sodium intake be limited to 1500 mg/day (NKDEP, 2011). This recommendation is consistent with the *Dietary Guidelines for Americans, 2010*, which suggest that people with CKD, hypertension, or diabetes limit sodium intake to 1500 mg/day. This represents a significant decrease in intake from the mean intake of 3330 mg/day among Americans aged 2 years and older (U.S. Department of Agriculture, Agricultural Research Service, 2010). Weight loss, if overweight, is also recommended to lower blood pressure.

Potassium

Normally, potassium consumed in excess of need is excreted in the urine. With loss of kidney function, potassium excretion is impaired, and hyperkalemia is a risk. Other factors that contribute to the risk of hyperkalemia include acidosis, catabolism, and the use of angiotensin-converting enzyme inhibitors (ACEIs) or angiotensin receptor blockers (ARBs) to control blood pressure. For all CKD stages, potassium allowance is based on the individual's serum potassium levels.

Phosphorus and Calcium

As kidney function deteriorates, the conversion of vitamin D to its active form is impaired, leading to alterations in the metabolism of calcium, phosphorus, and magnesium. Likewise, CKD progression leads to a gradual decline in phosphorus excretion, resulting in hyperphosphatemia, bone demineralization, and bone pain. Hyperphosphatemia, hypocalcemia, and low levels of active vitamin D stimulate parathyroid hormone (PTH) secretion, creating secondary hyperparathyroidism that further aggravates loss of bone mass and increases the risk that damaging deposits of calcium and phosphorus will form in the kidneys and other soft tissues such as the eyes, skin, heart, lungs, and blood vessels. Hyperphosphatemia increases the risk of death in both the general population and in people with CKD and may worsen the rate of CKD progression (Kovesdy and Kalantar-Zadeh, 2007). Correcting and preventing hyperphosphatemia is a major component of CKD management (Shinaberger et al., 2008).

Intake allowances are based on serum values; however, recommended levels of intake have not been established for either phosphorus or calcium (NKDEP, 2011). A low-phosphorus intake is relatively easy to achieve because phosphorus and protein share similar dietary sources, and protein intake is controlled. An adequate calcium intake can be difficult to achieve because restricted protein and phosphorus intakes only allow dairy products in limited amounts (e.g., ½ cup milk/day). Table 21.4 features the calcium, phosphorus, and protein content of selected foods. Secondary hyperparathyroidism is treated with a low-phosphorus diet, active vitamin D, and supplemental calcium.

Table 21.4 Calcium, Phosphorus, and Protein Content of Selected Foods

Item	Amount	Calcium (mg)	Phosphorus (mg)	Protein (g)
Grains				
White bread	1 slice	27	24	2
Whole wheat bread	1 slice	20	64	3
Long-grain rice	½ cup	10	81	3
Corn tortilla	1 med	44	79	1
Vegetables				
Artichoke, boiled	1 med	135	258	3
Kale, frozen, boiled	½ cup	90	18	2
Spinach, boiled	½ cup	122	50	3
Turnip greens, boiled	½ cup	99	21	1
Fruits				
Orange juice, calcium fortified	¾ cup	200	25	0
Avocado, raw	1 med	13	45	2
Dairy				
Skim	1 cup	302	247	8
2%	1 cup	297	232	8
Chocolate milk (with 1% milk)	1 cup	287	256	8
Low-fat fruit-flavored yogurt	1 cup	314	247	8
Cheddar cheese	1 oz	214	145	7
Meat and Beans				
Ground beef, broiled	3½ oz	12	191	27
Ham, cured, roasted	3½ oz	6	224	19
Chicken breast, roasted	½	13	196	27
Salmon, Chinook	3 oz	24	316	22
Refried beans, canned	½ cup	45	109	7
Great northern beans, canned	½ cup	70	178	7
Egg, poached	1	25	89	6
Almonds, blanched	1 oz	73	150	6
Peanut butter	2 tbsp	13	101	7
Sunflower seeds, dry roasted	1 oz	20	327	6

Vitamins and Minerals

There is little certainty about the vitamin needs of people with CKD (Steiber and Kopple, 2011). It is unclear whether vitamin metabolism is altered when GFR is >15 mL/min/1.73 m². What is known is that

- Vitamin intake may be inadequate secondary to anorexia or dietary restrictions. For instance, restrictions in potassium or phosphorus intake may limit foods high in water-soluble vitamins. Data from the Modification of Diet in Renal Disease study show that daily nutrient intake begins to decline when GFR is <60 mL/min/1.73 m² (Weiner et al., 2008).
- Certain medications may interfere with vitamin metabolism, particularly of vitamin B$_6$, folate, and possibly riboflavin.
- Vitamin deficiencies are common in people with advanced kidney disease who do not take supplements (Steiber and Kopple, 2011).

First and foremost, adequate calories and protein are recommended so that food sources of micronutrients are consumed. Specially formulated vitamin supplements are available with altered levels of certain vitamins for people with CKD because routine multivitamin preparations may provide too much of some vitamins (e.g., vitamin A) and too little of others (e.g., folic acid). In general (NKDEP, 2011),

- Supplements of riboflavin and vitamin B$_{12}$ may be necessary in patients on a low-protein diet (0.6 g/kg/day) because protein foods are sources of both of these vitamins.
- Medication/vitamin interactions may necessitate supplements of vitamin B$_6$.
- Supplements of thiamin and folic acid may be warranted.
- High doses of vitamin C (e.g., >30–60 mg/day) should not be taken.
- Data do not support routine supplementation with niacin and vitamins A, E, and K.
- The need for vitamin D is determined on an individual basis.
- Clients who are undergoing dialysis may develop a deficiency of zinc, which could contribute to anorexia and taste alterations. Supplements are recommended if a zinc deficiency is identified.
- Iron supplementation and erythropoietin are used to treat anemia of CKD. The risks and benefits of these treatments in CKD are not yet defined (Besarab and Coyne, 2010).

Nutrition Therapy During Dialysis

Diet for ESRD is complex and dynamic. The nutrient recommendations are used as a guideline in determining a patient's actual needs based on individual assessment. Protein, sodium, potassium, phosphorus, calcium, and fluid are all nutrients of concern (Table 21.5).

The protein allowance for patients treated with dialysis is 50% higher than the RDA to account for the loss of serum proteins and amino acids in the **dialysate**. Achieving this level of intake within the confines of other restrictions, especially phosphorus restriction, is difficult. Box 21.1 illustrates a menu at two different protein levels.

Calorie recommendations are 35 cal/kg for adults under 60 years of age and 30 to 35 cal/kg for those who are older. People who undergo peritoneal dialysis absorb a large amount of calories daily through the dialysate (approximately 340–680 cal/day), which needs to be considered. Calories from the dialysate impair the natural sense of hunger and generally prevent a fall in blood glucose levels between meals. Although they may look well fed, patients may actually have protein malnutrition (Beto and Bansal, 2004).

Dialysate: the dialysis solution used to extract wastes and fluid from the blood.

Table 21.5 Nutrient Recommendations for CKD Renal Replacement Therapy

Nutrient	Hemodialysis	Peritoneal Dialysis	Transplant
Protein (g/kg/day)	≥1.2; ≥50% HBV	≥1.2–1.3; ≥50% HBV	Initial: 1.3–1.5 Maintenance: 1.0
Calories (cal/kg/day)	35 if <60 years 30–35 if ≥60 years	35 if <60 years 30–35 if ≥60 years	Initial: 30–35 Maintenance: 25–30
Fat	Heart-healthy guidelines	Heart-healthy guidelines	Heart-healthy guidelines
Sodium (g/day)	1–3	2–4	Unrestricted; monitor effects of medication
Fluid (mL/day)	1000 + urine output	1500–2000 (monitor)	Generally unrestricted
Potassium (g/day)	2–3	3–4	Unrestricted; monitor effects of medication
Phosphorus (mg/day)	800–1000	800–1000	Generally unrestricted
Calcium (g/day)	≤2 from diet and medications	≤2 from diet and medications	1.2

Source: National Kidney Foundation. *Kidney Disease Outcomes Quality Initiative,* 2000, 2002, 2003; and Beto, J., & Bansal, V. (2004). Medical nutrition therapy in chronic kidney failure: Integrating clinical practice guidelines. *Journal of American Diet Association, 104,* 404–409.

When dialysis begins and protein allowance increases, phosphorus intake correspondingly increases, yet the recommendation is to limit intake to 800 to 1000 mg. People who adhere to a low-phosphorus diet are at risk of consuming an inadequate protein diet, which can lead to malnutrition and protein–energy wasting. A study by Shinaberger et al. (2008) concluded that the risk of controlling serum phosphorus by restricting dietary protein may outweigh the benefit of controlling phosphorus and may lead to greater mortality, especially in patients on maintenance hemodialysis. Phosphate binders, which decrease GI absorption of phosphorus and promote fecal excretion, allow for a higher protein (and phosphorus) intake. Phosphate binders, which must be taken with all meals and snacks, are necessary to control serum phosphorus levels for the majority of patients.

For people on hemodialysis, fluid allowance equals the volume of any urine produced plus 1000 mL. Fluid intake is monitored by weight gain: anuric hemodialysis patients should not gain more than approximately 2 pounds/day between treatments. For many patients on hemodialysis, limiting fluid intake is the biggest challenge. Teaching clients *why* the fluid restriction is important is only half the battle; teaching them *how* to control their intake and thirst is vital. Strategies to relieve thirst are listed in Box 21.2. Peritoneal dialysis patients usually have fewer problems with fluid retention.

Translating Recommendations into Meals

The diet for CKD is challenging; modifications can be numerous, extensive, and lifelong, and changes are frequent. It is a difficult task to design a meal plan that balances what the individual needs with what the individual can tolerate—and will accept. Getting the client

Box 21.1   Sample CKD Diet: Predialysis and with Dialysis

Sample CKD Predialysis (50 g Protein Diet)	Sample CKD with Dialysis (90 g Protein Diet)
Breakfast	
½ cup apricot nectar	½ cup apricot nectar
1 English muffin	1 English muffin
At least 1 tbsp margarine	1 tbsp margarine
Jelly	2 eggs fried in margarine
Coffee	Jelly
Sugar	1 cup coffee
Nondairy creamer	Sugar
	Nondairy creamer
Lunch	
Sandwich made with	Sandwich made with
2 oz turkey	4 oz turkey
2 slices whole wheat bread	2 slices whole wheat bread
Salad dressing	Salad dressing
Lettuce and 1 slice tomato	Lettuce and 1 slice tomato
1 small apple	1 small apple
½ cup low-fat milk	½ cup low-fat milk
Snack	
2 fruit roll-ups	
Dinner	
2 oz roast beef	4 oz roast beef
Low-sodium gravy	Low-sodium gravy
½ cup unsalted noodles with margarine	½ cup unsalted noodles with margarine
½ cup carrots with margarine	½ cup carrots
Lettuce, onions, cucumbers, green salad with olive oil and vinegar dressing	Lettuce, onions, cucumbers, green pepper salad with olive oil and vinegar dressing
⅛ blueberry pie	⅛ blueberry pie
Ginger ale	1 cup ginger ale
Snacks	
Carbonated beverages*	
Marshmallows, gumdrops, hard candy	Marshmallows, gumdrops, hard candy

*As allowed, depending on fluid needs.

to make permanent changes in eating habits and food choices can be an ongoing challenge. Box 21.3 lists strategies that may help promote dietary adherence.

A "choice" system, similar to the diabetic exchange system, may be used to help clients implement dietary restrictions. An individualized meal plan that corresponds as closely as possible to the client's food preferences and habits details the number of choices permitted from each list for each meal. Portion sizes are specified to help ensure relative consistency in nutrient intake. Table 21.6 shows choice lists with examples of representative foods. The composition and complexity of the choice list system differs with the type of treatment used (e.g., predialysis, hemodialysis, or peritoneal dialysis). For instance, people not receiving dialysis may not need to limit their intake of potassium and would be free to choose among low-, medium-, and high-potassium fruits and vegetables, whereas

Box 21.2   STRATEGIES TO RELIEVE THIRST

- Use ice or popsicles within the fluid allowance—very cold things are better at relieving thirst.
- Suck on hard candy or mints.
- Chew gum.
- Rinse your mouth without swallowing using refrigerated water.
- Rinse your mouth occasionally with refrigerated mouthwash.
- Suck on a lemon wedge.
- Eat bread with applesauce or jelly with margarine.
- Control blood glucose levels, as appropriate.
- Try frozen low-potassium fruit, such as grapes.
- Use small glasses instead of large ones.
- Apply petroleum jelly to the lips.

people undergoing hemodialysis may need to limit their intake of fruits and vegetables to those that are low in potassium. Despite the term "choice lists," selections can be severely limited. Tips for implementing nutrition therapy recommendations for CKD are featured in Box 21.4.

Kidney Transplantation

Kidney transplantation is a treatment option for people with ESRD. As with all major surgeries, the immediate postoperative diet is high in protein and calories to promote healing; nutrient needs gradually decrease after the initial postoperative period (see Table 21.5). Most dietary parameters are removed when the new kidney functions normally; side effects from immunosuppressant drugs may require some dietary modifications (Beto and Bansal, 2004). A lifelong commitment to a "healthy" eating is important to decrease the risk of obesity, hypertension, diabetes, and hyperlipidemia and maximize bone density.

Box 21.3   STRATEGIES THAT MAY HELP PROMOTE DIETARY ADHERENCE TO CKD DIET

- Provide positive messages about what to eat rather than emphasizing food restrictions.
- Encourage social support from family and friends.
- Foster the client's perception as successfully adhering to the plan. People who are more confident in their ability to adhere to the eating plan make better choices.
- Provide feedback on self-monitoring and laboratory data. Correlation of records with laboratory data enables the client to see cause and effect, reinforces the importance of nutrition therapy, and opens the door for problem solving.
- For clients who must restrict their intake of protein, encourage the use of low-protein breads, cereals, cookies, and pastas. Acceptability varies greatly among low-protein products, so if a client does not like one brand, it does not mean he or she will not like another.

Table 21.6 Choice Lists and Examples of Representative Foods

Choice Lists	Examples of Representative Foods
Animal protein foods	Beef, fish, eggs, poultry, shellfish
High-protein foods that are also high in sodium, potassium, and/or phosphorus	Cheese, dried peas and beans, milk, yogurt, tofu Canned tuna and salmon; cottage cheese; deli beef or turkey; processed meats, bacon, vegetarian burgers
Vegetables and fruit	
Low potassium	Cabbage, carrots, corn, eggplant, green beans, onions Apples, blueberries, grapes, pineapples, watermelon
Medium potassium	Asparagus, broccoli, celery, peas, turnips, zucchini Cantaloupe, mangoes, papaya, fresh peaches
High potassium	Avocado, Brussels sprouts, "greens," okra, potatoes, pumpkin, spinach, sweet potatoes, tomatoes, yams Apricots, bananas, nectarines, orange juice, prune juice
Milk and other high-phosphorus choices	Cheese, cooked dried peas and beans, oatmeal, milk, nuts, nut butters, soy milk, bran cereals, yogurt
Bread, cereal, and grain	Bagel, bread, pita, flour tortilla, low-sodium ready-to-eat cereals, pasta, rice, unsalted crackers
Bread, cereal, and grain with added sodium and phosphorus	Biscuits, cake, oatmeal, most ready-to-eat cereals, pancakes, waffles, pretzels
Fluids	Beverages, ice, soup, gelatin; ice cream and ice milk (each melt to ½ initial volume)
"Free" foods for calories	Gumdrops, hard candy, jelly, jelly beans, Life Savers, margarine, mayonnaise, sugar, syrup, vegetable oil, nondairy whipped topping

Source: Academy of Nutrition and Dietetics. (2012). Chronic kidney disease stage 5. Nutrition therapy for people on dialysis. In *Nutrition care manual.* Available at www.nutritioncaremanual.org. Accessed 7/6/12.

ACUTE KIDNEY INJURY

The sudden loss of renal function, previously known as acute renal failure, is now referred to as acute kidney injury (AKI). It is characterized by increases in serum creatinine and blood urea nitrogen levels. Urine output can be classified as anuria (<100 mL/day), oliguria (100–400 mL/day), or nonoliguria (>400 mL/day) (Kalista-Richards, 2011).

Among the many causes of AKI are shock, severe infection, trauma, medications, and obstruction. It is often part of multiple organ dysfunction in the critical care setting. Despite improvements in dialysis therapy and nutrition support, the mortality of AKI continues to be 50% to 60% (Brown, Compher, and the American Society for Parenteral and Enteral Nutrition [ASPEN] Board of Directors, 2010). The poor prognosis is related mainly to the degree of underlying illness and associated hypercatabolism. The primary focus of treatment is to treat the underlying disorder to prevent permanent renal damage.

Box 21.4   TIPS FOR IMPLEMENTING NUTRITION THERAPY FOR CKD

- Initially weigh or measure portion sizes and, thereafter, periodically spot-check portion sizes for accuracy because either too little or too much protein in the diet can cause uremic symptoms to return.
- Be sure to eat a good breakfast if appetite decreases as the day progresses, which may occur secondary to uremia.
- Limit meat intake to less than 5 to 6 oz/day for most men and less than 4 oz/day for most women. Think of meat as a side dish, not the main entrée.
- Spread protein allowance over the whole day instead of saving it all for one meal.
- Limit dairy products, including milk, yogurt, ice cream, and frozen yogurt, to ½ cup/day. Nondairy creamers are a low-phosphorus alternative, but they can be high in saturated fat.
- Limit cheese to 1 oz hard cheese per day or ⅓ cup cottage cheese per day.
- Limit high-phosphorus foods to one serving or less per day. High-phosphorus foods include beer, chocolate, cola, nuts, peanut butter, dried peas and beans, bran, bran cereals, and some whole grains.
- Do not add salt during cooking or at the table. Avoid processed foods, regular canned vegetables, convenience foods, and seasonings that contain salt (e.g., onion salt, lemon pepper, MSG).
- Eat heart healthy by choosing lean meats, nonfat milk and dairy products, trans fat–free margarines, and canola and olive oils.
- Try highly seasoned or strongly flavored foods if uremia has caused a change in the sense of taste.
- Eat a consistent intake of carbohydrate with regularly timed meals to control blood glucose levels, if appropriate.
- Seek physician approval before using any vitamin, mineral, or supplement.

Nutrition Therapy

It has not been proven that nutrition therapy for AKI promotes recovery of kidney function or improves survival, but it is likely that nutritional support is beneficial (Academy of Nutrition and Dietetics, 2012). The goal is to provide adequate amounts of calories, protein, and other nutrients to prevent or minimize malnutrition; however, the metabolic abnormalities that occur in hypercatabolic patients with AKI, such as accelerated protein breakdown, increased energy expenditure, and an inability to use protein and calories efficiently, make it difficult to achieve nutritional goals.

The American Society for Parenteral and Enteral Nutrition recommends enteral nutrition if the GI tract is functional and that intensive care unit patients with AKI receive a standard formula (Brown, Compher, and the ASPEN Board of Directors, 2010; McClave et al., 2009). Enteral formulas with low electrolyte profiles specifically designed for renal failure may be used if significant electrolyte abnormalities develop (McClave et al., 2009). Parenteral nutrition is used if it is the only effective means of providing adequate nutrition.

Ideally, calorie requirements are determined by indirect calorimetry. When that is not possible, an individualized assessment is recommended. Depending on the underlying stress and the patient's weight and nutrition status, calorie needs may range from 25 to 35 cal/kg/day or more, including calories provided through continuous renal replacement therapy (CRRT). Protein recommendations are controversial and vary with the type of renal replacement therapy used and the degree of catabolism. Protein should not be restricted as

Table 21.7 Nutrition Guidelines for Acute Kidney Injury

Nutrient	Recommendations	Factors That Impact Actual Allowance
Protein	1.5–2.5 g/kg	Degree of catabolism Renal function Approximate amino acid loss during CRRT is 10–15 g/day.
Calories	25–50 cal/kg	Degree of stress Nutritional status
Sodium	1.1–3.3 g/day	Serum sodium levels Blood pressure Edema Urinary losses (in diuretic phase) Use of dialysis
Potassium	2.0–3.0 g/day	Serum potassium levels Urinary losses (in diuretic phase)
Phosphorus	Individualized	Serum phosphorus levels
Calcium	Individualized	Serum calcium levels
Fluid	500 mL + urine output	Urine output Type of dialysis, if any

Source: Academy of Nutrition and Dietetics. (2012). Nutrition prescription for acute renal failure. In *Nutrition care manual.* Available at www.nutritioncaremanual.com. Accessed on 711/12; and McClave, S., Marteindale, R., Vanek, V., McCarthy, M., Roberts, P., Taylor, B., . . . Cresci, G. (2009). Guidelines for the provision and assessment of nutrition support therapy in the adult critically ill patient: Society of Critical Care Medicine (SCCM) and American Society for Parenteral and Enteral Nutrition (ASPEN). *Journal of Parenteral and Enteral Nutrition, 33,* 277–316.

a means to avoid or delay initiation of dialysis therapy (McClave et al., 2009). Serum levels of potassium, magnesium, phosphorus, and calcium are monitored. Table 21.7 summarizes nutrient recommendations and factors that influence nutrient needs.

KIDNEY STONES

Kidney stones form when insoluble crystals precipitate out of urine. They vary in size from sand-like "gravel" to large, branching stones, and although they form most often in the kidney, they can occur anywhere in the urinary system.

Approximately 75% of kidney stones are made of calcium oxalate; **hyperoxaluria** is considered to be a primary risk factor for this type of stone (Liebman and Al-Wahsh, 2011). The remaining stones are composed of calcium phosphate, uric acid, or **struvite**. Cystine (an amino acid) stones are rare and occur only in people with cystinuria, an autosomal recessive disorder.

Certain factors increase the risk of kidney stones, including dehydration or low urine volume, urinary tract obstruction, gout, chronic inflammation of the bowel, and intestinal bypass or ostomy surgery. A wide variety of dietary factors either promote or inhibit the formation of calcium oxalate kidney stones.

Fluid. A low fluid intake concentrates the urine, increasing the likelihood of chemicals precipitating out to form kidney stones—regardless of the composition of the stone. An adequate fluid intake helps keep urine dilute.

Oxalate. Oxalate is found in many plant foods, including nuts, fruit, vegetables, grains, and legumes. Normally, only 2% to 15% of **oxalate** consumed is absorbed (Liebman and

Hyperoxaluria: elevated levels of oxalate in the urine.

Struvite: magnesium ammonium phosphate crystals formed by the action of bacterial enzymes.

Oxalate: a salt of oxalic acid. Oxalate can form strong bonds with various minerals; when combined with calcium, it forms a nearly insoluble compound.

Al-Wahsh, 2011). People who have hyperoxaluria, known as "super absorbers," can absorb 50% more oxalate than nonstone formers (Reynolds, 2005). Hyperoxaluria can be caused by genetic disorders, chronic bowel inflammation, or a high-oxalate intake. Hyperoxaluria is more of a risk for stone formation than **hypercalciuria** (Mendonca et al., 2003).

People who form calcium oxalate stones are advised to limit their intake of oxalate (Box 21.5). Because **megadoses** of vitamin C increase both oxalate absorption and oxalate synthesis in people prone to calcium oxalate stones, daily doses should be limited to less than 2000 mg/day (Chai, Liebman, Kynast-Gales, and Massey, 2004).

Calcium. Dietary calcium favorably binds with dietary oxalate in the intestines, forming an insoluble compound that the body cannot absorb. When calcium intake is low, oxalate absorption and excretion increase, as does the risk of stone formation (Favus, 2011). A normal calcium intake consumed throughout the day is recommended to decrease the risk of stone formation. Optimal calcium intake can be attained while minimizing the risk of kidney stone formation by consuming dietary calcium and avoiding calcium supplements (Favus, 2011).

Protein. High intakes of animal protein increase urinary excretion of calcium, oxalate, and uric acid and reduce urinary pH (Seiner, Ebert, Nicolay, and Hesse, 2003). Protein intake in excess of the RDA is not recommended for people with a history of calcium oxalate kidney stones.

Sodium. A high-sodium intake promotes urinary calcium excretion by decreasing calcium reabsorption by the kidney (Seiner et al., 2003). Patients with hypercalciuria should limit their intake of sodium.

Nutrition Therapy

Box 21.5 lists nutrition strategies for decreasing the risk of calcium oxalate kidney stone formation; none are effective when used alone, yet nutrition therapy is considered the cornerstone in kidney stone management, whether or not medication is needed.

The DASH diet, which is high in fruits and vegetables, moderate in low-fat dairy products, and relatively low in animal protein, may offer a new potential approach to preventing kidney stones (Taylor, Fung, and Curhan, 2009). A study by Taylor et al. (2009) that examined the impact of a DASH-style diet on the incidence of kidney stones found that the diet is associated with a marked decrease in kidney stone risk despite its high-oxalate content. There may be several different mechanisms by which DASH is protective against kidney stones, including increasing calcium intake, increasing urinary citrate, or increasing urinary pH. The study data do not support the common practice of restricting dietary oxalate, particularly if that means a lower intake of fruits, vegetables, and whole grains.

Hypercalciuria: elevated levels of calcium in urine.

Megadoses: amounts at least 10 times greater than the DRI.

Box 21.5   **NUTRITION RECOMMENDATIONS FOR CALCIUM OXALATE KIDNEY STONES**

- Drink 3 to 4 quarts of fluid throughout the day, with most in the form of water.
- Avoid high-oxalate foods: peanuts, tree nuts (such as almonds, cashews, hazelnuts), soybeans, soy milk, wheat germ and wheat bran (including cereals), spinach, black tea, instant tea, rhubarb, beets, most dried beans (e.g., black, navy or great northern), chocolate, and sweet potatoes.
- Avoid large doses of supplemental vitamin C.
- Maintain adequate calcium intake (e.g., 3 servings/day) that is spread out over the day.
- Avoid high intakes of animal protein (e.g., >6 oz/day) and sodium (e.g., >2 g/day).

Source: National Kidney Foundation. (2012). *Diet and kidney stones.* Available at http://www.kidney.org/atoz/content/diet.cfm. Accessed on 7/11/12.

NURSING PROCESS: *Chronic Kidney Disease*

Carlos is 66 years old and has had type 2 diabetes for 20 years. He is 5 ft 7 in tall and weighs 172 pounds. His hemoglobin A1c is 8.2; he takes insulin twice a day. He has a history of hypertension and mild anemia and complains of sudden weight gain and "swelling." His blood urea nitrogen (BUN) and creatinine have been steadily increasing over the last several years, and his GFR is currently 63. During his last appointment, the doctor told Carlos to watch his protein intake and avoid salt. At this visit, Carlos' chief complaint is that he does not have an appetite anymore; he attributes his change in taste to not salting his food. The doctor has asked you to talk to Carlos about his diet.

Assessment

Medical–Psychosocial History	▪ Medical history including cardiovascular disease, hypertension, diabetes, and renal disease
	▪ Medications that affect nutrition such as diuretics, insulin, and lipid-lowering medications
	▪ Physical complaints such as fatigue, taste changes, anorexia, nausea, vomiting, diarrhea, muscular twitches, and muscle cramps
	▪ Psychosocial and economic issues such as living situation, cooking facilities, financial status, employment, and education
	▪ Understanding of the relationship between diet and renal function
	▪ Motivation to change eating style
Anthropometric Assessment	▪ Current height, weight, and body mass index (BMI)
	▪ Recent weight history
Biochemical and Physical Assessment	▪ Blood values of
	▪ BUN and creatinine
	▪ Sodium, potassium, and other electrolytes
	▪ Phosphorus and calcium
	▪ Glucose
	▪ Lipid profile
	▪ Hemoglobin and hematocrit
	▪ eGFR
	▪ Urinalysis for volume, urea, protein, etc.
	▪ Blood pressure
Dietary Assessment	▪ What kind of nutrition counseling have you had in the past?
	▪ How many meals and snacks do you usually eat?
	▪ What is a typical day's intake for you?
	▪ Do you follow a diet for diabetes? What gives you the most difficulty?
	▪ How is your appetite?
	▪ Do you have any food allergies or intolerances?
	▪ Do you have any feeding issues, such as difficulty chewing or swallowing?
	▪ What kind of protein do you eat most often? What is a typical serving size? Is it spread out over the day?

NURSING PROCESS: *Chronic Kidney Disease* (continued)

- Do you drink milk and, if so, how much per day?
- How successful were you "watching your protein and avoiding salt"?
- How often do you eat high-sodium foods, such as cold cuts, bacon, frankfurters, smoked meats, sausage, canned meats, chipped or corned beef, buttermilk, cheese, crackers, canned soups and vegetables, convenience products, pickles, and condiments?
- Do you use a salt substitute?
- Do you regularly eat fruits and vegetables? How many servings of each do you consume in an average day?
- How much fluid do you drink daily? What is your favorite beverage?
- Do you have any cultural, religious, and ethnic food preferences?
- Do you use vitamins, minerals, or nutritional supplements? If so, what, how much, and why do you use them?
- Do you drink alcohol?
- How often do you eat out?

Diagnosis

Possible Nursing Diagnosis

- Altered nutrition: eating less than the body needs r/t anorexia, taste changes, dietary restrictions

Planning

Client Outcomes

The client will

- Consume adequate calories to prevent weight loss
- Attain and maintain adequate nutritional status
- Experience improved appetite
- Practice self-management strategies especially self-monitoring protein and sodium intake
- Achieve normal or near-normal electrolyte levels
- Maintain adequate glucose control
- Achieve and maintain normal blood pressure
- Maintain normal urinary output
- Describe the rationale and principles of nutrition therapy for CKD and implement appropriate dietary changes
- Prevent further kidney damage

Nursing Interventions

Nutrition Therapy

Provide a 2000-calorie carbohydrate-controlled diet with 65 g protein and 1500 mg sodium, as ordered.

(continues on page 586)

NURSING PROCESS: *Chronic Kidney Disease* (continued)

Client Teaching	Instruct the client on
	1. The role of nutrition therapy in the treatment of CKD
	2. Eating plan essentials including
	▪ Limiting protein, emphasizing high-quality proteins, spreading protein allowance over the whole day
	▪ Consuming adequate calories
	▪ Limiting high-sodium foods, not adding salt during cooking or at the table
	▪ Using sodium-free seasonings and salt alternatives to improve the flavor of food
	3. Behavioral matters including
	▪ How to weigh and measure foods to ensure accurate portion sizes
	▪ Self-monitoring protein intake
	▪ Weighing oneself at approximately the same time every day with the same scale while wearing the same amount of clothing. Unexpected weight gain or loss should be reported to the physician.
	▪ That renal diet cookbooks are available to increase variety
	4. Changing eating attitudes
	▪ Learn to view the diet as an integral component of treatment and a means of life support
	▪ Strict adherence to the diet can improve the quality of life and decrease the workload on the kidneys

Evaluation

Evaluate and Monitor	
	▪ Monitor weight
	▪ Monitor lab values, blood pressure, and urine output
	▪ Monitor appetite
	▪ Evaluate food records, if available
	▪ Provide periodic feedback and reinforcement

 ## HOW DO YOU RESPOND?

Does cranberry juice prevent urinary tract infections? Cranberry has been found to be effective against urinary tract infections by preventing bacteria from adhering to the lining of the urinary tract, thereby promoting their excretion. However, the effects are transitory, so regular, perhaps more than twice daily, intake is necessary. Clients who are prone to urinary tract infections and like cranberry juice should be encouraged to consume it regularly. Cranberry juice appears more effective than cranberry capsules or tablets (Wang et al., 2012).

Are omega-3 fish oil supplements beneficial for people on hemodialysis? In addition to their beneficial effects on the heart, supplements of omega-3 fats may help benefit people on hemodialysis by preventing itching (uremic pruritus), decreasing vascular access graft thrombosis, and decreasing the dose of erythropoietin needed to maintain hemoglobin level within the goal range. The American Heart Association recommends people with or at risk of heart disease to consume 1 g of EPA and DHA per day, but people on dialysis may need as much as 2 g daily (Vergili, 2007). Because omega-3 fatty acids decrease platelet aggregation, clients should talk to their physician before using them, especially if they are taking anticoagulants. Fish oil supplements should be stored in the refrigerator to prevent rancidity.

CASE STUDY

Dorothea is a 72-year-old black woman who is 5 ft 5 in tall and weighs 149 pounds. She has coronary heart disease and a long-standing history of hypertension with progressive loss of kidney function. She recently started receiving hemodialysis and is gaining about 4 pounds between treatments. She has convinced herself that because she is on dialysis, she can eat and drink whatever she wants and "the machine will take care of it."

Yesterday, she ate the following:

Breakfast:	Grits with cheese
	Bacon
	Biscuit with butter
	Coffee
Lunch:	Hamburger on bun with ketchup and mustard
	Potato chips
	Banana
	Sweetened tea
Dinner:	Fried chicken
	Macaroni and cheese
	Collard greens
	Pound cake
	Sweetened tea

- What risk factors does Dorothea have for CKD?
- Based on her age, weight, and use of hemodialysis, what should the composition of her diet be (e.g., number of calories, grams of protein, grams of sodium)?
- Why is she gaining 4 pounds between treatments? What is a more reasonable goal? What would you suggest she do to achieve the goal?
- Evaluate her protein intake and recommend changes she could make to achieve her protein goals.
- What foods is she eating that are not heart healthy? What substitutions would you recommend?

- Evaluate her sodium intake and recommend changes she could make to limit her sodium intake.
- What foods is she eating that are high in potassium? What alternatives would you suggest?
- What foods is she eating that are high in phosphorus? Is her calcium intake adequate?
- What would you tell Dorothea about the use of dialysis and her theory about eating anything she wants?
- Which is the lesser risk: getting enough calories and protein by eating non–heart-healthy foods or adhering to the sodium and other restrictions but not getting enough calories and protein?

STUDY QUESTIONS

1. Which statement indicates the patient needs further instruction about diet for nephrotic syndrome?
   a. "I know I need to eat a high-protein diet to replace the protein lost in urine."
   b. "I need to limit my intake of saturated fat and cholesterol."
   c. "I should not use salt in cooking or at the table and avoid foods high in sodium such as processed foods, fast foods, convenience foods, condiments, and canned meat and vegetables."
   d. "I am going to try substituting soy protein for animal sources of protein because it may be better for me."

2. A client with predialysis CKD asks if it is okay that she saves all her meat allowance for her evening meal. Which of the following would be the nurse's best response?
   a. "You cannot have any meat on a predialysis diet."
   b. "It doesn't matter when you eat your meat allowance, so if you prefer to save it all for dinner, that is fine."
   c. "If you want to eat your meat allowance all at one time, it would be better to eat it for breakfast so that your body has all day to metabolize it."
   d. "It is best if you spread your meat allowance out over the whole day."

3. When developing a teaching plan for a client who is on dialysis, which of the following protein sources would the nurse suggest for a client who must also limit her intake of phosphorus?
   a. Beef
   b. Cheese
   c. Tofu
   d. Kidney beans

4. The nurse knows her instructions about preventing future calcium oxalate stones have been effective when the client verbalizes he should
   a. Avoid milk, cheese, and other sources of calcium.
   b. Take megadoses of vitamin C.
   c. Consume a normal amount of dietary calcium spread out over the course of the day.
   d. Eat a high-protein diet.

5. How do the protein recommendations for those with chronic kidney disease without diabetes differ from those who have diabetes?
   a. Protein is more restricted for people who do not have diabetes.
   b. Protein is more restricted for people who have diabetes.
   c. The protein recommendations do not differ for people with diabetes or without diabetes.
   d. There are no specific protein recommendations for people with diabetes because carbohydrates and fat are the priority concerns.

6. A client on hemodialysis asks if she can use popsicles to help relieve her thirst. Which of the following is the nurses' best response?
   a. "That's a great idea as long as you deduct the equivalent amount of fluid from your total daily fluid allowance."
   b. "Popsicles are empty calories. You are better off drinking just plain water."
   c. "Popsicles are great at relieving thirst, and because they are solid, they do not count as fluid, so you can eat them as desired."
   d. "Hot things are better at relieving thirst than cold things. Try small amounts of hot tea or coffee to relieve your thirst."

7. One of the factors that influence protein allowance during acute kidney injury is the individual's
   a. Level of activity
   b. Degree of catabolism
   c. Blood pressure
   d. Serum albumin concentration

8. The client asks if she will need to follow a diet after she recovers from her kidney transplant. Which of the following is the nurse's best response?
   a. "You will always have to limit protein and phosphorus intake to help preserve the health of the new kidney."
   b. "After recovery, all restrictions are lifted and you can eat anything you want."
   c. "You may need to modify some aspects of your diet because of side effects from the medications you will be taking, and you should continue to eat a heart-healthy diet to decrease the risks of diabetes, hypertension, heart disease, and obesity."
   d. "All the restrictions you followed before dialysis will resume after you recover from the transplant."

KEY CONCEPTS

- Loss of renal function profoundly affects metabolism, nutritional status, and nutritional requirements. The nutrients most affected are protein, calcium, phosphorus, vitamin D, fluid, sodium, and potassium.
- People with nephrotic syndrome lose protein, mostly albumin, in the urine. Hypo-albuminemia and hyperlipidemia are other characteristics. Protein intake should be limited to 0.8 to 1.0 g/kg/day, an amount consistent with the RDA for protein, to minimize protein loss in the urine. Sodium intake is limited; a fluid restriction is usually not necessary.
- Diet modifications for CKD are complex, unpalatable, and frequently adjusted according to the client's laboratory values and symptoms.
- Avoiding excess protein and limiting sodium are the cornerstones of nutrition therapy for slowing the progression of CKD. For people with diabetes, managing blood glucose levels may also slow CKD progression. A heart-healthy diet is recommended because the risk of cardiovascular disease is high in patients with CKD.
- There is a narrow margin of error regarding protein intake: too little protein results in body protein catabolism, which has the same effect as eating too much protein, namely, an increase in creatinine levels.
- A high-calorie diet is indicated whenever protein intake is restricted to ensure that the protein consumed will be used for specific protein functions, not for energy requirements.
- Usually, as renal function deteriorates, potassium and phosphorus intakes may be restricted.
- In patients with kidney disease, calcium metabolism is impaired because of faulty vitamin D metabolism, impaired intestinal absorption, and hyperphosphatemia as a result of loss of renal function. A high-calcium intake from food is not achievable when phosphorus is restricted.
- When dialysis is instituted, a high-protein intake is recommended to compensate for protein lost through the dialysate. Calories need to be adequate to spare protein.
- People on hemodialysis generally have more severe restrictions (e.g., fluid, sodium, potassium) than people on peritoneal dialysis.
- Clients who experience renal transplantation may need to alter their diets to lessen the side effects of immunosuppressant therapy. They should commit to a lifestyle of healthy eating to reduce the risk of diabetes, hypertension, obesity, and heart disease.

■ AKI represents an even greater nutritional challenge than CKD. Protein, sodium, potassium, phosphorus, and fluid are adjusted according to laboratory data, use of renal replacement therapy, renal function, and degree of catabolism.

■ Clients with a history of calcium oxalate kidney stones should consume 3 to 4 quarts of fluid daily, avoid megadoses of vitamin C, eat a normal calcium intake spread out over the day, and avoid foods high in oxalate.

Check Your Knowledge Answer Key

1. **TRUE** Early in the course of chronic kidney disease, limiting protein may help to preserve kidney function, but there are no guarantees and the optimal level of protein intake is not known.

2. **TRUE** Foods high in protein tend to be high in phosphorus. Other high-phosphorus foods include cola, chocolate, beer, bran, and bran cereal.

3. **FALSE** Although milk is an excellent source of high biologic value protein, it is high in phosphorus and thus can only be consumed in limited amounts (½ cup/day).

4. **FALSE** Although patients with CKD are at risk for hyperkalemia due to decreased potassium excretion, metabolic acidosis, and certain medications, hyperkalemia is usually not seen until CKD is advanced.

5. **TRUE** People with chronic renal disease tend to have accelerated atherosclerosis and may benefit from eating a heart-healthy diet—namely, less saturated fat, cholesterol, and trans fat.

6. **TRUE** Dialysis causes protein requirements to increase about 50% above normal because proteins and amino acids are lost in the dialysis.

7. **TRUE** People receiving peritoneal dialysis may absorb 100 to 200 g of glucose from the dialysate, which is 340 to 680 calories.

8. **FALSE** Weight gain between dialysis treatments reflects fluid retention. Excessive weight gain between dialysis treatments means the intake of sodium and fluid is too high, not that calorie intake is too high.

9. **FALSE** Most people with hypercalciuria should consume a normal calcium intake. Restricting calcium intake does not decrease the risk of calcium stones because it increases urinary oxalate concentration.

10. **FALSE** No single component of nutrition therapy, including increasing fluids, can effectively prevent kidney stones from forming.

Student Resources on thePoint

For additional learning materials, activate the code in the front of this book at
http://thePoint.lww.com/activate

Websites

American Association of Kidney Patients at **www.aakp.org**
American Kidney Fund at **www.kidneyfund.org**
National Institute of Diabetes and Digestive and Kidney Diseases at **www.niddk.nih.gov**
National Kidney and Urologic Diseases Information Clearinghouse (NKUDIC) at
   http://kidney.niddk.nih.gov
National Kidney Disease Education Program (NKDEP) at **www.nkdep.nih.gov/professionals/index.htm**
National Kidney Foundation at **www.kidney.org**
Nephron Information Center at **www.nephron.com**
Oxalosis and Hyperoxaluria Foundation at **www.ohf.org**

References

Academy of Nutrition and Dietetics. (2012). *Nutrition care manual.* Available at www.nutritioncaremanual.org. Accessed on 7/10/12.

Besarab, A., & Coyne, D. (2010). Iron supplementation to treat anemia in patients with chronic kidney disease. *Nature Reviews. Nephrology, 6,* 699–710.

Beto, J., & Bansal, V. (2004). Medical nutrition therapy in chronic kidney failure: Integrating clinical practice guidelines. *Journal of the American Dietetic Association, 104,* 404–409.

Brown, R., Compher, C., & the American Society for Parenteral and Enteral Nutrition Board of Directors. (2010). ASPEN clinical guidelines: Nutrition support in adult acute and chronic renal failure. *Journal of Parenteral and Enteral Nutrition, 34,* 366–377.

Burrowes, J. (2008). New recommendations for the management of diabetic kidney disease. *Nutrition Today, 43,* 65–69.

Centers for Disease Control and Prevention. (2010). *National chronic kidney disease fact sheet: General information and national estimates on chronic kidney disease in the United States.* Atlanta, GA: U.S. Department of Health and Human Services, Centers for Disease Control and Prevention. Available at www.cdc.gov/diabetes/pubs/pdf/kidney_Factsheet.pdf. Accessed on 6/27/12.

Chai, W., Liebman, M., Kynast-Gales, S., & Massey, L. (2004). Oxalate absorption and endogenous oxalate synthesis from ascorbate in calcium oxalate stone formers and in non-stone formers. *American Journal of Kidney Diseases, 44,* 1060–1069.

de Zeeuw, D., Remuzzi, G., Parving, H., Keane, W. F., Zhang, Z., Shahinfar, S., . . . Brenner, B. M. (2004). Proteinuria, a target for renoprotection in patients with type 2 diabetic nephropathy: Lessons from RENAAL. *Kidney International, 65,* 2309–2320.

Favus, M. (2011). The risk of kidney stone formation: The form of calcium matters. *American Journal of Clinical Nutrition, 94,* 5–6.

Gutekunst, L. (2010). Water, water everywhere, but what to drink? An update on hidden phosphorus in popular beverages. *Journal of Renal Nutrition, 20*(1), e1–e5. doi:10.1053/j.jm.2009.11.001

Kalista-Richards, M. (2011). The kidney: Medical nutrition therapy—Yesterday and today. *Nutrition in Clinical Practice, 26,* 143–150.

Kopple, J. (2008). Do low-protein diets retard the loss of kidney function in patients with diabetic nephropathy? *American Journal of Clinical Nutrition, 88,* 593–594.

Kovesdy, C., & Kalantar-Zadeh, K. (2007). Serum phosphorus and the risk of progression of chronic kidney disease. *Nephrology, Dialysis, and Transplantation, 22,* 3679–3680.

Levey, A. S., Adler, S., Caggiula, A. W., England, B. K., Greene, T., Hunsicker, L. G., . . . Teschan, P. E. (1996). Effects of dietary protein restriction on the progression of advanced renal disease in the Modification of Diet in Renal Disease Study. *American Journal of Kidney Diseases, 27,* 652–663.

Liebman, M., & Al-Wahsh, I. (2011). Probiotics and other key determinants of dietary oxalate absorption. *Advances in Nutrition, 2,* 254–260.

McClave, S., Martindale, R., Vanek, V., McCarthy, M., Roberts, P., Taylor, B., . . . Cresci, G. (2009). Guidelines for the provision and assessment of nutrition support therapy in the adult critically ill patient: Society of Critical Care Medicine (SCCM) and American Society for Parenteral and Enteral Nutrition (ASPEN). *Journal of Parenteral and Enteral Nutrition, 33,* 277–316.

Mendonca, C. O. G., Martini, L. A., Baxmann, A. C., Nishiura, J. L., Cuppari, L., Sigulem, D. M., & Heilberg, I. P. (2003). Effects of oxalate load on urinary oxalate excretion in calcium stone formers. *Journal of Renal Nutrition, 13,* 39–46.

Murphy, S., Xu, J., & Kochanek, K. (2012). *National vital statistics report 60(4). Deaths: Preliminary data for 2010.* Available at www.cdc.gov/nchs/data/nvsr/nvsr60/nvsr60_04.pdf. Accessed on 7/11/12.

National Kidney Disease Education Program. (2011). *Chronic kidney disease and diet: Assessment, management, and treatment. Treating CKD patients who are not on dialysis* (NIH Publication No. 11-7406). Washington, DC: USDHHS, NIDDK, NKDEP.

National Kidney Foundation. (2002). K/DOQI clinical practice guidelines for chronic kidney disease: Evaluation, classification, and stratification. *American Journal of Kidney Diseases, 39*(Suppl. 1), S1–S75.

Pan, Y., Guo, L., & Jin, H. (2008). Low-protein diet for diabetic nephropathy: A meta-analysis of randomized controlled trials. *American Journal of Clinical Nutrition, 88,* 660–666.

Reynolds, T. (2005). ACP best practice no. 181: Chemical pathology clinical investigation and management of nephrolithiasis. *American Journal of Clinical Pathology, 58,* 134–140.

Seiner, R., Ebert, D., Nicolay, C., & Hesse, A. (2003). Dietary risk factors for hyperoxaluria in calcium oxalate stone formers. *International Society of Nephrology, 63,* 1037–1043.

Shinaberger, C., Greenland, S., Kopple, J., Van Wyck, D., Mehrotra, R., Kovesdy, C. P., & Kalantar-Zadeh, K. (2008). Is controlling phosphorus by decreasing dietary protein intake beneficial or harmful in persons with chronic kidney disease? *American Journal of Clinical Nutrition, 88,* 1511–1518.

Steiber, A., & Kopple, J. (2011). Vitamin status and needs for people with stages 3–5 chronic kidney disease. *Journal of Renal Nutrition, 21,* 355–368.

Taylor, E., Fung, T., & Curhan, G. (2009). DASH-style diet associates with reduced risk for kidney stones. *Journal of the American Society of Nephrology, 20,* 2253–2259.

U.S. Department of Agriculture, Agricultural Research Service. (2010). Nutrient intakes from food: Mean amounts consumed per individual, by gender and age. What We Eat in American, NHANES 2007-2008. Available at www.ars.usda.gov/ba/bhnrc/fsrg. Accessed on 6/9/12.

Velasquez, M., & Bhathena, S. (2001). Dietary phytoestrogens: A possible role in renal disease protection. *American Journal of Kidney Diseases, 37,* 1056–1068.

Vergili, J. (2007). Are fish oil supplements right for you? *Kidney Times.* Available at http://www.kidneytimes.com/article.php?id=20071015191039. Accessed on 8/6/08.

Wang, C., Fang, C., Chen, N., Liu, S. S., Yu, P. H., Wu, T. Y., . . . Chen, S. C. (2012). Cranberry-containing products for prevention of urinary tract infections in susceptible populations. *Archives of Internal Medicine, 172,* 988–996.

Weiner, D., Tighiouart, H., Elsayed, E., Griffith, J. L., Salem, D. N., Levey, A. S., & Sarnak, M. J. (2008). The relationship between non-traditional risk factors and outcomes in individuals with stage 3 to 4 CKD. *American Journal of Kidney Disease, 51,* 212–223.

22 Nutrition for Patients with Cancer or HIV/AIDS

TRUE	FALSE		
☐	☐	**1**	People who are obese are at increased risk of several types of cancer.
☐	☐	**2**	Weight loss is an indicator of poor prognosis in people with cancer.
☐	☐	**3**	Clients who are adequately nourished may be better able to withstand the effects of cancer treatment.
☐	☐	**4**	Cachexia is directly related to the amount of calories consumed.
☐	☐	**5**	The appetite of clients with anorexia tends to improve as the day progresses.
☐	☐	**6**	Cancer survivors are urged to follow diet recommendations to reduce the risk of cancer in the future.
☐	☐	**7**	Lipodystrophy can be prevented with a low-fat diet.
☐	☐	**8**	Clients with HIV who are experiencing malabsorption always have diarrhea.
☐	☐	**9**	Clients with HIV/AIDS have problems with appetite and intake similar to those of cancer clients.
☐	☐	**10**	Nutritional counseling of clients with HIV/AIDS should include how to avoid foodborne illnesses.

LEARNING OBJECTIVES

Upon completion of this chapter, you will be able to

1 Evaluate a person's usual diet according to dietary recommendations to reduce the risk of cancer.
2 Summarize how cancer and cancer therapies affect nutritional status.
3 Give examples of ways to modify the diet to alleviate side effects of anorexia, nausea, fatigue, taste changes, mouth sores, dry mouth, and diarrhea.
4 Discuss three ways to increase a client's calorie and protein intake.
5 Calculate the calorie and protein requirements of a patient with cancer based on clinical status and weight.
6 Explain how HIV/AIDS affects nutritional status.
7 Compare cancer cachexia with HIV-related wasting.
8 Teach a person living with HIV/AIDS guidelines for a healthy diet.

Cancer and human immunodeficiency virus (HIV)/acquired immunodeficiency syndrome (AIDS) can cause devastating weight loss and malnutrition. Although nutrition therapy cannot cure either disease, it has the potential to maximize the effectiveness of drug therapy, alleviate the side effects of the disease and its treatments, and improve overall quality of life.

CANCER

Cancer, the second leading cause of death in the United States (Centers for Disease Control and Prevention [CDC], 2012), is a group name for more than 100 different diseases characterized by the uncontrolled growth of cells. Individual cancers differ in where they develop, how quickly they grow, the type of treatment they respond to, and how much they impact nutritional status.

The relationship between nutrition and cancer is multifaceted:

- One-third of all cancer deaths in the United States are related to dietary factors (World Cancer Research Fund [WCRF]/American Institute for Cancer Research [AICR], 2007), such as eating substances that may promote cancer or failing to eat foods that may protect against cancer. For instance, an estimated 14% to 20% of all cancer-related mortality in the United States is related to overweight and obesity (Calle, Rodriguez, Walker-Thurmond, and Thun, 2003). Conversely, a diet that provides a variety of fruits and vegetables, whole grains, and fish or poultry or is lower in red and processed meats is associated with a lower risk of developing certain cancers or dying from cancer (Kushi et al., 2012).
- The local effects of tumors, particularly those of the gastrointestinal (GI) tract, can impede eating. For instance, head and neck cancers can interfere with swallowing.
- Tumor-induced changes in metabolism can alter nutrient absorption or metabolism. Thus, it is possible for people with cancer to eat an adequate calorie intake and still lose weight.
- Cancer and cancer treatments can cause anorexia from a variety of factors, such as pain, depression/anxiety, early satiety, fatigue, nausea, loss of taste, sore mouth, dry mouth, thick saliva, or esophagitis. Anorexia can lead to weight loss, malnutrition, and poor prognosis.
- In addition to impairing intake, cancer treatments can alter nutrient intake, absorption, or need. While some effects may be relatively short term, such as the increased need for protein and calories to heal from surgery, others may be more long lasting, such as chronic dysphagia that may persist for years after treatment for head and neck cancer is completed.
- Adequate nutrition during the course of cancer treatment may improve tolerance to treatment, enhance immune function, aid in recovery, and maximize quality of life.
- Diet and lifestyle interventions can improve long-term outcomes for cancer survivors (Morey et al., 2009; Pierce et al., 2007).
- Palliative nutrition for terminally ill patients with cancer may improve quality of life and enhance well-being.

Nutrition in Cancer Prevention and Promotion

The WCRF's and AICR's (2007) second expert report, *Food, Nutrition, Physical Activity, and the Prevention of Cancer: A Global Perspective*, is the culmination of 5 years of rigorous and thorough review of the literature on diet and cancer. Contained within the report are the overriding guidelines to maintain a healthy weight, be physically active, and eat a mostly plant-based diet. The American Cancer Society (ACS) considered that report as well as subsequent comprehensive reviews when developing its most recent guidelines on nutrition and physical activity for cancer prevention (Kushi et al., 2012). The ACS guidelines (Table 22.1) are consistent with guidelines for cancer prevention issued by the WCRF/AICR as well as those from the

Table 22.1 ACS Guidelines on Nutrition and Physical Activity for Cancer Prevention

Guideline	Rationale
Achieve and maintain a healthy weight throughout life. ▪ Be as lean as possible throughout life without being underweight. ▪ Avoid excess weight gain at all ages. For those who are currently overweight or obese, losing even a small amount of weight has health benefits and is a good place to start. ▪ Engage in regular physical activity and limit consumption of high-calorie foods and beverages as key strategies for maintaining a healthy weight.	Some of the strongest links to cancer risk are excess body weight. There is convincing evidence that higher body fatness increases the risk of cancer of the esophagus, colon/rectum, postmenopausal breast, endometrium, and kidney (WCRF/AICR, 2007). Overweight and obesity probably increase the risk of gallbladder cancer and may be associated with an increased risk of cancer of the liver, non-Hodgkin lymphoma, multiple myeloma, cancer of the cervix, cancer of the ovary, and aggressive prostate cancer (Kushi et al., 2012). There are a few possible mechanisms by which fat may increase cancer risk: by increasing hormones that promote cancer cell growth; by promoting insulin resistance and hyperinsulinism, which increases the risk of certain cancers; or by promoting low levels of chronic inflammation, which can promote cancer cell growth and development (WCRF/AICR, 2007).
Adopt a physically active lifestyle. ▪ Adults should engage in at least 150 minutes of moderate-intensity or 75 minutes of vigorous-intensity activity each week, or an equivalent combination, preferably spread throughout the week. ▪ Children and adolescents should engage in at least 1 hour of moderate- or vigorous-intensity activity each day, with vigorous-intensity activity occurring at least 3 days each week. ▪ Limit sedentary behavior such as sitting, lying down, watching television, or other forms of screen-based entertainment. ▪ Doing some physical activity above usual activities, no matter what one's level of activity, can have many health benefits.	Physical activity may lower the risk of cancers of the breast, colon, and endometrium and advanced prostate cancer and may possibly lower the risk of pancreatic cancer (Kushi et al., 2012). Physical activity may help decrease cancer risk through its impact on sex hormones, insulin, prostaglandins, and immunity. Physical activity provides an added benefit of helping avoid excess body weight. Although the optimal intensity, duration, and frequency of physical activity needed to reduce the risk of cancer are not known, it is likely that activity in amounts higher than recommended may provide greater cancer risk reduction (Kushi et al., 2012). Evidence suggests that sitting time, independent of physical activity level, may contribute to the risk of various types of cancer. The health benefits of physical activity accumulate over a lifetime.
Consume a healthy diet, with an emphasis on plant foods. ▪ Choose foods and beverages in amounts that help achieve and maintain a healthy weight. ▪ Limit consumption of processed meat and red meat. ▪ Eat at least 2.5 cups of vegetables and fruits each day. ▪ Choose whole grains instead of refined grain products.	People who eat more processed and red meat, potatoes, refined grains, and sugar-sweetened beverages and foods are at higher risk for certain cancers (Kushi et al., 2012). Red and processed meats may increase the risk of colon and/or rectal cancer. People who eat a variety of vegetables and fruits, whole grains, and fish or poultry or less red and processed meats have a lower risk for developing certain cancers or dying from cancer. Fruits and vegetables may reduce the risk of cancers of the lung, mouth, pharynx, larynx, esophagus, stomach, and colorectum. A high fruit and vegetable intake is also associated with a lower risk of obesity, which impacts cancer risk. Whole grains may play a role in reducing the risk of GI cancers and may aid in weight control.
If you drink alcoholic beverages, limit consumption. ▪ Drink no more than 1 drink per day for women or 2 drinks per day for men.	Alcohol increases the risk of cancers of the mouth, pharynx, larynx, esophagus, liver, colorectum, and breast. It possibly increases the risk of pancreatic cancer. Alcohol can contribute to excess weight gain.

Source: Kushi, L., Doyle, C., McCullough, M., Rock, C. L., Demark-Wahnefried, W., Bandera, E. V., . . . Gansler, T. (2012). American Cancer Society guidelines on nutrition and physical activity for cancer prevention. *CA: A Cancer Journal for Clinicians, 62,* 30–67.

American Heart Association (Lichtenstein et al., 2006), American Diabetes Association (Bantle et al., 2008), and the *Dietary Guidelines for Americans, 2010* (U.S. Department of Agriculture and U.S. Department of Health and Human Services, 2010). All people, including cancer survivors, are urged to follow dietary recommendations to reduce the risk of cancer. See Chapter 8 for a comparison of nutrition guidelines to reduce the risk of cancer and other chronic diseases.

The Impact of Cancer on Nutrition

Cancer impacts nutrition through local effects caused by the tumor and by altering metabolism. It has been shown that at the time of diagnosis, 80% of patients with upper GI cancer and 60% of patients with lung cancer have already experienced significant weight loss, defined as a loss of at least 10% of body weight in 6 months (National Cancer Institute [NCI], 2011). Weight loss is an indicator of poor prognosis in people with cancer.

Local Tumor Effects

Local tumor effects occur when the tumor impinges on surrounding tissue, impairing its ability to function. The effects vary with the site and size of the tumor and are most likely to impact nutrition when the GI tract is involved (Table 22.2). GI obstruction can cause anorexia, dysphagia, early satiety, nausea, vomiting, pain, or diarrhea, leading to weight loss and malnutrition.

Metabolic Changes

Cancer Cachexia: a wasting syndrome associated with cancer characterized by progressive loss of body weight, fat, and **lean body mass**.

Lean Body Mass: the weight of the body minus the weight of fat.

A cascade of metabolic changes resulting from the effects of the tumor, the body's response, and the host–tumor interaction can lead to **cancer cachexia**, a complex multifactorial wasting syndrome (Donohoe, Ryan, and Reynolds, 2011). Tumor cells can produce proinflammatory and procachectic factors that stimulate inflammation and the breakdown of body protein and fat. The body responds with inflammatory and endocrine changes. The interplay between tumor and host leads to a systemic inflammatory response. The catabolic state is characterized by insulin resistance, decreased muscle protein synthesis, increased body protein turnover, and accelerated fat breakdown. Weight loss and anorexia occur, and cachexia results (NCI, 2011). Other signs and symptoms include reduced muscle strength, fatigue, and altered biochemistry, such as anemia and hypoalbuminemia

Table 22.2 Potential Local Effects of Cancer on Nutrition

Site	Potential Effects
Brain/CNS	Eating disabilities Chewing and swallowing difficulties
Head and neck	Difficulty in chewing and swallowing
Esophagus	Dysphagia related to obstruction Gastroesophageal reflux disease
Stomach	Early satiety, nausea, vomiting Impaired motility Obstruction, which may necessitate tube feeding or TPN
Bowel	Maldigestion and malabsorption Obstruction, which may necessitate tube feeding or TPN
Liver	Watery diarrhea related to an increase in serotonin, histamines, and other substances
Pancreas	Maldigestion and malabsorption Diabetes

CNS, central nervous system; TPN, total parenteral nutrition.

(Evans et al., 2008). Cachexia is associated with decreased quality of life, poor physical function, and poor prognosis.

The etiology of cancer cachexia is not completely understood. Cachexia appears to be unrelated to tumor size, type, or extent and occurs in both metastatic cancer and localized disease (NCI, 2011). It can develop in people who appear to have an adequate intake (NCI, 2011). Cachexia is believed to affect 60% to 80% of people with advanced cancer and has a mortality rate of 80% (von Haehling and Anker, 2010). People with GI cancers are at particular risk. Once wasting and weight loss begin, they are hard to reverse. Although some people respond to nutrition therapy, most do not experience a complete reversal of the syndrome, even with aggressive therapy (NCI, 2011). Medications may be used to stimulate appetite and promote weight gain associated with anorexia-cachexia syndrome, depending on the client's wishes, medical condition, and life expectancy (Table 22.3). Nutrition therapy, aimed at preserving lean muscle mass and fat stores, may improve quality of life and impact overall survival (NCI, 2011).

Table 22.3   Drugs Commonly Used for Anorexia-Cachexia Syndrome

Drug Category	Common Drugs Used	Comments
Progestational agents	Megestrol acetate	Promotes weight gain, but weight gain is primarily fat/water weight, not lean body tissue
Corticosteroids	Prednisolone	Stimulates appetite; studies show positive but short-term effects on appetite and quality of life but minimal or no effect on weight gain; risks limit suitability for long-term use
Cannabinoids	Dronabinol	Inconsistent evidence of effectiveness; has not shown superior benefit in promoting weight gain and appetite
Immunomodulatory agent	Thalidomide	Weight gain and increased lean body mass
Anabolic agents	Oxandrolone	Limited reports of successful appetite stimulation in cancer patients; increases lean body mass but only in people participating in resistance exercise
Antiserotonergic agent	Cyproheptadine hydrochloride	Minimal increase in appetite; no impact on progressive weight loss
Essential fatty acids	Omega-3 fatty acids (EPA/DHA)	Promote weight stabilization; no increase in lean body mass in clinical trials
Endocrine hormone	Melatonin	May slow weight loss; needs further study
Amino acids	Beta-hydroxy-beta-methylbutyrate (HMB) (a metabolite of leucine, glutamine, and arginine)	May decrease protein breakdown and loss of lean body mass in cachexia

Source: Academy of Nutrition and Dietetics. (2012). *Nutrition care manual.* Available at www.nutritioncaremanual.org. Accessed 7/19/12.

The Impact of Cancer Treatments

Cancer treatments include surgery, chemotherapy, radiation, immunotherapy, hemopoietic and stem cell transplantation, or a combination of therapies. Each treatment modality can contribute to progressive nutritional deterioration related to localized or systemic side effects that interfere with intake, increase nutrient losses, or alter metabolism. Nutritional therapy, used as an adjuvant to effective cancer therapy, helps to sustain the client through adverse side effects and may reduce morbidity and mortality. Conversely, inadequate nutrition can contribute to the incidence and severity of treatment side effects and increase the risk of infection, thereby reducing the chance for survival (Vigano, Watanabe, and Bruera, 1994).

Surgery

Surgery is often the primary treatment for cancer; approximately 60% of people diagnosed with cancer undergo some type of cancer-related surgery (NCI, 2011). People who are malnourished prior to surgery are at higher risk of morbidity and mortality. If time allows, nutritional deficiencies are corrected before surgery.

Postsurgical nutritional requirements increase for protein, calories, vitamin C, B vitamins, and iron to replenish losses and promote healing. Physiologic or mechanical barriers to good nutrition can occur depending on the type of surgery, with the greatest likelihood of complications arising from GI surgeries. Table 22.4 outlines potential side effects and complications incurred for various types of surgery.

Chemotherapy

Given alone or in combination, chemotherapy drugs damage the reproductive ability of both malignant and normal cells, especially rapidly dividing cells such as well-nourished cancer cells and normal cells of the GI tract, respiratory system, bone marrow, skin, and gonadal tissue. Cyclic administration of multiple drugs is given in maximum-tolerated doses.

The side effects of chemotherapy vary with the type of drug or combination of drugs used, dose, rate of excretion, duration of treatment, and individual tolerance. Chemotherapy side effects are systemic and, therefore, potentially more numerous than the localized effects seen with surgery or radiation. The most commonly experienced nutrition-related side effects are anorexia, taste alterations, early satiety, nausea, vomiting, mucositis/esophagitis, diarrhea, and constipation (NCI, 2011). Side effects increase the risk of malnutrition and weight loss, which may prolong recovery time between treatments. When subsequent chemotherapy treatments are delayed, successful treatment outcome is potentially threatened.

Radiation

Radiation causes cell death; particles of radioactive energy break chemical bonds, disrupting reproductive ability. Although radiation injures all rapidly dividing cells, it is most lethal for the poorly differentiated and rapidly proliferating cells of cancer tissue. Recovery from sublethal doses of radiation occurs in the interval between the first dose and subsequent doses. Normal tissue appears to recover more quickly from radiation damage than does cancerous tissue.

The type and intensity of radiation side effects depend on the type of radiation used, the site, the volume of tissue irradiated, the dose of radiation, the duration of therapy, and individual tolerance. Patients most at risk for nutrition-related side effects are those who have cancers of the head and neck, lungs, esophagus, cervix, uterus, colon, rectum, and pancreas (Table 22.5). Side effects usually develop around the second or third week of

Table 22.4 Potential Complications of Surgery

Type	Potential Complications
Head and neck resection	Impaired ability to speak, chew, salivate, swallow, smell, taste, and/or see Tube-feeding dependency
Esophagectomy or esophageal resection	Early satiety Regurgitation Fistula formation Stenosis Vagotomy → decreased stomach motility, decreased gastric acid production, diarrhea, steatorrhea
Gastric resection	Dumping syndrome: crampy diarrhea that develops quickly after eating, accompanied by flushing, dizziness, weakness, pain, distention, and vomiting Hypoglycemia Esophagitis Decreased gastric motility Fat malabsorption and diarrhea Deficiencies in iron, calcium, and fat-soluble vitamins Vitamin B_{12} malabsorption related to lack of intrinsic factor
Intestinal resection	Malnutrition related to generalized malabsorption Fluid and electrolyte imbalance Diarrhea Increased risk of renal oxalate stone formation and increased excretion of calcium Metabolic acidosis
Massive bowel resection	Steatorrhea Malnutrition related to severe generalized malabsorption Metabolic acidosis Dehydration
Ileostomy or colostomy	Fluid and electrolyte imbalance
Pancreatic resection	Generalized malabsorption Diabetes mellitus

treatment and then diminish 2 or 3 weeks after radiation therapy is completed. Some side effects may be chronic. Managing side effects helps improve intake and quality of life.

Immunotherapy

Immunotherapy seeks to enhance the body's immune system to help control cancer. The most common side effects include fever, which increases protein and calorie requirements, and nausea, vomiting, diarrhea, and fatigue. Left untreated, symptoms can cause weight loss and malnutrition, which impedes recovery.

Hemopoietic and Peripheral Blood Stem Cell Transplantation

Hemopoietic and stem cell transplants are preceded by high-dose chemotherapy and possibly total-body irradiation to suppress immune function and destroy cancer cells. Nutritional side effects arise from high-dose chemotherapy, total-body irradiation, and immunosuppressant medications, which are given before and after the procedure. Anorexia, taste alterations, nausea, vomiting, dry mouth, thick saliva, constipation, stomatitis, and esophagitis

Table 22.5 Potential Complications of Radiation

Area	Potential Complications
Head and neck	Altered or loss of taste (mouth blindness)
	Xerostomia (dry mouth)
	Thick salivary secretions
	Difficulty swallowing and chewing
	Loss of teeth
	Mucositis
	Stomatitis
Lower neck and midchest	Acute: esophagitis with dysphagia
	Delayed: fibrosis, esophageal stricture, dysphagia
	Nausea
	Edema
Abdomen and pelvis	Acute or chronic bowel damage can cause diarrhea, nausea, vomiting, enteritis, and malabsorption
	Bowel constriction, obstruction, or fistula formation
	Chronic blood loss from intestine and bladder
	Pelvic radiation can cause increased urinary frequency, urgency, and dysuria
Central nervous system	Nausea
	Dysgeusia

Neutropenia: abnormally low number of neutrophils in the blood, which increases the risk of infection.

may occur. Intestinal damage may cause severe diarrhea and malabsorption. Total parenteral nutrition (TPN) may be needed for 1 to 2 months after bone marrow transplantation.

When an oral diet resumes, a liquid diet restricted in lactose, fiber, and fat is given to minimize malabsorption and improve tolerance. Solid foods are gradually reintroduced. **Neutropenia** leaves the patient susceptible to infection, so precautionary measures must be taken to prevent foodborne illness (Box 22.1). Initially, most fresh fruit and vegetables

---

Box 22.1   Strategies to Reduce the Risk of Foodborne Illness

- Wash hands before and after handling food and eating and after using the restroom.
- Cook all meat, fish, and poultry to the well-done stage.
- Do not eat raw or undercooked eggs such as soft-boiled eggs, "over-easy" eggs, or Caesar salads with raw eggs in the dressing.
- Do not eat sushi, raw seafood, raw meats, or unpasteurized milk or dairy products.
- Do not drink water unless it is known to be safe.
- Refrigerate foods immediately after purchase.
- Avoid cross-contamination by using separate cutting boards and work surfaces for raw meats and poultry; keep work surfaces clean.
- Wash fruits and vegetables thoroughly in clean water.
- Do not use moldy or damaged fruits and vegetables.
- Thaw food in the refrigerator, never at room temperature.
- If the microwave is used to thaw frozen meat, cook the meat immediately after it is defrosted.
- Refrigerate leftovers immediately after eating; thoroughly reheat before eating.
- Discard leftovers after 24 hours.
- Keep hot foods >140°F and cold foods <40°F.
- Use expiration dates on food packaging to discard foods that may be unsafe to eat.
- Avoid salad bars and buffets when eating out.

and ground meats may be excluded to reduce the risk of foodborne illness. A high-protein, high-calorie, high-calcium diet is needed to counter the negative nitrogen and calcium balances caused by immunosuppressant medications.

Nutrition Therapy During Cancer Treatment

A "typical" cancer client does not exist. Whereas some clients present with weight loss and malnutrition at the time of cancer diagnosis, others are asymptomatic, and a substantial proportion are overweight or obese (Barrera and Demark-Wahnefried, 2009). The course of treatment may be aggressive or palliative; it may include surgery, chemotherapy, radiation, or a combination of treatments. The effect on nutritional status and intake may be mild or dramatic. Nutrition intake and status should be routinely monitored so nutrition therapy interventions can be adjusted accordingly. The goals of nutrition therapy for people being treated for cancer are to

- Manage weight. For normal-weight and underweight patients, the goal is to prevent weight loss. Preventing weight gain is appropriate for those who are overweight or obese; have certain hormonal cancers, such as prostate or breast cancer; and are treated with long-term, high-dose steroid therapy.
- Maintain lean body mass. Adequate protein and calories may help preserve lean body mass, muscle strength, and functional capacity.
- Prevent or reverse nutrient deficiencies. Food sources of nutrients are preferred over nutrient supplements.
- Maximize quality of life. Adequate nutrition may improve tolerance to treatment, improve immunocompetence, and promote wound healing.

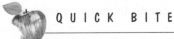

QUICK BITE

Selected high-calorie, high-protein nutritional formulas

	Calories (per 240 mL)	Protein (g/240 mL)
Ensure High-Protein	230	12
Boost	240	10
Boost High-Protein	240	15
Carnation Instant Breakfast (made with 8 oz whole milk)	300	12
Ensure Plus	360	13
Carnation Instant Breakfast Plus	375	12
Resource Shake Plus	480	15

Calories and Protein

Calories and protein are nutrients of concern given the impact metabolic changes and cancer treatments can have on nutritional status and that significant weight loss is linked to poor prognosis. Calorie needs may range from 25 to 30 cal/kg for nonambulatory or sedentary adults to 35 cal/kg or more for hypermetabolic or severely stressed patients. Protein needs range from 1.0 to 2.5 g/kg. Despite general guidelines for how much protein and calories may be needed, in practice, the challenge may be to simply get patients to eat enough to avoid weight loss. Strategies to maximize intake include getting the patient to

- Eat more food, which is not a realistic option for most people experiencing anorexia, nausea, or other side effects of cancer or cancer treatments.

Box 22.2   WAYS TO INCREASE THE PROTEIN AND CALORIE DENSITY OF FOODS

To Increase Protein and Calories
- Add skim milk powder to milk to make double-strength milk; chill well before serving.
- Use double-strength milk on hot or cold cereals and in scrambled eggs, soups, gravies, casseroles, milk shakes, and milk-based desserts.
- Substitute whole milk for water in recipes.
- Add grated cheese to soups, casseroles, vegetable dishes, rice, and noodles.
- Use peanut butter as a spread on slices of apple, banana, pear, crackers, or waffles; use as a filling for celery.
- Add finely chopped, hard-cooked eggs to sauces; add cream to soups and casseroles.
- Choose desserts made with eggs or milk such as sponge cake, angel food cake, custard, and puddings.
- Dip meat, poultry, and fish in eggs or milk and coat with bread or cereal crumbs before baking, broiling, or pan frying.
- Use yogurt as a topping for fruit, plain cakes, or other desserts; use in gravies and dips.

To Increase Calories
- Mix cream cheese with butter and spread on hot bread and rolls.
- Whenever possible, add butter to hot foods: breads, pancakes, waffles, soups, vegetables, potatoes, cooked cereal, rice, and pasta.
- Substitute mayonnaise for salad dressing in salads, eggs, casseroles, and sandwiches.
- Add dried fruit, nuts, or granola to desserts and cereal.
- Use whipped cream on pies, fruit pudding, gelatin, ice cream, and other desserts and in coffee, tea, and hot chocolate.
- Use marshmallows in hot chocolate, on fruits, and in desserts.
- Top baked potatoes, vegetables, and fruits with sour cream.
- Snack frequently on nuts, dried fruit, candy, buttered popcorn, cheese, granola, and ice cream.
- Use honey on toast, cereal, and fruit and in coffee and tea.

- Eat small, frequent snacks throughout the day rather than three meals. Smaller feedings are less overwhelming, especially when anorexia is an issue.
- Eat food that has been modified to be more protein and calorie dense. This approach can be effective if the client or caregiver understands how to increase the protein and calorie density of a variety of foods. Suggestions for increasing protein and calorie density appear in Box 22.2.
- Consume high-protein, high-calorie nutritional supplements, which may be the easiest and most consistent way to achieve a high-calorie, high-protein intake. They can be used as a supplement or replacement for solid food.
- A combination of the above.

Managing Nutrition-Related Symptoms

In a study of patients with advanced cancer, some degree of impairment in taste and/or smell was reported by 86% of patients, and approximately 50% reported that the impairment interfered with their enjoyment of eating (NCI, 2011). Patients may experience a decreased threshold for urea (bitter) and an increased threshold for sucrose (sweet), although these changes are not universal among all people with cancer. Poor appetite, nausea, early satiety, and impairments in taste and smell often occur together and are significantly linked to decreased calorie intake (NCI, 2011). Managing nutrition-related symptoms has the potential to improve calorie intake and maintain weight (Box 22.3).

Box 22.3   TIPS FOR MANAGING NUTRITION-RELATED PROBLEMS

Anorexia
- Overeat during "good" days.
- Eat a high-protein, high-calorie, nutrient-dense breakfast if appetite is best in the morning.
- Eat a small amount of food at set, frequent intervals, such as every 1–2 hours by the clock.
- Add extra protein and calories to food.
- Eat nutrient-dense foods first.
- Limit liquids with meals to avoid early satiety and bloating at mealtime.
- Use nutrition formulas (instant breakfast mixes, milk shakes, commercial supplements) in place of meals when appetite deteriorates or the client is too tired to eat.
- Make eating a pleasant experience by eating in a bright, cheerful environment, playing soft music, and enjoying the company of friends or family.
- Avoid strong food odors if they contribute to anorexia. Cook outdoors on a grill, serve cold foods rather than hot foods, or use takeout meals that do not need to be prepared at home. In the hospital, the tray cover should be removed before the tray is placed in front of the client so that food odors can dissipate.

Nausea
- Rinse mouth before and after eating.
- Eat frequently. Some people feel better by keeping a small amount of food in the stomach at all times.
- Slowly sip fluids throughout the day.
- Eat foods served cold, such as chicken salad instead of hot baked chicken or deli roast beef instead of pot roast.
- Eat high-carbohydrate, low-fat, easy-to-digest foods such as toast, crackers, yogurt, sherbet, cooked cereal, soft or canned fruits, watermelon, bananas, fruit juices, and angel food cake.
- Avoid fatty, greasy, fried, or strongly seasoned foods.
- Sit up for 1 hour after eating.
- Keep track of and avoid foods that cause nausea.
- Avoid eating 1–2 hours before chemotherapy or radiotherapy.
- Take antiemetics as prescribed even when symptoms are absent.

Fatigue
- Eat a hearty breakfast because fatigue may worsen as the day progresses.
- Engage in regular exercise if possible.
- Consume easy-to-eat foods that can be prepared with a minimal amount of effort, such as frozen dinners, takeout foods, sandwiches, instant breakfast mixes and liquid formulas, cheese and crackers, peanut butter on crackers, yogurt, and pudding.
- If weight loss isn't a problem, avoid overeating for energy. Excess weight worsens fatigue.
- Enlist the help of friends and family to provide meals.

(continues on page 604)

Box 22.3	Tips for Managing Nutrition-Related Problems (continued)

Taste Changes

- Use sugar-free lemon drops, gum, or mints to counter a metallic or bitter taste in the mouth.
- Brush your teeth or rinse with a mouthwash before eating.
- Eat small frequent meals.
- Use plastic utensils if food has a metallic taste.
- Experiment with tart foods such as citrus juices, cranberry juice, pickles, vinegar, or relishes to help overcome metallic taste.
- Eat meat with something sweet, such as pork with applesauce or turkey with cranberry sauce.
- Substitute poultry, eggs, cheese, and mild fish for beef and pork if they have a "bad," "rotten," or "fecal" taste.
- Add coffee to a sweet, milk-based beverage or buttermilk to a smoothie to cut sweetness.
- Avoid foods that are offensive; stick to those that taste good.
- Try new foods, such as lemon yogurt in place of strawberry.

Sore Mouth (Stomatitis)

- Practice good oral hygiene (thorough cleaning with a soft-bristle toothbrush or cotton swabs plus frequent mouth rinses with normal saline and water or baking soda and water). Commercial mouthwashes containing alcohol may irritate and burn the oral mucosa.
- Eat cold or room temperature foods.
- Eat soft, nonirritating foods that are easy to chew and swallow, such as bananas, applesauce, watermelon, canned fruit, cottage cheese, yogurt, mashed potatoes, macaroni and cheese, puddings, milkshakes, instant breakfast mixes, scrambled eggs, oatmeal, and other cooked cereals.
- Add gravy, broth, or sauces to increase the fluid content of foods, as appropriate.
- Cut food into small pieces.
- Numb the mouth with frozen bananas, ice chips, ice cream, or popsicles.
- Avoid spices, acidic foods, coarse foods, salty foods, alcohol, and smoking that can aggravate an already irritated oral mucosa.
- Consume high-calorie, high-protein drinks in place of traditional meals.
- Use a straw to drink liquids.
- Avoid wearing ill-fitting dentures.

Xerostomia (Dry Mouth)

- Use an alcohol-free mouth rinse before eating.
- Drink fluids with meals and all day long.
- Eat moist foods softened with gravies or sauces. Casseroles and stews are easier to eat than baked or roasted meats.
- Avoid dry, coarse foods.
- Avoid foods that stick to the roof of the mouth such as peanut butter.
- Avoid sugary food and beverages that promote dental decay.
- Drink high-calorie, high-protein liquids between meals.
- Stimulate saliva production with citrus fruits if tolerated, such as lemons, oranges, limes, and grapefruit.
- Consume frozen desserts, such as ice cream and frozen yogurt.

> **Box 22.3   Tips for Managing Nutrition-Related Problems** (continued)
>
> - Eating papaya may help break up "ropy" saliva.
> - Use ice chips and sugar-free hard candies and gum between meals to relieve dryness.
> - Use a straw to drink liquids.
> - Apply a moisturizer to the lips to help prevent drying.
> - Brush after every meal and snack.
>
> **Diarrhea**
> - Replace fluid and electrolytes with broth, soups, sports drinks, and canned fruit.
> - Drink at least 1 cup of liquid after each loose bowel movement.
> - Limit caffeine, hot or cold liquids, and high-fat foods because they aggravate diarrhea.
> - Avoid gassy foods and liquids such as dried peas and beans, cruciferous vegetables, carbonated beverages, and chewing gum.
> - Try foods high in pectin and other soluble fibers to slow transit time, such as oatmeal, cooked carrots, bananas, peeled apples, and applesauce.
> - Avoid sugar-free candy or gum containing sorbitol because it can contribute to osmotic diarrhea.
> - Unless tolerance to lactose has been confirmed, limit or avoid milk.

Enteral and Parenteral Nutrition Support

For both physiologic and psychological reasons, an oral diet is preferred whenever possible. When oral intake is inadequate or contraindicated, enteral or parenteral nutrition can nourish critically ill cancer patients. A client may be a candidate for nutrition support if one or more of the following criteria are met (NCI, 2011):

- Weight of less than 80% of ideal or a recent unintentional weight loss of more than 10% of usual weight
- Malabsorption of nutrients related to disease, short bowel syndrome, or cancer treatments
- Fistulas or draining abscesses
- Inability to eat or drink for more than 5 days
- Moderate or high nutritional risk as determined by nutritional screening or assessment
- Client or caregiver demonstrate competency in nutrition support for discharge planning

Although enteral nutrition (EN) therapy may prevent or treat malnutrition in people with cancer, it is not routinely used in well-nourished patients undergoing chemotherapy or surgery. EN is typically reserved for patients with certain types of cancer or for those whose treatment plan is in jeopardy because of malnutrition, such as patients undergoing chemoradiation to the head or neck. In this population, the early use of percutaneous endoscopic gastrostomy (PEG) tube feedings has been found to decrease weight loss, dehydration, malnutrition, and unplanned treatment interruptions (Academy of Nutrition and Dietetics, 2012). In addition, an arginine-enriched enteral formula given perioperatively to malnourished patients with head and neck cancer has been shown to improve long-term survival (Buijs et al., 2010). Likewise, for patients undergoing treatment for GI cancers, glutamine-enriched formulas have been shown to help maintain gut integrity and protect against damage from radiation and chemotherapy (NCI, 2011). For all other cases, the decision to use EN is individualized and should be limited to malnourished patients with a functional GI tract who are unable to consume an adequate intake of nutrients orally.

Parenteral nutrition (PN) can be a lifesaving therapy because it can deliver nutrients to patients who have a nonfunctional GI tract, such as those with obstruction, intractable nausea and/or vomiting, short bowel syndrome, or ileus (NCI, 2011). Other indications include severe diarrhea or malabsorption, severe mucositis or esophagitis, high-output GI fistula that cannot be bypassed by enteral intubation, and severe preoperative malnutrition. PN increases the risk of serious infectious, metabolic, and mechanical complications and should not be used for less than 5 days or in patients who are not hemodynamically stable. PN has not been shown to improve outcomes in end-of-life situations (McClave et al., 2009).

Palliative Nutrition Therapy

For clients with terminal cancer who are not being aggressively treated, nutrition therapy is an integral component of palliative care, with the goals of providing comfort and relieving side effects. Eating is encouraged as a source of pleasure, not as an adjunct to treatment. The client's requests and preferences are more important than the nutritional quality of the diet. Box 22.4 lists supportive measures for palliative nutrition therapy.

Nutrition for Cancer Survivors

The ACS and WCRF/AICR encourage cancer survivors to follow diet and lifestyle recommendations for cancer prevention—namely, maintain a healthy weight, be physically active, and eat a mostly plant-based diet (see Table 22.1). Data from observational studies of colorectal cancer survivors indicate that people who report a prudent diet (high in fruits, vegetables, whole grains, and low-fat dairy products) have improved overall survival and lower rates of colorectal recurrence and mortality than those who consume a typical Western diet (Meyerhardt et al., 2007). Likewise, cross-sectional data from breast and prostate cancer survivors show that diet quality during survivorship is significantly and positively associated with quality of life and physical functioning (Denmark-Wahnefried et al., 2004; Wayne et al., 2006). Although scientific evidence supporting nutrition recommendations for cancer survivors is currently limited (Robien and Denmark-Wahnefried, 2011), improving exercise and eating habits may reduce cancer recurrence as well as the risk of other chronic diseases.

Dietary Supplements

A study of cancer survivors found that more than 69% reported using dietary supplements after their diagnosis of cancer (Ferrucci, McCorkie, Smith, Stein, and Cartmel,

---

Box 22.4 SUPPORTIVE MEASURES FOR PALLIATIVE NUTRITION THERAPY

- Control unpleasant side effects, such as pain, constipation, nausea, vomiting, and heartburn, with medication.
- Respect the client's wishes regarding the level of nutritional support desired.
- Provide adequate mouth care to control dryness and thirst.
- Respect the client's personal tastes and preferences.
- Ensure a pleasant eating environment and serve attractive food.
- Serve food of appropriate textures.
- Use a team approach that includes physician, dietitian, and nurse.

2009). The most common reasons given for using supplements included "something they could do to help themselves" and "to boost their immune system." However, a majority of randomized controlled trials have not demonstrated a decrease in incidence or recurrence of cancer from nutrient supplementation (e.g., Lee et al., 2005; Wactawski-Wende et al., 2006). In some studies, supplements were found to increase the risk of cancer, such as an increased number of colorectal cancers in participants receiving folic acid in the Aspirin/Folate Polyp Prevention Study (Cole et al., 2007). Although routine vitamin and mineral supplements that provide 100% of the Dietary Reference Intake (DRI) are often recommended when intake is suboptimal, both the ACS and WCRF/AIRC recommend that cancer survivors obtain nutrients from food, not supplements (Kushi et al., 2012; WCRF/AIRC, 2007).

NUTRITION AND IMMUNODEFICIENCY

Nutritional status and immunity are interrelated.

- Good nutrition is important for immune system functioning. For instance, protein and various micronutrients are involved in the synthesis of enzymes, complement, antibodies, and other proteins important in immune system functioning. Malnutrition can impair immune system function and the ability to fight infection (Hughes and Kelly, 2006; Rasouli and Kern, 2008).
- Infection can impair nutritional status by causing inflammatory, hormonal, and immune responses that increase metabolic rate and nutrient requirements, promote loss of lean body tissue, cause anorexia, and alter nutrient storage and availability. Infections in the intestines can lead to diarrhea, malabsorption of nutrients, blood loss, and damage to the intestinal lining. Severe infection increases the risk of malnutrition.

Antiretroviral Therapy (ART): a combination of antiretroviral therapy medications that are typically used to control and reduce viral load.

HIV is a chronic infectious disease with acute episodes of opportunistic infection or malignancy (Kitahata, Tegger, Wagner, and Holmes, 2002). People who are well nourished and whose viral load is controlled are more likely to withstand the effects of HIV infection, possibly delaying the progression of HIV disease (Thomas and Mkandawire, 2006). Conversely, malnourished people with HIV infection, including those receiving **antiretroviral therapy (ART)**, have higher death rates than those who are well nourished (Mangili, Murman, Zampini, and Wanke, 2006). Appropriate body mass index (BMI) and body protein stores are correlated to the ability to survive HIV disease (Mocroft et al., 2007; Srasuebkul et al., 2009).

HIV-Associated Weight Loss and Wasting

HIV-related wasting syndrome, an AIDS-defining medical diagnosis, is defined by the CDC as unintentional weight loss of more than 10% of baseline weight plus either diarrhea or chronic weakness and fever for more than 30 days without a known cause (CDC, 1992). Shortcomings with this definition are that (1) it assumes that baseline weight, which may have been reported not measured, was the patient's usual or ideal weight and (2) the rate of weight loss is not considered (Mangili et al., 2006). Rapid or significant weight loss may be a risk even if BMI stays within the normal range (Mangili et al., 2006). In HIV wasting, there is a direct correlation between weight loss and death (Kotler, Tierney, Wang, and Pierson, 1989), although it has not been shown that wasting itself is the cause of death (Kosmiski, 2011).

Wasting causes a loss of both lean body mass and fat. Studies suggest that the type of weight loss in HIV-associated wasting varies with baseline body composition and that women may lose primarily fat, whereas men preferentially lose lean body mass until their body composition changes and then fat becomes preferentially lost (Academy of Nutrition and Dietetics, 2012). However, weight loss is a stronger predictor of death than loss of lean body mass, and baseline BMI is important; people with a baseline BMI ≥25 have a much lower risk of dying than those with a baseline BMI of <25, even though 25 is the beginning of the "overweight" range (Mangili et al., 2006).

When the AIDS epidemic began, severe malnutrition and weight loss were common. Despite major advances in the treatment and survival of people living with HIV and AIDS (PLHA), the incidence of wasting syndrome appears to have held steady (Siddiqui et al., 2009). Observations suggest that weight loss or wasting occurs in more than 30% of HIV-infected patients regardless of anti-HIV treatment (Mangili et al., 2006). Although ART has significantly improved morbidity and mortality related to HIV infection, it has not eliminated the issue of weight loss. All people who are HIV positive, including those treated with ART, are at risk for wasting.

Like cancer cachexia, the etiology of HIV-associated wasting is multifactorial and not completely understood. Contributing factors may be decreased intake related to nausea, anorexia, mouth infections, or fatigue. Diarrhea and malabsorption of nutrients decrease nutrient availability. Opportunistic infections or malignancies may also contribute to altered metabolism and weight loss, although they are not the major cause of wasting in PLHA. Excessive production of **cytokines** has also been implicated in HIV-associated weight loss. Although the majority of weight loss currently seen in PLHA cannot be explained, impaired intake and altered metabolism may be at least partially responsible.

Cytokines: a group name for more than 100 different proteins involved in immune responses; they are also critical for normal growth and development. Prolonged production of proinflammatory cytokines promotes hypercatabolism (hyper = excessive; catabolism = breaking down phase of metabolism).

Impaired Intake

Results from the Nutrition for Healthy Living Cohort study show that impaired intake among PLHA may be related to diet itself, GI symptoms, or malabsorption and GI dysfunction (Mangili et al., 2006). For instance,

- Men in the lowest CD4+ cell count percentile need the most calories per kilogram of body weight to maintain a lower BMI, yet their total daily calorie intake was not different than that of men of similar age in the general population. This suggests that nutritional need is high and intake falls short.
- Episodes of acute weight loss, defined as ≥5% of body weight, were associated with oral symptoms and difficulty swallowing but not anorexia. Even in the absence of an opportunistic infection, many people may have GI symptoms related to HIV infection or HIV medications that increase the risk of weight loss.
- Eighty-eight percent of the cohort had at least one abnormality in GI function, such as malabsorption. Because malabsorption can occur in the absence of diarrhea, malabsorption cannot be excluded on the basis of normal bowel patterns alone. Uncorrected, malabsorption can lead to malnutrition, wasting, and impaired quality of life.
- In many cases, socioeconomic factors, not clinical factors, may be blamed for poor intake. Almost 8% of participants did not have access to adequate food.

Changes in Metabolism

Viral Load: the level of virus or viral markers measured in the blood.

Resting energy expenditure (REE), the amount of calories used to fuel the involuntary activities of the body, increases in people with HIV/AIDS who are asymptomatic and untreated (Kosmiski, 2011). **Viral load** and ART have also been found to

Lipodystrophy: also called fat redistribution syndrome; a condition characterized by changes in body shape (loss of subcutaneous fat in the limbs, buttocks, and face and fat accumulation in the abdomen, back of neck and shoulders, and breast areas) and metabolism (increased resistance to insulin and abnormally high levels of blood cholesterol and triglycerides). Characteristics may occur separately or in any combination. Weight change is not always present.

independently increase REE (Roubenoff et al., 2002; Shevitz et al., 1999). Although the increase in REE may contribute to weight loss and wasting, the increase in REE is typically offset by a decrease in calories expended on physical activity (Kosmiski, 2011). Significant decreases in caloric intake may be a more important factor in weight loss than the increase in REE.

HIV **lipodystrophy** is a metabolic alteration characterized by changes in the distribution of body fat and metabolism. Most commonly, subcutaneous fat loss occurs in the face, extremities, and buttocks; fat accumulation may be seen at the back of the neck and trunk. These changes in body fat distribution do not necessarily cause a change in weight and may mask wasting to some extent. Lipodystrophy may also cause insulin resistance, hypertriglyceridemia, and excess fat in the liver and skeletal muscle and is associated with increased REE (Kosmiski, 2011). ART is implicated in its development, although the exact cause is not clear. Factors affecting risk include age, gender, genetics, length of time the patient has been HIV positive, and severity of the disease (Kressy, Wanke, and Gerrior, 2010). Lipodystrophy is not life threatening, but emotional distress caused by the significant changes in body shape and social stigmatization may cause clients to decrease or stop their ARTs because they are believed to be involved in its cause.

Nutrition Therapy

An individualized assessment determines the client's level of risk based on weight, weight change, changes in body composition, biochemical markers of malnutrition, clinical signs of malnutrition, dietary intake, and symptoms of HIV or side effects of treatment that impact intake or nutritional status. An individualized plan of care is designed that takes into account the client's socioeconomic, cultural, and ethnic background. Ideally, nutrition therapy begins before the client exhibits any symptoms of HIV disease even if intake appears adequate because the effectiveness of nutrition therapy may be limited once the client is ill enough to need hospital care.

Nutrition therapy for PLHA seeks to meet the client's nutrient needs, alleviate symptoms, and manage complications of the disease or medication intolerance. Although scientific knowledge about the role of nutrition in HIV is incomplete, it is apparent that the nutrient needs of PLHA differ from those of noninfected people, even before the onset of symptoms (e.g., weight loss). There are no unanimously agreed upon recommendations for calories or nutrients despite the universal goals of maintaining body weight and lean body mass. Tips for healthy eating with HIV are outlined in Box 22.5.

Box 22.5   HEALTHY EATING TIPS FOR PATIENTS WITH HIV

- Eat a diet rich in whole grains, vegetables, fruits, and legumes with lean sources of protein.
- Make at least half of all grain choices whole grains.
- Eat 5–6 servings, or approximately 3 cups/day, of a variety of fruits and vegetables.
- Choose skinless poultry, fish, extra-lean cuts of pork and beef, and low-fat milk and dairy products.
- Limit sweetened beverages and foods high in added sugar.
- Eat at least 1 serving/day of nuts, seeds, or legumes.
- Eat some carbohydrate, protein, and fat at each meal and snack.

Source: Woods, M., Potts, E., & Connors, J. (2010). *Building a high-quality diet.* Available at http://www.tufts.edu/med/nutrition-infection/hiv/health_high_quality_diet.html. Accessed on 8/18/08.

Calories

The World Health Organization (WHO) advisory group on nutrition and HIV issued recommendations in 2003 that suggested calorie intakes increase by 10% for asymptomatic clients so that body weight can be maintained despite the increase in REE (WHO, 2003). The report indicated that when HIV is symptomatic, calorie needs are estimated to increase by 20% to 30% above normal. A joint effort between the National Institute of Child Health and Human Development, the Office of AIDS Research of the National Institutes of Health, and the Department of Nutrition for Health and Development of the WHO recently created a working group (WG) to review those guidelines. The WG determined that an extra 10% increase in calories for asymptomatic patients is warranted but that there is limited evidence to support the recommendation of a 30% increase when HIV is symptomatic or the patient has an active infection (Raiten, Mulligan, Papathakis, and Wanke, 2011).

Calorie recommendations from HIV Research of the Nutrition Infection Unit at Tufts University School of Medicine are as follows (the "normal" healthy adult standard commonly used is 30 cal/kg) (Woods et al., 2010):

- 37 to 45 cal/kg if the client's weight is stable and there are no secondary infections
- 45 cal/kg if the client has an opportunistic infection
- 55 cal/kg if the client is losing weight

Protein

There is no evidence to indicate protein need increases in HIV-infected adults nor is there evidence to suggest that protein need does not increase (Raiten et al., 2011). Adding protein may be beneficial in maintaining or building lean body mass (American Dietetic Association, 2010). According to Woods et al. (2010), 1.2 to 2.0 g/kg/day of protein may be needed, an increase above the normal Recommended Dietary Allowance (RDA) of 0.8 g/kg/day. This recommendation translates to a rule-of-thumb guideline of 100 to 150 g/day for men and 80 to 100 g/day for women.

Fat

There is no evidence to support HIV-specific recommendations regarding the type or amount of fat for PLHA (Raiten et al., 2011). Because PLHA may have lipid abnormalities, a low–saturated fat diet, not a low–total fat diet, may be beneficial (see "Metabolic Alterations of Lipodystrophy"). A heart-healthy diet with monounsaturated fats and omega-3 fatty acids may help reduce the risk of cardiovascular disease.

Vitamins and Minerals

Observational studies suggest that low blood levels and inadequate intakes of some vitamins and minerals are associated with faster HIV disease progression and mortality (WHO, 2003). Nutrient deficiencies may occur from poor intake, malabsorption, infections, or diet–medication interactions. In general, dietary intake of micronutrients at RDA amounts is a reasonable recommendation for people with clinically stable disease (Forrester and Sztam, 2011). In some PLHA, short-term, high-dose multiple micronutrient supplementation may be beneficial, depending on the patient's nutritional status and immune status and the presence of coinfections (Forrester and Sztam, 2011). Evidence suggests potential harm from higher doses of selected micronutrients, especially of vitamin A and zinc in some populations (Raiten et al., 2011).

Enteral and Parenteral Nutrition Support

Clients who are unable to consume an adequate oral intake may require tube feeding for supplemental or complete nutrition. The same guidelines for use apply in HIV as in other populations, with extra attention to ensure sanitary conditions. The use of sterile water may be necessary for patients who have severe immune function impairments. PN is reserved for clients whose GI tract is nonfunctional. Hydrolyzed formulas consumed orally may be just as effective as PN in preventing weight loss in patients with severe malabsorption—with none of the risk associated with PN.

Manage Symptoms

Clients with HIV/AIDS may experience problems with appetite and intake similar to those of cancer clients. Nutrition therapy recommendations in Box 22.3 for managing nutrition-related problems are appropriate for PLHA as well as for people with cancer. As in the case of cancer, oral supplements are frequently used because they tend to leave the stomach quickly, are easy to consume, and provide significant quantities of calories and protein. Small frequent feedings (e.g., six to nine times daily) are encouraged.

Metabolic Alterations of Lipodystrophy

Nutrition therapy and exercise may help reverse some changes in body shape and improve the metabolic abnormalities of glucose intolerance, hypertriglyceridemia, and hypercholesterolemia. A Mediterranean diet low in saturated fat, refined sugar, and alcohol, and high in monounsaturated fats, fiber-rich whole grains, vegetables, and fruit may help to improve lipoprotein profiles and glucose tolerance. Fiber alone may help promote abdominal fat loss and improve insulin resistance. Resistance exercise, with or without an aerobic component, is recommended because it increases lean body mass and improves insulin resistance (Leyes, Martinez, and Forga Mde, 2008) and may also lower triglycerides and decrease abdominal fat (Kressy, Wanke, and Gerrior, 2010).

Food and Drug Interactions

Due to food–drug interactions, medication schedules and food restrictions are both complex and strict. Some clients stop ART because they are convinced that the drugs' side effects and complicated regimens are not worth the effort. Maximum effectiveness of drug therapy is dependent on compliance with the medication schedule and food restrictions. Table 22.6 lists drugs that should be taken on an empty stomach and those that need to be taken with food.

Food Safety

Because PLHA have compromised immune systems, steps should be taken to reduce the risk of foodborne illness (Fig. 22.1). Food safety strategies are listed in Box 22.1 (see Chapter 9 for more on foodborne illness).

Table 22.6 Single HIV/AIDS Medications and Timing of Food Intake

Generic Name (Brand Name)	Take with Food	Take on Empty Stomach	Take Without Regard to Food
Fusion inhibitor			
Enfuvirtide (Fuzeon)			√
Nucleoside reverse transcriptase inhibitors (NRTIs)			
Abacavir (Ziagen)			√
Didanosine (Videx)		√	
Emtricitabine (Emtriva)			√
Lamivudine (Epivir)			√
Stavudine (Zerit)			√
Tenofovir (Viread)	√		
Zalcitabine (Hivid)		√	
Zidovudine (Retrovir)			√ Do not take with high-fat meal.
Nonnucleoside reverse transcriptase inhibitors (NNRTIs)			
Delavirdine (Rescriptor)			√ Avoid alcohol.
Efavirenz (Sustiva)		√ Avoid alcohol.	
Etravirine (Intelence)	√		
Nevirapine (Viramune)			√
Rilpivirine (Endurant)	√		
Protease inhibitors			
Amprenavir (Agenerase)			√ Do not take with high-fat meal.
Atazanavir (Reyataz)	√		
Darunavir (Prezista)			√
Fosamprenavir (Lexiva)			√
Indinavir (Crixivan)			
Lopinavir (Kaletra)	√		
Nelfinavir (Viracept)	√ Take with fatty food		
Ritonavir (Norvir)	√		
Saquinavir (Invirase)	√ Take within 2 hours of a high-calorie, high-fat meal		
Tipranavir (Aptivus)	√ Take with high-fat meal		
Entry inhibitors			
Maraviroc (Selzentry)			√
Integrase inhibitors			
Raltegravir (Isentress)			√

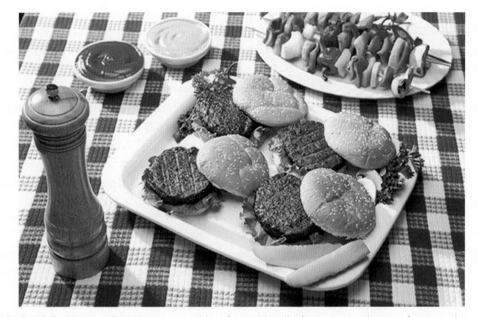

■ **FIGURE 22.1**   Cooking ground beef to 160° eliminates any danger from pathogenic bacteria such as *Escherichia coli*. (***Source:*** U.S. Department of Agriculture. Photo by Stephen Ausmus.)

NURSING PROCESS: *Cancer*

Karen is a 59-year-old former smoker who now calls herself a "health nut." She was recently diagnosed with lung cancer. She had surgery to remove her right lung and is receiving chemotherapy for cancerous "spots" on the left lung and stomach. She has lost 28 pounds and complains of nausea, vomiting, and a bad taste in her mouth. Because she has followed a healthy diet to prevent cancer for years, she is reluctant to now change her eating habits and eat more protein, fat, and calories. Right now she is eating mostly fruit, sherbet, and skim milk.

Assessment

Medical–Psychosocial History	▪ Medical history such as diabetes, heart disease, or hypertension
	▪ Types of drugs the client is receiving through chemotherapy; other prescribed medications that affect nutrition
	▪ Physician's goals and plan of treatment
	▪ Pattern of nausea and vomiting
	▪ Client's understanding of increased nutritional needs related to cancer and cancer therapies
	▪ Willingness to change her attitudes toward food and nutrition
	▪ Psychosocial and economic issues such as financial status, employment, and outside support system
	▪ Usual activity patterns
Anthropometric Assessment	▪ Height, current weight, usual weight
	▪ Rate of weight loss; percentage of usual body weight loss
	▪ BMI

(continues on page 614)

NURSING PROCESS: *Cancer* (continued)

Biochemical and Physical Assessment	▪ Laboratory data: prealbumin, serum electrolytes, any abnormal values
	▪ Nitrogen balance study, if available
	▪ General appearance/evidence of muscle wasting
Dietary Assessment	▪ How many daily meals and snacks are you eating?
	▪ What is a typical day's intake for you?
	▪ How is your appetite? When is your appetite the best?
	▪ What do you do to alleviate nausea?
	▪ How has your sense of taste changed? What do you do to cope with the changes?
	▪ Do you have any food allergies or intolerances?
	▪ Do you have any cultural, religious, or ethnic food preferences?
	▪ Do you use vitamins, minerals, or nutritional supplements?
	▪ Do you use liquid formulas, such as instant breakfast mixes or commercial products?
	▪ How much liquid do you consume in a day?
	▪ Do you use alcohol?

Diagnosis

Possible Nursing Diagnoses	▪ Altered nutrition: eating less than the body needs r/t nausea, vomiting, and taste changes secondary to cancer/cancer therapy as evidenced by 28-pound weight loss

Planning

Client Outcomes	The client will
	▪ Eat six to eight times daily
	▪ Add to the protein and calorie density of foods she eats
	▪ Drink at least 16 oz of a high-calorie, high-protein supplement daily
	▪ Switch from skim milk to whole milk, as tolerated
	▪ Verbalize interventions she will try to help alleviate nausea and taste alterations
	▪ Verbalize the importance of consuming adequate protein and calories and the role of fat in providing calories
	▪ Maintain present weight until chemotherapy is completed
	▪ Maintain/improve health status as evidenced by a prealbumin value within normal limits

Nursing Interventions

Nutrition Therapy	Provide regular diet as ordered with high-protein, high-calorie, in-between meal supplements

NURSING PROCESS: *Cancer* (continued)

Client Teaching	**Instruct the client**
	▪ That an adequate nutritional status reduces the side effects of treatment, may make cancer cells more receptive to treatment, and may improve quality of life; poor nutritional status may potentiate chemotherapeutic drug toxicity
	▪ That a preventative eating style is no longer appropriate; consuming adequate protein and calories (even fat calories) is the major priority
	Instruct the client on eating plan essentials, including
	▪ Protein sources the client may tolerate despite nausea and taste changes such as eggs, cheese, mild fish, nuts, dried peas and beans, milk shakes, eggnogs, puddings, ice cream, instant breakfast mixes, and commercial supplements
	▪ How to increase the protein and calorie density of foods eaten (see Box 22.2)
	▪ To eat small, frequent "meals" to help maximize intake but to avoid eating 12 hours before chemotherapy
	▪ To drink ample fluids 1–2 days before and after chemotherapy to enhance excretion of the drugs and to decrease the risk of renal toxicity
	Instruct the client on interventions to minimize nausea, such as
	▪ Eating foods served cold or at room temperature
	▪ Eating high-carbohydrate, low-fat foods such as toast, crackers, yogurt, sherbet, cooked cereal, soft or canned fruits, watermelon, bananas, fruit juices, and angel food cake
	▪ Avoiding fatty, greasy, fried, and strongly seasoned foods
	Instruct the client on behavior to help maximize intake, including
	▪ Viewing food as a medicine, rather than a social pleasure, that must be "taken" even when the desire to eat is lacking
	▪ Keeping track of and avoiding foods that cause nausea
	▪ Taking antiemetics as prescribed even when symptoms are absent
	▪ Sucking on sugarless hard candy during chemotherapy and using plastic utensils and dishes to mitigate the "bad taste" in her mouth
	▪ Avoiding anything that tastes unpleasant

Evaluation

Evaluate and Monitor	▪ Monitor weight
	▪ Monitor food intake records
	▪ Monitor management of side effects; suggest additional interventions as needed
	▪ Monitor laboratory values

HOW DO YOU RESPOND?

Why do cancer prevention recommendations suggest red meat intake be limited? Some of the most convincing evidence in the report issued by the WCRF/AICR (2007) is the link between red meat and colorectal cancer. The risk of colorectal cancer clearly rises when more than 18 oz per week of cooked red meat are eaten. The risk may be related to substances that occur naturally in red meat and substances that are produced when red meat is processed or cooked. Although more research is needed to fully explain the relationship between red meat and cancer, it is prudent to eat less red meat and processed meat and to avoid cooking red meat at high temperatures.

Doesn't canola oil cause cancer? The rumor that canola oil causes cancer stems from the fact that canola is derived from rapeseed. Rapeseed is naturally high in erucic acid, a fatty acid shown to be harmful to animals. However, in the 1970s, traditional plant breeding methods led to the creation of a low–erucic acid rapeseed, which is used to make canola oil. There are no human health risks associated with canola oil.

CASE STUDY

Steve is a 39-year-old male who has been HIV positive for 6 years. His waistline is expanding, and he blames that for his recent onset of heartburn. Based on a physical examination and insulin resistance, his doctor diagnosed lipodystrophy syndrome. Steve is 6 ft tall and weighs 190 pounds. His weight has been stable for the last several years, although he feels "fatter." He is on ART but is thinking of discontinuing the medication if it is the cause of his change in shape. He is willing to exercise but wants maximum benefit from minimum effort. He is also willing to change his eating habits but relies heavily on eating out. A typical day's intake is as follows:

Breakfast: A fast-food egg, bacon, and cheese sandwich on an English muffin
Hash browns
Large black coffee

Lunch: Double hamburger
French fries
Cola

Dinner: Grilled steak
Baked potato with sour cream
Water

Snacks: Chips

- Evaluate Steve's current weight. Would you recommend weight loss?
- How does Steve's weight impact heartburn and insulin resistance?
- How does his usual intake impact lipodystrophy, insulin resistance, and heartburn?
- What are Steve's nutrition-related problems? What nutrition therapy recommendations would you make?
- What would you tell Steve about exercise?
- What criteria would you monitor to evaluate the effectiveness of nutrition therapy?

STUDY QUESTIONS

1. The nurse knows her instructions about healthy eating to reduce the risk of cancer have been understood when the client states
   a. "If I follow those healthy eating guidelines, I will not get cancer."
   b. "To reduce the risk of cancer, I have to eat a vegetarian diet."
   c. "There is not enough known about diet and cancer to make informed choices about what to eat to reduce the risk of cancer."
   d. "A mostly plant-based diet may reduce the risk of cancer."

2. The nurse knows her instructions on how to reduce the risk of foodborne illness have been understood when the client states
   a. "It is okay to thaw food at room temperature as long as I cook it immediately after it is defrosted."
   b. "Leftovers are not safe to eat."
   c. "Fruits and vegetables do not need to be washed if I peel them or eat them after they are cooked."
   d. "All meat, fish, and poultry should be cooked to the well-done stage."

3. Which of the following strategies would the nurse suggest to help the client increase the protein density of his diet?
   a. Top baked potatoes with sour cream.
   b. Mix cream cheese with butter and spread on hot bread.
   c. Substitute milk for water in recipes.
   d. Add whipped cream to coffee.

4. Which of the following meals would be most appropriate for a patient whose only cancer treatment symptom that impacts intake is neutropenia?
   a. Baked macaroni and cheese with cooked green beans
   b. Cottage cheese and fresh fruit plate
   c. Soft cooked eggs with toast
   d. Caesar salad with Caesar salad dressing

5. The client asks what foods she can eat for protein because meat tastes "rotten" to her. Which of the following would be the nurse's best response?
   a. Cheese omelet, cold chicken sandwich, shrimp salad
   b. Vegetable soup, pulled-pork sandwich, meatloaf with gravy
   c. Spaghetti with meatballs, tacos, peanut butter and jelly sandwich
   d. Hot dogs, hamburgers, vegetable pizza

6. A client asks if it is okay to drink nutrition formulas in place of eating solid food because it seems to be the only thing she tolerates. Which of the following is the nurse's best response?
   a. "Nutrition formulas are okay to use as a supplement in your diet, but they do not provide enough nutrition to use them in place of a meal."
   b. "Nutrition formulas are rich in nutrients and can be used in place of meals if they are what you are able to tolerate best."
   c. "It is fine to rely on nutritional supplements but vary the brand to ensure you are getting adequate nutrition."
   d. "Nutrition formulas generally are too high in calories and protein to use in place of meals."

7. Which statement indicates the client with HIV needs further instruction about healthy eating?
   a. "Eating fat increases my chances of getting fat around my middle, so I am trying to choose all nonfat or low-fat food."
   b. "Eating carbs makes insulin resistance worse, so I am eating a very-low-carbohydrate diet."
   c. "Protein is the most important nutrient, so I am eating extra red meat at every meal."
   d. "Monounsaturated fats in olive oil, canola oil, nuts, and avocado are healthiest. I am eating more of them and less of other types of fats."

8. When should nutrition become part of the care plan for a client with HIV?
   a. Before the onset of symptoms
   b. When the client begins to lose weight
   c. After an acute episode of illness
   d. When weight loss is more than 5% of initial weight

KEY CONCEPTS

- Cancer is a group name for different diseases that differ in their impact on nutrition.
- As many as 30% of cancers may be related to dietary factors. Eating a plant-based diet, being physically active, and avoiding excess weight may reduce the risk of cancer.
- Tumors in the GI tract are more likely than other tumors to produce local effects that impact nutrition.
- Cancer may alter metabolism by causing glucose intolerance and insulin resistance, increasing energy expenditure, increasing protein catabolism, increasing fat catabolism, and increasing the use of fat for energy.
- Anorexia, a common problem in people with cancer, may lead to weight loss and malnutrition. Pain, depression/anxiety, early satiety, taste changes, fatigue, and nausea caused by cancer or its treatment may be contributing factors.
- Cancer cachexia is a progressive wasting syndrome characterized by preferential loss of lean body mass. Altered metabolism and anorexia are involved. The severity of cachexia is not directly related to calorie intake or tumor weight.
- Nutrition therapy may help sustain the client through adverse side effects of cancer treatments and may reduce morbidity and mortality.
- Requirements for protein, calories, vitamin C, B vitamins, and iron increase after surgery to replenish losses and promote healing. GI surgeries have the greatest chance of impacting nutrition.
- Unlike surgery and radiation, chemotherapy produces systemic side effects. Anorexia, nausea and vomiting, taste alterations, sore mouth or throat, diarrhea, early satiety, and constipation are the most common nutrition-related side effects of chemotherapy.
- Nutrition-related side effects from radiation are most likely to occur in people who have cancers of the head and neck, lungs, esophagus, cervix, uterus, colon, rectum, and pancreas.
- People who have bone marrow transplantation may need total parenteral nutrition (TPN) for 1 to 2 months or longer after the procedure.
- The goal of nutrition therapy for people being treated for cancer is to prevent weight loss (even in overweight patients) and maintain lean body mass. Avoiding unintentional weight gain is a goal for people who are overweight or obese at the time of

diagnosis and in those with certain hormonal cancers, such as breast and prostate cancers.

■ There are no validated parameters for determining the nutrition needs of patients with cancer. Generally, a high-calorie, high-protein diet with small frequent meals is recommended. The diet is modified to alleviate nutrition-related side effects.

■ Increasing the calorie and protein densities of the diet is generally more acceptable than increasing the volume of food served.

■ An oral diet is used whenever possible. Enteral and parenteral nutrition are options in specific situations.

■ Malnutrition may speed the progression from HIV disease to AIDS.

■ Weight loss and wasting remain common problems in PLHA, despite major advances in treatment and survival.

■ The cause of HIV-associated wasting is multifactorial. Impaired intake and altered metabolism may be at least partially responsible.

■ The exact nutritional requirements of PLHA are not known. Generally, calorie requirements increase 10% or more depending on the phase of the disease. There are no data to support an increased need for protein. Saturated fat, added sugars, and alcohol should be limited in cases of lipodystrophy syndrome.

■ PLHA may experience side effects similar to those of people with cancer. Nutrition therapy can help alleviate side effects to promote an adequate intake.

■ Drugs used for HIV/AIDS may interact with certain foods. Complex and strict dietary restrictions may be necessary to maximize drug effectiveness.

■ PLHA should practice food sanitation and safety to decrease the risk of foodborne illness.

Check Your Knowledge Answer Key

1. **TRUE** Convincing evidence links obesity with several types of cancer, such as pancreatic, kidney, and postmenopausal breast.

2. **TRUE** Weight loss is an indicator of poor prognosis in cancer patients.

3. **TRUE** Clients who are adequately nourished are better able to withstand the effects of cancer treatments.

4. **FALSE** Although anorexia can contribute to the development of cachexia, neither the incidence nor the severity of cachexia can be related directly to calorie intake.

5. **FALSE** The cancer patient's appetite is generally better in the morning and tends to deteriorate as the day progresses.

6. **TRUE** Cancer survivors are urged to follow diet recommendations to reduce the risk of cancer in the future.

7. **FALSE** A low-fat diet cannot prevent lipodystrophy, but following a Mediterranean-type diet that is low in saturated fat, added sugar, and alcohol may improve blood lipid levels and glucose tolerance. Fiber may promote loss of abdominal fat and improves insulin resistance.

8. **FALSE** Diarrhea does not necessarily accompany malabsorption caused by HIV infection. Malabsorption cannot be ruled out on the basis of bowel movements alone.

9. **TRUE** Patients with HIV/AIDS may experience problems related to appetite and intake similar to those of cancer patients.

10. **TRUE** The risk of foodborne infections in patients with HIV/AIDS can be reduced by educating them on food and water safety such as the importance of refrigerating foods, washing fruit and vegetables, and cooking meats thoroughly.

Websites

Websites related to cancer

American Botanical Council at **www.herbalgram.org**
American Cancer Society at **www.cancer.org**
American Institute for Cancer Research at **www.aicr.org**
American Society of Clinical Oncology at **www.asco.org**
National Cancer Institute at **www.cancer.gov**
National Center for Complementary and Alternative Medicine (NCCAM) at **www.nccam.nih.gov**
Oncology Nursing Society at **www.ons.org**

Websites related to HIV/AIDS

AIDS Education Global Information System (AEGIS) at **www.aegis.com**
AIDSinfo (A Service of the U.S. Department of Health and Human Services) at
    www.aidsinfo.nih.gov
Center for HIV Information from the University of California San Francisco School of Medicine at
    www.hivinsite.org
HIV Research of the Nutrition/Infection Unit at Tufts University School of Medicine at
    www.tufts.edu/med/nutrition-infection/hiv/
Health Resources and Services Administration (HRSA) HIV/AIDS Services at **http://hab.hrsa.gov**
National Institutes of Health, National Center for Complementary and Alternative Medicine at
    http://nccam.nih.gov

References

Academy of Nutrition and Dietetics. (2012). *Nutrition care manual.* Available at www.nutritioncaremanual.org. Accessed on 7/23/12.

American Dietetic Association. (2010). Position of the American Dietetic Association: Nutrition intervention and human immunodeficiency virus infection. *Journal of the American Dietetic Association, 110,* 1105–1119.

Bantle, J., Wylie-Rosett, J., Albright, A. L., Apovian, C. M., Clark, N. G., Franz, M. J., . . . Wheeler, M. L. (2008). Nutrition recommendations and the interventions for diabetes: A position statement of the American Diabetes Association. *Diabetes Care, 1*(Suppl. 1), S61–S78.

Barrera, S., & Demark-Wahnefried, W. (2009). Nutrition during and after cancer therapy. *Oncology, 23*(2, Suppl.), 15–21.

Buijs, N., van Bokhorst-de van der Schueren, M., Langius, A., Leemans, C. R., Kuik, D. J., Vermeulen, M. A., & Leeuwen, P. A. (2010). Perioperative arginine-supplemented nutrition in malnourished patients with head and neck cancer improves long-term survival. *American Journal of Clinical Nutrition, 92,* 1151–1156.

Calle, E., Rodriguez, C., Walker-Thurmond, K., & Thun, M. (2003). Overweight, obesity, and mortality from cancer in a prospectively studied cohort of US adults. *New England Journal of Medicine, 348,* 1625–1638.

Centers for Disease Control and Prevention. (1992). 1993 revised classification system for HIV infection and expanded surveillance case definition for AIDS among adolescents and adults. *Morbidity and Mortality Weekly Report, 41,* RR-17.

Centers for Disease Control and Prevention. (2012). Deaths: Preliminary data for 2010. National Vital Statistics Reports, 60(4). Available at http://www.cdc.gov/nchs/data/nvsr/nvsr60/nvsr60_04.pdf. Accessed 7/16/12.

Cole, B., Baron, J., Sandler, R., Haile, R. W., Ahnen, D. J., Bresalier, R. S., . . . Greenberg, E. R. (2007). Folic acid for the prevention of colorectal adenomas: A randomized clinical trial. *Journal of the American Medical Association, 297,* 2351–2359.

Denmark-Wahnefried, W., Clipp, E., Morey, M., Pieper, C. F., Sloane, R., Snyder, D. C., & Cohen, H. J. (2004). Physical function and associations with diet and exercise: Results of a cross-sectional survey among elders with breast or prostate cancer. *International Journal of Behavioral Nutrition and Physical Activity, 1,* 16.

Donohoe, C., Ryan, A., & Reynolds, J. (2011). Cancer cachexia: Mechanisms and clinical implications. *Gastroenterology Research and Practice, 2011,* 601434.

Evans, W., Morley, J., Argilés, J., Bales, C., Baracos V., Guttridge, D., . . . Anker, S. (2008). Cachexia: A new definition. *Clinical Nutrition, 27,* 793–799.

Ferrucci, L., McCorkie, R., Smith, T., Stein, K. D., & Cartmel, B. (2009). Factors related to the use of dietary supplements by cancer survivors. *Journal of Alternative and Complementary Medicine, 15,* 673–680.

Forrester, J., & Sztam, K. (2011). Micronutrients in HIV/AIDS: Is there evidence to change the WHO 2003 recommendations? *American Journal of Clinical Nutrition, 94*(Suppl.), 1683S–1689S.

Hughes, S., & Kelly, P. (2006). Interactions of malnutrition and immune impairment, with special reference to immunity against parasites. *Parasite Immunology, 18,* 577–588.

Kitahata, M., Tegger, M., Wagner, E., & Holmes, K. (2002). Comprehensive health care for people infected with HIV in developing countries. *British Medical Journal, 325,* 954–957.

Kosmiski, L. (2011). Energy expenditure in HIV infection. *American Journal of Clinical Nutrition, 94*(Suppl.), 1677S–1682S.

Kotler, D., Tierney, A., Wang, J., & Pierson, R. (1989). Magnitude of body cell mass depletion and the time of death from wasting with in AIDS. *American Journal of Clinical Nutrition, 50,* 444–447.

Kressy, J., Wanke, C., & Gerrior, J. (2010). *Lipodystrophy.* Available at www.tufts.edu/med/nutrition-infection/hiv/health_lipo.html. Accessed on 7/24/12.

Kushi, L., Doyle, C., McCullough, M., Rock, C. L., Demark-Wahnefried, W., Bandera, E. V., . . . Gansler, T. (2012). American Cancer Society guidelines on nutrition and physical activity for cancer prevention. *CA: A Cancer Journal for Clinicians, 62,* 30–67.

Lee, I., Cook, N., Gaziano, J., Gordon, D., Ridker, P. M., Manson, J. E., . . . Buring, J. E. (2005). Vitamin E in the primary prevention of cardiovascular disease and cancer. *Journal of the American Medical Association, 294,* 56–65.

Leyes, P., Martinez, E., & Forga Mde, T. (2008). Use of diet, nutritional supplements and exercise in HIV-infected patients receiving combination antiretroviral therapies: A systematic review. *Antiviral Therapy, 13,* 149–159.

Lichtenstein, A., Appel, L., Brands, M., Carnethon, M., Daniels, S., Franch, H. A., . . . Wylie-Rosett, J. (2006). Diet and lifestyle recommendations revision 2006: A scientific statement from the American Heart Association Nutrition Committee. *Circulation, 114,* 82–96.

Mangili, A., Murman, D. H., Zampini, A. M., & Wanke, C. A. (2006). Nutrition and HIV infection: Review of weight loss and wasting in the era of highly active antiretroviral therapy from the Nutrition for Healthy Living Cohort. *Clinical Infectious Diseases, 42,* 836–842.

McClave, S., Martindale, R., Vanek, V., McCarthy, M., Roberts, P., Taylor, B., . . . Cresci, G. (2009). Guidelines for the provision and assessment of nutrition support therapy in the adult critically ill patient: Society of Critical Care Medicine (SCCM) and American Society for Parenteral and Enteral Nutrition (ASPEN). *Journal of Parenteral and Enteral Nutrition, 33,* 277–316.

Meyerhardt, J., Niedzwiecki, D., Hollis, D., Saltz, L. B., Hu, F. B., Mayer, R. J., . . . Fuchs, C. S. (2007). Association of dietary patterns with cancer recurrence and survival in patients with stage III colon cancer. *Journal of the American Medical Association, 298,* 754–764.

Mocroft, A., Ledergerber, B., Zilmer, K., Kirk, O., Hirschel, B., Viard, J. P., . . . Lundgren, J. P. (2007). Short-term clinical disease progression in HIV-1-positive patients taking combination antiretroviral therapy: The EuroSIDA risk-score. *AIDS, 21,* 1867–1875.

Morey, M., Snyder, D., Sloan, R., Cohen, H. J., Peterson, B., Hartman, T. J., . . . Demark-Wahnefried, W. (2009). Effects of home-based diet and exercise on functional outcomes among older, overweight long-term cancer survivors: RENEW: A randomized controlled trial. *Journal of the American Medical Association, 301,* 1883–1891.

National Cancer Institute. (2011). *Nutrition in cancer care (PDQ).* Bethesda, MD: National Cancer Institute. Date last modified 11/30/11. Available at cancer.gov/cancertopics/pdq/supportivecare/nutrition/HealthProfessional. Accessed on 7/16/12.

Pierce, J., Natarajan, L., Caan, B., Parker, B. A., Greenberg, E. R., Flatt, S. W., . . . Stefanick, M. L. (2007). Influence of a diet very high in vegetables, fruit, and fiber and low in fat on prognosis following treatment for breast cancer: The Women's Healthy Eating and Living (WHEL) randomized trial. *Journal of the American Medical Association, 298,* 289–298.

Raiten, D., Mulligan, K., Papathakis, P., & Wanke, C. (2011). Executive summary: Nutritional care of HIV-infected adolescents and adults, including pregnant and lactating women: What do we know, what can we do, and where do we go from here? *American Journal of Clinical Nutrition*, *94*(Suppl.), 1667S–1676S.

Rasouli, N., & Kern, P. (2008). Adipocytokines and the metabolic complications of obesity. *Journal of Clinical and Endocrinology Metabolism*, *93*, 64–73.

Robien, K., & Denmark-Wahnefried, W. (2011). Evidence-based nutrition guidelines for cancer survivors: Current guidelines, knowledge gaps, and future research directions. *Journal of the American Dietetic Association*, *111*, 368–375.

Roubenoff, R., Grinspoon, S., Skolnik, P. R., Tchetgen, E., Abad, L., Spiegelman, D., . . . Gorbach, S. (2002). Role of cytokines and testosterone in regulating lean body mass and resting energy expenditure in HIV-infected men. *American Journal of Physiology Endocrinology Metabolism*, *283*, E138–E145.

Shevitz, A. H., Know, T. A., Spiegelman, D., Roubenoff, R., Gorbach, S. L., & Skolnik, P. R. (1999). Elevated resting energy expenditure among HIV-seropositive persons receiving high active antiretroviral therapy. *AIDS*, *12*, 1351–1357.

Siddiqui, J., Phillips, A., Freedland, E., Sklar, A. R., Darkow, T., & Harley, C. R. (2009). Prevalence and cost of HIV-associated weight loss in a managed care population. *Current Medical Research and Opinion*, *25*, 1307–1317.

Srasuebkul, P., Lim, P., Lee, M., Kumarasamy, N., Zhou, J., Sirisanthana, T., . . . Law, M. G. (2009). Short-term clinical disease progression in HIV-infected patients receiving combination antiretroviral therapy: Results from the TREAT Asia HIV observational database. *Clinical Infectious Diseases*, *48*, 940–950.

Thomas, A., & Mkandawire, S. (2006). The impact of nutrition on physiologic changes in persons who have HIV. *Nursing Clinics of North America*, *41*, 455–468.

U.S. Department of Agriculture & U.S. Department of Health and Human Services. (2010). *Dietary guidelines for Americans, 2010* (7th ed.). Available at www.health.gov/dietaryguidelines. Accessed on 7/16/12.

Vigano, A., Watanabe, S., & Bruera, E. (1994). Anorexia and cachexia in advanced cancer patients. *Cancer Surveillance*, *21*, 99–115.

von Haehling, S., & Anker, S. (2010). Cachexia is a major underestimated and unmet medical need: Facts and numbers. *Journal of Cachexia, Sarcopenia and Muscle*, *1*, 1–5.

Wactawski-Wende, J., Kotchen, J., Anderson, G., Assaf, A. R., Brunner, R. L., O'Sullivan, M. J., . . . Manson, J. E. (2006). Calcium plus vitamin D supplementation and the risk of colorectal cancer. *New England Journal of Medicine*, *354*, 684–696.

Wayne, S., Baumgartner, K., Baumgartner, R., Bernstein, L., Bowen, D. J., & Ballard-Barbash, R. (2006). Diet quality is directly associated with quality of life in breast cancer survivors. *Breast Cancer Research and Treatment*, *96*, 227–232.

Woods, M., Potts, E., & Connors, J. (2010). *Building a high-quality diet*. Available at www.tufts.edu/med/nutrition-infection/hiv/health_high_quality_diet.html. Accessed on 7/24/12.

World Cancer Research Fund/American Institute for Cancer Research. (2007). *Food, nutrition, physical activity, and the prevention of cancer: A global perspective*. Washington, DC: American Institute for Cancer Research.

World Health Organization. (2003). *Nutrient requirements for people living with HIV/AIDS*. Report of a technical consultation. Available at www.who.int/nutrition/publications/Content_nutrient_requirements.pdf. Accessed on 7/25/12.

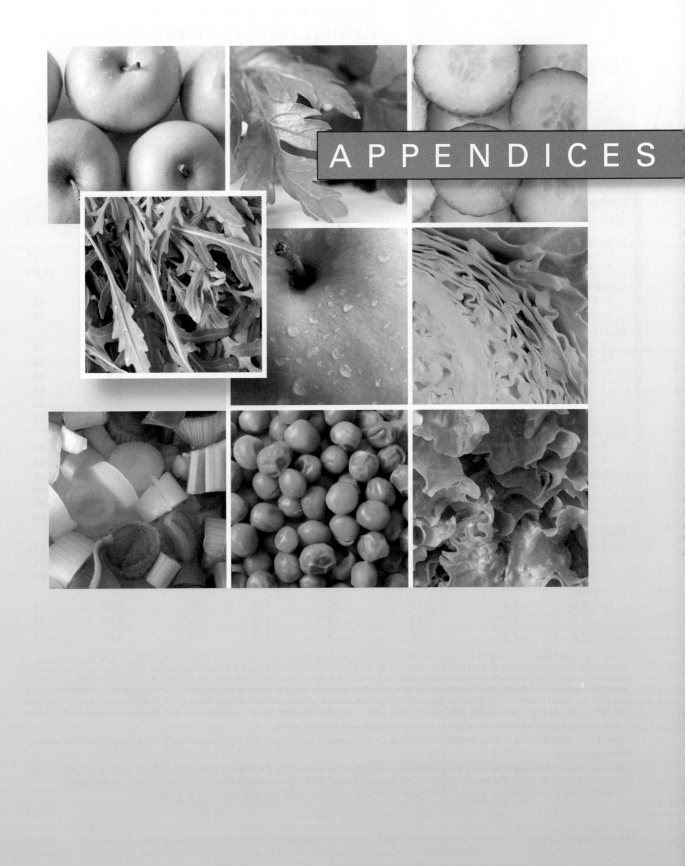

APPENDICES

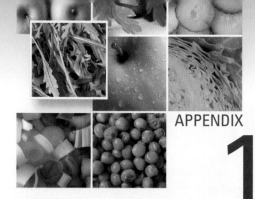

1

Dietary Reference Intakes (DRIs): Recommended Dietary Allowances and Adequate Intakes, Total Water and Macronutrients
Food and Nutrition Board, Institute of Medicine, National Academies

Life Stage Group	Total Water[a] (L/d)	Carbohydrate (g/d)	Total Fiber (g/d)	Fat (g/d)	Linoleic Acid (g/d)	α-Linolenic Acid (g/d)	Protein[b] (g/d)
Infants							
0–6 mo	0.7*	60*	ND	31*	4.4*	0.5*	9.1*
7–12 mo	0.8*	95*	ND	30*	4.6*	0.5*	**11.0+**
Children							
1–3 y	1.3*	**130**	19*	ND[c]	7*	0.7*	**13**
4–8 y	1.7*	**130**	25*	ND	10*	0.9*	**19**
Males							
9–13 y	2.4*	**130**	31*	ND	12*	1.2*	**34**
14–18 y	3.3*	**130**	38*	ND	16*	1.6*	**52**
19–30 y	3.7*	**130**	38*	ND	17*	1.6*	**56**
31–50 y	3.7*	**130**	38*	ND	17*	1.6*	**56**
51–70 y	3.7*	**130**	30*	ND	14*	1.6*	**56**
>70 y	3.7*	**130**	30*	ND	14*	1.6*	**56**
Females							
9–13 y	2.1*	**130**	26*	ND	10*	1.0*	**34**
14–18 y	2.3*	**130**	26*	ND	11*	1.1*	**46**
19–30 y	2.7*	**130**	25*	ND	12*	1.1*	**46**
31–50 y	2.7*	**130**	25*	ND	12*	1.1*	**46**
51–70 y	2.7*	**130**	21*	ND	11*	1.1*	**46**
>70 y	2.7*	**130**	21*	ND	11*	1.1*	**46**
Pregnancy							
14–18 y	3.0*	**175**	28*	ND	13*	1.4*	**71**
19–30 y	3.0*	**175**	28*	ND	13*	1.4*	**71**
31–50 y	3.0*	**175**	28*	ND	13*	1.4*	**71**
Lactation							
14–18 y	3.8*	**210**	29*	ND	13*	1.3*	**71**
19–30 y	3.8*	**210**	29*	ND	13*	1.3*	**71**
31–50 y	3.8*	**210**	29*	ND	13*	1.3*	**71**

Note: This table (taken from the DRI reports, see www.nap.edu) presents Recommended Dietary Allowances (RDA) in **bold type** or Adequate Intakes (AI) in ordinary type followed by an asterisk (*). An RDA is the average daily dietary intake level sufficient to meet the nutrient requirements of nearly all (97–98 percent) healthy individuals in a group. It is calculated from an Estimated Average Requirement (EAR). If sufficient scientific evidence is not available to establish an EAR, and thus calculate an RDA, an AI is usually developed. For healthy breastfed infants, the AI is the mean intake. The AI for other life stage and gender groups is believed to cover the needs of all healthy individuals in the group, but lack of data or uncertainty in the data prevent being able to specify with confidence the percentage of individuals covered by this intake.

[a] Total water includes all water contained in food, beverages, and drinking water.

[b] Based on g protein per kg of body weight for the reference body weight, e.g., for adults 0.8 g/kg body weight for the reference body weight.

[c] Not determined.

Sources: Dietary Reference Intakes for Energy, Carbohydrate, Fiber, Fat, Fatty Acids, Cholesterol, Protein, and Amino Acids (2002/2005); Dietary Reference Intakes for Water, Potassium, Sodium, Chloride, and Sulfate (2005). These reports may be accessed via http://www.nap.edu.

Reprinted with permission from the National Academies Press, Copyright 2005, National Academy of Sciences.

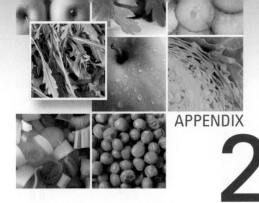

2

Dietary Reference Intakes (DRIs): Recommended Dietary Allowances and Adequate Intakes, Vitamins

Food and Nutrition Board, Institute of Medicine, National Academies

Life Stage Group	Vitamin A (μg/d)[a]	Vitamin C (mg/d)	Vitamin D (μg/d)[b,c]	Vitamin E (mg/d)[d]	Vitamin K (μg/d)	Thiamin (mg/d)
Infants						
0–6 mo	400*	40*	10*	4*	2.0*	0.2*
7–12 mo	500*	50*	10*	5*	2.5*	0.3*
Children						
1–3 y	**300**	**15**	**15**	**6**	30*	**0.5**
4–8 y	**400**	**25**	**15**	**7**	55*	**0.6**
Males						
9–13 y	**600**	**45**	**15**	**11**	60*	**0.9**
14–18 y	**900**	**75**	**15**	**15**	75*	**1.2**
19–30 y	**900**	**90**	**15**	**15**	120*	**1.2**
31–50 y	**900**	**90**	**15**	**15**	120*	**1.2**
51–70 y	**900**	**90**	**15**	**15**	120*	**1.2**
>70 y	**900**	**90**	**20**	**15**	120*	**1.2**
Females						
9–13 y	**600**	**45**	**15**	**11**	60*	**0.9**
14–18 y	**700**	**65**	**15**	**15**	75*	**1.0**
19–30 y	**700**	**75**	**15**	**15**	90*	**1.1**
31–50 y	**700**	**75**	**15**	**15**	90*	**1.1**
51–70 y	**700**	**75**	**15**	**15**	90*	**1.1**
>70 y	**700**	**75**	**20**	**15**	90*	**1.1**
Pregnancy						
14–18 y	**750**	**80**	**15**	**15**	75*	**1.4**
19–30 y	**770**	**85**	**15**	**15**	90*	**1.4**
31–50 y	**770**	**85**	**15**	**15**	90*	**1.4**
Lactation						
14–18 y	**1,200**	**115**	**15**	**19**	75*	**1.4**
19–30 y	**1,300**	**120**	**15**	**19**	90*	**1.4**
31–50 y	**1,300**	**120**	**15**	**19**	90*	**1.4**

Note: This table (taken from the DRI reports, see www.nap.edu) presents Recommended Dietary Allowances (RDA) in **bold type** or Adequate Intakes (AI) in ordinary type followed by an asterisk (∗). An RDA is the average daily dietary intake level sufficient to meet the nutrient requirements of nearly all (97–98 percent) healthy individuals in a group. It is calculated from an Estimated Average Requirement (EAR). If sufficient scientific evidence is not available to establish an EAR, and thus calculate an RDA, an AI is usually developed. For healthy breastfed infants, the AI is the mean intake. The AI for other life stage and gender groups is believed to cover the needs of all healthy individuals in the group, but lack of data or uncertainty in the data prevent being able to specify with confidence the percentage of individuals covered by this intake.

[a]As retinol activity equivalents (RAEs). 1 RAE = 1 μg retinol, 12 μg β-carotene, 24 μg α-carotene, or 24 μg β-cryptoxanthin. The RAE for dietary provitamin A carotenoids is two-fold greater than retinol equivalents (RE), whereas the RAE for preformed vitamin A is the same as RE.

[b]As cholecalciferol. 1 μg cholecalciferol = 40 IU vitamin D.

[c]In the absence of adequate exposure to sunlight.

[d]As α-tocopherol. α-Tocopherol includes *RRR*-α-tocopherol, the only form of α-tocopherol that occurs naturally in foods, and the *2R*-stereoisomeric forms of α-tocopherol (*RRR*-, *RSR*-, *RRS*-, and *RSS*-α-tocopherol) that occur in fortified foods and supplements. It does not include the *2S*-stereoisomeric forms of α-tocopherol (*SRR*-, *SSR*-, *SRS*-, and *SSS*-α-tocopherol), also found in fortified foods and supplements.

Riboflavin (mg/d)	Niacin (mg/d)[e]	Vitamin B_6 (mg/d)	Folate (μg/d)[f]	Vitamin B_{12} (μg/d)	Pantothenic Acid (mg/d)	Biotin (μg/d)	Choline (mg/d)[g]
0.3*	2*	0.1*	65*	0.4*	1.7*	5*	125*
0.4*	4*	0.3*	80*	0.5*	1.8*	6*	150*
0.5	6	0.5	150	0.9	2*	8*	200*
0.6	8	0.6	200	1.2	3*	12*	250*
0.9	12	1.0	300	1.8	4*	20*	375*
1.3	16	1.3	400	2.4	5*	25*	550*
1.3	16	1.3	400	2.4	5*	30*	550*
1.3	16	1.3	400	2.4	5*	30*	550*
1.3	16	1.7	400	2.4[h]	5*	30*	550*
1.3	16	1.7	400	2.4[h]	5*	30*	550*
0.9	12	1.0	300	1.8	4*	20*	375*
1.0	14	1.2	400[i]	2.4	5*	25*	400*
1.1	14	1.3	400[i]	2.4	5*	30*	425*
1.1	14	1.3	400[i]	2.4	5*	30*	425*
1.1	14	1.5	400	2.4[h]	5*	30*	425*
1.1	14	1.5	400	2.4[h]	5*	30*	425*
1.4	18	1.9	600[j]	2.6	6*	30*	450*
1.4	18	1.9	600[j]	2.6	6*	30*	450*
1.4	18	1.9	600[j]	2.6	6*	30*	450*
1.6	17	2.0	500	2.8	7*	35*	550*
1.6	17	2.0	500	2.8	7*	35*	550*
1.6	17	2.0	500	2.8	7*	35*	550*

[e]As niacin equivalents (NE). 1 mg of niacin = 60 mg of tryptophan; 0–6 months = preformed niacin (not NE).

[f]As dietary folate equivalents (DFE). 1 DFE = 1 μg food folate = 0.6 μg of folic acid from fortified food or as a supplement consumed with food = 0.5 μg of a supplement taken on an empty stomach.

[g]Although AIs have been set for choline, there are few data to assess whether a dietary supply of choline is needed at all stages of the life cycle, and it may be that the choline requirement can be met by endogenous synthesis at some of these stages.

[h]Because 10 to 30 percent of older people may malabsorb food-bound B_{12}, it is advisable for those older than 50 years to meet their RDA mainly by consuming foods fortified with B_{12} or a supplement containing B_{12}.

[i]In view of evidence linking folate intake with neural tube defects in the fetus, it is recommended that all women capable of becoming pregnant consume 400 μg from supplements or fortified foods in addition to intake of food folate from a varied diet.

[j]It is assumed that women will continue consuming 400 μg from supplements or fortified food until their pregnancy is confirmed and they enter prenatal care, which ordinarily occurs after the end of the periconceptional period—the critical time for formation of the neural tube.

Sources: *Dietary Reference Intakes for Calcium, Phosphorous, Magnesium, Vitamin D, and Fluoride* (1997). *Dietary Reference Intakes for Thiamin, Riboflavin, Niacin, Vitamin B_6, Folate, Vitamin B_{12}, Pantothenic Acid, Biotin, and Choline* (1998); *Dietary Reference Intakes for Vitamin C, Vitamin E, Selenium, and Carotenoids* (2000); *Dietary Reference Intakes for Vitamin A, Vitamin K, Arsenic, Boron, Chromium, Copper, Iodine, Iron, Manganese, Molybdenum, Nickel, Silicon, Vanadium, and Zinc* (2001); *Dietary Reference Intakes for Water, Potassium, Sodium, Chloride, and Sulfate* (2005); and *Dietary Reference Intakes for Calcium and Vitamin D* (2011). These reports may be accessed via http://www.nap.edu.

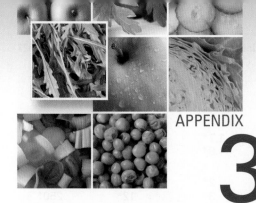

APPENDIX

3

Dietary Reference Intakes (DRIs): Recommended Dietary Allowances and Adequate Intakes, Elements
Food and Nutrition Board, Institute of Medicine, National Academies

Life Stage Group	Calcium (mg/d)	Chromium (μg/d)	Copper (μg/d)	Fluoride (mg/d)	Iodine (μg/d)	Iron (mg/d)	Magnesium (mg/d)	Manganese (mg/d)	Molybdenum (μg/d)	Phosphorus (mg/d)	Selenium (μg/d)	Zinc (mg/d)	Potassium (g/d)	Sodium (g/d)	Chloride (g/d)
Infants															
0–6 mo	200*	0.2*	200*	0.01*	110*	0.27*	30*	0.003*	2*	100*	15*	2*	0.4*	0.12*	0.18*
7–12 mo	260*	5.5*	220*	0.5*	130*	11	75*	0.6*	3*	275*	20*	3	0.7*	0.37*	0.57*
Children															
1–3 y	700	11*	340	0.7*	90	7	80	1.2*	17	460	20	3	3.0*	1.0*	1.5*
4–8 y	1,000	15*	440	1*	90	10	130	1.5*	22	500	30	5	3.8*	1.2*	1.9*
Males															
9–13 y	1,300	25*	700	2*	120	8	240	1.9*	34	1,250	40	8	4.5*	1.5*	2.3*
14–18 y	1,300	35*	890	3*	150	11	410	2.2*	43	1,250	55	11	4.7*	1.5*	2.3*
19–30 y	1,000	35*	900	4*	150	8	400	2.3*	45	700	55	11	4.7*	1.5*	2.3*
31–50 y	1,000	35*	900	4*	150	8	420	2.3*	45	700	55	11	4.7*	1.5*	2.3*
51–70 y	1,000	30*	900	4*	150	8	420	2.3*	45	700	55	11	4.7*	1.3*	2.0*
>70 y	1,200	30*	900	4*	150	8	420	2.3*	45	700	55	11	4.7*	1.2*	1.8*
Females															
9–13 y	1,300	21*	700	2*	120	8	240	1.6*	34	1,250	40	8	4.5*	1.5*	2.3*
14–18 y	1,300	24*	890	3*	150	15	360	1.6*	43	1,250	55	9	4.7*	1.5*	2.3*
19–30 y	1,000	25*	900	3*	150	18	310	1.8*	45	700	55	8	4.7*	1.5*	2.3*
31–50 y	1,000	25*	900	3*	150	18	320	1.8*	45	700	55	8	4.7*	1.5*	2.3*
51–70 y	1,200	20*	900	3*	150	8	320	1.8*	45	700	55	8	4.7*	1.3*	2.0*
>70 y	1,200	20*	900	3*	150	8	320	1.8*	45	700	55	8	4.7*	1.2*	1.8*
Pregnancy															
14–18 y	1,300	29*	1,000	3*	220	27	400	2.0*	50	1,250	60	12	4.7*	1.5*	2.3*
19–30 y	1,000	30*	1,000	3*	220	27	350	2.0*	50	700	60	11	4.7*	1.5*	2.3*
31–50 y	1,000	30*	1,000	3*	220	27	360	2.0*	50	700	60	11	4.7*	1.5*	2.3*
Lactation															
14–18 y	1,300	44*	1,300	3*	290	10	360	2.6*	50	1,250	70	13	5.1*	1.5*	2.3*
19–30 y	1,000	45*	1,300	3*	290	9	310	2.6*	50	700	70	12	5.1*	1.5*	2.3*
31–50 y	1,000	45*	1,300	3*	290	9	320	2.6*	50	700	70	12	5.1*	1.5*	2.3*

Note: This table (taken from the DRI reports, see www.nap.edu) presents Recommended Dietary Allowances (RDA) in **bold type** or Adequate Intakes (AI) in ordinary type followed by an asterisk (*). An RDA is the average daily dietary intake level sufficient to meet the nutrient requirements of nearly all (97–98 percent) healthy individuals in a group. It is calculated from an Estimated Average Requirement (EAR). If sufficient scientific evidence is not available to establish an EAR, and thus calculate an RDA, an AI is usually developed. For healthy breastfed infants, the AI is the mean intake. The AI for other life stage and gender groups is believed to cover the needs of all healthy individuals in the group, but lack of data or uncertainty in the data prevent being able to specify with confidence the percentage of individuals covered by this intake.

Sources: *Dietary Reference Intakes for Calcium, Phosphorous, Magnesium, Vitamin D, and Fluoride* (1997); *Dietary Reference Intakes for Thiamin, Riboflavin, Niacin, Vitamin B_6, Folate, Vitamin B_{12}, Pantothenic Acid, Biotin, and Choline* (1998); *Dietary Reference Intakes for Vitamin C, Vitamin E, Selenium, and Carotenoids* (2000); *Dietary Reference Intakes for Vitamin A, Vitamin K, Arsenic, Boron, Chromium, Copper, Iodine, Iron, Manganese, Molybdenum, Nickel, Silicon, Vanadium, and Zinc* (2001); *Dietary Reference Intakes for Water, Potassium, Sodium, Chloride, and Sulfate* (2005); and *Dietary Reference Intakes for Calcium and Vitamin D* (2011). These reports may be accessed via http://www.nap.edu.

Reprinted with permission from the National Academies Press, Copyright 2011, National Academy of Sciences.

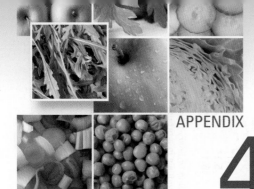

4 Answers to Study Questions

Chapter 1
1. a
2. d
3. b
4. b
5. b
6. d

Chapter 2
1. c
2. a
3. b
4. d
5. c
6. a
7. c
8. d

Chapter 3
1. a
2. b
3. d
4. d
5. c
6. a
7. c
8. a

Chapter 4
1. b
2. d
3. b
4. b
5. a
6. c
7. d
8. a

Chapter 5
1. b
2. c
3. c
4. c
5. d
6. b
7. c
8. a

Chapter 6
1. b
2. a
3. c
4. b
5. c
6. a
7. d
8. c

Chapter 7
1. c
2. b
3. c
4. b
5. c
6. b
7. a
8. b

Chapter 8
1. a
2. c
3. c
4. a
5. c
6. a
7. a
8. b

Chapter 9
1. b
2. c
3. c
4. d
5. a, c, d
6. c
7. a
8. a

Chapter 10
1. b
2. c
3. b
4. a, d, e
5. a, b, d, e
6. d
7. b
8. a

Chapter 11
1. b
2. a
3. b, d
4. c
5. b
6. a
7. a
8. c

Chapter 12
1. d
2. a
3. b
4. b
5. a, b, c
6. c
7. a
8. d

Chapter 13
1. d
2. c
3. a
4. b
5. a
6. a, b, c, d, e
7. c
8. a, c, d, e

Chapter 14
1. b
2. b
3. a
4. b, c, d
5. b
6. a
7. c
8. b

Chapter 15
1. b, c, d
2. d
3. c
4. a
5. b
6. a, b, c, d, e
7. a, b, d
8. c

Chapter 16
1. a
2. a
3. d
4. c
5. c
6. c
7. d
8. a

Chapter 17
1. a
2. a
3. c
4. b
5. b
6. b
7. d
8. d

Chapter 18
1. a
2. a
3. b
4. b
5. b
6. a
7. a
8. b

Chapter 19
1. c
2. d
3. d
4. d
5. a
6. b
7. c
8. a, b, c

Chapter 20
1. b
2. c
3. a
4. a
5. d
6. d
7. c
8. c

Chapter 21
1. a
2. d
3. a
4. c
5. a
6. a
7. b
8. c

Chapter 22
1. d
2. d
3. c
4. a
5. a
6. b
7. d
8. a

Index

Note: Page numbers followed by *b* indicate a box; those followed by *f*, an illustration; and those followed by *t*, a table.